Hemodynamics and Cardiology:
Neonatology Questions and Controversies

Hemodynamics and Cardiology

Neonatology Questions and Controversies

Series Editor

Richard A. Polin, M.D.
Professor of Pediatrics
College of Physicians and Surgeons
Columbia University
Director Division of Neonatology
Morgan Stanley Children's Hospital of New York-Presbyterian
Columbia University Medical Center
New York, New York

Other Volumes in the Neonatology Questions and Controversies Series

Hemodynamics and Cardiology
Neonatology Questions and Controversies

Cardiology Editor

Charles S. Kleinman, MD

Chief, Fetal Cardiology
Division of Pediatric Cardiology
The Center for Prenatal Pediatrics
Morgan Stanley Children's Hospital of New York-Presbyterian
Professor of Clinical Pediatrics in Obstetrics and Gynecology
Columbia University College of Physicians and Surgeons
Weill Medical College of Cornell University
New York, New York

Hemodynamics Editor

Istvan Seri, MD, PhD

Professor of Pediatrics
Keck School of Medicine, University of Southern California
Head, USC Division of Neonatal Medicine
Director, Center for Fetal and Neonatal Medicine
    and the Institute for Maternal-Fetal Health
Children's Hospital for Los Angeles and
    Women's and Children's Hospital, LAC+USC Medical Center
Los Angeles, California

Consulting Editor

Richard A. Polin, MD

Professor of Pediatrics
College of Physicians and Surgeons
Columbia University
Director Division of Neonatology
Morgan Stanley Children's Hospital of New York-Presbyterian
Columbia University Medical Center
New York, New York

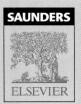

SAUNDERS

ELSEVIER

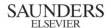

SAUNDERS
ELSEVIER

1600 John F. Kennedy Blvd.
Suite 1800
Philadelphia, PA 19103-2899

HEMODYNAMICS AND CARDIOLOGY: NEONATOLOGY QUESTIONS AND
CONTROVERSIES
ISBN-13: 978-1-4160-3162-8
Copyright © 2008 by Saunders, an imprint of Elsevier Inc.

Notice

Knowledge and best practice in this field are constantly changing. As new research and experience broaden our knowledge, changes in practice, treatment and drug therapy may become necessary or appropriate. Readers are advised to check the most current information provided (i) on procedures featured or (ii) by the manufacturer of each product to be administered, to verify the recommended dose or formula, the method and duration of administration, and contraindications. It is the responsibility of the practitioner, relying on their own experience and knowledge of the patient, to make diagnoses, to determine dosages and the best treatment for each individual patient, and to take all appropriate safety precautions. To the fullest extent of the law, neither the Publisher nor the Author assumes any liability for any injury and/or damage to persons or property arising out of or related to any use of the material contained in this book.

The Publisher

Library of Congress Cataloging-in-Publication Data

Hemodynamics and Cardiology: neonatology questions and controversies/
[edited by] Charles S. Klienman, Istvan Seri ; consulting editor,
Richard A. Polin.
    p. ; cm.
  ISBN 978-1-4160-3162-8

  1. Pediatric cardiology. 2. Newborn infants—Diseases. I. Klienman, Charles S. II. Seri,
Istvan, MD. III. Polin, Richard A, (Richard Alan), 1945-

  [DNLM: 1. Cardiovascular Diseases. 2. Infant, Newborn, Diseases. 3. Infant, Newborn.
4. Neonatology—methods. WS 290 C26758 2008]

RJ421.C26 2008

618.92′12—dc22

2007049316

Acquisitions Editor: Judith Fletcher
Developmental Editor: Lisa Barnes
Associate Developmental Editor: Bernard Buckholtz
Senior Project Manager: David Saltzberg
Design Direction: Karen O'Keefe-Owens

Printed China.

Last digit is the print number: 9   8   7   6   5   4   3   2   1

Contents

Contributors

Craig T. Albanese, MD, MBA
Professor of Surgery, Pediatrics and Obstetrics and Gynecology
Stanford University Medical Center, Stanford, California
John A. and Cynthia Fry Gunn Director of Surgical Services, and
Chief, Division of Pediatric Surgery
Lucile Packard Children's Hospital
Palo Alto, California
> *Fetal Cardiac Intervention*

Stefan Blüml, PhD
Associate Professor of Research Radiology
Keck School of Medicine
University of Southern California
Institute for Maternal Fetal Health
Children's Hospital Los Angeles
Los Angeles, California
> *Magnetic Resonance Imaging and Neonatal Hemodynamics*

Joel I. Brenner, MD
Director, Pediatric Cardiology
The Johns Hopkins Hospital
Baltimore, Maryland
> *Prevalence of Congenital Heart Disease*

Rowena G. Cayabyab, MD
Assistant Professor of Pediatrics
USC Division of Neonatal Medicine
Department of Pediatrics
Women's and Children's Hospital
LAC+USC Medical Center and
Children's Hospital Los Angeles
Keck School of Medicine
University of Southern California
Los Angeles, California
> *Clinical Presentations of Systemic Inflammatory Response in Term and Preterm Infants*

Jonathan M. Chen, MD
Associate Professor of Cardiothoracic Surgery
Weill Medical College of Cornell University
Director, Pediatric Cardiac Surgery
New York Presbyterian Hospital
New York, New York
Cardiac Surgery in the Neonate with Congenital Heart Disease

Cynthia H. Cole, MD, MPH
Director of Research
Beth Israel Deaconess Medical Center
Boston, Massachusetts
The Preterm Neonate with Relative Adrenal Insufficiency and Pressor Resistance

Ryan R. Davies, MD
Resident in Cardiothoracic Surgery
Division of Cardiothoracic Surgery
Department of Surgery
Columbia University
New York Presbyterian Hospital
New York, New York
The Preterm Neonate with Relative Adrenal Insufficiency and Pressor Resistance

Mary T. Donofrio, MD, FAAP, FACC, FASE
Associate Professor of Pediatrics
Pediatric Cardiology
George Washington University
Director of the Fetal Heart Program
Co-Director of Echocardiography
Children's National Heart Institute
Children's National Medical Center
Washington, District of Columbia
Impact of Congenital Heart Disease and Surgical Intervention on Neurodevelopment

William D. Engle, MD
Associate Professor of Pediatrics
University of Texas Southwestern Medical Center
Dallas, Texas
Definition of Normal Blood Pressure Range: the Elusive Target

Nicholas J. Evans, DM, MRCPCH

Clinical Associate Professor
Department of Neonatal Medicine
Royal Prince Alfred Hospital and
The University of Sydney
Sydney, Australia

Functional Echocardiography in the Neonatal Intensive Care Unit

Mark Friedberg, MD

Associate Professor in Pediatrics
University of Toronto
Cardiologist
Department of Pediatric Cardiology
The Hospital for Sick Children
Toronto, Canada

Fetal Cardiac Intervention

Philippe S. Friedlich, MD, MS Epi, MBA

Section Head, CHLA Operations
Medical Director, Neonatal and Infant Critical Care Unit
The Center for Fetal & Neonatal Medicine
Children's Hospital Los Angeles
Associate Professor of Pediatrics
Keck School of Medicine
University of Southern California
Los Angeles, California

Shock in the Surgical Neonate

Carl P. Garabedian, MD

Clinical Associate Professor
University of Washington School of Medicine
Seattle, Washington
Director of Pediatric Catherization Lab
Sacred Heart Medical Center and Children's Hospital
Spokane, Washington

Neonatal Interventional Catheterizations

Gorm Greisen, MD, PhD

Head, Department of Neonatology, Rigshopitalet
Professor of Pediatrics
University of Copenhagen
Copenhagen, Denmark

Autoregulation of Vital and Nonvital Organ Blood Flow in the Preterm and Term Neonate and Use of Organ Blood Flow Assessment in the Diagnosis and Treatment of Neonatal Shock

Frank L. Hanley, MD

Professor, Cardiothoracic Surgery
Stanford University Medical Center
Stanford California
Director, Children's Heart Center
Cardiothoracic Surgery
Lucile Packard Children's Hospital
Palo Alto, California
Fetal Cardiac Intervention

William E. Hellenbrand, MD

Professor of Clinical Pediatrics
Columbia University
Chief, Pediatric Cardiology
Morgan Stanley Children's Hospital New York-Presbyterian
New York, New York
Neonatal Interventional Catheterizations

Charles S. Kleinman, MD

Chief, Fetal Cardiology
Division of Pediatric Cardiology
The Center for Prenatal Pediatrics
Morgan Stanley Children's Hospital of New York-Presbyterian
Professor of Clinical Pediatrics in Obstetrics and Gynecology
Columbia University College of Physicians and Surgeons
Weill Medical College of Cornell University
New York, New York
Impact of Prenatal Diagnosis on the Management of Congenital Heart Disease

Martin Kluckow, MBBS, PhD

Senior Lecturer in Neonatology
University of Sydney
Senior Neonatologist
Department of Neonatal Medicine
Royal North Shore Hospital
Sydney, Australia
The Very Low Birth Weight Neonate During the First Postnatal Day

Heather S. Lipkind, MD

Assistant Professor
Obstetrics, Gynecology and Reproductive Science Maternal
Fetal Medicine
Yale University School of Medicine
New Haven, Connecticuit
Obstetric Management of Fetuses with Congenital Heart Disease

Ralph S. Mosca, MD

Chief, Pediatric Cardiac Surgery
Division of Cardiothoracic Surgery
Department of Surgery
Columbia University
New York Presbyterian Hospital
New York, New York

Cardiac Surgery in the Neonate with Congenital Heart Disease

Shahab Noori, MD

Assistant Professor of Pediatrics
Neonatal Perinatal Medicine
Department of Pediatrics
University of Oklahoma College of Medicine
Neonatologist
The Children's Hospital
Oklahoma City, Oklahoma

The Etiology, Pathophysiology and Phases of Neonatal Shock and the Very Low Birth Weight Neonate with a Hemodynamically Significant Ductus Arteriosus During the First Postnatal Week

David Osborn, MBBS, MMed (Clin Epi), FRACP, PhD

Clinical Associate Professor
Neonatologist
Royal Prince Alfred Newborn Care
Royal Prince Alfred Hospital
Sydney, Australia

Evidence-based Evaluation of the Management of Neonatal Shock

Ashok Panigrahy, MD

Assistant Professor of Neuroradiology
Keck School of Medicine
University of Southern California
Neuroradiologist
Department of Radiology
Institute for Maternal Fetal Health
Children's Hospital Los Angeles
Los Angeles, California

Magnetic Resonance Imaging and Neonatal Hemodynamics

Beth Feller Printz, MD, PhD

Assistant Professor of Clinical Pediatrics in Radiology
Department of Pediatrics
Columbia University
Assisant Atending
Division of Pediatric Cardiology
Department of Pediatrics
Morgan Stanley Children's Hospital of New York-Presbyterian
New York, New York

MRI Evaluation of the Neonate with Congenital Heart Disease

Jan M. Quaegebeur, MD

Chief, Pediatric Cardiac Surgery
Chief, Congenital Heart Center
Division of Cardiothoracic Surgery
Department of Surgery
Columbia University
New York Presbyterian Hospital
New York, New York

Cardiac Surgery in the Neonate with Congenital Heart Disease

Vadiyala Mohan Reddy, MD

Associate Professor
Cardiothoracic Surgery
Stanford University Medical Center
Stanford, California
Chief, Division of Pediatric Cardiac Surgery
Cardiothoracic Surgery
Lucile Salter Packard Children's Hospital
Palo Alto, California

Fetal Cardiac Intervention

Jack Rychik, MD

Associate Professor of Pediatrics
University of Pennsylvania School of Medicine
Director, Fetal Heart Program
Cardiac Center of the Children's Hospital of Philadelphia
Philadelphia, Pennsylvania

The Twin-Twin Transfusion Syndrome: Evolving Concepts

Istvan Seri, MD, PhD

Professor of Pediatrics
Keck School of Medicine, University of Southern California
Head, USC Division of Neonatal Medicine
Director, Center for Fetal and Neonatal Medicine
and the Institute for Maternal-Fetal Health
Children's Hospital Los Angeles and
Women's and Children's Hospital, LAC+USC Medical Center
Los Angeles, California

The Etiology, Pathophysiology, and Phases of Neonatal Shock,
The Very Low Birth, Weight Neonate During the First Postnatal Day,
The Very Low Birth Weight Neonate with A Hemodynamically Significant
Ductus Arteriosus During the First Postnatal Week, Clinical Presentations of
Systemic Inflammatory Response in Term and Preterm Infants, and Shock
in the Surgical Neonate

Cathy E. Shin, MD, FACS, FAAP

Assistant Professor of Clinical Surgery
Keck School of Medicine, University of Southern California and
Children's Hospital Los Angeles
Los Angeles, California

Shock in the Surgical Neonate

Norman H. Silverman, MD, DSc, (Med) FACC, FASE

Professor of Pediatrics
Division of Pediatric Cardiology
The Roma and Marvin Auerback Scholar in Pediatric Cardiology
Director, Pediatric and Fetal Echocardiography Laboratories
Lucile Packard Children's Hospital
Palo Alto, California
Fetal Cardiac Intervention

Lynn L. Simpson, MD

Associate Professor of Obstetrics and Gynecology
Columbia University College of Physicians and Surgeons
Director, OB/GYN Ultrasound
Medical Director, Center for Prenatal Pediatrics
Program Director, Maternal-Fetal Medicine Fellowship
New York Presbyterian Hospital
New York, New York
Obstetric Management of Fetuses with Congenital Heart Disease

Caterina Tiozzo, MD

Neonatologist
Department of Pediatrics
University of Padua
Padua, Italy
Shock in the Surgical Neonate

Suresh Victor, MRCPCH, PhD

Clinical Lecturer and Honorary Consultant Neonatologist
Maternal and Fetal Health Research Group
Faculty of Medical and Human Sciences
University of Manchester
Manchester, United Kingdom
Near-infrared Spectroscopy and its Use for the Assessment of Tissue Perfusion in the Neonate

A. Michael Weindling, MA, MD, BSc, FRCP, FRCPCH, Hon FRCA

Professor of Perinatal Medicine
University of Liverpool
Consultant Neonatologist
Liverpool Women's Hospital
Liverpool, United Kingdom
Near-infrared Spectroscopy and its Use for the Assessment of Tissue Perfusion in the Neonate

Series Foreword

Learn from yesterday, live for today, hope for tomorrow. The important thing is not to stop questioning.

ALBERT EINSTEIN

"The art and science of asking questions is the source of all knowledge."

THOMAS BERGER

In the mid-1960s W.B. Saunders began publishing a series of books focused on the care of newborn infants. The series was entitled *Major Problems in Clinical Pediatrics*. The original series (1964-1979) consisted of ten titles dealing with problems of the newborn infant (*The Lung and its Disorders in the Newborn infant* edited by Mary Ellen Avery, *Disorders of Carbohydrate Metabolism in Infancy* edited by Marvin Cornblath and Robert Schwartz, *Hematologic Problems in the Newborn* edited by Frank A. Oski and J. Lawrence Naiman, *The Neonate with Congenital Heart Disease* edited by Richard D. Rowe and Ali Mehrizi, *Recognizable Patterns of Human Malformation* edited by David W. Smith, *Neonatal Dermatology* edited by Lawrence M. Solomon and Nancy B. Esterly, *Amino Acid Metabolism and its Disorders* edited by Charles L. Scriver and Leon E. Rosenberg, *The High Risk Infant* edited by Lula O. Lubchenco, *Gastrointestinal Problems in the Infant* edited by Joyce Gryboski and *Viral Diseases of the Fetus and Newborn* edited by James B. Hanshaw and John A. Dudgeon. Dr. Alexander J. Schaffer was asked to be the consulting editor for the entire series. Dr. Schaffer coined the term "neonatology" and edited the first clinical textbook of neonatology entitled *Diseases of the Newborn*. For those of us training in the 1970s, this series and Dr. Schaffer's textbook of neonatology provided exciting, up-to-date information that attracted many of us into the subspecialty. Dr. Schaffer's role as "consulting editor" allowed him to select leading scientists and practitioners to serve as editors for each individual volume. As the "consulting editor" for *Neonatology Questions and Controversies*, I had the challenge of identifying the topics and editors for each volume in this series. The six volumes encompass the major issues encountered in the neonatal intensive care unit (newborn lung, fluid and electrolytes, neonatal cardiology and hemodynamics, hematology, immunology and infectious disease, gastroenterology and neurology). The editors for each volume were challenged to combine discussions of fetal and neonatal physiology with disease pathophysiology and selected controversial topics in clinical care. It is my hope that this series (like *Major Problems in Clinical Pediatrics*) will excite a new generation of trainees to question existing dogma (from my own generation) and seek new information through scientific investigation. I wish to congratulate and thank each of the volume editors (Drs. Bancalari, Oh, Guignard, Baumgart, Kleinman, Seri, Ohls, Yoder, Neu and Perlman) for their extraordinary effort and finished products. I also wish to acknowledge Judy Fletcher at Elsevier, who conceived the idea for the series and who has been my "editor and friend" throughout my academic career.

Richard A. Polin, MD

Preface

Cardiovascular compromise is a presenting finding in a significant number of symptomatic preterm and term neonates during the neonatal period. Yet, timely diagnosis of neonatal circulatory compromise is hampered by the limitations in our ability to appropriately assess systemic and organ blood flow in the neonate and by our limited understanding of the impact of congenital heart disease, prematurity or extra-cardiac illness on the hemodynamic changes occurring during normal postnatal circulatory transition. As a result, treatment of cardiovascular compromise especially in neonates without congenital heart disease has rarely been based on a thorough understanding of the underlying pathophysiology. Instead, these neonates are uniformly treated with volume boluses followed by the administration of vasopressors and/or inotropes with little regard to the etiology, phase or pathophysiology of neonatal shock. It is not surprising therefore that there is no evidence demonstrating that treatment of shock in neonates without congenital heart disease improves mortality or clinically meaningful short- and long-term outcomes. As for neonates with suspected or prenatally diagnosed ductal dependent congenital heart disease, the initial approach is based on some evidence as maintenance of ductal patency and maneuvers to decrease oxygen consumption in these patients improves survival.

This book consists of two major sections. The section on *congenital heart disease* discusses the most recent information on the approach to diagnosis and management of neonates with certain forms of congenital heart disease.

The focus of pediatric cardiologists involved in the care of neonates with critical hemodynamic compromise has changed during the past decades. Rather than reactive, responding to severe manifestations of hypoxemia and ischemia that are already manifest, efforts have focused on the potential for identifying, in advance of delivery, the fetuses most likely to have cardiovascular difficulty transitioning to independent extrauterine existence. The section on *fetal hemodynamics* discusses the diagnosis and obstetrical management of fetuses with structural heart disease. There is discussion of autoregulation of fetal blood flow, and the potential impact of such autoregulation on the development of the brain and long-term neurocognitive results. The hemodynamic ramifications of twin-to-twin transfusion syndrome are discussed, as a review of the syndrome itself, and as a means of assessing cardiovascular responses to altered pre- and afterload. This may serve as a foundation for the understanding of, and the formulation of new intrauterine treatments. The role of catheter treatment of the fetus and of the neonate is reviewed, with the role of the postnatal catheterization laboratory having changed from a diagnostic to a largely therapeutic venue reviewed. An effort is made to summarize the role of fetal echocardiography in altering the management and outcome for these babies upon review of a three-decade-long experience with fetal diagnosis and treatment.

The section on *neonatal hemodynamics* first addresses the pathophysiology of neonatal shock, the autoregulation of vital and non-vital organ blood flow and the controversies surrounding the definition of normal blood pressure in the neonatal patient population. The most recent advances in our approach to the diagnosis of neonatal shock are then discussed including the use of functional

Section I

Pathophysiology of Neonatal Shock

Chapter 1

Etiology, Pathophysiology, and Phases of Neonatal Shock

Shahab Noori, MD • Istvan Seri, MD, PhD

Definition and Stages of Neonatal Shock
Hypovolemia
Myocardial Dysfunction
Abnormal Vasoregulation
Adrenal Insufficiency
Summary
References

As adequate organ perfusion depends on maintenance of cardiac output and systemic vascular resistance (SVR), diminished cardiac output and abnormal SVR result in decreased organ perfusion. However, the impact of the changes in cardiac output and SVR on blood pressure is less predictable because blood pressure is the product of the interaction between cardiac output (systemic blood flow) and SVR (blood pressure = SVR × flow). Therefore, changes in blood pressure may reflect changes in cardiac output (systemic blood flow), SVR, or both. In the mature cardiovascular system, blood pressure remains normal if flow has dropped significantly to the nonvital organs as long as SVR is elevated and vital organ perfusion is maintained (compensated shock; see below). Conversely, blood pressure may be at the lower end of the normal range yet systemic blood flow is maintained if SVR is reduced as long as perfusion pressure to organs provides appropriate driving force to flow. Due to these complex interactions, the use of blood pressure as the sole indicator of normal circulation may not be sufficient to adequately assess the cardiovascular status and simultaneous measurement of systemic perfusion and thus organ blood flow may be necessary.

This is especially true for preterm and term neonates during the period of immediate postnatal adaptation. In these patients, immaturity of the cardiovascular system and the complexities associated with the circulatory transition to extrauterine life limit our ability to determine the normal blood pressure range and thus the use of blood pressure alone to accurately assess the cardiovascular status. However, continuous assessment of systemic perfusion by means other than measurement of blood pressure is not available for neonates. Therefore, in addition to following changes in blood pressure, the neonatologist is left to rely on rather insensitive and somewhat nonspecific indirect signs of organ perfusion such as prolonged capillary refill time (CRT), increased peripheral-to-core temperature difference, low urine output and/or lactic acidosis when attempting to assess systemic blood flow and tissue perfusion in the neonatal patient population, especially during the transitional period.

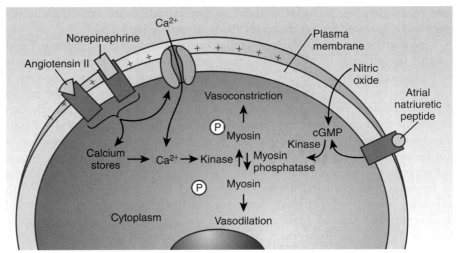

FIGURE 1-3 Regulation of vascular smooth-muscle tone. The steps involved in vasoconstriction and vasodilation are shown in blue and red, respectively. Phosphorylation (P) of myosin is the critical step in the contraction of vascular smooth muscle. The action of vasoconstrictors such as angiotensin II and norepinephrine result in an increase in cytosolic calcium concentration, which activates myosin kinase. Vasodilators such as atrial natriuretic peptide and nitric oxide activate myosin phosphatase and, by dephosphorylating myosin, cause vasorelaxation. The plasma membrane is shown at resting potential (plus signs). The abbreviation cGMP denotes cyclic guanosine monophosphate. *Adapted with permission from Landry DW and Oliver JA. N Engl J Med. 2001;345:588–595.*

hydrogen ion and lactate concentrations, activates K_{ATP} channels resulting in vasodilation and increases in tissue oxygen delivery to compensate for the initiating tissue hypoxia (33).

As mentioned earlier, a large number of vasodilators and vasoconstrictors exert their effects through K_{ATP} channels. For instance, increases in atrial natriuretic peptide (ANP), adenosine, and nitric oxide production, as seen in septic shock, can activate K_{ATP} channels (33,34). Therefore, it has been suggested that K_{ATP} channels play a crucial role in pathogenesis of the vasodilatory shock seen in sepsis. Indeed, animal studies have demonstrated an improvement in blood pressure following administration of a K_{ATP} channel blocker (35,36). However, a recent small human trial failed to show any benefit of the administration of the K_{ATP} channel inhibitor glibenclamide in adults with septic shock (37). Although there are problems with the methodology (38) and the sample size in this study (37), the results cast some doubt on the extent of K_{ATP} channel involvement at least in milder forms of septic shock in adults.

Eicosanoids are derived from cell membrane phospholipids via metabolism of arachidonic acid by cyclooxygenase or lipoxygenase. Different types of eicosanoids have different effects on vascular tone. For example, prostacyclin and prostaglandin E_2 are vasodilators while thromboxane A_2 is a potent vasoconstrictor. Apart from their involvement in the physiologic regulation of vascular tone, these paracrine and autocrine factors play a role in the pathogenesis of shock. Indeed, both human and animal studies have shown a beneficial cardiovascular effect of cyclooxygenase inhibition in septic shock (39,40). In addition, compared with the wild type, rats deficient in essential fatty acids, and thus unable to produce significant amounts of eicosanoids, are less susceptible to endotoxic shock. However, the role of eicosanoids in the pathogenesis of shock is more complex as some studies suggest that the administration and not inhibition of some of these factors has a beneficial effect in shock. For example, administration of PGI_2, PGE_1, and PGE_2 improves cardiovascular status in animals with hypovolemic shock (41,42). Another layer of complexity in this matter is reflected by the observation that the production of both vasodilator and vasoconstrictor prostanoids is increased in shock (43,44).

Endogenous nitric oxide (NO) also plays an important role in the physiologic regulation of vascular tone. Normally, NO is produced in vascular endothelial cells by the enzyme endothelial NO synthase (eNOS). NO then diffuses to the smooth muscle cell and triggers the production of cGMP, a second messenger, which in turn activates myosin phosphatase, a key enzyme in the process of muscle relaxation.

In septic shock, endotoxin and cytokines such as tumor necrosis factor α (TNFα) increase the expression of inducible NO synthase (iNOS) (45–48). Studies in animals and humans have shown that NO level significantly increases in various forms of shock especially in septic shock. (49,50). The excessive production of NO by the up-regulated iNOS then leads to sustained pathological vasodilation with hypotension and vasopressor resistance. Because of its role in pathogenesis of shock, many studies have looked at the NO production pathway as a potential target of therapeutic intervention. However, the approach of using nonselective inhibitors of NO production in septic shock caused significant side effects and increased mortality (51–53). These deleterious effects were likely due to the inhibition of not only iNOS but also eNOS. As mentioned earlier, eNOS plays an important role in the physiologic regulation of vascular tone. Subsequently, the use of a selective iNOS inhibitor was shown to result in improvements in hypotension and reduction in lactic acidosis (54). Whether selective the use of an iNOS inhibitor would be beneficial in neonatal shock is not known at present.

Recently, there has been a renewed interest in role of vasopressin in the pathophysiology of vasodilatory shock (55,56). Although in postnatal life this hormone is primarily involved in the physiologic regulation of osmolarity and fluid homeostasis, there is accumulating evidence suggesting that decreased production and end-organ effectiveness of vasopressin play a role in the pathogenesis of vasodilatory shock. Vasopressin exerts its vascular effects through the stimulation of the V_1 receptors with the V_{1a} receptor subtype being expressed in vessels of all the vascular beds while the V_{1b} subtype is only present in the pituitary gland. The renal effects of vasopressin are mediated through V_2 receptors present in the distal tubules and collecting ducts.

As opposed to the role of vasopressin in the physiologic regulation of fetal vascular tone, during postnatal life and under physiologic conditions, the low serum vasopressin levels contribute little if any to the maintenance of vascular smooth muscle tone. However, under pathologic conditions, such as in shock, the decrease in the blood pressure is mitigated by rising hormone levels. With progression of the cardiovascular compromise, vasopressin levels usually decline possibly due to depletion of vasopressin stores. This then leads to further loss of vascular tone contributing to the development of refractory hypotension (57). Indeed, recent reports on the effectiveness of vasopressin administration in reversing refractory hypotension support the role of vasopressin in the pathophysiology of vasodilatory shock (58,59). Interestingly, the vasoconstrictor effects of vasopressin in the different vascular beds appear to be dose-dependent (60).

Excessive production of NO and activation of K_{ATP} channels are some of the mechanisms discussed earlier in pathogenesis of vasodilatory shock. Under these circumstances, vasopressin also inhibits NO-induced cGMP production and inactivates K_{ATP} channels. In addition, vasopressin induces the release of calcium from the sarcoplasmic reticulum and augments the vasoconstrictive effects of norepinephrine. Thus, via these complex cardiovascular effects, vasopressin opposes the actions of some of the cellular mechanisms of vasodilatory shock and may be of therapeutic importance in selected cases.

ADRENAL INSUFFICIENCY

Among other functions, the adrenal glands play a crucial role in maintaining cardiovascular homeostasis. Mineralocorticoids exert their effects on intravascular volume through regulation of extracellular sodium concentration. In the case of mineralocorticoid deficiency such as the salt-wasting type of congenital adrenal hyperplasia, renal loss of sodium and the resultant volume depletion lead to a decrease in blood volume and eventually cardiac output and result in the development of shock. Glucocorticoids primarily exert their physiologic cardiovascular effects by enhancing the vascular and cardiac responsiveness to endogenous catecholamines. The rapid rise of blood pressure in the early postnatal period has been attributed to maturation of vascular smooth muscle and its response to endogenous catecholamines, the decrease in the production of vasodilatory hormones prevalent in fetal life, changes in expression of vascular angiotensin II receptor subtypes, and accumulation of elastin and collagen in large arteries (61–63). Glucocorticoids may also play a role in the developmental increase in blood pressure by enhancing expression of angiotensin II receptors and collagen synthesis in the vascular wall (64). Given the importance of corticosteroids (gluco- and mineralocorticoids) in cardiovascular stability, it is not surprising that the deficiency of these hormones has been implicated in pathogenesis of shock and the development of vasopressor/inotrope resistance.

Preterm infants are born with an immature hypothalamus–pituitary–adrenal axis. It has been suggested that preterm infants are only capable of producing enough gluco- and mineralocorticoids to meet their metabolic demand and growth while they are not stressed. When critically ill, however, they may not be able to mount an adequate stress response; a condition referred to as *relative adrenal insufficiency*. Although a growing body of literature supports this concept, the exact cause of relative adrenal insufficiency remains unclear.

Hanna and coworkers (65) demonstrated a normal response to both corticotrophin releasing hormone (CRH) and ACTH stimulation tests in extremely low birth weight (ELBW) infants. They concluded that failure of adequate stress response in some sick preterm neonates may be related to the inability of extremely premature brain to recognize stress or because of inadequate hypothalamic secretion of CRH. In contrast, Ng and collaborators (66) reported a severely reduced cortisol but normal ACTH response to human CRH in premature infants with vasopressor/inotrope-resistant hypotension. Using CRH stimulation test, the same group of investigators also studied the characteristics of pituitary–adrenal response in a large group of VLBW infants (67). Compared to normotensive infants, hypotensive VLBW neonates requiring vasopressor/inotropes had higher ACTH but lower cortisol responses. These data suggest that even in VLBW preterm infants, the pituitary gland is mature enough to mount an adequate ACTH response and that the primary problem of relative adrenal insufficiency might be the inability of the adrenal glands to adequately increase gluco- and mineralocorticoid production in response to increased ACTH production.

While absolute adrenal insufficiency is a rare diagnosis in the neonatal period, there is accumulating evidence that relative adrenal insufficiency is a rather common entity especially in VLBW infants. Relative adrenal insufficiency is often defined as a low total serum cortisol level considered inappropriate for the degree of severity of the patient's illness. However, there is no agreement on what this level might be. In the adult, various cortisol levels have been proposed to define relative adrenal insufficiency. However, for the purpose of hormone replacement therapy, a cortisol level below 15 μg/dL is usually considered diagnostic for relative adrenal insufficiency in the adult (68). As for the neonatal patient population, some investigators have suggested a cutoff value of 5 μg/dL while others have been using the 15 μg/dL cutoff value recommended for adults for making the presumptive diagnosis of relative adrenal insufficiency in neonates (69,70). However, the use of an arbitrary single serum cortisol level to define relative adrenal insufficiency may not be appropriate in the neonatal period primarily because there is a large variation in serum cortisol levels in neonates (65,67,71–77). In addition, both gestational and postnatal age affect serum cortisol levels as there is an inverse relationship between serum cortisol levels and gestational and postnatal age at least up to three months after birth (78–81). Another important point to consider is that free rather than bound serum cortisol is the active form of the hormone. As most cortisol is bound to corticosteroid binding globulin and albumin in the circulation, variations in the concentration of these binding proteins may have a significant impact on the concentration of the biologically active form (i.e. free cortisol) (82). Conversely, total serum cortisol levels may change without any changes in the concentration of free cortisol (82). Under physiologic circumstances, the ratio of free-to-total serum cortisol is also different in adults from that in neonates as in adults free cortisol constitutes about 10% of total serum cortisol while in neonates this number is 20 to 30% (78). In addition, critical illness affects the percentage of free cortisol present in the serum as, at least in critically ill adults, the percentage of free cortisol can be almost three times as high as in healthy subjects (82). Recently, Ng et al. (67) showed a correlation between serum cortisol level and the lowest blood pressure registered in the immediate postnatal period in VLBW infants. They also demonstrated that this finding was independent of gestational age and that serum cortisol levels inversely correlated with the maximum and cumulative doses of vasopressor/inotropes. Yet, despite these correlations, they found an overlap in serum cortisol levels between normotensive and hypotensive VLBW infants. This finding makes it difficult to clearly define a serum cortisol level below which adrenal insufficiency can be diagnosed.

In addition to cardiovascular instability, immaturity of the hypothalamus–pituitary–adrenal axis has also been linked to susceptibility to common complications of prematurity such as PDA and bronchopulmonary dysplasia (BPD) (72,83,84). Given the role of glucocorticoids in the regulation of blood pressure and cardiovascular homeostasis, it is not surprising that adrenal insufficiency is commonly suspected as the cause of hypotension especially in VLBW neonates with vasopressor/inotrope-resistant hypotension. However, findings of a recent study suggest that relative adrenal insufficiency may also be common in near-term and term infants as more than half of near-term and term neonates receiving mechanical ventilation and vasopressor/inotrope support were found to have serum cortisol levels below 15 μg/dL (70). Interestingly, recent findings suggest that certain conditions such as congenital diaphragmatic hernia predispose term neonates to adrenal insufficiency (85). However, as mentioned above, even greater proportions of preterm neonates have low serum cortisol levels. For example, Korte and associates (69) showed that 76% of ill VLBW infants have cortisol levels less than 15 μg/dL. Finally, the recent demonstration of improvements in the cardiovascular status and normalization of the blood pressure in response to low-dose corticosteroid administration lends further support to the role of adrenal insufficiency in pathogenesis of neonatal hypotension especially in the preterm infant (66,86–92).

Downregulation of Adrenergic Receptors

With prolonged stimulation of receptors, and exposure to agonists, receptors first become desensitized and then downregulated. This process has been extensively studied in cardiovascular β- and α-adrenergic receptors. Initially, desensitization of receptor signaling occurs within seconds to minutes of ligand-induced activation of the receptor. This process involves phosphorylation of the cytosolic loops of the receptor resulting in conformational changes in receptor structure. This, in turn, leads to uncoupling of the receptor from its G-protein. If stimulation continues, reversible endocytosis of the intact receptor takes place. However, if the ligand–receptor interaction continues for hours, downregulation of the receptor occurs via activation of a lysosomal pathway resulting in the degradation of the receptor molecule. Recovery from down-regulation requires synthesis of new receptor molecules, a process that likely takes many hours and is up-regulated by the genomic actions of glucocorticoids (89,93–95).

Down-regulation of cardiovascular adrenergic receptors has recently been implicated in the pathogenesis of vasopressor/inotrope-resistant hypotension. The repeatedly documented improvement in the cardiovascular status of patients with refractory hypotension following steroid administration provides indirect evidence for the involvement of receptor down-regulation in the development of vasopressor/inotrope resistance. In addition, it shows the clinical relevance and applicability of basic research conducted on the genomic actions of glucocorticoids on the regulation of cardiovascular adrenergic receptor expression (94,95). Interestingly, vasopressor requirement decreases within 6 to 12 h following corticosteroid administration (Fig. 1-4A and 1-4B), the time thought to be necessary for biosynthesis of new receptors (89,90). However, it is important to point out that the beneficial steroidal effects on the cardiovascular system are not limited to adrenergic receptor up-regulation. Other genomic and nongenomic steroidal mechanism of actions exerted by gluco- or mineralocorticoids include the inhibition of iNOS synthesis, up-regulation of myocardial angiotensin II receptors, increases in

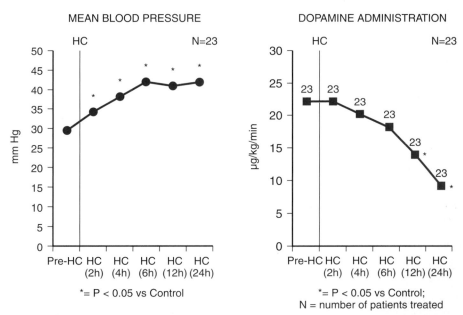

FIGURES 1-4A and 1-4B The increase in mean blood pressure and the decrease in dopamine requirement in response to low-dose hydrocortisone (HC) treatment in preterm infants with vasopressor-resistant hypotension. *Adapted with permission from Seri I, et al. Pediatrics 2001;107:1070–1074.*

cytosolic calcium availability in vascular smooth muscle and myocardial cells, inhibition of the degradation and reuptake of norepinephrine and epinephrine, and inhibition of prostacyclin production (89,96–98).

While down-regulation of cardiovascular adrenergic receptors is well described in adults, and many clinical observations support its occurrence in neonates, a recent animal study has questioned the presence of this phenomenon in the cardiovascular system in the early neonatal period. Autman and colleagues (99) studied the effects of acute and chronic stimulation of β-adrenergic receptors in newborn rats. They found that neonatal β-adrenergic receptors are inherently capable of desensitization in some but not all tissues. For instance, while β-adrenergic receptors in the liver were rapidly desensitized, β-agonists did not elicit desensitization in neonatal cardiac β-adrenergic receptors and the adenyl cyclase signaling pathway. Further research is required to address this area of developmental cardiovascular physiology.

SUMMARY

This chapter has reviewed the etiology, clinical phases, presentation, and pathophysiology of neonatal shock with special focus on the findings of clinical and translational studies in the area of developmental hemodynamics. Although much has been learned over the past years about the pathophysiology of neonatal shock, clinical application of the knowledge gained from these studies remains limited primarily because of the lack of large, well-designed, randomized clinical trials investigating the effects of the pathogenesis-driven treatment modalities on neonatal mortality and short- and long-term morbidity.

REFERENCES

1. Seri I. Circulatory support of the sick newborn infant. In Seminars in Neonatology: Perinatal Cardiology, vol. 6. Levene MI, Evans N, Archer N, eds. London, WB Saunders, 2001:85–95.
2. Nuntnarumit P, Yang W, Bada-Ellzey HS. Blood pressure measurements in the newborn. Clin Perinatol 1999;26:981–996.
3. Zubrow AB, Hulman S, Kushner H, Falner B. Determinants of blood pressure in infants admitted to neonatal intensive care units: a prospective multicenter study. J Perinatol 1995;15:470–479.
4. Munro MJ, Walker AM, Barfield CP. Hypotensive extremely low birth weight infants have reduced cerebral blood flow. Pediatrics 2004;114:1591–1596.
5. Victor S, Marson AG, Appleton RE, Beirne M, Weindling AM. Relationship between blood pressure, cerebral electrical activity, cerebral fractional oxygen extraction, and peripheral blood flow in very low birth weight newborn infants. Pediatr Res 2006;59:314–319.
6. Tsuji M, Saul JP, du Plessis A, Eichenwald E, Sobh J, Crocker R, Volpe JJ. Cerebral intravascular oxygenation correlates with mean arterial pressure in critically ill premature infants. Pediatrics 2000;106:625–632.
7. Tyszczuk L, Meek J, Elwell C, Wyatt JS. Cerebral blood flow is independent of mean arterial blood pressure in preterm infants undergoing intensive care. Pediatrics 1998;102:337–341.
8. Kissack CM, Garr R, Wardle SP, Weindling AM. Cerebral fractional oxygen extraction in very low birth weight infants is high when there is low left ventricular output and hypocarbia but is unaffected by hypotension. Pediatr Res 2004;55:400–405.
9. Seri I, Evans J. Controversies in the diagnosis and management of hypotension in the newborn infant. Curr Opin Pediatr 2001;13:116–123.
10. Al-Aweel I, Pursley DM, Rubin LP, Shah B, Weisberger S, Richardson DK. Variations in prevalence of hypotension, hypertension, and vasopressor use in NICUs. J Perinatol 2001;21:272–278.
11. Bauer K, Linderkamp O, Versmold HT. Systolic blood pressure and blood volume in preterm infants. Arch Dis Child, Fetal Neonatal Edn 1994;70:F230–F231.
12. Barr PA, Bailey PE, Sumners J, Cassady G. Relation between arterial blood pressure and blood volume and effect of infused albumin in sick preterm infants. Pediatrics 1977;60:282–289.
13. Wright IM, Goodall SR. Blood pressure and blood volume in preterm infants. Arch Dis Child, Fetal Neonatal Edn 1994;70:F230–F231.
14. Gill AB, Weindling AM. Randomised controlled trial of plasma protein fraction versus dopamine in hypotensive very low birthweight infants. Arch Dis Child 1993;69:284–287.
15. Lundstrom K, Pryds O, Greisen G. The haemodynamic effects of dopamine and volume expansion in sick preterm infants. Early Hum Dev 2000;57:157–163.
16. Anderson PA. The heart and development. Semin Perinatol 1996;20:482–509.

17. Noori S, Seri I. Pathophysiology of newborn hypotension outside the transitional period. Early Hum Dev 2005;81:399–404.
18. Rowland DG, Gutgesell HP. Noninvasive assessment of myocardial contractility, preload, and afterload in healthy newborn infants. Am J Cardiol 1995;75:818–821.
19. Kluckow M, Evans N. Low superior vena cava flow and intraventricular haemorrhage in preterm infants. Arch Dis Child, Fetal Neonatal Edn 2000;82:F188–F194.
20. Kehrer M, Blumenstock G, Ehehalt S, Goelz R, Poets C, Schoning M. Development of cerebral blood flow volume in preterm neonates during the first two weeks of life. Pediatr Res 2005;58:927–930.
21. Noori S, Friedlich P, Seri I. Pathophysiology of neonatal shock. In Fetal and Neonatal Physiology. third edn. Polin RA, Fox WW, Abman S, eds. Philadelphia, WB Saunders, 2003:772–782.
22. Reuss ML, Rudolph AM. Distribution and recirculation of umbilical and systemic venous blood flow in fetal lambs during hypoxia. third edn. J Dev Physiol 1980;2:71–84.
23. Davies JM, Tweed WA. The regional distribution and determinants of myocardial blood flow during asphyxia in the fetal lamb. Pediatr Res 1984;18:764–767.
24. Kuhnert M, Seelbach-Goebel B, Butterwegge M. Predictive agreement between the fetal arterial oxygen saturation and scalp pH: results of the German multicenter study. Am J Obstet Gynecol 1998;178:330–335.
25. Gunes T, Ozturk MA, Koklu SM, Narin N, Koklu E. Troponin-T levels in perinatally asphyxiated infants during the first 15 days of life. Acta Paediatr 2005;94:1638–1643.
26. Trevisanuto D, Picco G, Golin R, et al. Cardiac troponin I in asphyxiated neonates. Biol Neonate 2006;89:190–193.
27. Gaze DC, Collinson PO. Interpretation of cardiac troponin measurements in neonates – the devil is in the details. Biol Neonate 2006;89:194–196.
28. Szymankiewicz M, Matuszczak-Wleklak M, Hodgman JE, Gadzinowski J. Usefulness of cardiac troponin T and echocardiography in the diagnosis of hypoxic myocardial injury of full-term neonates. Biol Neonate 2005;88:19–23.
29. Walther FJ, Siassi B, Ramadan NA, Wu PY. Cardiac output in newborn infants with transient myocardial dysfunction. J Pediatr 1985;107:781–785.
30. Barberi I, Calabro MP, Cordaro S, et al. Myocardial ischaemia in neonates with perinatal asphyxia. Electrocardiographic, echocardiographic and enzymatic correlations. Eur J Pediatr 1999;158:742–747.
31. Seri I, Noori S. Diagnosis and treatment of neonatal hypotension outside the transitional period. Early Hum Dev 2005;81:405–411.
32. Landry DW, Oliver JA. The pathogenesis of vasodilatory shock. N Engl J Med 2001;345:588–595.
33. Quayle JM, Nelson MT, Standen NB. ATP-sensitive and inwardly rectifying potassium channels in smooth muscle. Physiol Rev 1997;77:1165–1232.
34. Murphy ME, Brayden JE. Nitric oxide hyperpolarizes rabbit mesenteric arteries via ATP-sensitive potassium channels. J Physiol 1995;486:47–58.
35. Vanelli G, Hussain SN, Dimori M, Aguggini G. Cardiovascular responses to glibenclamide during endotoxaemia in the pig. Vet Res Commun 1997;21:187–200.
36. Gardiner SM, Kemp PA, March JE, Bennett T. Regional haemodynamic responses to infusion of lipopolysaccharide in conscious rats: effects of pre- or post-treatment with glibenclamide. Br J Pharmacol 1999;128:1772–1778.
37. Warrillow S, Egi M, Bellomo R. Randomized, double-blind, placebo-controlled crossover pilot study of a potassium channel blocker in patients with septic shock. Crit Care Med 2006;34:980–985.
38. Oliver JA, Landry DW. Potassium channels and septic shock. Crit Care Med 2006;34:1255–1257.
39. Fink MP. Therapeutic options directed against platelet activating factor, eicosanoids and bradykinin in sepsis. J Antimicrob Chemother 1998;41:81–94.
40. Arons MM, Wheeler AP, Bernard GR, et al. Effects of ibuprofen on the physiology and survival of hypothermic sepsis. Ibuprofen in Sepsis Study Group. Crit Care Med 1999;27:699–707.
41. Feuerstein G, Zerbe RL, Meyer DK, Kopin IJ. Alteration of cardiovascular, neurogenic, and humoral responses to acute hypovolemic hypotension by administered prostacyclin. J Cardiovasc Pharmacol 1982;4:246–253.
42. Machiedo GW, Warden MJ, LoVerme PJ, Rush BF Jr. Hemodynamic effects of prolonged infusion of prostaglandin E1 (PGE1) after hemorrhagic shock. Adv Shock Res 1982;8:171–176.
43. Reines HD, Halushka PV, Cook JA, Wise WC, Rambo W. Plasma thromboxane concentrations are raised in patients dying with septic shock. Lancet 1982;2:174–175.
44. Ball HA, Cook JA, Wise WC, Halushka PV. Role of thromboxane, prostaglandins and leukotrienes in endotoxic and septic shock. Intensive Care Med 1986;12:116–126.
45. Rubanyi GM. Nitric oxide and circulatory shock. Adv Exp Med Biol 1998;454:165–172.
46. Liu S, Adcock IM, Old RW, Barnes PJ, Evans TW. Lipopolysaccharide treatment in vivo induces widespread tissue expression of inducible nitric oxide synthase mRNA. Biochem Biophys Res Commun 1993;196:1208–1213.
47. Taylor BS, Geller DA. Molecular regulation of the human inducible nitric oxide synthase (iNOS) gene. Shock 2000;13:413–424.
48. Titheradge MA. Nitric oxide in septic shock. Biochim Biophys Acta 1999;1411:437–455.
49. Doughty L, Carcillo JA, Kaplan S, Janosky J. Plasma nitrite and nitrate concentrations and multiple organ failure in pediatric sepsis. Crit Care Med 1998;26:157–162.
50. Carcillo JA. Nitric oxide production in neonatal and pediatric sepsis. Crit Care Med 1999;27:1063–1065.

51. Barrington KJ, Etches PC, Schulz R, et al. The hemodynamic effects of inhaled nitric oxide and endogenous nitric oxide synthesis blockade in newborn piglets during infusion of heat-killed group B streptococci. Crit Care Med 2000;28:800–808.

52. Mitaka C, Hirata Y, Ichikawa K, et al. Effects of nitric oxide synthase inhibitor on hemodynamic change and O2 delivery in septic dogs. Am J Physiol 1995;268(5 Pt 2):H2017–H2023.

53. Grover R, Zaccardelli D, Colice G, Guntupalli K, Watson D, Vincent JL. An open-label dose escalation study of the nitric oxide synthase inhibitor, N(G)-methyl-L-arginine hydrochloride (546C88), in patients with septic shock. Glaxo Wellcome International Septic Shock Study Group. Crit Care Med 1999;27:913–922.

54. Mitaka C, Hirata Y, Yokoyama K, Makita K, Imai T. A selective inhibitor for inducible nitric oxide synthase improves hypotension and lactic acidosis in canine endotoxic shock. Crit Care Med 2001;29:2156–2161.

55. Rozenfeld V, Cheng JW. The role of vasopressin in the treatment of vasodilation in shock states. Ann Pharmacother 2000;34:250–254.

56. Robin JK, Oliver JA, Landry DW. Vasopressin deficiency in the syndrome of irreversible shock. J Trauma 2003;54:S149–S154.

57. Landry DW, Oliver JA. The pathogenesis of vasodilatory shock. N Engl J Med 2001;345:588–595.

58. Landry DW, Levin HR, Gallant EM, et al. Vasopressin deficiency contributes to the vasodilation of septic shock. Circulation 1997;95:1122–1125.

59. Liedel JL, Meadow W, Nachman J, Koogler T, Kahana MD. Use of vasopressin in refractory hypotension in children with vasodilatory shock: five cases and a review of the literature. Pediatr Crit Care Med 2002;3:15–18.

60. Malay MB, Ashton JL, Dahl K, et al. Heterogeneity of the vasoconstrictor effect of vasopressin in septic shock. Crit Care Med 2004;32:1327–1331.

61. Cox BE, Rosenfeld CR. Ontogeny of vascular angiotensin II receptor subtype expression in ovine development. Pediatr Res 1999;45:414–424.

62. Kaiser JR, Cox BE, Roy TA, Rosenfeld CR. Differential development of umbilical and systemic arteries. I. ANG II receptor subtype expression. Am J Physiol 1998;274:R797–R807.

63. Bendeck MP, Langille BL. Rapid accumulation of elastin and collagen in the aortas of sheep in the immediate perinatal period. Circ Res 1991;69:1165–1169.

64. Leitman DC, Benson SC, Johnson LK. Glucocorticoids stimulate collagen and noncollagen protein synthesis in cultured vascular smooth muscle cells. J Cell Biol 1984;98:541–549.

65. Hanna CE, Keith LD, Colasurdo MA, et al. Hypothalamic pituitary adrenal function in the extremely low birth weight infant. J Clin Endocrinol Metab 1993;76:384–387.

66. Ng PC, Lam CWK, Fok TF, et al. Refractory hypotension in preterm infants with adrenocortical insufficiency. Arch Dis Child, Fetal Neonatal Edn 2001;84:F122–F124.

67. Ng PC, Lee CH, Lam CWK, Ma KC, Chan IH, Wong E. Transient adrenocortical insufficiency of prematurity and systemic hypotension in very low birthweight infants. Arch Dis Child, Fetal Neonatal Edn 2004;89:F119–F126.

68. Cooper MS, Stewart PM. Corticosteroid insufficiency in acutely ill patients. N Engl J Med 2003;348:727–734.

69. Korte C, Styne D, Merritt TA, Mayes D, Wertz A, Helbock HJ. Adrenocortical function in the very low birth weight infant: improved testing sensitivity and association with neonatal outcome. J Pediatr 1996;128:257–263.

70. Fernandez E, Schrader R, Watterberg K. Prevalence of low cortisol value in term and nearterm infants with vasopressor-resistant hypotension. J Perinatol 2005;25:114–118.

71. Hingre RV, Gross SJ, Hingre KS, Mayes DM, Richman RA. Adrenal steroidogenesis in very low birth weight preterm infants. J Clin Endocrinol Metab 1994;78:266–270.

72. Watterberg KL, Scott SM. Evidence of early adrenal insufficiency in babies who develop bronchopulmonary dysplasia. Pediatrics 1995;95:120–125.

73. Jett PL, Samuels MH, McDaniel PA, et al. Variability of plasma cortisol levels in extremely low birth weight infants. J Clin Endocrinol Metab 1997;82:2921–2925.

74. Hanna CE, Jett PL, Laird MR, Mandel SH, LaFranchi SH, Reynolds JW. Corticosteroid binding globulin, total serum cortisol, and stress in extremely-low-birth-weight infants. Am J Perinatol 1997;14:201–204.

75. Ng PC, Wong GWK, Lam CWK, et al. The pituitary–adrenal responses to exogenous human corticotropin-releasing hormone in preterm, very low birth weight infants. J Clin Endocrinol Metab 1997;82:797–799.

76. Procianoy RS, Cecin SKG, Pinheiro CEA. Umbilical cord cortisol and prolactin levels in preterm infants; Relation to labour and delivery. Acta Paediatr Scand 1983;72:713–716.

77. Terrone DA, Smith LG, Wolf EJ, Uzbay LA, Sun S, Miller RC. Neonatal effects and serum cortisol levels after multiple courses of maternal corticosteroids. Obstet Gynecol 1997;90:819–823.

78. Rokicki W, Forest MG, Loras B, Bonnet H, Bertand J. Free cortisol of human plasma in the first three months of life. Biol Neonate 1990;57:21–29.

79. Wittekind CA, Arnold JD, Leslie GI, Luttrell B, Jones MP. Longitudinal study of plasma ACTH and cortisol in very low birth weight infants in the first 8 weeks of life. Early Hum Dev 1993;33:191–200.

80. Goldkrand JW, Schulte RL, Messer RH. Maternal and fetal plasma cortisol levels at parturition. Obstet Gynecol 1976;47:41–45.

81. Scott SM, Watterberg KL. Effect of gestational age, postnatal age, and illness on plasma cortisol concentrations in premature infants. Pediatr Res 1995;37:112–116.

82. Hamrahian AH, Oseni TS, Arafah BM. Measurements of serum free cortisol in critically ill patients. N Engl J Med 2004;350:1629–1638.

83. Watterberg KL, Scott SM, Backstrom C, Gifford KL, Cook KL. Links between early adrenal function and respiratory outcome in preterm infants: airway inflammation and patent ductus arteriosus. Pediatrics 2000;105:320–324.

84. Watterberg KL, Gerdes JS, Cole CH, et al. Prophylaxis of early adrenal insufficiency to prevent bronchopulmonary dysplasia: a multicenter trial. Pediatrics 2004;114:1649–1657.

85. Pittinger TP, Sawin RS. Adrenocortical insufficiency in infants with congenital diaphragmatic hernia: a pilot study. J Pediatr Surg 2000;35:223–225.

86. Helbock HJ, Insoft RM, Conte FA. Glucocorticoid-responsive hypotension in extremely low birth weight newborns. Pediatrics 1993;92:715–717.

87. Fauser A, Pohlandt F, Bartmann, Gortner L. Rapid increase of blood pressure in extremely low birth weight infants after a single dose of dexamethasone. Eur J Pediatr 1993;152:354–356.

88. Gaissmaier RE, Pohlandt F. Single dose dexamethasone treatment of hypotension in preterm infants. J Pediatr 1999;134:701–705.

89. Seri I, Tan R, Evans J. Cardiovascular effects of hydrocortisone in preterm infants with pressor-resistant hypotension. Pediatrics 2001;107:1070–1074.

90. Noori S, Siassi B, Durand M, Acherman R, Sardesai S, Ramanathan R. Cardiovascular effects of low-dose dexamethasone in very low birth weight neonates with refractory hypotension. Biol Neonate 2006;89:82–87.

91. Noori S, Friedlich P, Wong P, Ebrahimi M, Siassi B, Seri I. Hemodynamic changes after low-dose hydrocortisone administration in vasopressor-treated preterm and term neonates. Pediatrics 2006;118:1456–66.

92. Ng PC, Lee CH, Bnur FL, et al. A double-blind, randomized, controlled study of a "stress dose" of hydrocortisone for rescue treatment of refractory hypotension in preterm infants. Pediatrics 2006;117:367–375.

93. Tsao P, von Zastrow M. Downregulation of G protein-coupled receptors. Curr Opin Neurobiol 2000;10:365–369.

94. Davies AO, Lefkowitz RJ. Regulation of beta-adrenergic receptors by steroid hormones. Annu Rev Physiol 1984;46:119–130.

95. Hadcock JR, Malbon CC. Regulation of beta adrenergic receptor by permissive hormones: gluco-corticoids increase steady-state levels of receptor mRNA. Proc Natl Acad Sci USA 1988;85:8415–8419.

96. Radomski MW, Palmer RMJ, Moncada S. Glucocorticoids inhibit the expression of an inducible, but not the constitutive, nitric oxide synthase in vascular endothelial cells. Proc Natl Acad Sci USA 1990;87:10043–10047.

97. Wehling M. Specific, nongenomic actions of steroid hormones. Annu Rev Physiol 1997;59:365–393.

98. Segar JL, Bedell K, Page WV, Mazursky JE, Nuyt AM, Robillard JE. Effect of cortisol on gene expression of the renin–angiotensin system in fetal sheep. Pediatr Res 1995;37:741–746.

99. Auman JT, Seidler FJ, Tate CA, Slotkin TA. Are developing beta-adrenoceptors able to desensitize? Acute and chronic effects of beta-agonists in neonatal heart and liver. Am J Physiol Regul Integr Comp Physiol 2002;283:R205–R217.

Chapter 2

Autoregulation of Vital and Nonvital Organ Blood Flow in the Preterm and Term Neonate

Gorm Greisen, MD, PhD

Regulation of Arterial Tone

Blood Flow to the Brain

Blood Flow to Other Organs

Distribution of Cardiac Output in the Healthy Human Neonate

Mechanisms Governing the Redistribution of Cardiac Output in the Fetal "Dive" Reflex

Distribution of Cardiac Output in the Shocked Newborn

Other Scenarios

References

In most organs the principal role of perfusion is to provide substrates for cellular energy metabolism, with the final purpose of maintaining normal intracellular concentrations of the high-energy phosphate metabolites adenosine triphosphate (ATP) and phosphocreatine (PCr). The critical substrate is usually oxygen. Accordingly, organ blood flow is regulated by the energy demand of the given tissue. For instance in the brain, during maximal activation by seizures, cerebral blood flow increases 3-fold while in the muscle during maximal exercise, blood flow increases up to 8-fold. In addition, some organs such as the brain, heart, and liver have higher baseline oxygen and thus blood flow demand than others. Finally, in the skin, perfusion may be considerably above the metabolic needs as the increase in skin blood flow plays an important role in thermoregulation. Indeed, during heating, skin blood flow may increase by as much as 4-fold without any increase in energy demand.

In the developing organism metabolic requirements are increased by as much as 40%. Since growth requires generation of new protein and fat, energy metabolism and, in particular, tissue oxygen requirement are not increased as much.

When blood flow is failing there are several lines of defense mechanisms before the tissue is damaged. First, more oxygen is extracted from the blood. Normal oxygen extraction is about 30%, resulting in a venous oxygen saturation of 65 to 70%. Oxygen extraction can increase up to 50 to 60%, resulting in a venous oxygen saturation of 40 to 50%, which corresponds to a venous, i.e. end-capillary, oxygen tension of 3 to 4 kPa. This is the critical value for oxygen tension for driving the diffusion of molecular oxygen from the capillary into the cell and to the mitochondrion (Fig. 2-1). Second, microvascular anatomy and the pathophysiology of the

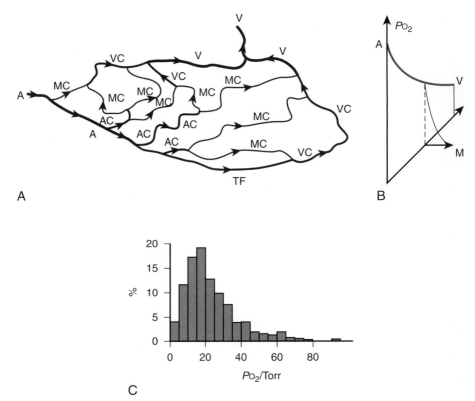

FIGURE 2-1 (A) Draft of a capillary network. (B) A three-dimensional graph illustrating the Po_2 gradients from the arterial (A) to the venous (V) end of the capillaries and the radial gradient of Po_2 in surrounding tissue to the mitochondrion (M). Y-axis: Po_2; X-axis: distance along the capillary (typically 1000 μm); Z-axis: distance into tissue (typically 50 μm). (C) The wide distribution of tissue Po_2 as recorded by microelectrode. Y-axis: frequency of measurements; X-axis: Po_2. Po_2 values in tissue are typically 10 to 30 Torr (1.5 to 4.5 kPa), but range from near-arterial levels to near zero. The cells with the lowest Po_2 determine the ischemic threshold, i.e. the most remote cells at the venous end of capillaries. Microvascular factors, such as capillary density, and distribution of blood flow among capillaries are very important for oxygen transport to tissue. Microvascular factors are not discussed in this chapter.

underlying disease process are both important for the final steps of oxygen delivery to tissue. When the cell senses oxygen insufficiency, its function is affected as growth stops, organ function fails, and finally cellular and thus organ survival are threatened (Fig. 2-2). Ischemia is the term used for inadequate blood flow to maintain appropriate cellular function and integrity. Since there are several steps in the cellular reaction to oxygen insufficiency, more than one ischemic threshold may be defined.

The immature mammal is able to "centralize" blood flow during periods of stress. This pattern of flow distribution is often called the "dive reflex", since it is qualitatively similar to the adaptation of circulation in seals during diving, a process that allows sea mammals to stay under water for 20 min or more. Blood flow to the skin, muscle, kidneys, liver, and other nonvital organs is reduced to spare the oxygen reserve for the vital organs: the brain, heart, and adrenals. This reaction is relevant during birth with the limitations on placental oxygen transport imposed by uterine contractions and has been studied intensively in the fetal lamb. It has the potential of prolonging passive survival at a critical moment in the individual's life. For comparison, the "fight-or-flight" response of the mature terrestrial mammal supports sustained maximal muscle work.

Blood flows toward the point of lowest resistance. While flow velocities in the heart are high enough to allow kinetic energy of the blood to play an additional role, this role is minimal in the peripheral circulation. Organs and tissues are

FIGURE 2-2 **The lines of defense against oxygen insufficiency**. First, when blood pressure falls, autoregulation of organ blood flow will reduce vascular resistance and keep blood flow nearly unaffected. If the blood pressure falls below the lower limit of the autoregulation, or if autregulation is impaired by vascular pathology or immaturity, blood flow to the tissue falls. At this point, oxygen extraction increases from each milliliter of blood. The limit of this compensation is when the minimal venous oxygen saturation, or rather the minimal end-capillary oxygen tension has been reached. This process is determined by microvascular factors as illustrated in Fig. 2-1. When the limits of oxygen extraction have been reached, the marginal cells resort to anaerobic metabolism (increase glucose consumption to produce lactate) to meet their metabolic needs. If this is insufficient, oxygen consumption decreases as metabolic functions related to growth and to organ function are shut down. However, in vital organs, such as the brain, heart, and adrenal glands, loss of function is life threatening. In nonvital organs, development may be affected if this critical state is long lasting. Acute cellular death by necrosis occurs only when vital cellular functions break down and membrane potentials and integrity cannot be maintained.

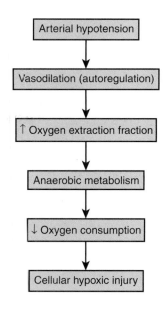

perfused in parallel and the blood flow through the tissue is the result of the pressure gradient from artery to vein, the so-called perfusion pressure. Vascular resistance is due to the limited diameter of blood vessels, particularly the smaller arteries and arterioles, and blood viscosity. Regulation of organ blood flow takes place by modifying arterial diameter, i.e. by varying the tone of the smooth muscle cells of the arterial wall. Factors that influence vascular resistance are usually divided into four categories: blood pressure, chemical (Pco_2 and Po_2), metabolic (functional activation), and neurogenic. Most studies have been done on cerebral vessels. The account below therefore refers to cerebral vessels from mature animals, unless stated otherwise.

REGULATION OF ARTERIAL TONE

The Role of Conduit Arteries in Regulating Vascular Resistance

It is usually assumed that the arteriole – the precapillary muscular vessel with a diameter of 20 to 150 μm – is the primary determinant of vascular resistance and the larger arteries are more or less considered as passive conduits. However, this is not the case. For instance, in the adult cat the pressure in the small cerebral arteries (150 to 200 μm) is only 50 to 60% of the aortic pressure (1). Thus, the reactivity of the entire muscular arterial tree is of relevance in regulating organ blood flow and the role of the pre-arteriolar vessels is likely more important in the newborn than in the adult. First, the smaller body size translates to smaller conduit arteries. The resistance is proportional to length but inversely proportional to the diameter to the power of four. Therefore the conduit arteries of the newborn will make an even more important contribution to the vascular resistance. Second, conduit arteries in the newborn are very reactive. The diameter of the carotid artery increases by 75% during acute asphyxia in term lambs, whereas the diameter of the descending aorta decreases by 15% (2). The latter change may just reflect a passive elastic reaction to the decreased blood pressure, whereas the former indicates active vasodilation translating into reduced vascular tone. For comparison, flow-induced vasodilatation in the forearm in adults is in the order of 5% or so. As resistance is proportional to the diameter to the power of four, the findings in asphyxiated lambs indicate a roughly 90% reduction of the arterial component of the cerebrovascular resistance with a near doubling of the arterial component of

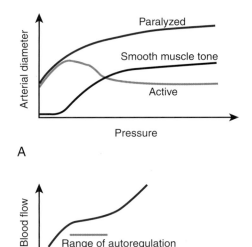

FIGURE 2-3 Increasing pressure leads to progressive dilatation of a paralyzed artery. As pressure increases more, the elastic capacity is exhausted and vasodilation decreases as collagen restricts further dilation limiting risk of rupture (A). A certain range of pressures is associated with a proportional variation in smooth muscle tone. The precise mechanism of this mechano-chemical coupling is not known but it is endogenous to all vascular smooth muscle cells. As a result, in an active artery, the diameter varies inversely with pressure over a certain range. This phenomenon represents at the basis arterial "autoregulation" (B).

vascular resistance in the lower body. Incidentally, these observations also suggest that blood flow velocity as recorded from conduit arteries by Doppler ultrasound may be potentially misleading in the neonatal patient population.

Arterial Reaction to Pressure (Autoregulation)

Smooth-muscle cells of the arterial wall contract in response to increased intravascular pressure in the local arterial segment to a degree that more than compensates for the passive stretching of the vessel wall by the increased pressure. The net result is that arteries constrict when pressure increases and dilate when pressure drops. This phenomenon is called the autoregulation of blood flow (Fig. 2-3) and the cellular mechanisms of this process are now better understood. Vessel wall constriction constitutes an intrinsic myogenic reflex and is independent of endothelial function. Rather, pressure induces an increase in the smooth muscle cell membrane potential, which regulates vascular smooth muscle cell activity through the action of voltage-gated calcium channels. Although the precise mechanism of the mechano-chemical coupling is unknown, the calcium signal is modulated in many ways (3). It is beyond the scope of this chapter to discuss the modulation of the calcium signal in detail. Suffice it to mention that phospholipases and activation of protein kinase C are involved, and, at least in the rat middle cerebral artery, the arachidonic acid metabolite 20-HETE has also been implicated (4). Furthermore, a different modulation of intracellular calcium concentration by alternative sources such as the calcium-dependent K^+ channels also exists. The role of the different K^+ channels in modifying smooth cell membrane potential may, at least in part, explain the various arterial responses to pressure in different vascular beds. These vascular bed-specific responses result in the unique blood flow distribution between vital and nonvital organs (5).

Interaction of Autoregulation and Hypoxic Vasodilatation

As described above, arterial smooth muscle tone is affected by a number of factors, all contributing to determine the incident level of vascular resistance. Among the vasodilators, hypoxia is one of the more potent and physiologically relevant factors.

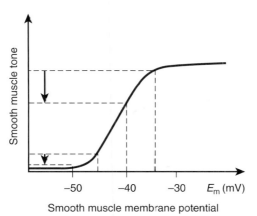

Smooth muscle membrane potential

FIGURE 2-4 The relationship between smooth muscle cell membrane potential (E_m) and tone. Pressure affects smooth muscle tone through membrane potential. Increased pressure increases membrane potential (i.e. makes it less negative), whereas decreased pressure induces hyperpolarization (membrane potential more negative). Hyperpolarization induces relaxation and hence vasodilatation. The modifying effect of hypoxia is illustrated by the dashed lines and arrows. At high membrane potential (−35 mV), a decrease in membrane potential by 5 mV induces a marked reduction in muscular tone. Thus, at high pressures hypoxemia can be compensated by vasodilatation. However, at low membrane potential (hyperpolarization) a similar hypoxia-induced decrease in membrane potential has much less effect on muscular tone. This predicts that at low blood pressure, hypoxemia cannot be well compensated by increased blood flow. Many other factors may influence muscle tone by modifying membrane potential, and the magnitude of effects can be predicted to be interdependent.

Vascular reactivity to O_2 depends, in part, on intact endothelial function ensuring appropriate local nitric oxide (NO) production. Hypoxia also induces tissue lactic acidosis. The decreased pH constitutes a point of interaction between the O_2 reactivity and the CO_2 reactivity (see below). In addition, hypoxia decreases smooth-muscle membrane potential by the direct and selective opening of both the calcium-activated and ATP-sensitive K^+ channels in the cell membrane (6). In the immature brain, adenosine is also an important regulator of the vascular response to hypoxia (7). The cellular response to hypoxia is independent of the existing intravascular pressure (8). However, at lower pressures, the decrease in membrane potential only leads to minimal further arterial dilation because, at low vascular tone, the membrane potential/muscular tone relationship is outside the steep part of the slope (Fig. 2-4). In other words, at low perfusion pressures the dilator pathway has already been near maximally activated. Therefore in a hypotensive neonate, a superimposed hypoxic event cannot be appropriately compensated due to the low perfusion pressure. The end-result is tissue hypoxia–ischemia with the potential of causing irreversible damage to organs especially to the brain.

Interaction of Autoregulation and P_{CO_2}

Arteries and arterioles constrict with hypocapnia and dilate with hypercapnia. The principal part of this reaction is mediated through changes in pH, i.e. H^+ concentration. Perivascular pH has a direct effect on the membrane potential of arterial smooth muscle cells since the extracellular H^+ concentration is one of the main determinants of the potassium conductance of the plasma membrane in arterial smooth muscle cells regulating the outward K^+ current (6). Therefore when the pH decreases, the K^+ outflow from the vascular smooth muscle cell increases, resulting in hyperpolarization of the cell membrane and thus vasodilatation. Furthermore, increased, extracellular and, to a lesser degree, intracellular H^+ concentrations reduce the conductance of the voltage-dependent calcium channels further enhancing vasorelaxation (9).

Hypercapnic vasodilatation is reduced by up to 50% when NO synthase (NOS) activity is blocked in the brain of the adult rat (10). The hypercapnic response is restituted by the addition of an NO donor (11). This finding suggests that unhindered local NO production is necessary for the pH to exert its vasoregulatory effects. It has recently been suggested that, although the calcium-activated and ATP-sensitive K^+ channels play the primary role in the vascular response to changes in P_{CO_2}, the function of these channels is regulated by local NO production (12).

The role of prostanoids (13,14) in mediating the vascular response to P_{CO_2} is less clear. The fact that indomethacin abolishes the normal cerebral (or other organ) blood flow–CO_2 response in preterm infants (15) is likely a direct effect of the drug independent of its inhibitory action on prostanoid synthesis. This notion is supported by the finding that ibuprofen is devoid of such effects on the organ blood flow–CO_2 response (16).

INTERACTION OF AUTOREGULATION AND FUNCTIONAL ACTIVATION (METABOLIC BLOOD FLOW CONTROL)

Several mechanisms operate to match local blood flow to metabolic requirements, including changes in pH, local production of adenosine, ATP and NO, and local neural mechanisms. In muscle it appears that there is not a single factor dominating, since the robust and very fast coupling of activity and blood flow is almost unaffected by blocking any of these mechanisms one by one (17). In brain, astrocytes may be the central cites of regulation of this response in the neurovascular unit via their perivascular end-feet (18) and by utilizing many of the above-listed cellular mechanisms such as changes in K^+ ion flux and local production of prostanoids, ATP, and adenosine. Among these cellular regulators, adenosine has been proposed to play a principal role (19). Adenosine works by regulating the activity of the calcium-activated and ATP-sensitive K^+ channels.

Flow-mediated Vasodilatation

Endothelial cells sense flow by shear stress, and produce NO in reaction to high shear stress at high flow velocities. NO diffuses freely, and reaches the smooth-muscle cell underneath the endothelium. NO acts on smooth-muscle K^+ channels using cyclic GMP as the secondary messenger and then a series of intermediate steps. Since NO is a vasodilator, the basic arterial reflex to high flow is vasodilation. Thus, when a tissue is activated (e.g. a muscle contracts), the local vessels first dilate, as directed by the mechanisms of the metabolic flow control described earlier, and blood flow increases. This initial increase in blood flow is then sensed in the conduit arteries through the shear-stress-induced increase in local NO production and vascular resistance is further reduced allowing flow to increase yet again. The action remains local as the generated NO diffusing into the bloodstream is largely inactivated by hemoglobin.

The Sympathetic Nervous System

Epinephrine in the blood originates from the adrenal glands, whereas norepinephrine is produced by the sympathetic nerve endings and the extra-adrenal chromafin tissue. Sympathetic nerves are present in nearly all vessels located in the adventitia and on the smooth muscle cells. Adrenoreceptors are widely distributed in the cardiovascular system, located on smooth muscle and endothelial cells. Several different adrenoreceptors exist; alpha-1 receptors with at least three subtypes are present primarily in the arteries and the myocardium, while alpha-2, beta-1, and beta-2 receptors are expressed in all types of vessels and the myocardium. In the arteries and veins alpha-receptor stimulation causes vasoconstriction, and beta-receptor stimulation results in vasodilatation. Both alpha- and beta-adrenoreceptors are frequently expressed in the membrane of the same cell. Therefore, the response of the given cell to epinephrine or norepinephrine depends on the relative abundance of the receptor types expressed (20). Of clinical importance is the regulation of the expression of the cardiovascular adrenergic receptors by corticosteroids, the high incidence of relative adrenal insufficiency in preterm neonates and critically ill term infants, the role of gluco- and mineralo-corticoids in maintaining the sensitivity of the cardiovascular system to endogenous and exogenous catecholamines and the down-regulation of the cardiovascular adrenergic receptors in response to increased release of endogenous catecholamines or administration of exogenous catecholamines in critical illness (21–23). Typically, arteries and arterioles of the skin, gut, and muscle constrict in response to increases in endogenous catecholamine production, whereas those of the heart and brain either do not constrict or dilate (see below). The response also depends on the resting tone of the given vessel. Furthermore, the sensitivity of a vessel to circulating norepinephrine may be less than the sensitivity to norepinephrine produced by increased sympathetic nerve activity, since alpha-1 receptors may be particularly abundant in the membrane regions close to the nerve terminals. The signaling pathways of the adrenoreceptors are complex and dependent on the receptor subtype. Activation of alpha-adrenoreceptors generally results in vasoconstriction mediated by increased release of calcium from intracellular stores as a first step, while beta-receptor induced vasodilation is mediated by increased cyclic AMP generation. However, the system is far more complex and, among other mechanisms, receptor activation-associated changes in K^+ conductance and local NO synthesis are also involved. Finally, the sympathetic nervous system is activated during hypoxia, hypotension, or hypovolemia via stimulation of different chemo- and baroreceptors in vessel walls and the vasomotor centers in the medulla. Activation of the sympathetic nervous system plays a central role in the cardiovascular response to stress and it is the mainstay of the dive reflex response during hypoxia–ischemia.

Humoral Factors in General Circulation

A large number of endogenous vasoactive factors other than those mentioned earlier also play a role in the extremely complex process of organ blood flow regulation such as angiotensin-II, arginine–vasopressin, vasointestinal peptide, neuropeptide gamma, and endothelin-1. However, none of these vasoactive factors has been shown to have a significant importance in isolation under normal conditions except for the role of angiotensin-II in regulating renal microhemodynamics.

Summary

In summary, a great many factors have an input and interact to define the degree of contraction of the vascular smooth muscle cells and hence regulate arterial and arteriolar tone (Fig. 2-4). Although many details are unknown, especially in the developing immature animal or human, the final common pathways appears to involve the smooth-cell membrane potential, cytoplasmic calcium concentration, and the calcium/calmodulin myosin light-chain kinase-mediated phosphorylation of the regulatory light chains of myosin resulting in the interaction of actin and myosin (Fig. 2-5). However, the complexity of the known factors and their interplay as well as the differences in the response among the different organs are

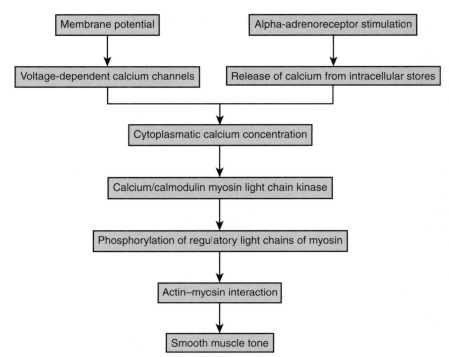

FIGURE 2-5 A scheme of the pathway from smooth muscle cell membrane potential and alpha-adrenoreceptor stimulation to changes in muscle tone.

overwhelming and no simple or unifying principle of vascular tone regulation has gained a foothold. Indeed, the complexity predicts that vascular tone and reactivity in a particular arterial segment in a particular tissue may differ markedly from that in other segments or other tissues. Unfortunately, the insights are as yet insufficient to allow any quantitative predictions for different organs or vascular tree segments.

BLOOD FLOW TO THE BRAIN

Brain injury is common in newborn infants. It can occur rapidly, is frequently irreversible, and rarely, in itself, prevents survival. Injury to no other organs in the neonatal period has the same clinical importance as the other organs have a better capacity to recover even from severe hypoxic–ischemic damage. Disturbances in blood flow and inflammation have been proposed as the major factors in the development of neonatal brain injury.

Autoregulation of Cerebral Blood Flow in the Immature Brain

Pressure–flow autoregulation has been widely investigated in the immature cerebral vasculature since the original observation of direct proportionality of cerebral blood flow (CBF) to systolic blood pressure in a group of neonates during stabilization after birth (24).

An adequate autoregulatory plateau, shifted to the left to match the lower perinatal blood pressure, has been demonstrated in several animal species shortly after birth, including dogs (25,26), lambs (27,28), and rats (29). In fetal lambs, autoregulation is not present at 0.6 gestation but is functional at 0.9 gestation (30). The lower threshold of the autoregulation is developmentally regulated and it is closer to the normal resting systemic blood pressure at 0.75 gestation compared to 0.9 gestation (31). Thus, in the more immature subject there is less vasodilator reserve, which limits the effectiveness of CBF autoregulation at earlier stages of development.

In newborn lambs, autoregulation could be completely abolished for 4 to 7 h by 20 min of hypoxemia with arterial oxygen saturations about 50% (32).

Unfortunately, the response of CBF autoregulation to pathological conditions and the impact of immaturity on the process are much less well investigated in the human neonate. The reason for this is that studies with controlled manipulation of blood pressure over a significant range cannot be performed for obvious reasons. However, observational studies of global CBF in stable neonates without evidence of major brain injury suggest that autoregulation is intact (33–38). More recently, in a group of premature neonates of 24 to 34 weeks' gestation (median gestational age, 27.5 weeks) absolute cerebral blood flow was measured by near-infrared spectroscopy (NIRS) using the oxygen transient method and the findings in 14 hypotensive subjects (mean blood pressure < 30 mm Hg) were compared with those in 16 patients with mean blood pressures of 30 mm Hg or more. CBF was 13.9 vs. 12.3 mL/100 g/min, suggesting that the lower pressure-threshold of autoregulation in these babies was below 30 mm Hg (39). In a group of 13 extremely preterm babies with a median gestational age of 24 weeks (60% of gestation) CBF measured by NIRS was found to be very low at 6.7 mL/100 g/min (range, 4.4 to 11 mL/100 g/min). However, there was no association between CBF and mean blood pressure in these patients suggesting that autoregulation in the human may develop earlier than in the lamb (40). These latter findings were supported by another study using NIRS to estimate fractional oxygen extraction by the jugular venous occlusion method in very preterm babies as fractional oxygen extraction in 14 babies of 27 weeks' gestation and with a mean arterial blood pressure of 25 mm Hg did not differ from that in the controls (41). In contrast to this finding, evidence of absent autoregulation has been found in term infants under pathological conditions such as following severe birth asphyxia and in preterm infants preceding major germinal layer hemorrhage (36,38,42).

Based on imaging of flow using single photon emission computed tomography (SPECT) during arterial hypotension in 24 preterm infants with persistently normal brain ultrasound it has been suggested that CBF to the periventricular white matter may be selectively reduced at blood pressures below 30 mm Hg (43). Although these data support the notion that the periventricular white matter represents a "watershed area," the statistical relation in this study was based on differences among different infants and thus there may be alternative explanations for the findings. However, in support of the findings of this study, a recent study using NIRS to assess absolute CBF in very preterm neonates during the first postnatal day found some evidence for the lower threshold of the autoregulatory curve being around 29 mm Hg (44).

In conclusion, the lower threshold for CBF autoregulation may be around 30 mm Hg or somewhat below and autoregulation can be assumed to operate in most newborn infants, even the most immature. When blood pressure falls below the threshold, CBF will fall more than proportionally due to the elastic reduction in vascular diameter. However, significant blood flow is believed to be present until the blood pressure is below 20 mm Hg.

Effect of Carbon Dioxide on CBF Autoregulation

Changes in carbon dioxide tension (P_{CO_2}) have more pronounced effects on CBF than on blood flow in other organs due to the presence of the blood–brain barrier. The blood–brain barrier is an endothelium with tight junctions, which does not allow HCO_3^- to pass through readily. The restricted diffusion of HCO_3^- means that hypercapnia decreases pH in the perivascular space in the brain more readily than elsewhere in blood were the buffering is more effective due to the presence of hemoglobin. This difference in response to a change in P_{CO_2} continues until HCO_3^- equilibrates over the course of hours.

In normocapnic adults small acute changes in arterial P_{CO_2} ($Pa,_{CO_2}$) result in a change in CBF by 30% per kPa (4% per mm Hg $Pa,_{CO_2}$). Similar reactivity has been demonstrated in the normal human neonate by venous occlusion plethysmography (45,46) and in stable preterm ventilated infants without major germinal layer hemorrhage by using the ^{133}Xe clearance technique (35). However, $Pa,_{CO_2}$ reactivity is less than 30% per kPa during the first 24 h (36).

Contrary to the vasodilation induced by increases in the $Pa,_{CO_2}$, a hyperventilation-related decrease in $Pa,_{CO_2}$ causes hypocapnic cerebral vasoconstriction and has been found to be associated with brain injury in preterm (35,47,48) but not in term infants (49) or adults. It is an open question whether hypocapnia alone can cause ischemia, or if it works in combination with other factors, such as hypoxemia, hypoglycemia, the presence of high levels of cytokines, sympathetic activation, or seizures.

Metabolic Control of Blood Flow to the Brain

CBF, estimated by venous occlusion plethysmography, is increased during active sleep as compared to quiet sleep (50–52). Using the ^{133}Xe clearance method in preterm infants of 32 to 35 weeks' postmenstrual age, Greisen et al. (53) found that global CBF increased in the wake state compared to quiet or active sleep. Thus, there is flow-metabolism coupling even before term gestation in the brain. This finding is further supported by the documented increase in CBF seen during seizure activity and by the strong relation between CBF and blood hemoglobin concentration (33,37).

Recently, the cerebrovascular response to functional activation by visual stimulation has been studied by magnetic resonance imaging (MRI) (54,55) and NIRS (56). The findings suggest a non-existent or inconsistent response in infants before term or within the first weeks after birth. The authors explained their findings by the presence of underdeveloped visual cortical projections even at term. Recent studies on the cerebrovascular response to sensorimotor stimulation using functional MRI also found an inconsistent pattern of responses in former very preterm and preterm neonates at near-term postmenstrual age (57,58). These findings can also be explained by the developmentally regulated delay in the maturation of the sensorimotor cortex.

Cerebrovenous oxygen saturation was entirely normal (64% ± 5%) as estimated by NIRS and jugular occlusion technique in 11 healthy, term infants three days after birth (59). This indicates that there is a balance between blood flow and cerebral oxygen consumption at term. The average value of global CBF measured by ^{133}Xe clearance in 11 preterm, healthy infants during the first postnatal week was 20 mL/100 g/min (34). However, the contrast between flow to gray and white matter is high compared to the findings in immature animals (60).

Adrenergic Mechanisms Affecting CBF Autoregulation

Based on findings of animal studies, the sympathetic system appears to play a greater role affecting CBF and its autoregulation in the perinatal period compared to later in life (61–65). This finding has been attributed to the relative immaturity of the nitric oxide-induced vasodilatory mechanisms during early development (66). The adrenergic effect results, at least in part, to enhanced constriction of conduit arteries.

A rare study of human neonatal arteries *in vitro* (obtained post-mortem from preterm neonates with gestational age of 23 to 34 weeks) showed basal tone and a pressure–diameter relation quite similar to those seen in adult pial arteries (67). The neonatal arteries, however, were significantly more sensitive to exogenous norepinephrine and electrical field activation of adventitial sympathetic nerve fibers and had a much higher sympathetic nerve density (68) compared to those in the adult pial arteries (69).

The Effect of Medications

Indomethacin reduces CBF in experimental animals, adults, and preterm neonates (70). As mentioned earlier, a loss of the normal CBF–CO_2 reactivity has also been demonstrated in preterm infants (15). The crucial question concerning the use of indomethacin in preterm neonates and its effect of CBF is whether indomethacin reduces CBF to ischemic levels resulting in brain injury. Interestingly, although indomethacin decreases the incidence of severe peri-intraventricular hemorrhage (PIVH), this early effect does not translate to better long-term neurodevelopmental outcomes (71). This raises the possibility that the indomethacin-induced global decrease in CBF may represent a double-edged sword. Contrary to indomethacin, ibuprofen does not have significant cerebrovascular effects (16,72). However, it is not known whether the use of ibuprofen for the treatment of patent ductus arteriosus (PDA) results in improved long-term neurodevelopmental outcome compared to indomethacin.

Among the methylxanthines, aminophylline reduces CBF and $Pa,_{CO_2}$ in experimental animals, adults, and preterm infants (73) but caffeine has less effect on CBF (71). Methylxanthines are potent adenosine receptor antagonists. However, it is not entirely clear whether the reduction of CBF is the direct effect of methylxanthines, a result of the decrease in $Pa,_{CO_2}$, or a combination of these two actions.

Dopamine increases blood pressure and thereby may affect CBF. However, it does not appear to have a selective (dilatory) effect on brain vessels (75,76).

In babies with blood pressure over 30 mm Hg, dopamine infusion at 0.3 mg/kg/h was effective in increasing arterial blood pressure and left ventricular output, and did not increase CBF (77). In babies with hypotension, however, a positive pressure–flow relation was found at 1.9% per mm Hg (CI, 0.8 to 3.0) (78) and 6% per mm Hg (44). It is unclear whether the discrepancy between the findings of these two studies and those cited above (75,76) can be explained by the presence or absence of hypotension, by the statistical uncertainty of small studies, or by differences in the methodology and the clinical status of the patients.

Ischemic Thresholds in the Brain

In the newborn puppy, $Sv,_{O_2}$ may decrease from 75 to 40% without provoking significant lactate production (79). The exact minimum value of "normal" $Sv,_{O_2}$ depends, among others, on the oxygen dissociation curve. Therefore, it may be affected by changes in pH and the proportion of fetal hemoglobin present in the blood.

In the cerebral cortex of the adult baboon and man, the threshold of blood flow sufficient to maintain tissue integrity depends on the duration of the low flow. For instance, if the low flow lasts for a few hours, the limit of minimal CBF to maintain tissue integrity is around 10 mL/100 g/min (80). In acute localized brain ischemia, blood flow may remain sufficient to maintain structural integrity but fail to sustain electrical activity; a phenomenon called "border zone" or "penumbra" (81). Indeed, in progressing ischemia electrical failure is a warning for the development of permanent tissue injury. In the adult human brain cortex, electrical function ceases at about 20 mL/100 g/min of blood flow, while in the subcortical gray matter and brainstem of the adult baboon the blood flow threshold is around 10 to 15 mL/100 g/min (82).

The threshold values of CBF for neonates are not known. However, in view of the low resting levels of CBF and the comparatively longer survival in total ischemia or anoxia, neonatal CBF thresholds are likely to be considerably below 10 mL/100 g/min. Indeed, in ventilated preterm infants visual evoked responses were unaffected at global CBF levels below 10 mL/100 g/min corresponding to a cerebral oxygen delivery of 50 μmol/100 g/min (35,83).

However, low CBF and cerebral oxygen delivery estimated by ^{133}Xe clearance carry a risk of later death, cerebral atrophy, or neurodevelopmental deficit (84–87).

As mentioned earlier though, the lower limit of acceptable CBF is unknown in the neonate and it is also unclear whether treatment modalities aimed at increasing CBF can improve the outcome.

Periventricular white matter is believed to be particularly vulnerable to hypoxic–ischemic injury especially in preterm infants. However, the pathogenesis of white matter injury is likely to be more complex as interactions among decreased perfusion and increased cytokine production and oxidative damage have recently been postulated to be of importance. The only direct evidence indicating that periventricular leukomalacia (PVL) is primarily a hypoxic–ischemic lesion comes from the findings identifying hyperventilation with the associated cerebral vasoconstriction as a robust risk factor for PVL and cerebral palsy.

BLOOD FLOW TO OTHER ORGANS

Based on studies on the distribution of cardiac output in term fetal lambs and newborn piglets, the typical abdominal organ blood flow appears to be around 100 to 350 mL/100 g/min (88,89). In the fetus, abdominal organ blood flow is higher than in the newborn with the exception of the intestine.

Kidney

The adult kidneys constitute 0.5% of body weight but represent 25% of resting cardiac output, making them the most richly perfused organ of the body. In the newborn, although the kidneys are relatively larger, they receive less blood flow probably due to the immature renal function. Renal arteries display appropriate autoregulation with a lower threshold adjusted to the prevailing lower blood pressure (90). In addition to structural immaturity, high levels of circulating vasoactive mediators such as angiotensin-II, vasopressin, and endogenous catecholamines explain the relatively low renal blood flow in the immediate postnatal period. Indeed, after alpha-adrenergic receptor blockade, renal nerve stimulation results in increased blood flow. To counterbalance the renal vasoconstriction and increased sodium reabsorption caused by the above-mentioned hormones, the neonatal kidney is more dependent on the local production of vasodilatory prostaglandins compared to later in life. This explains why indomethacin, a cyclooxygenase (COX) inhibitor, readily reduces renal blood flow and urinary output in the neonate but not in the euvolemic child or adult. Interestingly, the renal side effects of another COX inhibitor, ibuprofen, are less pronounced in the neonate (91). Finally, dopamine increases renal blood flow at a dose with minimal effect on blood pressure (75).

Liver

The liver is a large organ that has a double blood supply with blood originating from the stomach and intestines through the portal system and also from the hepatic branch of the celiac artery through the hepatic artery. The proportion of blood flow from these sources in the normal adult is 3:1, respectively. Hepatic vessels are richly innervated with sympathetic and parasympathetic nerves. The hepatic artery constricts in response to sympathetic nerve stimulation and exogenous norepinephrine while the response of the portal vein is less well characterized. Angiotensin-II is a potent vasoconstrictor of the hepatic vascular beds. During the first days after birth, a portion of the portal blood flow remains shunted past the liver through the ductus venosus until it closes. Portal liver blood flow in lambs is 100 to 150 mL/100 g/min during the first postnatal day and increases to over 200 mL/100 g/min by the end of the first week (92).

Stomach and Intestines

The stomach and intestines are motile organs, and variation in intestinal wall tension influences vascular resistance (93). For example, stimulation of sympathetic nerves results in constriction of the intestinal arteries and arterioles and in the relaxation of the intestinal wall. Thus, the effects on vascular resistance and intestinal wall tension are opposite. Furthermore, a number of gastrointestinal hormones and paracrine substances such gastrin, glucagon, and cholecystokinin dilate intestinal vessels likely contributing to the increase in intestinal blood flow during digestion. Local metabolic coupling also contributes to the digestion-associated increase in intestinal blood flow. Intestinal blood flow also shows well-developed autoregulation, and responses to sympathetic nerve stimulation, exogenous catecholamines and angiotensin-II similar to that of the other abdominal organs in the immature animal.

DISTRIBUTION OF CARDIAC OUTPUT IN THE HEALTHY HUMAN NEONATE

If the heart fails to increase cardiac output to maintain systemic blood pressure, a selective and marked increase in the flow to one organ can in principle compromise blood flow to other organs ("steal" phenomenon). No single organ of critical importance is large in itself at birth (Table 2-1).

Blood Flow to the Upper Part of the Body

Blood flow to various organs differs considerably at the resting state. The data from recent Doppler flow volumetric studies allows some comparisons for the upper part of the body in healthy term infants. Blood flow to the brain, defined as the sum of the blood flowing through the two internal carotid and two vertebral arteries, corresponds to 18 mL/100 g/min using a mean brain weight of 385 g for the term infant. This blood flow is close to what is expected from the data on CBF in the literature assessed by NIRS and ^{133}Xe clearance (Table 2-2).

Blood Flow to the Lower Part of the Body

Lower-body blood flows are less well studied in the human neonate. In a recent study in ELBW infants with no ductal shunt and a cardiac output of 200 mL/kg/min, aortic blood flow was found to be 90 mL/kg/min at the level of the diaphragm (94). Although this finding is in good agreement with the data by Kluckow and

Table 2-1	Organ Weights in Term** and Extremely Low Birth Weight Neonates**	
	BODY WEIGHT (g)	
Organ or Tissue	**3500**	**1000**
Brain	411 (12%)	143 (15%)
Heart	23 (1%)	8 (1%)
Liver	153 (4%)	47 (5%)
Kidney	28 (1%)	10 (1%)
Fat	23%*	<5%

Data from Charles and Smith (105).
*Data from Uthaya et al. (106).
**Total body water is around 75% and 85–90% of body weight in term neonates and extremely low birth weight neonates, respectively.

Vessel	n	Age	Flow (mL/kg/min)	Flow (mL/min)	Reference
Vertebral arteries	22	39–40 (weeks)	–	19*	Kehrer et al. (105)
Internal carotid arteries			–	51*	
Right common carotid	21	Day 1–3	17.7	117**	Sinha (106)
Superior vena cava	14	Day 1	76	258	Kluckow and Evans (95)
Ascending aorta			147	500	

Table 2-2 Volumetric Blood Flow by Doppler Ultrasound Measurement for the Upper Part of the Body in Healthy Term Infants

In the study by Kehrer et al. (105) newborn infants born at term were mixed with former preterm infants reaching 39–40 postmenstrual weeks.
*Values for sum of right and left.
**Value multiplied by 2 for comparison.

Evans (95) showing that approximately 50% of left ventricular output returns through the superior vena cava (SVC) in preterm neonates, some caution is warranted because most preterm infants enrolled in the studies on SVC blood flow measurements had a PDA.

The data on individual abdominal organ flows in neonates are less current but available with a renal blood flow (right+left) of 21 mL/kg/min (96), a superior mesenteric artery blood flow of 43 mL/kg/min (97), and a celiac artery blood flow of 70 mL/kg/min (98). In the study by Agata et al. (98), the results were divided by two to account for the parabolic arterial flow profile. However, since the sum of these abdominal organ blood flows exceeds the blood flow in the descending aorta and since blood flow from other organ systems in the lower body such as bones, muscle, and skin have not been taken into consideration, it is clear that blood flows to the abdominal organs have been overestimated in the neonate. The reasons for this discrepancy are unclear but they may, at least in part, be related to the use of less sophisticated color Doppler equipment using lower ultrasound frequencies in the studies performed in the early 1990s. In terms of perfusion rate, the renal blood flow of 21 mL/min/kg body weight transforms to 210 mL/min/100 g kidney weight. Again, this is higher than that expected from studies using hippuric acid clearance (99). Taking all these findings into consideration, it is reasonable to conclude that normal organ flow in the human neonate is likely to be comparable to that in different animal species and is around 100 to 300 mL/100 g/min. For comparison, lower limb blood flow in the human infant has been estimated by NIRS and the venous occlusion technique to be around 3.5 mL/100 g/min (100).

In summary, cardiac output is distributed approximately equally to the upper and lower body in the normal healthy newborn infant at gestational ages from 28 to 40 weeks. It may come as a surprise to many readers that only 25 to 30% of the blood flow to the upper part of the body goes to the brain, whereas the abdominal organs can be assumed to account for the largest part of the blood flow to the lower part of the body. Although good estimates of abdominal organ perfusion rates are not available, they appear to be higher than the perfusion rate of the brain. Therefore, a relative hyperperfusion of the abdominal organs could result in an significant "steal" of cardiac output from the brain.

MECHANISMS GOVERNING THE REDISTRIBUTION OF CARDIAC OUTPUT IN THE FETAL "DIVE" REFLEX

Aerobic Diving

The diving reflex of sea mammals occurs within the "aerobic diving limit," that is, without hypoxia severe enough to lead to the production of lactic acid. The key components are reflex bradycardia mediated through the carotid chemoreceptors and the vagal nerve, reflex vasoconstriction of the vascular beds of "nonvital" organs, and recruitment of blood from the spleen. All of this results in a reduced cardiac output, a dramatically increased circulation time, and hence a lag between tissue oxygen consumption and CO_2 production (101).

Reactions to Hypoxia

Similarly, the immediate reaction to hypoxia in the perinatal mammal is bradycardia and peripheral vasoconstriction. Since the reaction to fetal distress is of great clinical interest, it has been extensively studied in the fetal lamb. The response to fetal distress is qualitatively similar but quantitatively different among the different modes of induction of fetal distress such as maternal hypoxemia, graded reduction of umbilical blood flow, repeated or graded reduction or complete arrest of uterine blood flow, and reduction of fetal blood volume (102). Among the vital organs, adrenal blood flow increases in all situations and, whereas the typical response also includes an increase in the blood flow to the heart and the brain, this is not the case when fetal distress is caused by reduction of fetal blood volume (heart) or the arrest of uterine blood flow (brain). As for the nonvital organs, although the typical response is a reduction in blood flow to the gut, liver, kidneys, muscle, and skin, this is not the case when fetal distress is caused by the graded reduction of umbilical blood flow. The fetal circulation is unique and significantly different from the circulation following the transitional adaptation of the newborn and includes the presence of the umbilical vascular bed, the shunting of oxygenated umbilical venous blood past the liver through the ductus venosus, and streaming of this blood through the foramen ovale to the left side of the heart and upper part of the body. These peculiar features may explain some of the above-described differences between fetal and postnatal hemodynamic responses to stress.

Modifying Effects

Preterm lambs appear less able to produce a strong epinephrine and norepinephrine response to stress and the blood pressure rise is accordingly less than at term (102). Since carotid sinus denervation does not abolish the redistribution of cardiac output, supplementary mechanisms must be operational in the fetus (103). Indeed, at least in the later phase (after 15 min) of the hemodynamic response, the renin–angiotensin system seems to play an important role. Importantly, recent findings indicate that a systemic inflammatory response significantly interferes with the redistribution of cardiac output during arrest of uterine blood flow in the fetal sheep and compromises cardiac function and the chance of successful resuscitation (104). This hemodynamic response to inflammation in the fetal sheep appears to be, at least in part, regulated by locally generated NO as it could be prevented by the administration of the non-selective NO synthase inhibitor, L-NAME.

DISTRIBUTION OF CARDIAC OUTPUT IN THE SHOCKED NEWBORN

The Term Neonate with Low Cardiac Output

The pale gray, yet awake term baby with poor systemic perfusion due to congenital heart disease resulting in decreased cardiac output (systemic blood flow) may be the best example for the operation of efficient cardiovascular centralization mechanisms in the human newborn. This baby may have very low central venous oxygen saturation, but will still produce urine, have bowel motility, and, in the initial phase of the cardiovascular compromise, a normal blood lactate. There is little we may be able to do – short of the appropriate cardiac surgical procedure – to help this baby improve the distribution of the limited systemic blood flow. Attempts to increase blood pressure or, conversely, to reduce cardiac afterload may, in fact, interfere with the precarious blood flow distribution and lead to further decreases in blood flow to the organs despite "normal" blood pressure readings, or to a decrease in perfusion pressure resulting in further impairment in tissue perfusion, respectively. In this situation, treatment resulting in increased systemic blood flow without decreasing the perfusion pressure is the only appropriate approach.

The Very Preterm Neonate During Immediate Postnatal Adaptation

In the very preterm neonate with poor systemic perfusion during the period of immediate postnatal transition with the fetal channels still open, the situation is likely to be different. This baby may present with a better color and capillary refill suggesting appropriate peripheral perfusion. Yet, motor activity is likely to be reduced, urinary output low, and blood lactate slightly high. Based on the findings discussed earlier, this baby may have immature and insufficient adrenergic mechanisms to rely on for maintaining sufficient perfusion pressure to the vital organs. In addition, owing to the immaturity of the myocardium, this patient may initially be unable to adapt to the sudden increase in the systemic vascular resistance following separation from the placenta. Regulation of CBF and the sensitivity of the cerebral arteries and arterioles are likely also affected by the immaturity. This would result in the presence of a very narrow CBF autoregulatory plateau and, due to the enhanced expression of alpha-adrenergic receptors during early development, an increased vasoconstrictive response to the administration of exogenous sympathomimetic amines resulting in further decreases in CBF despite improvement in the blood pressure. Again, maintenance of both an appropriate systemic blood flow and perfusion pressure must be the goal of the intervention (see Section III, Chapter 8).

OTHER SCENARIOS

Other scenarios relevant to the neonatologist are shock due to low peripheral vascular resistance in sepsis and loss of blood volume. The inflammatory vascular pathology associated with infection cannot be directly treated, and the effectiveness of available supportive treatment modalities of the critically ill septic neonate has not been systematically studied. In addition, microvascular pathophysiology, oxygen radical damage and disturbances in the oxidative metabolism may be as important as the issues of distribution of blood flow. In contrast, the clinical problem and management associated with loss of blood volume are simpler as long as it is recognized in a timely manner.

REFERENCES

1. Heistad DD. What is new in cerebral microcirculation. Landis award lecture. Microcirculation 2001;8:365–375.
2. Malcus P, Kjellmer I, Lingman G, Marsal K, Thiringer K, Rosén K. Diameters of the common carotid artery and aorta change in different directions during acute asphyxia in the fetal lamb. J Perinat Med 1991;19:259–267.
3. Hill MA, Zou H, Potocnik SJ, Meininger GA, Davis MJ. Invited Review: Arteriolar smooth muscle mechanotransduction: Ca2 signaling pathways underlying myogenic reactivity. J Appl Physiol 2001;91:973–983.
4. Gebremedin A, Lange AR, Lowry TF, et al. Production of 20-HETE and its role in autoregulation of cerebral blood flow. Circ Res 2000;87:60–65.

5. Dora KA. Does arterial myogenic tone determine blood distribution in vivo? Am J Physiol Heart Circ Physiol 2005;289:1323–1325.

6. Pearce WJ, Harder DR. Cerebrovascular smooth muscle and endothelium. In Neurophysiological Basis of Cerebral Blood Flow Control: An Introduction. Mraovitch S, Sercombe R, eds. London, John Libbey & Co, 1996:153–158.

7. Pearce WJ. Hypoxic regulation of the fetal cerebral circulation. J Appl Physiol 2006;100:731–738.

8. Liu Y, Harder DR, Lombard JH. Interaction of myogenic mechanisms and hypoxic dilation in rat middle cerebral arteries. Am J Physiol Heart Circ Physiol 2002;283:H2276–H2281.

9. Aalkjær C, Poston L. Effects of pH on vasular tension. Which are the important mechanisms? J Vasc Res 1996;33:347–359.

10. Wang Q, Pelligrino DA, Baughman VL, Koeng HM, Albrecht RF. The role of neuronal nitric oxide synthetase in regulation of cerebral blood flow in normocapnia and hypercapnia in rats. J Cereb Blood Flow Metab 1995;15:774–778.

11. Iadecola C, Zhang F. Permissive and obligatory roles of NO in cerebrovascular responses to hypercapnia and acethylcholine. Am J Physiol 1996;271:R990–1001.

12. Lindauer U, Vogt J, Schuh-Hofer S, Dreier JP, Dirnagl U. Cerebrovascular vasodilation to extraluminal acidosis occurs via combined activation of ATP-sensitive and Ca2+-activated potassium channels. J Cereb Blood Flow Metab 2003;23:1227–1238.

13. Wagerle LC, Mishra OP. Mechanism of CO2 response in cerebral arteries of the newborn pig: role of phospholipase, cyclooxygenase, and lipooxygenase pathways. Circ Res 1988;62:1019–1026.

14. Rama GP, Parfenova H, Leffler CW. Protein kinase Cs and tyrosine kinases in permissive action of prostacyclin on cerebrovascular regulation in newborn pigs. Pediatr Res 1996;41:83–89.

15. Edwards AD, Wyatt JS, Ricardsson C, Potter A, Cope M, Delpy DT, Reynolds EOR. Effects of indomethacin on cerebral haemodynamics in very preterm infants. Lancet 1992;i:1491–1495.

16. Patel J, Roberts I, Azzopardi D, Hamilton P, Edwards AD. Randomized double-blind controlled trial comparing the effects of ibobrufen with indomethacin on cerebral hemodynamics in preterm infants with patent ductus arteriosus. Pediatr Res 2000;47:36–42.

17. Clifford PS, Hellsten Y. Vasodilatory mechanisms in contracting skeletal muscle. J Appl Physiol 2004;97:393–403.

18. Koehler RC, Gebremedhin D, Harder DR. Role of astrocytes in cerebrovascular regulation. J Appl Physiol 2006;100:307–317.

19. Phillis JW. Adenosine and adenine nucleotides as regulators of cerebral blood flow: roles of acidosis, cell swelling, and KATP channels. Crit Rev Neurobiol 2004;16:237–270.

20. Guimaraes S, Moura D. Vascular adrenoreceptors: an update. Pharm Rev 2001;53:319–356.

21. Seri I, Tan, R, Evans J. The effect of hydrocortisone on blood pressure in preterm neonates with vasopressor-resistant hypotension. Pediatrics 2001;107:1070–1074.

22. Watterberg KL. Adrenal insufficiency and cardiac dysfunction in the preterm infant. Pediatr Res 2002;51:422–424.

23. Noori S, Seri I. Pathophysiology of newborn hypotension outside the transitional period. Early Hum Dev 2005;81:399–404.

24. Lou HC, Lassen NA, Friis-Hansen B. Low cerebral blood flow in hypotensive perinatal distress. Acta Neurol Scand 1977;56:343–352.

25. Hernandez MJ, Brennan RW, Bowman GS. Autoregulation of cerebral blood flow in the newborn dog. Brain Res 1980;184:199–201.

26. Pasternak JF, Groothuis DR. Autoregulation of cerebral blood flow in the newborn beagle puppy. Biol Neonate 1985;48:100–109.

27. Tweed WA, Cote J, Pash M, Lou H. Arterial oxygenation determines autoregulation of cerebral blood flow in the fetal lamb. Pediatr Res 1983;17:246–249.

28. Papile LA, Rudolp AM, Heyman MA. Autoregulation of cerebral blood flow in the preterm fetal lamb. Pediatr Res 1985;19:59–161.

29. Pryds A, Pryds O, Greisen G. Cerebral presure autoregulation and vasoreactivity in the newborn rat. Pediatr Res 2005;57:294–298.

30. Helau S, Koehler RC, Gleason CA, Jones MD, Traystman RJ. Cerebrovascular autoregulation during fetal development in sheep. Am J Physiol Heart Circ Physiol 1994;266:H1069–H1074.

31. Müller T, Löhle M, Schubert H, et al. Developmental changes in cerebral autoregulatory capacity in the fetal sheep parietal cortex. J Physiol 2002;539:957–967.

32. Tweed WA, Cote J, Lou H, Gregory G, Wade J. Impairment of cerebral blood flow autoregulation in the newborn lamb by hypoxia. Pediatr Res 1986;20:516–519.

33. Younkin DP, Reivich M, Jaggi JL, Obrist WD, Delivoria-Papadopoulos M. The effect of haematocrit and systolic blood pressure on cerebral blood flow in newborn infants. J Cereb Blood Flow Metab 1987;7:295–299.

34. Greisen G. Cerebral blood flow in preterm infants during the first week of life. Acta Paediatr Scand 1986;75:43–51.

35. Greisen G, Trojaborg W. Cerebral blood flow, PaCO2 changes, and visual evoked potentials in mechanically ventilated, preterm infants. Acta Paediatr Scand 1987;76:394–400.

36. Pryds O, Greisen G, Lou H, Friis-Hansen B. Heterogeneity of cerebral vasoreactivity in preterm infants supported by mechanical ventilation. J Pediatr 1989;115:638–645.

37. Pryds O, Andersen G E, Friis-Hansen B. Cerebral blood flow reactivity in spontaneously breathing, preterm infants shortly after birth. Acta Paediatr Scand 1990;79:391–396.

38. Pryds O, Greisen G, Lou H, Friis-Hansen B. Vasoparalysis is associated with brain damage in asphyxiated term infants. J Pediatr 1990;117:119–125.

39. Tyszczuk L, Meek J, Elwell C, Wyatt JS. Cerebral blood flow is independent of mean arterial blood pressure in preterm infants undergoing intensive care. Pediatrics 1998;102:337–341.

40. Noone MA, Sellwood M, Meek JH, Wyatt JS. Postnatal adaptation of cerebral blood flow using near infrared spectroscopy in extremely preterm infants undergoing high-frequency oscillatory ventilation. Acta Paediatr 2003;92:1079–1084.

41. Wardle SP, Yoxall CW, Weindling AM. Determinants of cerebral fractional oxygen extraction using near-infrared spectroscopy in preterm neonates. J Cereb Blood Flow Metab 2000;20:272–279.

42. Milligan DWA. Failure of autoregulation and intraventricular haemorrhage in preterm infants. Lancet 1980;i:896–899.

43. Børch K, Greisen G. Regional cerebral blood flow during hypotension and hypoxemia in preterm infants (abstract). Pediatr Res 1997;42:389–399.

44. Munro MJ, Walker AM, Barfield CP. Hypotensive extremly low birth weight infants have reduced cerebral blood flow. Pediatrics 2004;114:1591–1596.

45. Leahy FAN, Cates D, MacCallum M, Rigatto H. Effect of CO2 and 100% O2 on cerebral blood flow in preterm infants. J Appl Physiol 1980;48:468–472.

46. Rahilly PM. Effects of 2% carbon dioxide, 0.5% carbon dioxide, and 100% oxygen on cranial blood flow of the human neonate. Pediatrics 1980;66:685–689.

47. Calvert SA, Hoskins EM, Fong KW, Forsyth SC. Atiological factors associated with the development of periventricular leucomalacia. Acta Paediatr Scand 1987;76:254–259.

48. Graziani LJ, Spitzer AR, Mitchell DG, Merton DA, Stanley CS, Robinson N, McKee L. Mechanical ventilation in preterm infants: Neurosonographic and developmental studies. Pediatrics 1992;90:515–522.

49. Ferrara B, Johnson DE, Chang P-N, Thompsom TR. Efficacy and neurologic outcome of profound hypocapneic alkalosis for the treatment of persistent pulmonary hypertension in infancy. J Pediatr 1984;105:457–461.

50. Milligan DWA. Cerebral blood flow and sleep state in the normal newborn infant. Early Hum Develop 1979;3:321–328.

51. Rahilly PM. Effects of sleep state and feeding on cranial blood flow of the human neonate. Arch Dis Child 1980;55:265–270.

52. Mukhtar AI, Cowan FM, Stothers JK. Cranial blood flow and blood pressure changes during sleep in the human neonate. Early Hum Develop 1982;6:59–64.

53. Greisen G, Hellstrom-Westas L, Lou H, Rosen I, Svenningsen NW. Sleep-waking shifts and cerebral blood flow in stable preterm infants. Pediatric Research 1985;19:1156–1159.

54. Born P, Leth H, Miranda MJ, et al. Visual activation in infants and young children studied by functional magnetic resonance imaging. Pediatr Res 1998;44:578–583.

55. Martin E, Joeri P, Loenneker T, et al. Visual processing in infants and children studied using functional MRI. Pediatr Res 1999;46:135–140.

56. Meek JH, Firbank M, Elwell CE, et al. Regional hemodynamic responses to visual stimulation in awake infants. Pediatr Res 1998;43:840–843.

57. Erberich GS, Friedlich P, Seri I, Nelson, DM, Bluml S. Brain activation detected by functional MRI in preterm neonates using an integrated radiofrequency neonatal head coil and MR compatible incubator. Neuroimage 2003;20:683–692.

58. Erberich SG, Panigrahy A, Friedlich P, Seri I, Nelson MD, Gilles FH. Somatosensory lateralization in the newborn brain. Neuroimage 2006;29:155–161.

59. Buchvald FF, Keshe K, Greisen G. Measurement of cerebral oxyhaemoglobin saturation and jugular blood flow in term healthy newborn infants by near-infrared spectroscopy and jugular venous occlusion. Biol Neonate 1999;75:97–103.

60. Børch K, Greisen G. Blood flow distribution in the normal human preterm brain. Pediatr Res 1998;43:28–33.

61. Hernandez MJ, Hawkins RA, Brennan RW. Sympathetic control of regional cerebral blood flow in the asphyxiated newborn dog. In Cerebral Blood Flow, Effects of Nerves and Neurotransmitters. Heistad DD, Marcus ML, eds. New York, Elsevier, 1982:359–366.

62. Hayashi S, Park MK, Kuelh TJ. Higher sensitivity of cerebral arteries isolated from premature and newborn baboons to adrenergic and cholinergic stimulation. Life Sciences 1984;35:253–260.

63. Wagerle LC, Kumar SP, Delivoria-Papadopoulos M. Effect of sympathetic nerve stimulation on cerebral blood flow in newborn piglets. Pediatric Research 1986;20:131–135.

64. Kurth CD, Wagerle LC, Delivoria-Papadopoulos M. Sympathetic regulation of cerebral blood flow during seizures in newborn lambs. Am J Physiol 1988;255:H563–H568.

65. Goplerud JM, Wagerle LC, Delivoria-Papadopoulos M. Sympathetic nerve modulation of regional cerebral blood flow during asphyxia in newborn piglets. Am J Physiol 1991;260:H1575–H1580.

66. Wagerle LC, Moliken W, Russo P. Nitric oxide and alpha-adrenargic mechanisms modify contractile responses to norepinephrine in ovine fetal and newborn cerebral arteries. Pediatr Res 1995;38:237–242.

67. Bevan RD, Vijayakumaran E, Gentry A, Wellman T, Bevan JA. Intrinsic tone of cerebral artery segments of human infants between 23 weeks of gestation and term. Pediatr Res 1998;43:20–27.

68. Bevan R, Dodge J, Nichols P, Poseno T, Vijayakumaran E, Wellman T, Bevan JA. Responsiveness of human infant cerebral arteries to sympathetic nerve stimulation and vasoactive agents. Pediatr Res 1998;44:730–739.

69. Bevan RD, Dodge J, Nichols P, Penar PL, Walters CL, Wellman T, Bevan JA. Weakness of sympathetic neural control of human pial compared with superficial temporal arteries reflects low innervation density and poor sympathetic responsiveness. Stroke 1998;29:212–221.

70. Pryds O, Greisen G, Johansen K. Indomethacin and cerebral blood flow in preterm infants treated for patent ductus arteriosus. Eur J Pediatr 1988;147:315–316.

71. Schmidt B, Davis P, Moddemann D, et al., and Trial of Indomethacin Prophylaxis in Preterms Investigators. Long-term effects of indomethacin prophylaxis in extremely-low-birth-weight infants. N Engl J Med 2001;344:1966–1972.

72. Mosca F, Bray M, Lattanzio M, Fumagalli M, Tosetto C. Comparative evaluation of the effects of indomethacin and ibuprofen on cerebral perfusion and oxygenation in preterm infants with patent ductus arteriosus. J Pediatr 1997;131:549–554.

73. Pryds O, Schneider S. Aminophylline induces cerebral vasoconstriction in stable, preterm infants without affecting the visual evoked potential. European Journal of Pediatrics 1991;150:366–369.

74. Lundstrøm KE, Larsen PB, Brendstrup L, Skov L, Greisen G. Cerebral blood flow and left ventricular output in spontaneously breathing, newborn preterm infants treated with caffeine or aminophylline. Acta Paediatr 1995;84:6–9.

75. Seri I, Abbasi S, Wood DC, Gerdes JS. Regional hemodynamic effects of dopamine in the sick preterm neonate. J Pediatr 1998;133:728–734.

76. Zhang J, Penny DJ, Kim NS, Yu VY, Smolich JJ. Mechanisms of blood pressure increase induced by dopamine in hypotensive preterm neonates. Arch Dis Child 1999;81:F99–F104.

77. Lundstrøm KE, Pryds O, Greisen G. The haemodynamic effect of dopamine and volume expansion in sick preterm infants. Early Hum Develop 2000;57:157–163.

78. Jayasinghe D, Gill AB, Levene MI. CBF reactivity in hypotensive and normotensive preterm infants. Pediatr Res 2003;54:848–853.

79. Reuter JH, Disney TA. Regional cerebral blood flow and cerebral metabolic rate of oxygen during hyperventilation in the newborn dog. Pediatric Research 1986;20:1102–1106.

80. Jones TH, Morawetz RB, Crowell RM, et al. Thresholds of focal cerebral ischaemia in awake monkeys. J Neurosurg 1981;54:773–782.

81. Astrup J. Energy-requiring cell functions in the ischaemic brain. J Neurosurg 1982;56:482–497.

82. Branston NM, Ladds A, Symon L, Wang AD. Comparison of the effects of ischaemia on early components of somatosensory evoked potentials in brainstem, thalamus, and cerebral cortex. J Cereb Blood Flow Metab 1984;4:68–81.

83. Pryds O, Greisen G. Preservation of single flash visual evoked potentials at very low cerebral oxygen delivery in sick, newborn, preterm infants. Pediatr Neurol 1990;6:151–158.

84. Lou HC, Skov H. Low cerebral blood flow: a risk factor in the neonate. J Pediatr 1979;95:606–609.

85. Ment RL, Scott DT, Lange RC, Ehrenkrantz RA, Duncan CC, Warshaw JB. Postpartum perfusion of the preterm brain: relationship to neurodevelopmental outcome. Childs Brain 1983;10:266–272.

86. Pryds O. Low neonatal cerebral oxygen delivery is associated with brain injury in preterm infants. Acta Paediatr 1994;83:1233–1236.

87. Krageloh-Mann I, Toft P, Lunding J, Andresen J, Pryds O, Lou HC. Brain lesions in preterms: origin, consequences and compensation. Acta Paediatrica 1999;88:897–908.

88. Fujimori K, Honda S, Sanpei M, Sato A. Effects of exogenous big endothelin-1 on regional blood flow in fetal lambs. Obstet Gynecol 2005;106:818–823.

89. Powell RW, Dyess DL, Collins JN, et al. Regional blood flow response to hypothermia in premature, newborn, and neonatal piglets. J Pediatr Surg 1999;34:193–198.

90. Jose PA, Haramati A, Fildes RD. Postnatal maturation of renal blood flow. In Fetal and Neonatal Physiology. Polin RA, Fox WW, eds. Philadephia, WB Saunders, 1998:1573–1578.

91. Pezzati M, Vangi V, Biagiotti R, Bertini G, Cianciulli D, Rubaltelli FF. Effects of indomethacin and ibuprofen on mesenteric and renal blood flow in preterm infants with patent ductus arteriosus. J Pediatr 1999;135:733–738.

92. Rudolph CD, Rudolph AM. Fetal and postnatal hepatic vasculature and blood flow. In Fetal and Neonatal Physiology. Polin RA, Fox WW, eds. Philadephia, WB Saunders, 1998:1442–1449.

93. Clark DA, Miller MJS. Development of the gastrointestinal circulation in the fetus and newborn. In Fetal and Neonatal Physiology. Polin RA, Fox WW, eds. Philadephia, WB Saunders, 1998:929–933.

94. Shimada S, Kasai T, Hoshi A, Murata A, Chida S. Cardiocirculatory effects of patent ductus arteriosus in extremely-low-birth-weight infants with respiratory distress syndrome. Pediatr Int 2003;45:255–262.

95. Kluckow M, Evans N. Superior vena cava flow. A novel marker of systemic blood flow. Arch Dis Child 2000;82:F182–187.

96. Visser MO, Leighton JO, van de Bor M, Walther FJ. Renal blood flow in the neonate: quantitation with color and pulsed Doppler ultrasound. Radiology 1992;183:441–444.

97. Van Bel F, van Zwieten PH, Guit GL, Schipper J. Superior mesenteric artery blood flow velocity and estimated volume flow: duplex Doppler US study of preterm and term neonates. Radiology 1990;174:165–169.

98. Agata Y, Hiraishi S, Misawa H, et al. Regional blood flow distribution and left ventricular output during early neonatal life: a quantitative ultrasonographic assessment. Pediatr Res 1994;36:805–810.

99. Yao LP, Jose PA. Developmental renal hemodynamics. Pediatr Nephrol 1995;9:632–637.

100. Bay-Hansen R, Elfving B, Greisen G. Use of near infrared spectroscopy for estimation of peripheral venous saturation in newborns: comparison with co-oximetry of central venous blood. Biol Neonate 2002;82:1–8.

101. Stephenson R. Physiological control of diving behaviour in the Weddell seal *Leptonychotes weddelli*: a model based on cardiorespiratory control theory. J Exp Biol 2005;208:1971–1991.

I PATHOPHYSIOLOGY OF NEONATAL SHOCK

102. Jensen A, Garnier Y, Berger R. Dynamics of fetal circulatory responses to hypoxia and asphyxia. Eur J Obstet Gynecol Reprod Biol 1999;84:155–172.
103. Green LR, McGarrigle HHG, Bennet L, Hanson MA. Angiotensin II and cardiovascular chemo-reflex responses to acute hypoxia in late gestation fetal sheep. J Physiol 1998;507:857–867.
104. Coumans ABC, Garnier Y, Supcun S, Jensen AM, Berger R, Hasaart THM. Nitric oxide and fetal organ blood flow during normoxia and hypoxemia in endotoxin-treated fetal sheep. Obstet Gynecol 2005;105:145–155.
105. Kehrer M, Krägeloh-Mann L, Goelz R, Schöning M. The development of cerebral perfusion in healthy preterm and term neonates. Neuropediatrics 2003;34:281–286.
106. Sinha AK, Cane C, Kempley ST. Blood flow in the common carotid artery in term and perterm infants: reproducibility and relation to cardiac output. Arch Dis Child 2006;91:31–35.
107. Charles AD, Smith NM. Perinatal postmortem. In Roberton's Textbook of Neonatology. Rennie JM, ed. Beijing, Elsevier, 2005:1207–1215.
108. Uthaya S, Bell J, Modi N. Adipose tissue magnetic resonance imaging in the newborn. Horm Res 2004;62(Suppl 3):1430–1438.

Chapter 3

Definition of Normal Blood Pressure Range: The Elusive Target

William D. Engle, MD

Case Study

Measuring Blood Pressure

Normative Data for Blood Pressure in Neonates

Adjuncts to Blood Pressure Measurement in the Diagnosis of Compromised Circulatory Function

Clinical Factors that may Affect Blood Pressure

Conclusions

References

Few aspects of the management of high-risk neonates have generated as much controversy as the assessment of blood pressure, and this is particularly true of preterm neonates. The approach to this problem may differ greatly among various institutions and between clinicians within a given center. The variation may relate to training, but it is also is related to a need for further data that would provide the clinician with a better understanding of the relationship between blood pressure and outcome.

CASE STUDY

An 820 g male infant was born at 27 weeks' gestation. The pregnancy was complicated by placenta previa, and delivery was by cesarean section (C/S) after preterm, premature rupture of membranes, and subsequent onset of labor. There was no significant vaginal bleeding. The infant was apneic initially but he responded well to positive-pressure ventilation. He developed retractions and grunting, and was intubated. Apgars were 5 and 8.

In the neonatal intensive care unit (NICU), the chest X-ray (CXR) was consistent with surfactant defficiency (respiratory distress syndrome, RDS), and he received surfactant replacement therapy. Subsequently, the Fi_{O_2} requirement to maintain oxygen saturation in the 88 to 94% range decreased from 0.70 to 0.30, and ventilatory pressures were weaned appropriately. Attempts to place an umbilical artery catheter (UAC) were unsuccessful; an umbilical venous catheter (UVC) was placed. He was begun on a dextrose and amino acid solution at 60 mL/kg/day and ampicillin and gentamicin were given. The hematocrit was 47% and serum glucose was 97 to 125 mg/dL.

Mean blood pressure on admission was 31 mm Hg (determined by oscillometry). At 2 h of postnatal life, mean blood pressure had decreased to 25 mm Hg. Heart rate varied between 135 and 160 bpm. The infant was moving spontaneously, and capillary refill time was ~2 s. He had not voided.

This case is similar to those seen frequently in any NICU: the very small neonate who seems to be doing fairly well from a cardiorespiratory standpoint, but whose mean blood pressure engenders acute discomfort in the staff. Various issues involving whether or how to treat the blood pressure in the very low birth weight (VLBW) neonate during the immediate postnatal period are discussed in Section III, Chapter 8. Here we might ask:

1. Should a preterm neonate who requires mechanical ventilation, and in whom a UAC is unsuccessful, have a peripheral arterial line?
2. If so, should this be attempted immediately after the failed UAC attempt, or only after it appears that the blood pressure will be a problem?
3. What evidence is available to determine when a "problem" blood pressure exists?
4. What is the role of heart rate, capillary refill time, urine output, and other nonspecific indicators of the cardiovascular status in the decision-making process as one attempts to determine whether or not this is an adequate blood pressure?

To address these questions, this chapter reviews the (1) methods of measurement of blood pressure, (2) normative values for blood pressure in preterm and term neonates, (3) clinical assessments used often in conjunction with blood pressure measurement, and (4) clinical factors that can influence blood pressure.

MEASURING BLOOD PRESSURE

It is appropriate to ask why there is so much attention paid to assessment of blood pressure. Clearly, the primary issue regarding possible hypotension in neonates is the concern that impaired central nervous system perfusion may lead to ischemic damage (1,2). Arterial pressure is determined by two factors: the propulsion of blood by the heart and the resistance to flow of this blood through the blood vessels (3). Thus, *flow = pressure/resistance* and, consequently, *pressure = flow × resistance.* In the case of the systemic circulation, the left ventricle serves as the pump, which generates sufficient pressure to overcome vascular resistance and create systemic arterial flow and maintain appropriate perfusion pressure in the organs. From a clinical standpoint, blood flow resulting in adequate tissue perfusion is the variable of critical interest, and disturbances of perfusion represent some position on the continuum of the complex disorder of shock (3). However, since it is not practical to measure flow routinely, and resistance can only be calculated but not measured, we rely greatly on blood pressure determinations to gauge the adequacy of cardiac output and systemic perfusion. It is obvious from the above equations that significant changes in vascular resistance might result in changes in blood flow (and thus changes in tissue perfusion) without recognizable alterations in blood pressure. This suggests that blood pressure is not the only physiologic variable of primary interest. This issue becomes even more complicated in the transitional circulation of the VLBW neonate with shunting across the fetal channels, where neither mean blood pressure nor cardiac output alone is necessarily a good predictor of systemic blood flow (4).

The "gold standard" for determination of blood pressure in the critically ill neonate is a direct continuous reading from an indwelling arterial line, and generally this method is used whenever arterial access is available. The ability to measure blood pressure non-invasively (5) represents a major advance in neonatal care, although a major drawback associated with these methods is the inability to obtain continuous measurements. Detailed recent reviews of blood pressure measurement and monitoring in the neonate are available (6,7).

Direct Measurement of Blood Pressure

Using a catheter–transducer fluid-filled system, blood pressure is measured directly most frequently by utilizing a UAC with its tip in the thoracic or distal aorta or a catheter placed in a peripheral, usually radial or posterior tibial, artery. The purpose of this section is to point out common issues related to direct measurement of blood pressure in neonates. For a more extensive review of direct measurement of blood pressure, the reader is referred to several excellent publications (6–9).

The first direct measurement of blood pressure was made in the eighteenth century and is credited to Hales (8,10). He attached a long vertical tube to a cannula that was inserted into the crural artery of a horse (8), and demonstrated reduction in blood pressure following hemorrhage. Subsequent development of the U-shaped mercury manometer by Poiseuille (7) allowed the measuring equipment to be reduced in size.

A wave can be defined as a traveling disturbance carrying energy (7), and characterized by frequency, intensity or amplitude, direction, and velocity. The pressure pulse is a complex waveform that is dependent on site of measurement (see below). It should be noted that the speed of the pressure pulse greatly exceeds that of the actual blood flow (11), and the fundamental frequencies of the pressure pulse bear little relationship to the repetition rate of the initiating event (7). The pressure pulse should not be confused with the pulse pressure, which refers to the difference between systolic and diastolic blood pressure.

The system used for continuous, direct blood pressure monitoring in today's NICU generally is referred to as "under-damped and second order" (7). Instead of a column of mercury, modern systems for measuring blood pressure have several components, the most important of which is the transducer. The transducer converts mechanical energy (pressure) to electrical energy (current or voltage). Compared with older strain gauge pressure transducers, today's transducers have a silicon chip, and they are inexpensive, accurate, and disposable (12). The transducer must be positioned at the level of the catheter opening, and correctly "zeroing" the system (stopcock connected to transducer open to atmospheric pressure) is a critical step in obtaining accurate blood pressure values. This process should be performed at least every 12 h to ensure the accuracy of blood pressure measurements over time. The pressure measured by the transducer has three components: $P = P_s + P_k + P_r$, where P_s is the static component, P_k is the kinetic component, and P_r is the reference level component (13). Although P_s is not influenced by catheter type, with an end-hole catheter the P_k component can be increased by 5 to 7 mm Hg (during systole) compared with the pressure obtained with a side-hole catheter (13). P_r will be zero if the transducer is placed at the level of the catheter opening, as noted above.

An ideal pressure-monitoring system should reflect the pressure pulse accurately so that the monitor waveform is similar to that at the site of measurement (7), and to do this it must have an appropriate frequency response. A method for determining the resonant frequency and damping coefficient has been described by Gardner (9). Systems in clinical use generally have a resonant frequency of 15 to 25 Hz and a coefficient of 0.1 to 0.4 (6).

Generally, direct readings of blood pressure in the neonate are considered to be accurate, although several problems may occur. A small-diameter catheter may cause the systolic reading to be low. Excessive damping secondary to the introduction of small air bubbles or clots into the system may result in decreased systolic but increased diastolic readings (6,13). Since mean blood pressure, which is considered more reflective of perfusion pressure than systolic or diastolic pressure, has generally been considered to be unaffected by damping, this potential inaccuracy may not be a significant clinical problem. However, Cunningham et al. (14) reported that damping (defined as a sudden reduction of pulse pressure by more than 8 mm Hg or complete loss of the systolic and diastolic differential) also may affect mean blood pressure. In 24% of damping episodes studied, the difference was ≥4.1 mm Hg (14).

Conversely, as the pressure pulse travels from aortic root to peripheral arteries, amplification of some components may occur (6), and somewhat counterintuitively, measured systolic pressure may be higher in the dorsalis pedis or radial artery versus the aorta (7). This is caused by a gradual increase in impedance as the pressure pulse travels distally through more narrow channels, and the observed waveform may appear narrower and taller than observed more proximally. Diastolic and mean blood pressure are less affected by this phenomenon, but mean blood pressure calculated using the formula "diastolic pressure plus one-third of pulse pressure" will be falsely high (6). Generally, the difference is not clinically significant, and a very strong correlation between blood pressures obtained via umbilical and peripheral artery catheters was reported by Butt and Whyte (15).

Gevers et al. (16) studied arterial blood pressure waveforms (radial and posterior tibial) in critically ill neonates using a high-fidelity catheter tip-transducer system. Radial artery waveforms resembled those observed in adult proximal aorta rather than adult radial artery, and posterior tibial waveforms resembled those of the adult femoral artery, rather than those of the adult posterior tibial artery. The authors postulated that the observed "central appearance" was secondary to the close proximity of the radial and posterior tibial arteries to the aorta and femoral artery, respectively, due to the small and short limbs of the neonate.

Although direct measurement of blood pressure is considered the gold standard and generally is felt to be the most appropriate method for monitoring a critically ill neonate (see below), it is important to minimize distortions if one is to obtain accurate values. Use of tubing that is as short as possible, large-bore, stiff, and non-compliant as well as minimizing the number of stopcocks and manifolds will help in this regard (17).

Non-invasive Measurement of Blood Pressure

Manufacturers of non-invasive blood pressure monitors must provide accuracy data to the FDA before they may be marketed (18). Guidelines followed in generating this data must conform to the requirements of the American National Standard for Manual, Electronic, or Automated Sphygmomanometers (ANSI/ AAMI SPIO). The mean difference of paired comparisons between direct and non-invasive methods must be within ±5 mm Hg with a standard deviation ≤ 8 mm Hg (19). In considering studies that have examined agreement between invasive and non-invasive methods, it is important to consider the impact of more recent technological improvements. For example, Nelson et al. (20) found that an improved algorithm for the DINAMAP MPS[TM] oscillometric device resulted in agreement that met the standards noted above.

All non-invasive techniques for estimating blood pressure analyze changes in blood flow (17) and, since direct methods measure pressure, one would not necessarily expect the results obtained with non-invasive and direct methods to be identical. Of the common non-invasive techniques (palpation, auscultation, Doppler, and oscillometry), oscillometry is used most often (21). An additional method that utilizes a photoelectric principle and provides a continuous arterial waveform through a finger cuff also has been described (22,23). The Finapres

(FINger Arterial PRESsure) method uses a photoplethysmographic system applied to the finger and provides a continuous beat-to-beat waveform. Because the cuff is too large for a neonate, in both studies the investigators placed the finger cuff around the wrist of the baby. One of the studies (22) found considerable differences between Finapres and umbilical arterial blood pressure measurements, and concluded that Finapres is not reliable in estimating absolute values of blood pressure. However, because of accurate estimation of beat-to-beat changes of blood pressure values, the authors concluded that Finapres provides a non-invasive tool for investigating autonomic cardiovascular regulation in neonates (22). A discussion of basic principles of non-invasive blood pressure measurement in infants has been published recently (18).

The measurement of blood pressure by oscillometry was first described by Marey in 1876 (7), and Ramsey reported the use of an automated instrument based on the oscillometric technique (Dinamap, Critikon, Tampa, FL) in 1979 (24). This device is able to measure cuff oscillations at given pressures as sensed by a pressure transducer; systolic pressure is the pressure at which cuff oscillation begins to increase as the cuff is deflated. Mean pressure is the lowest cuff pressure at which oscillometric amplitude is maximum, and diastolic pressure is the pressure at which the amplitude of cuff oscillations stops decreasing (6).

The agreement between blood pressure values obtained directly and by oscillometry has generally been good (24–31). However, some investigators have found that the agreement is poor, and suggested that non-invasive techniques are not sufficiently accurate for routine use (32). Of course, when comparing direct and non-invasive methods, it is important to ensure accuracy of the reference method by performing dynamic calibration (frequency response and damping coefficient) for each infant (18). However, this exercise is not always noted (17).

One well-documented reason for lack of agreement with intra-arterial blood pressure may be use of an inappropriate cuff size when performing oscillometric measurements. Sonesson and Broberger (33) reported that mean blood pressure was overestimated with a cuff width to arm circumference ratio of 0.33 to 0.42. Accuracy improved with a ratio of 0.44 to 0.55. In the study by Kimble et al. (25), the appropriate cuff width-to-arm circumference ratio was 0.45 to 0.70 (Fig. 3-1). Clark et al. (34) reported that the ideal ratio was 0.40, although few neonates were included, and blood pressure was obtained using a mercury sphygmomanometer. In a study of 15 preterm infants, Wareham et al. (35) reported a strong correlation

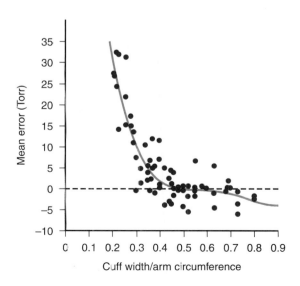

FIGURE 3-1 A non-linear regression analysis comparing error (Dinamap minus intra-arterial) with cuff width to arm circumference ratio. Each point represents the average of 10 determinations with the same cuff in a given patient. *Kimble KJ, Darnall RA Jr, Yelderman M, Ariagno RL, Ream AK. An automated oscillometric technique for estimating mean arterial pressure in critically ill newborns. Anesthesiology 1981;54:423–425, Fig. 1. Used with permission from Lippincott Williams & Wilkins.*

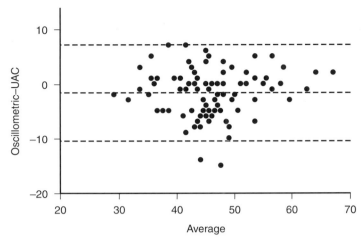

FIGURE 3-2 Differences between oscillometric and arterial mean blood pressure measurements plotted against average values of two measurements. Central dashed line represents mean difference; two outlying dashed lines represent ± 2 SDs. UAC indicates umbilical artery catheter. *Wareham JA, Haugh LD, Yeager SB, Horbar JD. Prediction of arterial blood pressure in the premature neonate using the oscillometric method. AJDC 1987;141:1108–1110, Fig. 4. Used with permission,* British Publishing Group Ltd.

between oscillometric and arterial blood pressure, but with 95% prediction intervals. The differences are particularly apparent when the data are displayed in a Bland–Altman plot (Fig. 3-2). In this study, cuff width for each infant was selected according to the manufacturer's recommendations. Briassoulis (36) compared oscillometric and arterial catheter determinations in six preterm neonates. Agreement between the two methods was poor and did not vary significantly with use of a larger cuff.

It is of concern that several investigators have found that blood pressure determined by oscillometry overestimates directly obtained blood pressure, since this relationship might lead to failure to treat hypotensive neonates. As noted above (33), this overestimation might be due to a cuff that is too small. In a study of 12 VLBW neonates, Diprose et al. (37) reported that the oscillometric method overestimated blood pressure in hypotensive infants. Cuff width-to-arm circumference ratios were not reported in this study (although the authors commented that the cuffs actually may have been too large because of the relatively small size of the patients), and data regarding mean blood pressure were not included. Fanaroff and Wright (38) reported that mean blood pressure during the first 48 postnatal hours, determined by the oscillometric technique, exceeded direct readings by about 3 mm Hg; however, cuff size was not reported. Others also have reported a tendency for oscillometric determinations to exceed direct measurements (39). In the study by Wareham et al. (35), diastolic blood pressure was overestimated by the oscillometric method, but systolic and mean blood pressure were underestimated.

Studies comparing blood pressure measurements from upper versus lower limbs have produced conflicting results (40–44). In term neonates, Park and Lee (45) observed no difference in blood pressure between arm and calf. Piazza et al. (46) compared upper and lower limb systolic blood pressure in term neonates in the first 24 h and found that higher readings in the upper versus lower limb were more common than vice versa. However, higher readings in the lower limb were sufficiently common (28%) for these investigators to conclude that either possibility should be considered normal. In subsequent follow-up of 25 of the study neonates up to three years of age, systolic blood pressure was higher in the lower extremities in 24/25.

More recently, Cowan et al. (47) determined arm and calf blood pressure in term neonates in active and quiet sleep during the first five postnatal days. The increase in blood pressure during this period was greater in the arm than in the calf, and calf blood pressure appeared to be more dependent on sleep state than did arm blood pressure. Subsequently, Kunk and McCain (48) studied 65 preterm neonates with mean birth weight of 1629 g. During days one to five, there were no significant differences in systolic, diastolic, and mean blood pressures between arm and calf, although arm blood pressures consistently were slightly higher. On day seven, there was a significant difference with arm > calf for systolic blood pressure by an average of 2.7 mm Hg.

Nwankwo et al. (21) studied a standard blood pressure measurement protocol to determine the effect of state, startle response to cuff inflation, and infant position. Using the Dinamap oscillator, they observed slightly higher pressures in the supine position and with the first of three successive blood pressure recordings. Variability of blood pressure determinations using the standard protocol was less than when blood pressure was recorded by nursing staff. These investigators emphasized the importance of a rest period following cuff application and a standardized approach in blood pressure measurement (21).

Papadopoulos et al. (49) compared three oscillometric devices [Dinamap 8100 (Critikon), SpaceLabs M90426 (SpaceLabs Medical) and the Module HP M1008B (Hewlett-Packard; HP)] to a simulator. The Dinamap and SpaceLabs readings were in good agreement with the reference method, whereas mean errors for systolic and diastolic blood pressure with the HP device were 21 and 15 mm Hg, respectively.

Pichler et al. (50) compared two commonly used oscillometric systems, the HP-Monitor CMS Model 68 S with Module HP M1008B and the Dinamap 8100. By Bland–Altman analysis, it was shown that mean blood pressure determined by the Dinamap was significantly higher than with the HP. This study is difficult to interpret since direct determination of blood pressure was not made for comparison. However, it does point out that results in non-invasive determination of blood pressure may be dependent on the system used by a particular NICU.

More recently, Dannevig et al. (51) compared blood pressure obtained with three different monitors (Dinamap Compact, Criticare Model 506 DXN2, and Hewlett-Packard Monitor with the HP MI008B Module) with determinations made with an invasive system (Hewlett-Packard). Twenty neonates (birth weight 531 to 4660 g) were studied during the first postnatal week. Difference between oscillometric and invasive pressures (measurement deviance) was related to two factors: (1) size of infant and (2) monitoring system. In smaller infants, the non-invasively measured value tended to be too high, and as arm circumference increased, measurement deviance decreased with all monitors. The Hewlett-Packard gave lower pressure readings than either the Criticare or Dinamap (Fig. 3-3); Criticare and Dinamap tended to show too high a value in the smallest infants, while Hewlett-Packard tended to give too low a value in the larger infants. These investigators concluded that blood pressure should preferably be measured invasively in severely ill neonates and preterm infants.

While caution in the interpretation of indirectly obtained blood pressure measurements is prudent, the clinical usefulness of this technique has been demonstrated. In many instances, the trend in blood pressure in a particular infant is of critical importance, and the exact absolute value may be of less relevance. Fortunately, those critically ill neonates in whom decisions regarding treatment of possible hypotension need to be made are the patients most likely to have arterial access. When the most frequently used site for direct access (umbilical artery) is not available, as in the case presented at the beginning of this chapter, direct access via a peripheral artery should be attempted.

The best method for routine non-invasive blood pressure measurement is the oscillometric method, and the sophisticated bedside cardiorespiratory monitoring systems in current use allow the clinician to monitor blood pressure at set intervals and display the results on the same screen that shows heart rate, oxygen saturation, and so forth. As noted above, use of the proper cuff size is critical. Although differences among various oscillometric monitors have been demonstrated, at

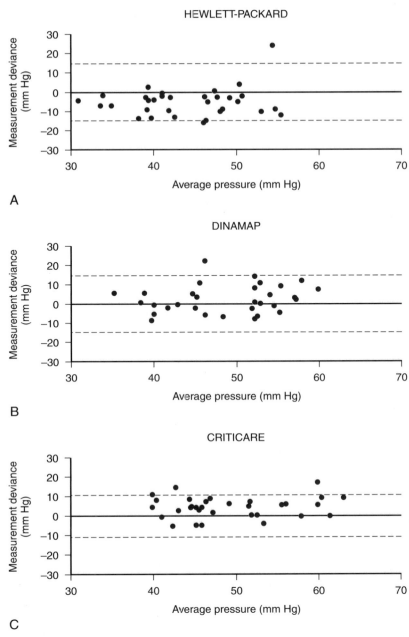

FIGURE 3-3 Bland–Altman plots comparing invasively measured arterial blood pressure and measurements obtained with three oscillometric devices (Dinamap™, Criticare™, Hewlett-Packard™). *Dannevig I, Dale HC, Liestol K, Lindemann R. Blood pressure in the neonate: three non-invasive oscillometric pressure monitors compared with invasively measured blood pressure. Acta Paediatr 2005;94:191–196, Fig. 1. Used with permission from Taylor & Francis.*

this time there does not seem to be conclusive evidence to favor a particular monitor system over all others.

NORMATIVE DATA FOR BLOOD PRESSURE IN NEONATES

The establishment of normal values for blood pressure in newborn infants has been attempted by numerous investigators, and there is fairly good agreement in the results reported from various institutions (52). In most (but not all) studies, blood pressure is higher in larger, more mature infants, and there is an increase in blood pressure with increasing postnatal age (6,15,53–70). Small for gestational age (SGA) infants may have lower blood pressure than larger babies of comparable gestational age (56,70–72), although comparable blood pressure values also have been reported (73). It should be noted that "normative values" may be influenced by management protocols within a given institution. Also, most studies have not determined that the "physiologic range" for blood pressure is occurring simultaneously with normal organ blood flow (74,75). Kluckow and Evans (75,76) reported a weak correlation between mean blood pressure and superior vena cava (SVC) blood flow used for the assessment of systemic blood flow in preterm infants < 32 weeks' gestation during the first two postnatal days when shunting across the fetal channels prevents the use of the left ventricular output as the measure of systemic blood flow. Conversely, Munro et al. (77) reported that ELBW neonates who were hypotensive during the first postnatal days had lower cerebral blood flow than normotensive neonates.

Although in 1963 Moss and Duffie (78) reported that blood pressure was higher in preterm versus term neonates, this finding could not be confirmed. The report by Kitterman et al. (71) in 1969 was one of the earliest studies of blood pressure in neonates, and these results were used widely in neonatal intensive care units. However, this study included only nine patients with birth weights ≤1500 g. Bucci et al. (56) measured systolic blood pressure indirectly using a xylol-pulse indicator instrument. These investigators developed a regression equation for systolic blood pressure that included birth weight, gestational age, and postnatal age in 189 neonates with birth weight 860 to 2300 g, gestational age 25 to 41 weeks, and postnatal age 3 to 96 h:

$$SPB = 23.20 + 8.13\chi_w + 0.503\chi_{GA} + 0.226\chi_{PA} - 0.00160\chi_{PA}^2$$

where χ_w is body weight (in kg), χ_{GA} is gestational age (GA) (in weeks), χ_{PA} is postnatal age (in hours), and systolic blood pressure (SBP) is in mm Hg.

The study published by Versmold et al. (72) in 1981 included 16 stable neonates with birth weights 610 to 980 g (eight infants were small for gestational age); blood pressure during the first 12 postnatal hours was measured directly through an umbilical artery catheter. Despite this report, which demonstrated that the 95% confidence limits for mean blood pressure ranged from 24 to 44 mm Hg, the value of 30 mm Hg has been widely adopted as a critical lower limit for acceptable blood pressure in preterm neonates. This notion was based on findings suggesting that the lower limit of the cerebral blood flow autoregulatory curve was around 30 mm Hg (77,79) and that neonates with mean arterial pressures <30 mm Hg had a high likelihood of developing central nervous system pathology (see below). Subsequently, Watkins et al. (80) reported that the 10th percentile for mean blood pressure for a baby with a birth weight of 600 g was below 30 mm Hg until 72 h postnatal (Table 3-1). Similar low values for extremely preterm neonates were reported by Nuntnarumit et al. (6) (Fig. 3-4). This figure demonstrates clearly the striking differences in mean blood pressure between term and preterm neonates, but with parallel increases occurring over the first 72 h postnatal. Interestingly, following an initial decrease during the first 6 to 12 postnatal hours, cerebral blood flow also increases after delivery in both term and preterm neonates (81). However, the initial decrease is more dramatic in the VLBW patient population, and it is during the ensuing period of rapid improvement in cerebral blood flow (reperfusion) that peri-intraventricular hemorrhage PIVH) occurs (75). Tan (82,83) also has studied both term and preterm neonates, and found that the differences between awake and asleep blood pressure values seen in term neonates were not observed in VLBW neonates.

In 1999, Lee et al. (67) demonstrated that the lower 95% confidence interval for mean blood pressure was even lower than reported by Versmold et al. (72), with

Table 3-1   Variation of Mean Blood Pressure* with Birth Weight at 3 to 96 h Postnatal Age

Birth weight (g)	TIME (h) POSTNATAL AGE								
	3	12	24	36	48	60	72	84	96
500	35/23	36/24	37/25	38/26	39/28	41/29	42/30	43/31	44/33
600	35/24	36.25	37/26	39/27	40/28	41/29	42/31	44/32	45/33
700	36/24	37/25	38/26	39/28	42/29	42/30	43/31	44/32	45/34
800	36/25	37/26	39/27	40/28	41/29	42/31	44/32	45/33	46/34
900	37/25	38/26	39/27	40/29	42/30	43/31	44/32	45/34	47/35
1000	38/26	39/27	40/28	41/29	42/31	43/32	45/33	46/34	47/35
1100	38/27	39/27	40/29	42/30	43/31	44/32	45/34	46/35	48/36
1200	39/27	40/28	41/29	42/30	43/32	45/33	46/34	47/35	48/37
1300	39/28	40/29	41/30	43/31	44/32	45/33	46/35	48/36	49/37
1400	40/28	41/29	42/30	43/32	44/33	46/34	47/35	48/36	49/38
1500	40/29	42/30	43/31	44/32	45/33	46/35	48/36	49/37	50/38

*Numbers refer to average MBP/tenth percentile for MBP.
From: Watkins AMC, West CR, Cooke RWI. Blood pressure and cerebral haemorrhage and ischaemia in very low birthweight infants. Early Hum Develop 1989;19:103–110, Figure 2. Used with permission from Elsevier Ltd.

values of 20 to 23 mm Hg observed in the 500 to 800 g infants. These authors cautioned against treatment for a low blood pressure value alone unless there are co-existing signs of hypoperfusion, such as poor capillary return, oliguria, and metabolic acidosis (see below).

In 1983 Adams et al. (84) reported findings of a study of continuously recorded blood pressure in 15 infants with birth weight ≤1500 g, utilizing a system capable of measuring and storing 60 data points each minute. When a linear regression analysis of hourly mean blood pressure as a function of postnatal age was calculated, these investigators found significant correlations for gestational age and birth weight with the slopes and intercepts of the linear equations. While these authors noted that the relatively steep rise in mean blood pressure in the less mature infants may be a predisposing factor in the development of intraventricular hemorrhage, it should be noted that birth weight was ≥1180 g in 13/15 neonates. Subsequently, Cunningham et al. (85) performed continuous recordings of blood pressure and noted cyclical variation with hypertensive "waves." They postulated that this blood pressure instability might predispose to intraventricular hemorrhage (86). Cunningham et al. (87) subsequently reported mean blood pressure ranges in 232 very low birth weight neonates. Intraventricular hemorrhage (IVH) was

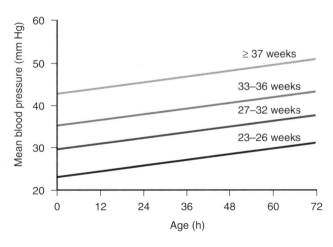

FIGURE 3-4 Mean blood pressure in neonates with gestational ages of 23 to 43 weeks (*n* = 103, neonates admitted to NICU). The graph shows the predicted mean blood pressure during the first 72 h of life. Each line represents the lower limit of 80% confidence interval (two-tail) of mean blood pressure for each gestational age group; 90% of infants for each gestational age group will be expected to have a mean blood pressure value equal to or above the value indicated by the corresponding line, the lower limit of the confidence interval. *Nuntnarumit P, Yang W, Bada-Ellzey HS. Blood pressure measurements in the newborn. Clin Perinatol 1999;26:981–996, Fig. 3. Used with permission from Elsevier.*

associated with low blood pressure on the day IVH was noted or on the day before. Periventricular leukomalacia (PVL) was not associated with blood pressure.

In neonates with gestational age 24 to 28 weeks, Dimitriou et al. (88) observed blood pressure rhythms (circadian and ultradian) on postnatal day two but not on day seven. They concluded that this observation was secondary to lingering maternal influence rather than an endogenous "clock." Gemelli et al. (89) observed circadian rhythm of blood pressure at four days postnatal in males but not in females. The highest values were in the morning between 0600 and 0900. These authors emphasized the importance of physiological variances in correct clinical assessment.

Shortland et al. (58) studied 32 VLBW neonates and reported higher mean blood pressures in infants with birth weight ≥ 1251 g versus those with birth weight <1250 g. No relationship between blood pressure and postnatal age (days one to six) was observed in infants in the latter group, while a significant correlation ($r = 0.34$, $P < 0.005$) between mean blood pressure and postnatal age was found in those with birth weight ≥ 1251 g.

Emery and Greenough (90) measured blood pressure in VLBW neonates over the first 28 postnatal days. A significant relationship between mean blood pressure and postnatal age was observed in infants who later developed and did not develop chronic lung disease ($r = 0.94$, $P < 0.02$, and $r = 0.92$, $P < 0.05$, respectively). When a correction was made for birth weight, it was determined by these investigators that blood pressure was higher after day one and throughout the neonatal period in the neonates later developing chronic lung disease.

In two reports, Hegyi et al. described blood pressure ranges in preterm infants in the immediate postnatal period (91) and in the first postnatal week (92). Soon after birth, 20 to 50% of those neonates with low Apgar scores had blood pressure values below the 5th percentile for healthy infants. Of note, in healthy infants, as well as in those who received mechanical ventilation and in those whose mothers were hypertensive, the limits of systolic and diastolic blood pressure were found to be independent of birth weight and gestational age. In the latter study (92), blood pressure increased steadily during the first week of life. However, no relationships between blood pressure variables and birth weight, gender, or race were observed.

In a retrospective study, Cordero et al. (93) examined mean arterial pressure in 101 neonates with birth weight ≤ 600 g during the first 24 postnatal hours. Mean arterial pressure was similar at birth in stable and unstable neonates, but subsequent increases over the first 24 h were less in the unstable group, despite a greater incidence of therapy for hypotension (Fig. 3-5). These authors considered that failure of mean arterial pressure to increase between 3 and 6 h postnatal and a mean arterial pressure of ≤ 28 mm Hg at 3 h postnatal to be a reasonable predictor of the need for therapy for hypotension. It should be noted that mean gestational age was 27 versus 25 weeks in the stable and unstable groups, respectively.

Zubrow et al. (63) reported the findings of a large multicenter study conducted by the Philadelphia Neonatal Blood Pressure Study Group. In this investigation, systolic and diastolic blood pressure was significantly correlated with birth weight gestational age, and post-conceptional age. In each of four gestational age groups, systolic and diastolic blood pressure was significantly correlated with postnatal age over the first five days of life.

Le Flore et al. (69) studied 116 VLBW neonates during the first 72 postnatal hours. Mean blood pressure increased 38% during this period ($r = 0.96$). Increases in blood pressure in infants with birth weight ≤ 1000 g are shown in Fig. 3-6. There was a similar increase in blood pressure in the neonates with birth weight 1001 to 1500 g. However, mean blood pressure in the smaller infants was ~20% less than in the larger infants throughout the study.

The Joint Working Group of the British Association of Perinatal Medicine (94) has recommended that mean arterial blood pressure, in mm Hg, should be

36 *STABLE* ELBW INFANTS

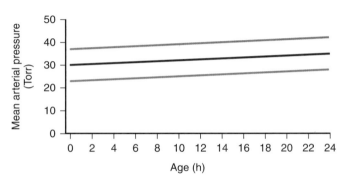

65 *UNSTABLE* ELBW INFANTS

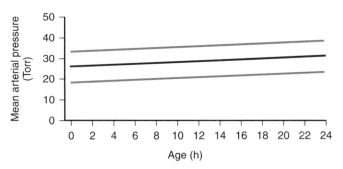

FIGURE 3-5 Regression lines and 80% confidence limits: 531 MAP readings (stable), MAP = (0.237 × hours) + 29.90; 1066 MAP readings (unstable), MAP = (0.196 × hours) + 25.74. MAP indicates mean arterial pressure. *Cordero L, Timan CJ, Waters HH, Sachs LA. Mean arterial pressures during the first 24 h of life in ≤600 gram birth weight infants. J Perinatol 2002;22:348–353, Fig. 1. Used with permission from Nature Publishing Group.*

maintained at or above the gestational age of the infant in weeks during the immediate postnatal period. In light of the above studies this approach seems to have merit (95), but further investigation will be required to establish its safety and efficacy. Of course, whether one considers the acceptable blood pressure to be the gestational age in weeks or a value higher than the 10th percentile for gestational age or birth weight, it is important to remember that being born at a very early gestation represents an abnormal situation, and that having a blood pressure in the "normal" range relative to one's peers does not guarantee that this is a safe situation. A patient using crutches may be able to walk at a speed that is at the 50th percentile for all patients on crutches, but this does not ensure safety in crossing a busy street. Using a value for mean blood pressure that was below gestational age as criteria for hypotension, Pellicer et al. (96) observed improved cerebral intravascular oxygenation following treatment with dopamine or epinephrine in VLBW neonates during the first postnatal day. These findings suggest that mean arterial blood pressures at or below gestational age in VLBW neonates during the first postnatal day are below the autoregulatory blood pressure range for cerebral blood flow. Indeed, the recent findings of Munro et al. (97) suggest that a mean blood pressure of <30 mm Hg remains a useful clinical benchmark (79). Conversely, normal cerebral electrical function may be observed in VLBW neonates when the blood pressure is quite low (98), and a lack of correlation between mean blood pressure and cerebral fractional oxygen extraction has been reported during the first postnatal day (99). Interestingly, recent findings from the same group also suggest that electrical brain activity may be affected at mean arterial blood pressures at or below 23 to 24 mm Hg in VLBW neonates during the first postnatal day (100). However, one should remember that a likely temporally functional impairment does not necessarily equate to a negative impact on brain development or damage to brain structure just as fainting does not indicate that brain damage has necessarily occurred.

FIGURE 3-6 Change in systolic blood pressure (SBP) (A), diastolic blood pressure (DBP) (B), and mean blood pressure (MBP) (C) in neonates ≤ 1000 g birth weight (n = 36) during the initial 72 h postnatal. Lines represent means and 95% confidence intervals (P < 0.0001). Equations for lines of best fit were: SBP = 0.17x + 43.2; DBP = 0.13x + 25.8; MBP = 0.14x + 32.9. In each instance, the y-intercept was significantly lower (P < 0.001) than the value for comparable lines of best fit in infants with birth weights 1001–1500 g; however, no significant differences in slopes for the lines of best fit were observed between the two birth weight groups. LeFlore JL, Engle WD, Rosenfeld CR. Determinants of blood pressure in very low birth weight neonates: lack of effect of antenatal steroids. Early Hum Dev 2000;59:37–50, Fig. 2. Used with permission from Elsevier.

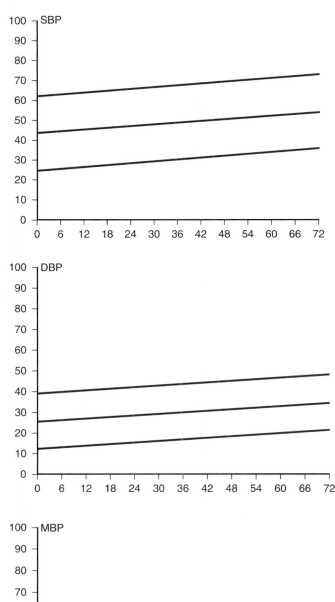

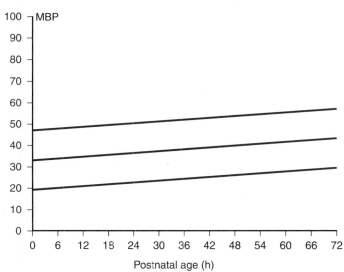

Clearly, more studies relating blood pressure, organ flow, and subsequent outcome are needed especially in the VLBW patient population during the first postnatal days when most of the severe central nervous system pathology may develop. With regard to the case described to at the beginning of the chapter, if this infant's mean blood pressure had been stable in the low-to-mid 30s, it would seem reasonable to continue with frequent oscillometric determinations.

The mechanism for the gradual rise in blood pressure during the first postnatal week is unknown. We previously reported that urinary prostaglandin E_2 and plasma 6-keto-prostaglandin $F_{1\alpha}$ (stable metabolite of prostacyclin) decreased during the first three postnatal days in preterm neonates (101). This could result in a rise in vascular tone and increased vascular reactivity (102,103). However, the hormonal mechanisms of the postnatal cardiovascular adaptation are more complex than could be explained by changes in one hormone or paracrine system alone as, for instance, the concomitant decrease in catecholamine and vasopressin levels would favor lower blood pressures. Indeed, more recently it has been reported that vascular smooth muscle protein expression and contractility demonstrate functional maturation during development (104,105). Thus, the rise in blood pressure during the fetal–neonatal transition may reflect decreases in the activity and synthesis of vasodilators, which are critical to fetal survival, as well as intrinsic changes in vascular smooth muscle function occurring prior to and following birth, both of which appear to be developmentally regulated. Hemodynamic adjustment of the immature myocardium to the relatively high resistance imposed suddenly at the time of birth plays a role as well (4).

In summary, blood pressure is lower in preterm versus term neonates on the first postnatal day, and there is a direct relationship between blood pressure and gestational age over a broad range of maturity at birth. This difference persists through the first week of life, as relatively parallel increases in blood pressure are observed in all gestational age groups. Blood pressure continues to increase in preterm and term infants during the first four postnatal months, and when systolic and diastolic blood pressure are plotted against weight, the slopes for VLBW neonates are greater than those observed in low birth weight neonates or those with normal birth weight (65).

ADJUNCTS TO BLOOD PRESSURE MEASUREMENT IN THE DIAGNOSIS OF COMPROMISED CIRCULATORY FUNCTION

Perkin and Levin (106) have described three stages of shock, and it is important to remember that in the initial or compensated stage there may be no or minimal derangement in blood pressure (107). Indirect evidence of changes in nonvital organ perfusion during the compensated phase of shock include oliguria, prolonged capillary refill (greater than 3 s), excessive temperature gradient between surface and core, tachypnea, tachycardia, and pallor (108). In the uncompensated phase, blood pressure and vital (brain, heart, and adrenal glands) organ perfusion also decrease. Clinical observations of the indirect signs of organ perfusion are important, but can be misleading when used in isolation, especially during the immediate postnatal transition of the VLBW neonate. These signs are most helpful when used together and in conjunction with continuous or frequent blood pressure determinations.

Urine Output

The presence of normal urine output is considered to be an indicator of adequate circulatory function, and might suggest that a blood pressure that appears to be marginal is, in fact, physiologic for that neonate. Conversely, decreased urine output is often cited as evidence that there is circulatory inadequacy and that blood pressure may be too low. These assessments assume, of course, that fluid administration is sufficient, intrinsic renal function is normal, and the impact of the normally high levels of vasopressin and catecholamines on renal function immediately after delivery have been taken into consideration. In addition, there are pathological situations in which concern regarding hypotension is high, e.g. neonates with a hypoxic–ischemic insult, but in whom the kidneys often have sustained significant damage (109). In this case, the ability to assess urine output as an indicator of cardiovascular function is lost.

As referred to above, the other significant problem with quantification of urine output in the clinical decision-making process regarding possible hypotension is that low urine output is physiologic in the first day or so following birth. Accordingly, in some normal term and preterm infants, the first void may not occur until 24 h after delivery (110). Unfortunately, this period coincides with a time of great concern, particularly in preterm neonates, for hypotension and possible organ hypoperfusion, particularly of the central nervous system (4).

Despite these concerns, low urine output (assuming accurate assessment and/or collection) may be an important clinical indicator of circulatory compromise, particularly if there has been previous normal and stable output. If intake has not changed, and the environment is the same (e.g. the patient has not been moved from an incubator to a radiant warmer), then a significant decrease in urine output probably indicates a circulatory problem that needs to be addressed. It is important to remember that at this stage (compensated shock), the blood pressure may be normal because of distribution of organ blood flow to the vital organs, with decreased blood flow to the kidneys as well as other nonvital vascular beds (106). Conversely, the presence of normal urine output is evidence in favor of adequate circulation.

Metabolic Acidosis

Metabolic acidosis often is considered in a somewhat similar light as oliguria, i.e. in its absence there is a tendency to assume that the circulatory status is normal. With inadequate tissue perfusion, tissue hypoxia ensues, and lactic acid is produced. Although sometimes subtle, most clinicians regard development of metabolic acidosis (in a patient whose pulmonary gas exchange is adequate) as an ominous finding that supports the presence of circulatory inadequacy.

Occasionally, peripheral perfusion is so poor that lactate is formed but not "mobilized" to the general circulation and the site of blood gas determination. When this is the case, the clinician often has findings other than metabolic acidosis (e.g. very low blood pressure) to help with the diagnosis of circulatory insufficiency.

Finally, the clinician must differentiate anion-gap (lactic) acidosis from non-anion-gap (bicarbonate wasting) acidosis in the neonate. This is of particular importance in the VLBW patient population where renal bicarbonate wasting due to renal tubular immaturity is the rule rather than the exemption. Therefore, only following the changes in base deficit may not be sufficient for the indirect assessment of the hemodynamic status, and measurement of serum lactate levels may be indicated when the status of tissue perfusion is unclear.

Hyperkalemia

Kluckow and Evans (111) examined the relationship between low systemic blood flow (as estimated by SVC blood flow) and early changes in serum potassium in preterm neonates. The mean minimum blood flow was significantly lower in those neonates who became hyperkalemic versus those with normokalemia, and a rate of rise of serum potassium greater than 0.12 mmol/L/h in the first 12 h predicted a low flow state with 93% accuracy. This interesting observation deserves further study, but it provides the clinician with another tool for overall assessment of cardiovascular stability. However, the complexity of the regulation of the distribution of total body potassium between the intra- and extracellular compartments (primarily determined by the functional maturity and activity of the sodium–potassium ATPase) and that of the function of the immature kidneys warrants cautiousness when using the changes in serum potassium levels as supporting or refuting evidence of poor systemic perfusion in the neonate, especially during the period of immediate postnatal adaptation.

Heart Rate

The association of tachycardia with shock is a classic observation frequently made in combat situations and in civilians with severe trauma and blood loss. For the neonate, an increase in heart rate is the most effective way to increase cardiac output, since the ability to increase stroke volume is somewhat limited. Thus, one might assume that tachycardia is a reliable sign of hypotension and circulatory inadequacy, however it is important to note that most hypotensive neonates are not hypovolemic, particularly in the early postnatal period (112).

Problems with the use of heart rate to indicate hypotension are many, however. Firstly, there is a wide range of normal for heart rate (113). Secondly, there are many factors other than hypotension that cause a neonate to be tachycardic, such as hunger, pain, agitation, elevated body temperature, excessive noise levels, and pharmacologic agents. Heart rate was lower in lambs whose mothers received betamethasone (114). Thirdly, a neonate with hypotension also may be hypoxic, and the typical response of the neonate (unlike the older child or adult) to hypoxia is a vagally mediated decrease in the heart rate. Also, if myocardial damage has occurred and is responsible for the observed hypotension, the heart may not be able to maintain a sustained increase in rate. In a recent study of preterm neonates, systemic blood flow and heart rate were not significantly correlated (75).

Despite these issues, assessment of heart rate may be useful and should be considered in the neonate with suspected hypotension. A clear increase from a previously stable baseline, in the absence of others factors causing tachycardia, should suggest that a measured blood pressure that seems to be marginal may truly represent significant circulatory compromise.

Capillary Refill Time and Central–peripheral Temperature Difference

Capillary refill time (CRT) has been studied extensively in neonates, children, and adults, and is an assessment that tends to provoke strong emotions among those who either do or do not consider it useful clinically (115–117). The CRT is determined by blanching an area of skin and measuring the elapsed time until baseline color returns. The test was described originally by Beecher et al. (118) in 1947, was part of the Trauma Score (119,120), and is used as a tool in life support programs, including Pediatric Advanced Life Support. Numerous studies of CRT have determined that age, ambient and skin temperature, anatomical site of measurement, and duration of pressure influence the value obtained (121,122).

Wodey et al. (123) studied 100 neonates who required intensive care and found no correlation between CRT and shortening fraction, left atrial diameter/aortic diameter ratio, blood pressure, or heart rate. However, a significant correlation between CRT and cardiac index was observed. LeFlore and Engle (124) studied

Table 3-2   Relationship Between CPTd and CRT and Other Parameters at 3 and 10 h Postnatal Age

CPTd or CRT	Sn	Sp	PPV	NPV	LR+	LR−
CPTd ≥2°C						
3 h	29 (15–42)	78 (65–90)	20 (8–32)	85 (74–96)	1.29	0.92
10 h	41 (27–55)	66 (52–79)	41 (27–55)	66 (52–79)	1.19	0.90
All observations	40 (32–48)	69 (61–77)	23 (16–30)	83 (77–90)	1.30	0.87
CRT ≥3 s						
3 h	54 (45–63)	79 (72–86)	23 (16–31)	93 (89–98)	2.55	0.58
10 h	59 (50–68)	75 (67–82)	51 (42–60)	80 (73–87)	2.33	0.55
All observations	55 (50–60)	80 (76–84)	33 (29–38)	91 (88–94)	2.78	0.56
CRT ≥4 s						
3 h	38 (30–47)	93 (88–97)	38 (30–47)	93 (88–97)	5.24	0.66
10 h	26 (18–33)	97 (93–100)	77 (70–84)	74 (67–82)	7.44	0.77
All observations	29 (24–33)	96 (94–98)	55 (50–60)	88 (85–91)	6.84	0.75

Values in parentheses are 95% confidence intervals.

LR+, Positive likelihood ratio; LR−, negative likelihood ratio; NPV, negative predictive value; PPV, positive predictive value; Sn, sensitivity; Sp, specificity.

Data from: Osborn DA, Evans N, Kluckow M. Clinical detection of low upper body blood flow in very premature infants using blood pressure, capillary refill time, and central-peripheral temperature difference. Arch Dis Child, Fetal Neonatal Ed 2004;89):F168–F173, Table 3. Used with permission from BMJ Publishing Group.

healthy term newborns at 1 to 4 h after delivery. Brief (1 to 2 s) and extended (3 to 4 s) pressure was applied at various anatomic sites. Although an inverse relationship between CRT and blood pressure would be expected, this was not observed. In several instances, a highly significant direct relationship was observed, suggesting that vasoactive substances present in the early post-delivery period caused increased vascular resistance, increased blood pressure and prolonged CRT.

Osborn et al. (125) studied the ability of CRT, central–peripheral temperature difference (CPTd) ≥2 °C and blood pressure to detect low SVC flow in neonates < 30 weeks' gestation. Results for CPTd and CRT are shown in Table 3-2. Sensitivity improved to 78% when mean blood pressure < 30 mm Hg and central CRT ≥ 3 s were used in combination. Tibby et al. (126) found that neither CRT nor CPTd correlated well with any hemodynamic variables in post-cardiac surgery children.

Measurement of CRT has become a routine part of physical examination. Its use should be accompanied by an appreciation of its limitations. The use of CPTd, a test not performed as frequently as CRT, has similar limitations.

CLINICAL FACTORS THAT MAY AFFECT BLOOD PRESSURE

As discussed above, it appears that birth weight, gestational age, and postnatal age are significant determinants of blood pressure in the VLBW neonate. Additional demographic and clinical variables that may influence blood pressure in this high-risk population are reviewed below. Clinical situations associated with severe alterations in blood pressure, such as blood loss, asphyxia, and sepsis, are discussed elsewhere in this book.

Maternal Age and Blood Pressure

In a large study (Project Viva, Harvard Vanguard Medical Associates), Gillman et al. (127) observed a direct relationship between maternal age and newborn systolic blood pressure. In 96% of neonates, blood pressure was measured before 72 h postnatal age. In a mixed linear regression model, systolic blood pressure in newborns (mean gestational age 39.7 weeks) increased by 0.8 mm Hg for each increase of five years in maternal age, even after controlling for potentially confounding factors. Maternal blood pressure was also a strong independent predictor of newborn blood pressure. For every 10 mm Hg rise in third trimester maternal systolic blood pressure, newborn systolic blood pressure increased by 0.9 mm Hg (127).

Route of Delivery

Faxelius et al. (128) compared sympathoadrenal activity and peripheral blood flow in term infants delivered vaginally and by cesarean section. Peripheral vascular resistance was higher both at birth and at 2 h postnatal in the vaginally delivered infants, corresponding to higher catecholamine concentrations. However, in this relatively small study ($n = 24$) mean blood pressures were similar between the groups. More recently, Agata et al. (129) reported significantly higher catecholamine concentrations in vaginally delivered infants versus those delivered by cesarean section; left ventricular output and its regional distribution showed a similar pattern in the two groups. Pohjavuori and Fyhrquist (130) found an association between cord blood arginin vasopressin (AVP) and adrenocorticotropin hormone (ACTH) levels, route of delivery, and blood pressures. Vaginally delivered infants had the highest blood pressures and AVP and ACTH levels, followed by those delivered by cesarean section with labor and then those delivered by elective cesarean section. These studies (128–130) were performed in term neonates; in VLBW infants (69) blood pressures were similar in infants delivered vaginally versus those delivered by cesarean section. Likewise in the study noted above by Zubrow et al. (63), stepwise multiple linear regression analysis did not identify route of delivery as a significant determinant of blood pressure variation in preterm neonates. Breech delivery has been associated with blood pressure in the lower range of normal (131). Finally, the amount of placental transfusion (as well as postnatal transfusion) may affect blood pressure (132).

Patent Ductus Arteriosus

Cardiovascular effects of patent ductus arteriosus (PDA) in preterm lambs were studied by Clyman et al. (133) in a model in which ductal size could be regulated. Highly significant decreases in diastolic blood pressure were observed with any size left-to-right ductal shunt, while systolic blood pressure did not change with a small shunt and changed only slightly with either moderate or large shunt.

Ratner et al. (134) studied 34 preterm infants of whom 17 developed clinically significant PDA. These investigators noted that diastolic blood pressure <28 mm Hg was suggestive of the presence of PDA. While diastolic blood pressure was significantly decreased in the PDA group from the first postnatal day, of note, systolic blood pressure was lower after the second day only. Blood pressures were similar to those in the non-PDA group following ligation of the PDA.

Evans and Moorcraft (135) found similar blood pressures with or without PDA in infants with birth weight 1000 to 1500 g. However, in those with birth weight <1000 g, mean, systolic, and diastolic blood pressures were lower in infants with PDA versus those without PDA. Furthermore, these hemodynamic effects could be demonstrated well before the PDA became clinically apparent. These authors cautioned against the use of volume expanders and/or inotropic agents in this population, since these treatments might be counterproductive if the etiology of the hypotension were a hemodynamically significant but clinically silent PDA. Furthermore, volume expansion appears to be a risk factor for development of a symptomatic PDA in VLBW neonates (136,137). It is apparent that problems with low blood pressure related to PDA, especially diastolic blood pressure, may result in inadequate perfusion of many organs secondary to the "vascular steal" phenomenon (138). Management of this clinical problem is, of course, best directed at closure of the PDA rather than at increasing the blood pressure by other means.

Apnea

Circulatory changes resulting from apnea in the neonate have been summarized by Miller and Martin (139). The initial decrease in heart rate is accompanied by a rise in pulse pressure, usually secondary to an increase in systolic pressure, occasionally accompanied by a fall in diastolic pressure (140). These events presumably are secondary to increased filling volume associated with bradycardia which leads to enhanced stroke volume in accordance with Starling's law. As the severity of apnea and bradycardia increases, blood pressure may decrease, along with a fall in cerebral blood flow velocity (141). Thus, during prolonged apnea, cerebral perfusion may decrease significantly, placing the infant at risk for brain injury.

Respiratory Support

Infants with severe respiratory distress syndrome (RDS) may have lower blood pressure than that observed in premature neonates without RDS or in infants with less severe RDS (142,143). An association in infants with RDS between marked fluctuations in arterial blood pressure and fluctuating cerebral blood-flow velocity has been demonstrated (144); the association between this pattern and intraventricular hemorrhage (IVH) may be mediated as much by alterations on the venous side of the cerebral circulation as by alterations on the arterial side (144,145). In a study in which a lower coefficient of variation of systolic blood pressure was observed, blood pressure fluctuation actually was lower in infants who developed IVH (146). Also, an association between acute hypocarbia and marked systemic hypotension has been reported (147). This association places infants at very high risk for central nervous system injury.

Three aspects of respiratory management in preterm neonates might be expected to have an effect on blood pressure: (1) use of increased airway pressures, given either by constant positive airway pressure (CPAP) or conventional or high-frequency ventilation, (2) suctioning of the airway, and (3) instillation of an exogenous surfactant preparation into the airway. Holzman and Scarpelli (148) reported no effect of positive end-expiratory pressure (PEEP) on mean arterial pressure in normal dogs. In neonates, Yu and Rolfe (149) observed no change in mean arterial pressure with or without CPAP. In some studies in which systemic blood pressure did not fall despite high airway pressures (150,151), it was shown that an increase in systemic vascular resistance occurred. Kluckow and Evans (76) and Evans and Kluckow (152) observed a highly significant negative influence of mean airway pressure on mean blood pressure in preterm neonates requiring mechanical ventilation. Similarly, Skinner et al. (153) reported a negative correlation between systemic blood pressure and mean airway pressure in 33 preterm neonates with hyaline membrane disease. Decreases in blood pressure fluctuations during mechanical ventilation may be achieved through use of various methods of synchronized mechanical ventilation as shown by Hummler et al. (154).

Perlman and Volpe (155) studied 35 intubated preterm neonates undergoing routine suctioning. Mean blood pressure increased during suctioning in all but one patient, and these investigators concluded that the observed increases in cerebral blood flow velocity and intracranial pressure were directly related to the increased blood pressure. Perry et al. (61) reported that blood pressure elevations were temporally related to suctioning and other procedures, and they associated systolic blood pressure above a "stability boundary" with increased risk for PIVH.

Omar et al. (156) studied blood pressure responses to care procedures (suctioning, chest auscultation and physiotherapy, mouth rinsing, diaper changing, and naso-gastric feeding) in 22 ventilated, preterm infants. In general, blood pressure responses were biphasic, with a decrease in blood pressure followed by a greater and longer-lasting increase.

Numerous investigators have studied physiologic effects of surfactant instillation in neonates, and differences in these reports may be secondary to dosing, technique of administration, adjustments in ventilator settings to avoid significant changes in P_{CO_2} levels, or other factors (6,157–161). In most studies, any effects on blood pressure were transient. There may be greater hemodynamic effects associated with natural surfactant preparations, perhaps related to their generally more rapid pulmonary effects and greater ability to release local vasoactive mediators when compared with artificial surfactant preparations (6,159,161).

Antenatal Steroids

Infusion of cortisol into the sheep fetus results in increased arterial pressure and decreased blood volume (162). Stein et al. (163) observed that neonatal sheep who received hydrocortisone prenatally had increased cardiovascular function despite a marked attenuation in the anticipated surge of plasma catecholamine concentrations and a decrease in epinephrine secretion rate. Adenyl cyclase activity in myocardial tissue was increased (163).

Several reports have suggested that neonatal blood pressure is higher in preterm infants whose mothers received antenatal steroids to hasten fetal lung maturity (164,165). This finding would not be unexpected, since previous studies have suggested that sick preterm neonates may have relative adrenocorticosteroid insufficiency (166–168), and successful treatment with hydrocortisone or dexamethasone of hypotension refractory to conventional therapies has been documented (169–174).

Kari et al. (164) performed a randomized, controlled trial to study whether prenatal dexamethasone improves the outcome of preterm neonates who receive exogenous surfactant. While neonates whose mothers received dexamethasone tended to have higher mean arterial blood pressure during the first three postnatal days, this relationship was less clear when adjustment for birth weight was made, in which case a significant difference in blood pressure was noted only 2 h following the initial dose of surfactant. Subsequently, Moise et al. (165) studied the amount of blood pressure support required by extremely preterm infants (23 to 27 weeks' gestation) whose mothers did or did not receive antenatal steroids. Infants not exposed to antenatal steroids had lower mean blood pressures from 16 to 48 h postnatally. Furthermore, the use of dopamine was increased in the infants not exposed to antenatal steroids. Garland et al. (175) linked the reduction in severe IVH observed in infants whose mothers received antenatal steroids to normal blood pressures in those infants. More recently, Demarini et al. (176) reported that mean blood pressures during the first 24 h postnatal were increased in VLBW infants whose mothers received antenatal steroids, and that volume expansion and vasopressor support were decreased in those infants. These findings in human neonates have been supported by studies in lambs (114) and baboons (177,178).

Conversely, LeFlore et al. (69) reported no differences in blood pressures in 116 VLBW neonates whose mothers did or did not receive antenatal steroids. Similar results were obtained by Omar et al. (179) and Cordero et al. (93). Mantaring and Ostrea (180) reported a tendency for higher mean blood pressure in infants ≥1000 g whose mothers received antenatal steroids but a tendency for lower mean blood pressure in infants <1000 g who were exposed to antenatal steroids. Leviton et al. (181) found no difference in the incidence of lowest mean blood pressure <30 mm Hg in infants whose mothers did or did not receive a complete course of antenatal glucocorticoid prophylaxis. Recently, Dalziel et al. (182) reported that blood pressure at six years of age did not differ between children exposed prenatally to betamethasone and those not exposed.

Other Indicators of Changes in Circulatory Function

Maternal smoking may be associated with increased diastolic blood pressure in the neonate (64). Beratis et al. (183) reported that both systolic and diastolic blood pressure were increased in infants of mothers who smoked, that there was a direct relationship between neonatal blood pressure and the number of cigarettes smoked, and that the effect could persist for at least 12 months. Although maternal hypertension may be a factor associated with higher neonatal blood pressure, this is not consistently reported (69,91,92,180,184–186). Cocaine exposure *in utero* has been shown to be associated with increased blood pressure on the first day of life in term neonates (187,188) and increased circulating catecholamine concentrations have been demonstrated (189,190). Mean arterial pressure was unchanged, but arterial pressure variability was decreased with both pancuronium and pethidine (meperidine) (191); while fentanyl and midazolam may cause hypotension in neonates. In a recent study, Simons et al. (192) concluded that overall mean blood pressures were similar in ventilated neonates who received morphine versus placebo. Numerous studies have demonstrated that blood pressure may increase (145) as well as decrease (193) with pneumothorax. Seizure activity may have variable effects on blood pressure (145). Finally, increased neonatal blood pressure has been documented in infants with chronic lung disease who receive dexamethasone therapy (194,195).

CONCLUSIONS

Recent studies have broadened our knowledge of the complex processes controlling fetal and neonatal blood pressure. Clinical studies in VLBW neonates have provided normative data for blood pressure, especially in the first few postnatal days, and have demonstrated that many of the more immature preterm infants have mean blood pressures in the 20 to 25 mm Hg range especially during the first postnatal day. On the other hand, as noted above, having a blood pressure in the "normal range" does not necessarily guarantee that it is safe. Adjunctive assessments such as urine output and CRT may be helpful, particularly when considered together, but the clinician at the bedside often faces a difficult dilemma in weighing the risks and benefits of therapy for presumed low blood pressure. Further outcome-based studies are needed to address the issue of confirmation of acceptable cardiovascular status in preterm and term neonates adjusted for gestational and postnatal age.

REFERENCES

1. Lou HC, Skov H, Psych C, Pedersen H. Low cerebral blood flow: a risk factor in the neonate. J Pediatr 1979;95:606–609.
2. Kopelman AE. Blood pressure and cerebral ischemia in very low birth weight infants. J Pediatr 1990;116:1000–1002.
3. Guyton AC, Hall JE. Textbook of Medical Physiology, 9th edn Philadelphia, WB Saunders, 1996.
4. Kluckow M. Low systemic blood flow and pathophysiology of the preterm transitional circulation. Early Human Dev 2005;81:429–437.
5. Emery EF, Greenough A. Assessment of non-invasive techniques for measuring blood pressure in preterm infants of birthweight less than or equal to 750 grams. Early Human Dev 1993;33:217–222.
6. Nuntnarumit P, Yang W, Bada-Ellzey HS. Blood pressure measurements in the newborn. Clin Perinatol 1999;26:981–996.

7. Darnall RA. Blood-pressure monitoring. In Physiological Monitoring and Instrument Diagnosis in Perinatal and Neonatal Medicine. Brans Y, Hay WJ, eds. Cambridge, Cambridge University Press, 1995:246–266.

8. O'Rourke MF. What is blood pressure? Am J Hypertens 1990;3:803–810.

9. Gardner RM. Direct blood pressure measurement – dynamic response requirements. Anesthesiology 1981;54:227–236.

10. Hales S. Statistical Essay Containing Haemastatics London, Innys & Mamby, 1733.

11. Park MK, Robotham JL, German VF. Systolic pressure amplification in pedal arteries in children. Crit Care Med 1983;11:286–289.

12. Lotze A, Rivera O, Walton DM. Blood pressure monitoring. In Atlas of Procedures in Neonatology. MacDonald MG, Ramasethu J, eds., 3rd edn Philadelphia, Lippincott Williams and Wilkins, 2002:51–59.

13. Weindling AM. Blood pressure monitoring in the newborn. Arch Dis Child 1989;64:444–447.

14. Cunningham S, Symon AG, McIntosh N. Changes in mean blood pressure caused by damping of the arterial pressure waveform. Early Hum Devel 1994;36:27–30.

15. Butt WW, Whyte H. Blood pressure monitoring in neonates: comparison of umbilical and peripheral artery catheter measurements. J Pediatr 1984;105:630–632.

16. Gevers M, Hack WW, Ree EF, Lafeber HN, Westerhof N. Arterial blood pressure wave forms in radial and posterior tibial arteries in critically ill newborn infants. J Dev Physiol 1993;19:179–185.

17. Darnall RA, Jr. Noninvasive blood pressure measurement in the neonate. Clin Perinatol 1985;12:31–49.

18. Stebor AD. Basic principles of noninvasive blood pressure measurement in infants. Adv Neonatal Care 2005;52:52–261.

19. Association for the Advancement of Medical Instrumentation. American National Standard: Manual, Electronic, or Automated Sphygmomanometers, ANSI/AAMI SP10, ANSI, Arlington, VA, 2002

20. Nelson RM, Stebor AD, Groh CM, Timoney PM, Theobald KS, Friedman BA. Determination of accuracy in neonates for non-invasive blood pressure device using an improved algorithm. Blood Press Monit 2002;7:123–129.

21. Nwankwo MU, Lorenz JM, Gardiner JC. A standard protocol for blood pressure measurement in the newborn. Pediatrics 1997;99:E10.

22. Andriessen P, Schoffelen RL, Berendsen RC, et al. Noninvasive assessment of blood pressure variability in preterm infants. Pediatr Res 2004;55:220–223.

23. Ramsey M, III. Noninvasive automatic determination of mean arterial pressure. Med Biol Eng Comput 1979;17:11–18.

24. Drouin E, Gournay V, Calamel J, Mouzard A, Roze J-C. Feasibility of using finger arterial pressure in neonates. Arch Dis Child 1997;77:F139–F140.

25. Kimble KJ, Darnall RA, Jr, Yelderman M, Ariagno RL, Ream AK. An automated oscillometric technique for estimating mean arterial pressure in critically ill newborns. Anesthesiology 1981;54:423–425.

26. Lui K, Doyle PE, Buchanan N. Oscillometric and intra-arterial blood pressure measurements in the neonate: a comparison of methods. Aust Paediatr J 1982;18:32–34.

27. Colan SD, Fujii A, Borow KM, MacPherson D, Sanders SP. Noninvasive determination of systolic, diastolic, and end-systolic blood pressure in neonates, infants, and young children: comparison with central aortic pressure measurements. Am J Cardiol 1983;52:867–870.

28. Park MK, Menard SM. Accuracy of blood pressure measurement by the dinamap monitor in infants and children. Pediatr 1987;79:907–914.

29. Friesen RH, Lichtor JL. Indirect measurement of blood pressure in neonates and infants utilizing an automatic noninvasive oscillometric monitor. Anesth Analg 1981;60:742–745.

30. Pilossoff V, Schober JG, Peters D, Buhlmeyer K. Non-invasive oscillometric measurement of systolic, mean and diastolic blood pressure in infants with congenital heart defects after operation. A comparison with direct blood pressure measurements. Eur J Pediatr 1985;144:324–330.

31. Cullen PM, Dye J, Hughes DG. Clinical assessment of the neonatal Dinamap 847 during anesthesia in neonates and infants. J Clin Monit 1987;3:229–234.

32. Pellegrini-Caliumi G, Agostino R, Nodari S, Maffei G, Moretti C, Bucci G. Evaluation of an automatic oscillometric method and of various cuffs for the measurement of arterial pressure in the neonate. Acta Paediatr Scand 1982;71:791–797.

33. Sonesson S-E, Broberger U. Arterial blood pressure in the very low birthweight neonate. Acta Paediatr Scand 1987;76:338–341.

34. Clark JA, Lieh-Lai MW, Sarnaik A, Mattoo TK. Discrepancies between direct and indirect blood pressure measurements using various recommendations for arm cuff selection. Pediatrics 2002;110:920–923.

35. Wareham JA, Haugh LD, Yeager SB, Horbar JD. Prediction of arterial blood pressure in the premature neonate using the oscillometric method. AJDC 1987;141:1108–1110.

36. Briassoulis G. Arterial pressure measurement in preterm infants. Crit Care Med 1986;14:735–738.

37. Diprose GK, Evans DH, Archer LNJ, Levene MI. Dinamap fails to detect hypotension in very low birthweight infants. Arch Dis Child 1986;61:771–773.

38. Fanaroff AA, Wright E. Profiles of mean arterial blood pressure (MAP) for infants weighing 501–1500 grams. Pediat Res 1990;27:205A.

39. Chia F, Ang AT, Wong TW, et al. Reliability of the Dinamap non-invasive monitor in the measurement of blood pressure of ill Asian newborns. Clin Pediatr (Philadelphia) 1990;29:262–267.

40. Goldring D, Wohltmann H. Flush method for blood pressure determinations in newborn infants. J Pediatr 1952;40:285–289.

41. Moss AJ, Liebling W, Dams FH. The flush method for determining blood pressures in infants. II. Normal values during the first year of life. Pediatrics 1958;21:950–957.

42. de Swiet M, Peto J, Shinebourne EA. Difference between upper and lower limb blood pressure in normal neonates using Doppler technique. Arch Dis Child 1974;49:734–735.

43. Forfar JO, Kibel MA. Blood pressure in the newborn estimated by the flush method. Arch Dis Child 1956;31:126–130.

44. Uhari M, Isotalo H, Kauppinen R, Kouvalainen K. Difference between upper and lower limb blood pressure in newborns. Acta Paediatr Scand 1981;70:941–942.

45. Park MK, Lee DH. Normative arm and calf blood pressure values in the newborn. Pediatrics 1989;83:240–243.

46. Piazza SF, Chandra M, Harper RG, Sia CG, McVicar M, Huang H. Upper- vs lower-limb systolic blood pressure in full-term normal newborns. Am J Dis Child 1985;139:797–799.

47. Cowan F, Thoresen M, Walloe L. Arm and leg blood pressures – are they really so different in newborns? Early Hum Dev 1991;26:203–211.

48. Kunk R, McCain GC. Comparison of upper arm and calf oscillometric blood pressure measurement in preterm infants. J Perinatol 1996;16(2 Pt 1):89–92.

49. Papadopoulos G, Mieke S, Elisaf M. Assessment of the performances of three oscillometric blood pressure monitors for neonates using a simulator. Blood Press Monit 1999;4:27–33.

50. Pichler G, Urlesberger B, Reiterer F, Gradnitzer E, Muller W. Non-invasive oscillometric blood pressure measurement in very-low-birthweight infants: a comparison of two different monitor systems. Acta Paediatr 1999;88:1044–1045.

51. Dannevig I, Dale HC, Liestol K, Lindemann R. Blood pressure in the neonate: three non-invasive oscillometric pressure monitors compared with invasively measured blood pressure. Acta Paediatr 2005;94:191–196.

52. Engle WD. Blood pressure in the very low birth weight neonate. Early Hum Dev 2001;62:97–130.

53. Pipkin FB, Smales ORC. Blood pressure and angiotensin II in the newborn. Arch Dis Child 1975;50:330.

54. Goodman HG, Cumming GR, Raber MB, Abbasi S. Photocell oscillometer for measuring systolic pressure in newborn. Am J Dis Child 1962;103:152–159.

55. Levison H, Kidd BSL, Gemmell PA, Swyer PR. Blood pressure in normal full-term and premature infants. Am J Dis Child 1966;111:374–379.

56. Bucci G, Scalamandre A, Savignoni PG, Mendicini M, Picece-Bucci S. The systemic systolic blood pressure of newborns with low weight. Acta Paediatr Scand 1972;229:5–26.

57. Ingelfinger JR, Powers L, Epstein MF. Blood pressure norms in low-birth-weight infants: birth through 4 weeks. Pediat Res 1983;17:319A.

58. Shortland DB, Evans DH, Levene MI. Blood pressure measurements in very low birth weight infants over the first week of life. J Perinat Med 1988;16:93–97.

59. Hulman S, Edwards R, Chen YQ, Polansky M, Falkner B. Blood pressure patterns in the first three days of life. J Perinatol 1991;11:231–234.

60. Spinazzola RM, Harper RG, de Soler M, Lesser M. Blood pressure values in 500- to 750-gram birthweight infants in the first week of life. J Perinatol 1991;11:147–151.

61. Perry EH, Bada HS, Ray JD, Korones SB, Arheart K, Magill HL. Blood pressure increases, birth weight-dependent stability boundary, and intraventricular hemorrhage. Pediatrics 1990;85:727–732.

62. D'Souza SW, Janakova H, Minors D, et al. Blood pressure, heart rate, and skin temperature in preterm infants: associations with periventricular haemorrhage. Arch Dis Child 1995;72:F162–F167.

63. Zubrow AB, Hulman S, Kushner H, Falkner B. Determinants of blood pressure in infants admitted to neonatal intensive care units: a prospective multicenter study. J Perinatol 1995;15:470–479.

64. O'Sullivan MJ, Kearney PJ, Crowley MJ. The influence of some perinatal variables on neonatal blood pressure. Acta Paediatr 1996;85:849–853.

65. Georgieff MK, Mills MM, Gomez-Marin O, Sinaiko AR. Rate of change of blood pressure in premature and full term infants from birth to 4 months. Pediatr Nephrol 1996;10:152–155.

66. Alves JGB, Vilarim JND, Figueiroa JN. Fetal influences on neonatal blood pressure. J Perinatol 1999;19:593–595.

67. Lee J, Rajadurai VS, Tan KW. Blood pressure standards for very low birthweight infants during the first day of life. Arch Dis Child, Fetal Neonatal Ed 1999;81:F168–F170.

68. Hindmarsh PC, Brook CGD. Evidence for an association between birth weight and blood pressure. Acta Paediatr 1999;428:66–69.

69. LeFlore JL, Engle WD, Rosenfeld CR. Determinants of blood pressure in very low birth weight neonates: lack of effect of antenatal steroids. Early Hum Dev 2000;59:37–50.

70. Gupta JM, Scopes JW. Observations on blood pressure in newborn infants. Arch Dis Child 1965;40:637–644.

71. Kitterman JA, Phibbs RH, Tooley WH. Aortic blood pressure in normal newborn infants during the first 12 hours of life. Pediatrics 1969;44:959–968.

72. Versmold HT, Kitterman JA, Phibs RH, Gregory GA, Toley WH. Aortic blood pressure during the first 12 hours of life in infants with birth weight 610 to 4,220 grams. Pediatrics 1981;67:607–613.

73. Strambi M, Vezzosi P, Buoni S, Berni S, Longini M. Blood pressure in the small-for-gestational age newborn. Minerva Pediatr 2004;56:603–610.

74. Seri I, Evans J. Controversies in the diagnosis and management of hypotension in the newborn infant. Curr Opin Pediatr 2001;13:116–123.

75. Kluckow M, Evans N. Low superior vena cava flow and intraventricular haemorrhage in preterm infants. Arch Dis Child, Fetal Neonatal Ed 2000;82:F188–F194.

76. Kluckow M, Evans N. Relationship between blood pressure and cardiac output in preterm infants requiring mechanical ventilation. J Pediatr 1996;129:506–512.

77. Munro MJ, Walker AM, Barfield CP. Hypotensive extremely low birth weight infants have reduced cerebral blood flow. Pediatrics 2004;114:1591–1596.

78. Moss AJ, Duffie ER, Jr. Emmanouilides G. Blood pressure and vasomotor reflexes in the newborn infant. Pediatrics 1963;32:175–179.

79. Miall-Allen VM, de Vries LS, Whitelaw AGL. Mean arterial blood pressure and neonatal cerebral lesions. Arch Dis Child 1987;62:1068–1069.

80. Watkins AMC, West CR, Cooke RWI. Blood pressure and cerebral haemorrhage and ischaemia in very low birthweight infants. Early Hum Develop 1989;19:103–110.

81. Kehrer M, Blumenstock G, Ehehalt S, Goelz R, Poets C, Schoning M. Development of cerebral blood flow volume in preterm neonates during the first two weeks of life. Pediatr Res 2005;58:927–930.

82. Tan KL. Blood pressure in full-term healthy neonates. Clin Pediatr (Philadelphia) 1987;26:21–24.

83. Tan KL. Blood pressure in very low birth weight infants in the first 70 days of life. J Pediatr 1988;112:266–270.

84. Adams MA, Pasternak JF, Kupfer BM, Gardner TH. A computerized system for continuous physiologic data collection and analysis: initial report on mean arterial blood pressure in very low-birth-weight infants. Pediatrics 1983;71:23–30.

85. Cunningham S, Deere S, McIntosh N. Cyclical variation of blood pressure and heart rate in neonates. Arch Dis Child 1993;69:64–67.

86. Goddard J, Lewis RM, Armstrong DL, Zeller RS. Moderate, rapidly induced hypertension as a cause of intraventricular hemorrhage in the newborn beagle model. J Pediatr 1980;96:1057–1060.

87. Cunningham S, Symon AG, Elton RA, Zhu C, McIntosh N. Intra-arterial blood pressure reference ranges, death and morbidity in very low birthweight infants during the first seven days of life. Early Hum Dev 1999;56:151–165.

88. Dimitriou G, Greenough A, Kavvadia V, Mantagos S. Blood pressure rhythms during the perinatal period in very immature, extremely low birthweight neonates. Early Hum Dev 1999;56:49–56.

89. Gemelli M, Manganaro R, Mami C, Rando F, De LF. Circadian blood pressure pattern in full-term newborn infants. Biol Neonate 1989;56:315–323.

90. Emery EF, Greenough A. Neonatal blood pressure levels of preterm infants who did and did not develop chronic lung disease. Early Hum Develop 1992;31:149–156.

91. Hegyi T, Carbone MT, Anwar M, et al. Blood pressure ranges in premature infants. I. The first hours of life. J Pediatr 1994;124:627–633.

92. Hegyi T, Anwar M, Carbone MT, et al. Blood pressure ranges in premature infants: II. The first week of life. Pediatrics 1996;97:336–342.

93. Cordero L, Timan CJ, Waters HH, Sachs LA. Mean arterial pressures during the first 24 hours of life in < or = 600-gram birth weight infants. J Perinatol 2002;22:348–353.

94. Report of a Joint Working Group of the British Association of Perinatal Medicine and the Research Unit of the Royal College of Physicians. Development of audit measures and guidelines for good practice in the management of neonatal respiratory distress syndrome. Arch Dis Child 1992;67:1221–1227.

95. Seri I, Noori S. Diagnosis and treatment of neonatal hypotension outside the transitional period. Early Hum Dev 2005;81:405–411.

96. Pellicer A, Valverde E, Elorza MD, et al. Cardiovascular support for low birth weight infants and cerebral hemodynamics: a randomized, blinded, clinical trial. Pediatrics 2005;115:1501–1512.

97. Munro MJ, Walker AM, Barfield CP. Preterm circulatory support is more complex than just blood pressure: in reply. Pediatrics 2005;115:1115–1116.

98. Weindling AM, Bentham J. Blood pressure in the neonate. Acta Paediatr 2005;94:138–140.

99. Kissack CM, Garr R, Wardle SP, Weindling AM. Cerebral fractional oxygen extraction in very low birth weight infants is high when there is low left ventricular output and hypocarbia but is unaffected by hypotension. Pediatr Res 2004;55:400–405.

100. Victor S, Marson AG, Appleton RE, Beirne M, Weindling AM. Relationship between blood pressure, cerebral electrical activity, cerebral fractional oxygen extraction, and peripheral blood flow in very low birth weight newborn infants. Pediatr Res 2006;59:314–319.

101. Engle WD, Arant BS, Jr, Wiriyathian S, Rosenfeld CR. Diuresis and respiratory distress syndrome: physiologic mechanisms and therapeutic implications. J Pediatr 1983;102:912–917.

102. Joppich R, Scherer B, Weber PC. Renal prostaglandins: relationship to the development of blood pressure and concentrating capacity in pre-term and full term healthy infants. Eur J Pediatr 1979;132:253–259.

103. Joppich R, Hauser I. Urinary prostacyclin and thromboxane A_2 metabolites in preterm and full-term infants in relation to plasma renin activity and blood pressure. Biol Neonate 1982;42:179–184.

104. Chern J, Kamm KE, Rosenfeld CR. Smooth muscle myosin heavy chain isoforms are developmentally regulated in male fetal and neonatal sheep. Pediatr Res 1995;38:697–703.

105. Arens Y, Chapados RA, Cox BE, Kamm KE, Rosenfeld CR. Differential development of umbilical and systemic arteries. II. Contractile proteins. Am J Physiol, Regul Integr Comp Physiol 1998;274:R1815–R1823.

106. Perkin RM, Levin DL. Shock in the pediatric patient. Part I. J Pediatr 1982;101:163–169.

107. Noori S, Seri I. Pathophysiology of newborn hypotension outside the transitional period. Early Hum Dev 2005;81:399–404.

108. Faix RG, Pryce CJE. Shock and hypotension. In Neonatal Emergencies. Donn SM, Faix RG, eds. Mount Kisco, NY, Futura Publishing, 1991:371–385.

109. Myers BD, Moran SM. Hemodynamically mediated acute renal failure. N Engl J Med 1986;314:97–105.

110. Clark DA. Times of first void and first stool in 500 newborns. Pediatrics 1977;60:457–459.

111. Kluckow M, Evans N. Low systemic blood flow and hyperkalemia in preterm infants. J Pediatr 2001;139:227–232.

112. Seri I. Inotrope, lusitrope, and pressor use in neonates. J Perinatol 2005;25(Suppl 2):S28–S30.

113. Garson AJ, Smith RJ, Moak J. Tachyarrhythmias. In Fetal and Neonatal Cardiology. Long W, ed. Philadelphia, WB Saunders, 1990:511–518.

114. Smith LM, Ervin MG, Wada N, Ikegami M, Polk DH, Jobe AH. Antenatal glucocorticoids alter postnatal preterm lamb renal and cardiovascular responses to intravascular volume expansion. Pediatr Res 2000;47:622–627.

115. Baraff LJ. Capillary refill: is it a useful clinical sign? Pediatrics 1993;92:723–724.

116. Harris GD, Saavedra JM, Finberg L. Capillary refill? Pediatrics 1994;94(2, Pt 1):240.

117. Saavedra JM, Harris GD, Li S, Finberg L. Capillary refilling (skin turgor) in the assessment of dehydration. Am J Dis Child 1991;145:296–298.

118. Beecher HK, et al. The internal state of the severely wounded man on entry to the most forward hospital. Recent Advances in Surgery 1947;22:672–681.

119. Champion HR, Sacco WJ, Hannan DS, Lepper RL, Atzinger ES, Copes WS, et al. Assessment of injury severity: the triage index. Crit Care Med 1980;8:201–208.

120. Champion HR, Sacco WJ, Carnazzo AJ, Copes W, Fouty WJ. Trauma score. Crit Care Med 1981;9:672–676.

121. Gorelick MH, Shaw KN, Baker MD. Effect of ambient temperature on capillary refill in healthy children. Pediatrics 1993;92:699–702.

122. Schriger DL, Baraff L. Defining normal capillary refill: variation with age, sex, and temperature. Ann Emerg Med 1988;17:932–935.

123. Wodey E, Pladys P, Betremieux P, Kerebel C, Ecoffey C. Capillary refilling time and hemodynamics in neonates: a Doppler echocardiographic evaluation. Crit Care Med 1998;26:1437–1440.

124. LeFlore JL, Engle WD. Capillary refill time is an unreliable indicator of cardiovascular status in term neonates. Adv Neonatal Care 2005;5:147–154.

125. Osborn DA, Evans N, Kluckow M. Clinical detection of low upper body blood flow in very premature infants using blood pressure, capillary refill time, and central–peripheral temperature difference. Arch Dis Child, Fetal Neonatal Ed 2004;89:F168–F173.

126. Tibby SM, Hatherill M, Murdoch IA. Capillary refill and core-peripheral temperature gap as indicators of haemodynamic status in paediatric intensive care patients. Arch Dis Child 1999;80:163–166.

127. Gillman MW, Rich-Edwards JW, Rifas-Shiman SL, Lieberman ES, Kleinman KP, Lipshultz SE. Maternal age and other predictors of newborn blood pressure. J Pediatr 2004;144:240–245.

128. Faxelius G, Lagercrantz H, Yao A. Sympathoadrenal activity and peripheral blood flow after birth: comparison in infants delivered vaginally and by cesarean section. J Pediatr 1984;105:144–148.

129. Agata Y, Hiraishi S, Misawa H, et al. Hemodynamic adaptations at birth and neonates delivered vaginally and by cesarean section. Biol Neonate 1995;68:404–411.

130. Pohjavuori M, Fyhrquist F. Vasopressin, ACTH and neonatal haemodynamics. Acta Paediatr Scand Suppl 1983;305:79–83.

131. Holland WW, Young IM. Neonatal blood pressure in relation to maturity, mode of delivery, and condition at birth. Br Med J 1956;2:1331–1333.

132. Peltonen T. Placental transfusion – advantage and disadvantage. Eur J Pediatr 1981;137:141–146.

133. Clyman RI, Mauray F, Heymann MA, Roman C. Cardiovascular effects of patent ductus arteriosus in preterm lambs with respiratory distress. J Pediatr 1987;111:579–587.

134. Ratner I, Perelmuter B, Toews W, Whitfield J. Association of low systolic and diastolic blood pressure with significant patent ductus arteriosus in the very low birth weight infant. Crit Care Med 1985;13:497–500.

135. Evans N, Moorcraft J. Effect of patency of the ductus arteriosus on blood pressure in very preterm infants. Arch Dis Child 1992;67:1169–1173.

136. Furzan JA, Reisch J, Tyson JE, Laird P, Rosenfeld CR. Incidence and risk factors for symptomatic patent ductus arteriosus among inborn very-low-birth-weight infants. Early Hum Develop 1985;12:39–48.

137. Mouzinho AI, Rosenfeld CR, Risser R. Symptomatic patent ductus arteriosus in very-low-birth-weight infants: 1987–1989. Early Hum Develop 1991;27:65–77.

138. Alverson DC, Eldridge MW, Johnson JD, et al. Effect of patent ductus arteriosus on left ventricular output in premature infants. J Pediatr 1983;102:754–757.

139. Miller MJ, Martin RJ. Pathophysiology of apnea of prematurity. In Fetal and Neonatal Physiology. 2nd edn, Polin RA, Fox WW, eds. Philadelphia, WB Saunders, 1998:1129–1143.

140. Girling DJ. Changes in heart rate, blood pressure, and pulse pressure during apnoeic attacks in newborn babies. Arch Dis Child 1972;47:405–410.

141. Perlman JM, Volpe JJ. Episodes of apnea and bradycardia in the preterm newborn: impact on cerebral circulation. Pediatr 1985;76:333–338.

142. Cabal LA, Larrazabal C, Siassi B. Hemodynamic variables in infants weighing less than 1000 grams. Clin Perinatol 1986;13:327–338.

143. Korvenranta H, Kero P, Valimaki I. Cardiovascular monitoring in infants with respiratory distress syndrome. Biol Neonate 1983;44:138–145.

144. Perlman JM, McMenamin JB, Volpe JJ. Fluctuating cerebral blood-flow velocity in respiratory-distress syndrome. N Engl J Med 1983;309:204–209.

145. Volpe JJ Neurology of the Newborn, 3rd edn. Philadelphia, WB Saunders, 1995:172–207.

146. Miall-Allen VM, de Vries LS, Dubowitz LM, Whitelaw AG. Blood pressure fluctuation and intra-ventricular hemorrhage in the preterm infant of less than 31 weeks' gestation. Pediatrics 1989;83:657–661.

147. Jacobs MM, Phibbs RH. Prevention, recognition, and treatment of perinatal asphyxia. Clin Perinatol 1989;16:785–807.

148. Holzman BH, Scarpelli EM. Cardiopulmonary consequences of positive end-expiratory pressure. Pediat Res 1979;13:1112–1120.

149. Yu VYH, Rolfe P. Effect of continuous positive airway pressure breathing on cardiorespiratory function in infants with respiratory distress syndrome. Acta Paediatr 1977;66:59–64.

150. Maayan C, Eyal F, Mandelberg A, Sapoznikov D, Lewis BS. Effect of mechanical ventilation and volume loading on left ventricular performance in premature infants with respiratory distress syndrome. Crit Care Med 1986;14:858–860.

151. Hausdorf G, Hellwege H-H. Influence of positive end-expiratory pressure on cardiac performance in premature infants: a doppler-echocardiographic study. Crit Care Med 1987;15:661–664.

152. Evans N, Kluckow M. Early determinants of right and left ventricular output in ventilated preterm infants. Arch Dis Child 1996;74:F88–F94.

153. Skinner JR, Boys RJ, Hunter S, Hey EN. Pulmonary and systemic arterial pressure in hyaline membrane disease. Arch Dis Child 1992;67:366–373.

154. Hummler H, Gerhardt T, Gonzalez A, Claure N, Everett R, Bancalari E. Influence of different methods of synchronized mechanical ventilation on ventilation, gas exchange, patient effort, and blood pressure fluctuations in premature neonates. Pediatr Pulmonol 1996;22:305–313.

155. Perlman JM, Volpe JJ. Suctioning in the preterm infant: effects on cerebral blood flow velocity, intracranial pressure, and arterial blood pressure. Pediatrics 1983;72:329–334.

156. Omar SY, Greisen G, Ibrahim MM, Youssef AM, Friis-Hansen B. Blood pressure responses to care procedures in ventilated preterm infants. Acat Paediatr Scand 1985;74:920–924.

157. Cowan F, Whitelaw A, Wertheim D, Silverman M. Cerebral blood flow velocity changes after rapid administration of surfactant. Arch Dis Child 1991;66:1105–1109.

158. Segerer H, van Gelder W, Angenent WM, et al. Pulmonary distribution and efficacy of exogenous surfactant in lung-lavaged rabbits are influenced by the instillation technique. Pediat Res 1993;34:490–494.

159. Chan JO, Moglia BA, Reeves IV, Kim AH, Darrow KA, Seaton JF, et al. Cardiorespiratory and stress hormone responses during first dose surfactant administration in neonates with RDS. Pediatr Pulmonol 1994;17:246–249.

160. Schipper JA, Mohammad GI, van Straaten HLM, Koppe JG. The impact of surfactant replacement therapy on cerebral and systemic circulation and lung function. Eur J Pediatr 1997;156:224–227.

161. Moen A, Yu X-Q, Almaas R, Curstedt T, Saugstad OD. Acute effects on systemic circulation after intratracheal instillation of Curosurf or Survanta in surfactant-depleted newborn piglets. Acta Paediatr 1998;87:297–303.

162. Wood CE, Cheung CY, Brace RA. Fetal heart rate, arterial pressure, and blood volume responses to cortisol infusion. Am J Physiol, Regul Integ Comp Physiol 1987;253:R904–R909.

163. Stein HM, Oyama K, Martinez A, et al. Effects of corticosteroids in preterm sheep on adaptation and sympathoadrenal mechanisms at birth. Am J Physiol, Endocrinol Metab 1993;264:E763–E769.

164. Kari MA, Hallman M, Eronen M, et al. Prenatal dexamethasone treatment in conjunction with rescue therapy of human surfactant: a randomized placebo-controlled multicenter study. Pediatrics 1994;93:730–736.

165. Moise AA, Wearden ME, Kozinetz CA, Gest AL, Welty SE, Hansen TN. Antenatal steroids are associated with less need for blood pressure support in extremely premature infants. Pediatrics 1995;95:845–850.

166. Colasurdo AA, Hanna CE, Gilhooly JT, Reynolds JW. Hydrocortisone replacement in extremely premature infants with cortisol insufficiency. Clin Res 1989;37180A.

167. Watterberg KL, Scott SM. Evidence of early adrenal insufficiency in babies who develop broncho-pulmonary dysplasia. Pediatrics 1995;95:120–125.

168. Hanna CE, Jett PL, Laird MR, Mandel SH, LaFranchi SH, Reynolds JW. Corticosteroid binding globulin, total serum cortisol, and stress in extremely low-birth-weight infants. Am J Perinatol 1997;14:201–214.

169. Tantivit P, Subramanian N, Garg M, Ramanathan R, deLemos RA. Low serum cortisol in term newborns with refractory hypotension. J Perinatol 1991;19:352–357.

170. Derleth DP. Extraordinary response to dexamethasone therapy for hypotension in a premature newborn: a case report. Pediatr Res 1992;31:200A.

171. Fauser A, Pohlandt F, Bartmann P, Gortner L. Rapid increase of blood pressure in extremely low birth weight infants after a single dose of dexamethasone. Eur J Pediatr 1993;152:354–356.

172. Helbock HJ, Insoft RM, Conte FA. Glucocorticoid-responsive hypotension in extremely low birth weight newborns. Pediatrics 1993;92:715–717.

173. Ramanathan R, Siassi B, Sardesai S, deLemos R. Dexamethasone versus hydrocortisone for hypotension refractory to high dose inotropic agents and incidence of candida infection in extremely low birth weight infants. Pediatr Res 1996;39240A.

174. Gaissmaier RE, Pohlandt F. Single-dose dexamethasone treatment of hypotension in preterm infants. J Pediatr 1999;134:701–705.

175. Garland JS, Buck R, Leviton A. Effect of maternal glucocorticoid exposure on risk of severe intraventricular hemorrhage in surfactant-treated preterm infants. J Pediatr 1995;126:272–279.

176. Demarini S, Dollberg S, Hoath SB, Ho M, Donoan EF. Effects of antenatal corticosteroids on blood pressure in very low birth weight infants during the first 24 hours of life. J Perinatol 1999;19:419–425.

177. Smith LM, Altamirano AK, Ervin MG, Seidner SR, Jobe AH. Prenatal glucocorticoid exposure and postnatal adaptation in premature newborn baboons ventilated for six days. Am J Obstet Gynecol 2004;191:1688–1694.

178. Ervin MG, Seidner SR, Leland MM, Ikegami M, Jobe AH. Direct fetal glucocorticoid treatment alters postnatal adaptation in premature newborn baboons. Am J Physiol 1998;274(4, Pt 2)R1169–R1176.

179. Omar SA, DeCristofaro JD, Agarwal BI, LaGamma EF. Effects of prenatal steroids on water and sodium homeostasis in extremely low birth weight neonates. Pediatrics 1999;104:482–488.

180. Mantaring JV, Ostrea EM. Effect of perinatal factors on blood pressure in preterm neonates. Pediatr Res 1996;39228A.

181. Leviton A, Kuban KC, Pagano M, Allred EN, Van ML. Antenatal corticosteroids appear to reduce the risk of postnatal germinal matrix hemorrhage in intubated low birth weight newborns. Pediatrics 1993;91:1083–1088.

182. Dalziel SR, Liang A, Parag V, Rodgers A, Harding JE. Blood pressure at 6 years of age after prenatal exposure to betamethasone: follow-up results of a randomized, controlled trial. Pediatrics 2004;114:e373–e377.

183. Beratis NG, Panagoulias D, Varvarigou A. Increased blood pressure in neonates and infants whose mothers smoked during pregnancy. J Pediatr 1996;128:806–812.

184. Woodbury RA, Robinow M, Hamilton WF. Blood pressure studies on infants. Am J Physiol 1938;122:472–479.

185. Cabal LA, Reed J, Miller F, Hodgman JE. Elevated blood pressure in infants of pre-eclamptic mothers. Pediatr Res 1981;15459A.

186. Miller FC, Read JA, Cabal L, Siassi B. Heart rate and blood pressure in infants of preeclamptic mothers during the first hour of life. Crit Care Med 1983;11:532–535.

187. van de Bor M, Walther FJ, Ebrahimi M. Decreased cardiac output in infants of mothers who abused cocaine. Pediatrics 1990;85:30–32.

188. van de Bor M, Walther FJ, Sims ME. Increased cerebral blood flow velocity in infants of mothers who abuse cocaine. Pediatrics 1990;85:733–736.

189. Mirochnick M, Meyer J, Cole J, Herren T, Zuckerman B. Circulating catecholamine concentrations in cocaine-exposed neonates: a pilot study. Pediatrics 1991;88:481–485.

190. Ward SLD, Schuetz S, Wachsman L, et al. Elevated plasma norepinephrine levels in infants of substance-abusing mothers. AJDC 1991;145:44–48.

191. Miall-Allen VM, Whitelaw AGL. Effect of pancuronium and pethidine on heart rate and blood pressure in ventilated infants. Arch Dis Child 1987;62:1179–1180.

192. Simons SHP, van Dijk M, van Lingen RA, et al. Randomized controlled trial evaluating effects of morphine on plasma adrenaline/noradrenaline concentrations in newborns. Arch Dis Child, Fetal Neonatal Ed 2005;90:F36–F40.

193. Zak LK, Donn SM. Thoracic air leaks. In Neonatal Emergencies. Donn SM, Faix RG, eds. Mount Kisco, NY, Futura, 1991:311–325.

194. Ng PC. The effectiveness and side effects of dexamethasone in preterm infants with bronchopulmonary dysplasia. Arch Dis Child 1993;68(3, Spec No):330–336.

195. Marinelli KA, Burke GS, Herson VC. Effects of dexamethasone on blood pressure in premature infants with bronchopulmonary dysplasia. J Pediatr 1997;130:594–602.

Diagnosis of Neonatal Shock

Chapter 4

Use of Organ Blood Flow Assessment in the Diagnosis and Treatment of Neonatal Shock

Gorm Greisen, MD, PhD

Doppler Ultrasound

Near-Infrared Spectroscopy

Magnetic Resonance Imaging

The Kety–Schmidt Method

^{133}**Xe Clearance**

Single Photon Emission Computed Tomography

Stable Xenon-Enhanced Computed Tomography

Positron Emission Tomography

Other Methods

Conclusion

References

This chapter describes the methods available to assess organ blood flow in the neonate, and discusses their strengths, weaknesses, and sources of errors. Most detail is given on Doppler ultrasound and near-infrared (NIR) spectroscopy, since these are the most practical methods, they have been used at the bedside, and are likely to produce new research data in the near future. The measurement of cerebral blood flow (CBF) is described first and in more detail, since this is where most of the experience is. A brief section at the end then addresses the experience with assessment of blood flow to other organs.

Organ blood flow is usually expressed in mL/min, as this is the most descriptive unit when an organ is supplied from a single artery and/or drained via a single vein. Indeed, in animal experimentation the simplest method to measure blood flow to an organ is to drain the venous outflow into a calibrated container. The description of blood flow in mL/min has been used to judge the flow to an organ expressed as a fraction of cardiac output. Whether this fraction changes during development or under pathological conditions such as hypoxia, arterial hypotension, and/or low cardiac output states are important and clinically relevant questions in the field of developmental physiology and pathophysiology. Finally, to allow comparison among groups of infants of different gestational age and thus body weight, it is useful to normalize blood flow for body weight and express it as mL/min/kg.

However, organ blood flow can also be expressed in mL/100 g tissue/min. This measure may refer to an organ as a whole or to a specific region or compartment in a given organ, depending on the method of measurement. The simplest methods to assess organ blood flow use Fick's principle for inert tracers: "Flow equals the rate of change in tissue concentration of tracer divided by the arterio-venous concentration difference of the tracer." This measure is especially useful to assess the flow in relation to metabolism and organ function.

It is important to emphasize that blood flow is a complex and dynamic variable. Aside from physiologic fluctuations in organ blood flow governed by the changes in functional activity and thus the metabolic demand of a given organ, blood flow may significantly change within seconds under pathological conditions such as with abrupt changes in blood pressure or the onset of hypoxia. In addition, blood flow may vary from one part of an organ to the other as during functional activation, or during stress, the distribution may change markedly.

For several decades authors on perinatal circulation have been pointing out the need to consider blood flow, rather than only arterial blood pressure. Therefore, thoughtful neonatal practice would include the use of indirect measures of blood flow, such as skin color, peripheral–core temperature difference, capillary refill time, urine output, and lactic acidosis. Unfortunately, these indirect signs of tissue perfusion either lack sensitivity and specificity (i.e. peripheral–core temperature difference, capillary refill time) or do not represent the changes in the hemodynamic status in a timely manner (i.e. urine output and lactic acidosis).

As for the methods available for the more direct assessment of organ blood flow in neonates, very few units routinely utilize these tools. Why is this so?

There are four main reasons why assessment of organ blood flow has not been done routinely in the clinical practice. First, none of the many methods which have been tried in research settings has achieved broader application because none satisfies the requirements in terms of ease, precision, accuracy, non-invasiveness, and cost. In reality, therefore, no method is truly available to clinicians who want to upgrade their clinical practice. Methods using standard equipment (such as ultrasound) require much skill, while the ones which in principle are "push-button" methods require special instruments and validation. Second, no method has truly sufficient precision. For research, a method of measurement is considered appropriate if it is unbiased. By analysis of results from groups of subjects it is still possible to achieve statistically significant results. For clinical use, however, it is absolutely necessary that a single measurement is sufficiently precise. Third, research on organ blood flow in neonates has focused on physiology and pathophysiology and done little in the way of defining the clinical benefit of having measures of blood flow in ill infants. This means that there is only little incentive for the clinician to overcome the difficulties presented above. Finally, as with the now routine direct measurement of arterial blood pressure, ideally organ blood flow should be monitored continuously and expressed as absolute flow (mL/min). To date, none of the methods come even close to this requirement.

DOPPLER ULTRASOUND

Doppler ultrasound to assess changes in CBF was first used in neonates in 1979 (1). As clinical and research interest focussed on CBF during this time, several methods, including Doppler ultrasound, were introduced to assess blood flow to the brain of the neonate. The use of Doppler ultrasound for functional echocardiography in the neonate is described in Section II, Chapter 5 in detail.

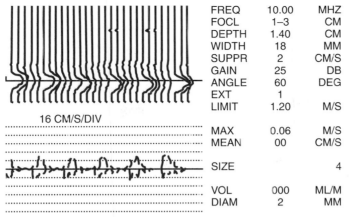

FREQ	10.00	MHZ
FOCL	1–3	CM
DEPTH	1.40	CM
WIDTH	18	MM
SUPPR	2	CM/S
GAIN	25	DB
ANGLE	60	DEG
EXT	1	
LIMIT	1.20	M/S
MAX	0.06	M/S
MEAN	00	CM/S
SIZE		4
VOL	000	ML/M
DIAM	2	MM

16 CM/S/DIV

FIGURE 4-1 Output from a prototype Doppler instrument with multiple gates built in the late 1980s. The vertical lines represent the mean velocity detected in each of the 128 gates every 50 ms. Together the 128 gates span 18 mm, i.e. approximately 0.15 mm is covered by each. The probe was placed on the neck of a newborn infant to measure flow in the common carotid artery. The vertical line is 1.4 cm under the skin. The flow profile is parabolic as expected and steeper during systole. From the flow profile, the diameter can be estimated to be approximately 3 mm at 60° angle of insonation. This is the principle behind color-coded Doppler ultrasound. As a result of the speed of data processing, new instruments have the Doppler information as part of the two-dimensional ultrasound image. The vessel diameter is then read from the color image by the investigator using electronic calipers. Two principles can be used to estimate mean flow velocity for volumetric Doppler. The sample volume is set so that the entire vessel is covered. The machine can weigh the received mixture of frequency shifts (i.e. velocities) by their intensity, i.e. by the mass of erythrocytes flowing at each velocity. However, intensity is not a perfect measure of mass and not all ultrasound transducers produce homogenous sonification of the entire vessel. Alternatively, the maximum velocity can be used and divided by a factor of 2. This corresponds to equality of the volume of a parabola with a cylinder of half the height. Maximum frequency is normally well measured, but the method will fail if the flow profile is not parabolic.

The Doppler Principle

According to the Doppler principle, the frequency shift of the reflected sound (the "echo") is proportional to the velocity of the reflector. Since erythrocytes in blood reflect ultrasound, blood flow velocity can be measured based on simple physics. This equation states that the frequency shift equals the flow velocity multiplied by the emitted frequency divided by the speed of sound in the tissue. However, there are several factors that need to be taken into consideration and corrected for with the use of the Doppler principle. First, the apparent velocity has to be corrected for the angle between the blood vessel and the ultrasound beam. Second, it should be kept in mind that multiple frequencies are detected when performing an ultrasound study of a vessel, since the flow velocity decreases from the center of the stream toward the vessel wall. In addition, even the vessel wall itself contributes to the signal and the velocity is pulsating in nature, as it is faster in systole than in diastole (Fig. 4-1).

The First Instruments

The instruments of the 1970s and early 1980s were continuous wave (with no resolution of depth, with no image, and a crude mean frequency shift estimator). Finding an arterial signal was done blindly, using general anatomical knowledge and an audible signal with the frequency shift in the 50 to 500 Hz range while searching for the loudest pulsating signal with the highest pitch. This left the angle and the true spatial average undetermined, and therefore the scale of measurement uncertain. Indices of pulsatility (resistance index: [(peak systolic flow velocity − end diastolic flow velocity)/end diastolic flow velocity] and pulsatility index: [(peak systolic flow velocity − end diastolic flow velocity)/mean flow velocity]) were often used since these indices are independent of the angle of insonation.

Indices of Pulsatility

Indices of pulsatility reflect downstream resistance to flow and pulsatility in the umbilical artery has achieved great clinical importance in fetal monitoring (2). In newborn infants, however, the resistance index in the anterior cerebral artery was only weakly associated with cerebral blood flow as measured by ^{133}Xe clearance (3). In addition, further, more sophisticated modeling revealed that arterial blood pressure pulsatility and arterial wall compliance are as important determinators of the indices of pulsatility as is the downstream resistance (4). In summary, Doppler data on resistance indices may be valid and have often been corroborated by other methods, but could be imprecise and heavily biased. In an elegant paper, however, the pulsatility index was shown to carry independent prognostic ability in term infants with neonatal hypoxic–ischemic encephalopathy (5).

Blood Flow Velocity

With the technical advances in the 1980s, duplex scanning combining imaging and Doppler, range-gating limiting flow detection to a small sample volume, and frequency analysis allowing proper maximum and mean frequency shift estimation became available and contributed to more reliable measurement of blood flow velocity. However, this still left the question of accurate determination of the arterial caliber unanswered. This is an important point, as the calculation of absolute organ blood flow in mL/min equals flow velocity (cm/s) multiplied by arterial cross-sectional area (cm^2). The inability to accurately measure the arterial cross-sectional area precludes comparison from one infant to another, one organ to another and, in essence, from one state to another, since arterial caliber varies dynamically in the immature individual (6,7). In summary, although improved techniques now allow more accurate and precise measurement of flow velocity, it is still uncertain if this has really improved the value of this modality, since measurement of absolute blood flow is more informative that determination of blood flow velocity alone.

Volumetric Measurements

This last hurdle to absolute, volumetric measurement of flow has been addressed using ultrasound imaging to measure arterial cross-sectional area as part of the method. In large-diameter vessels this can be now used quite accurately. For instance, to measure left and right ventricular output, the diameter of the ascending aorta and the pulmonary trunk, respectively, need to be precisely determined. The diameter of these two major vessels is 6 to 10 mm, and an error of 0.5 mm on the first generation of duplex scanners translated to a reproducibility of 10 to 15%. Recently, for measurement of superior vena cava (SVC) flow at the vessel's entry into the right atrium with a diameter of 3 to 6 mm, reproducibility of SVC flow of 14% was reported using a 7 MHz transducer (8). With the advent of color-coded imaging and the use of higher ultrasound frequencies, volumetric measurement of distributary arteries have also become possible in the newborn. For instance, measurement of blood flow in the right common carotid artery with a diameter of 2 to 3 mm was reported to have a reproducibility of 10 to 15% using a 15 MHz transducer (9), while that in both internal carotid and both vertebral arteries with diameters of 1 to 2 mm was found to be 7% for the sum of the blood flows in the four arteries using a 10 MHz transducer (10).

NEAR-INFRARED SPECTROSOPY

NIR spectroscopy is also discussed in Section II, Chapter 6. Transillumination of the head of small animals is possible using NIR spectroscopy and the first clinical research use of this technology was carried out in newborns (11). Quantitative spectroscopy was subsequently performed in 1986 (12). Over the following years a large number of papers on NIR spectroscopy in newborns have been published.

Geometry

The newborn infant's head is ideally suited for NIR spectroscopy. The overlying tissues are relatively thin, which ensures that the signal is dominated by brain tissue including both the white and gray matter. NIR spectroscopy recordings can be performed with the light applied to one side of the head and received on the other side (*transmission mode*) in the low-birth-weight infant with biparietal diameters from 6 to 8 cm. In this situation a large part of the brain is included in the measurement, and the results may be interpreted as assessment of "global" brain blood flow. Larger babies can only be investigated with the emitting and receiving fibers in an angular arrangement (*reflection mode*), usually with both optodes on the same side of the head. In this situation a smaller volume of brain tissue between the optodes is investigated. This may be chosen on purpose, also in smaller babies, to obtain "regional" results. With a shorter interoptode distance, blood flow in a narrow and shallow tissue volume is investigated with a relatively larger fraction of extracerebral tissues. Therefore, interoptode distances of less than 3 cm are not recommended.

Algorithms and Wavelength

Several different types of NIR spectroscopy instruments have been used. The number of wavelengths used has also varied from two to six. With the use of different wavelengths, the mathematical algorithms used to separate the signals of oxyhemoglobin (O_2Hb), deoxyhemoglobin (HHb), and the cytochrome aa3 oxidase difference signal (Cyt.ox), have differed (13). This may have had an impact of our ability to appropriately analyze the differences in the findings among the different papers, particularly among those published earlier, as some of the differences may have been due to differences in the NIR spectroscopy methodology applied.

Pathlength

The pathlength of light traversing the tissue must be known to calculate concentrations, i.e. to measure quantitatively. The pathlength in tissue exceeds the geometrical distance between the optodes by a factor of 3 to 6 and this factor is named the differential pathlength factor (DPF). Correct estimation of pathlength is one of the basic problems in NIR spectroscopy as it varies up to 20% among infants. Although instruments exist which allow direct measurement of pathlength, these are not commonly used.

Quantification of Cerebral Blood Flow

Measurement of blood flow by NIR spectroscopy is based on Fick's principle (14) and utilizes a rapid change in arterial oxyhemoglobin used as the intravascular tracer. By using the change in the oxygenation index (OI) observed after a small sudden change in the arterial concentration of oxygen, CBF (in mL/100 g/min) can be calculated as $CBF = \Delta OI/(k \times \int Sa,o_2 \times dt)$, where OI is measured in units of μmol/L, and

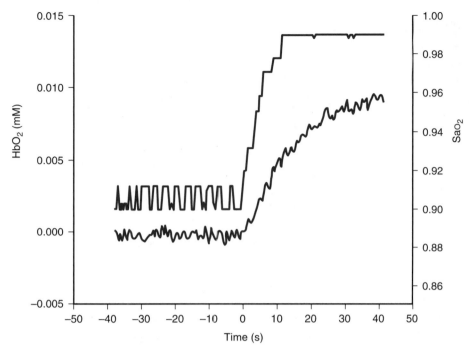

FIGURE 4-2 Measurement of CBF by NIR spectroscopy in a newborn infant. Arterial saturation (as monitored by a pulse oximeter) is stable at 90 to 91% until F_{I,O_2} is increased. Within a few seconds the arterial saturation rises to 95% and above. The rise in cerebral concentration of oxyhemoglobin is slower due to the time it takes for the more highly oxygenated arterial blood to fill the vascular bed of the brain. By restricting the analysis to the first 6 to 8 s as it is assumed that the venous saturation is still unchanged, a simplified version of the Fick's principle can be used. NIR spectroscopy using an intravascular tracer and measuring over a few seconds gives results of "global" cerebral blood flow similar to the result obtained with the use of ^{133}Xe clearance. Xenon is a diffusible tracer equilibrating between blood and tissue. Wash-out is much slower and measurements are made over 8 to 15 min.

$k = \text{Hgb} \times 1.05 \times 100$. Hgb is blood hemoglobin in mmol/L (tetraheme), Sa_{O_2} is given in %, and t is time, in min (Fig. 4-2).

Assumptions

The method of measuring CBF rests on several assumptions. First, during measurement CBF, cerebral blood volume (CBV), and oxygen extraction are assumed to be constant. Second, the period of measurement must be less than the cerebral transit time (approximately 10 s). Finally, this method of CBF measurement also has significant practical limitations For instance, in infants with severe lung disease, Sa_{O_2} may be fixed at a low level despite administration of oxygen, whereas in infants with normal lungs, Sa_{O_2} is near 100% in room air. Although this problem could be overcome by using air–nitrogen mixtures and then switching to room air, results of such experiments have not been reported. In addition, there are significant ethical considerations when using a hypoxic gas mixture in healthy newborns even if for only a brief period of time.

Reproducibility and Validation

Measurements of blood flow with NIR spectroscopy have a reported reproducibility of 17 to 24% and have been validated against ^{133}Xe clearance in sick newborns. These comparisons constitute important direct external validation of NIR spectroscopy in the brain of human neonates. The agreement between the two methods was found to be acceptable (15,16).

Indocyanine Green as an Alternative Tracer

A dye, indocyanine green, given by intravenous injection, has been used in place of oxygen utilizing a special fiber-optic instrument to measure intra-arterial indocyanine green concentration (17). The results were similar but the reproducibility of this technique was better (15%) than that of conventional NIR spectroscopy. Recently, an improvement of this method has also been proposed, using a convolution algorithm to account for venous outflow and a non-invasive pulse dye-densitometer for measurement of arterial indocyanine green concentration. Although the findings are encouraging in piglets (18), this newest method has not yet been applied in human infants. Similarly to the conventional NIR spectroscopy methodology, where the sensitivity of the pulse oximeter presents one of the technical problems, the pulse dye-densitometer is the major technical limitation of the NIR spectroscopy method using indocyanine green as the tracer molecule.

Trend Monitoring of Hemoglobin Signals

In principle, NIR spectroscopy allows on-line trending of changes in O_2Hb and HHb, and hence those of total hemoglobin (tHb). Total hemoglobin, the sum of $[O_2Hb]$ and $[HHb]$, is proportional to changes in cerebral blood volume (CBV), which in turn can be used as a surrogate measure of CBF. The appropriateness of this assumption, however, has only been established for reactions to changes in arterial CO_2 tension (19). Furthermore, constant optode distance is crucial in trend monitoring and if the head circumference changes even by a fraction of a millimeter as a result of change in CBV or brain water content, the trends are significantly biased. In addition, minor changes in the optode–skin contact induce large transients in the signal and/or baseline shifts. Despite these limitations, several investigators have successfully accomplished trend monitoring.

The Hemoglobin Difference, or Oxygenation Index

The difference between $[O_2Hb]$ and $[HHb]$ is called Hbdiff and, when divided by a factor of two, it is known as the oxygenation index (OI). The Hbdiff is an indicator of the mean oxygen saturation of the hemoglobin in all types of blood vessels in the tissue. This measure has been shown to change appropriately in many experimental models and clinical studies, but has important limitations. First, in terms of interpretation, it is not known how much of the signal originates from blood in the arteries, capillaries, or veins. Data in piglets suggest that the arterial-to-venous ratio is about 1:2 (20). The signal can also be seriously confounded by concomitant changes in tHb, as tHb affects the amount of blood distributed in the arterial, capillary or venous compartments. Finally, the lack of a fixed zero-point makes it impossible to specify a threshold for intervention or even an alarm level for clinical use.

Quantification of Hemoglobin-oxygen Saturation

Three different principles are being used in second-generation instruments to measure hemoglobin–oxygen saturation in absolute terms without manipulation of $Fi_{,O_2}$ or using another tracer like a dye. With spatially resolved spectroscopy, the detection of the transmitted light at two or more different distances from the light emitting optode allows monitoring of the ratio of absolute $[O_2Hb]$ to $[tHb]$, i.e. the hemoglobin saturation. The hemoglobin saturation measured by this method is called the tissue oxygenation index (TOI) (21). This measure is the weighted average of arterial, capillary, and venous blood oxygenation, and hence cannot easily be validated. The measurement depends on the tissue being optically homogeneous, which is unlikely to be the case. Nevertheless, TOI values near cerebrovenous values have been found, and appropriate changes in TOI have been documented with changes in arterial oxygen saturation and arterial $P\text{CO}_2$. As the signal-to-noise ratio is not as good as that of OI, TOI is less useful for quantifying the response to rapid therapeutic interventions. The other two principles are time-resolved spectroscopy, which detects the time-of-flight of very short light pulses (22), and phase shift spectroscopy, which detects the phase shift and phase modulation of a continuous frequency-modulated source of light (23). With the use of these two methods it is also possible to estimate the absolute concentrations of O_2Hb and HHb, and from these to calculate TOI.

Bias of the Tissue Oxygenation Index

TOI, similar to OI (see above), cannot be compared directly to any other measurement because it represents the findings in a mixture of blood in the arteries, capillaries, and veins. Interestingly, though, TOI has recently been validated on the head of young infants with heart disease during cardiac catheterization (24). In this study, across a TOI range of 40 to 80%, the mean value was almost identical to oxygen saturation in jugular venous blood as measured by co-oximetry. This suggests a significant negative bias as, in addition to venous blood, the TOI also represents arterial and capillary blood. In addition, TOI has not been compared to any other measures of venous saturation in preterm or term neonates, not even internal consistency of TOI with Sv,O_2 measured by NIRS during obstruction of venous outflow has been reported.

Precision of the Tissue Oxygenation Index

In the study in young infants with heart disease (24), while the mean difference was negligible, limits of agreement of individual measurements were as wide as −12 to +11%. Since co-oximetry is very precise, this variation represents an estimate of the error of TOI. Using the same commercial instrument in newborns and young infants, the limits of agreement after optode replacement were found to be −17 to +17% (25). In preterm or term neonates, the variation associated with replacement of the optodes could fully account for this poor precision (26). Therefore, it is conceivable that the main reason for the significant variability of TOI lies in the small anatomical differences between the different positions of the optodes causing the assumption of scatter isotropy to fail. For comparison, arterial hemoglobin oxygen saturation can be measured by pulseoximetry with limits of agreement of ±6%.

Importance of the Low Precision of the Tissue Oxygenation Index

TOI is a surrogate measure of cerebrovenous saturation. This important physiological variable is tightly regulated with the normal values being between 60 and 70%. During hypoxemia, or cerebral ischemia, when CBF decreases without a change in cerebral oxygen consumption, cerebrovenous saturation falls. Hence, cerebrovenous saturation is a useful measure of the sufficiency of cerebral perfusion. However, the major technical problem is that for instance a 30% decrease in the CBF will only lead to a drop from 70 to 60% in the cerebrovenous oxygen saturation, which is well within the limits of the error of measurement.

MAGNETIC RESONANCE IMAGING

Although magnetic resonance imaging (MRI) is discussed in detail in Section II, Chapter 7 the present chapter reviews the basics of methodology. The nucleus hydrogen is stable but magnetically asymmetric and hence behaves like a magnetic dipole. Subjected to a strong magnetic field (0.2 to 3 T), it will tend to align with the field (longitudinal magnetization), in the sense that it rotates around the direction of the magnetic field. This rotation (called precession, like a spinning top) occurs at a frequency proportional to the strength of the magnetic field. Exposed to a pulse of electromagnetic energy of proportional frequency at a 90° angle of the field, the rotation may be synchronized resulting in transverse magnetization and a decrease in the longitudinal magnetization. After the pulse, the synchrony continues and re-emits electromagnetic energy for some time. Imaging depends on the gradients in the magnetic field, which makes a particular frequency specific to a specific plane. By the use of gradients in the X, Y, and Z plane, a three-dimensional reconstruction is possible. Image contrast comes from the fact that tissues differ according to the chemical and physical constitution of their hydrogen nuclei.

Measurement of Blood Flow

Blood flow is essentially moving water, i.e. moving hydrogen nuclei, which tend to cause loss of signal. In the simplest way, global CBF may be estimated by imaging the four arteries on the neck and multiplying their cross-sectional area with the blood flow velocity, estimated by the loss of magnetization caused by fresh blood (water) flowing into the plane of imaging. This procedure, however, is more complex than the use of ultrasound with and is likely to be less precise.

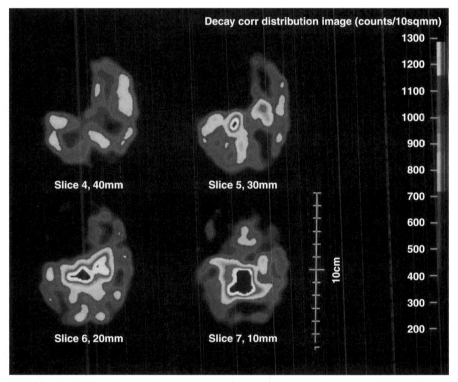

FIGURE 4-3 Flow images in a near-term newborn infant with a large right frontal subdural hematoma. The four slices are axial at 10, 20, 30, and 40 mm above the orbito-meatal line. The images show no measurable flow to the entire right frontal lobe. Furthermore, flow is high in the central parts of the brain and also appears to be higher in cortex compared to the white matter. However, the latter is not well illustrated due to limited spatial resolution (nominally 8 mm FWHM for this image). The image was made by HMPAO, a "chemical microsphere" labeled with ^{99m}Tc given intravenously. The HMPAO fixes in tissue during the first pass. The image really is just the distribution of the tracer, i.e. of bolus distribution. To translate such an image to flow, in addition to linearization, an estimate of arterial input is required. The latter is very difficult to achieve for HMPAO, but it is easier for some other tracers.

17. Patel J, Marks K, Roberts I, et al. Measurement of cerebral blood flow in newborn infants using near infrared spectroscopy with indocyanine green. Pediatr Res 1998;43:34–39.

18. Brown DW, Picot PA, Naeini JG, Springett R, Delpy DT, Lee TY. Quantitative near infrared spectroscopy measurement of cerebral hemodynamics in newborn piglets. Pediatr Res 2002;51:564–570.

19. Pryds O, Greisen G, Skov L, Friis-Hansen B. The effect of PaCO2 induced increase in cerebral blood volume and cerebral blood flow in mechanically ventilated, preterm infants. Comparison of near infra-red spectrophotometry and 133Xenon clearance. Pediatr Res 1990;27:445–449.

20. Brun NC, Moen A, Borch K, Saugstad OD, Greisen G. Near-infrared monitoring of cerebral tissue oxygen saturation and blood volume in newborn piglets. Am J Physiol 1997;273:H682–H686.

21. Suzuki S, Takasaki S, Ozaki T, Kobayashi Y. A tissue oxygenation monitor using NIR spatially resolved spectroscopy. SPIE 1999;3597:582–592.

22. Ijichi S, Kusaka T, Isobe K, Kawada K, Imai T. Quantification of cerebral hemoglobin as a function of oxygenation using near-infrared time-resolved spectroscopy in a piglet model of hypoxia. J Biomed Optics 2005;10:024–026.

23. Zhao J, Ding HS, Hou XL, Zhou CL, Chance B. In vivo determination of the optical properties of infant brain using frequency-domain near-infrared spectroscopy. J Biomed Opt 2005;10:024–028.

24. Nagdyman N, Fleck T, Schubert S, Ewert P, Peters B, Lange PE, Abdul-Khaliq H. Comparison between cerebral tissue oxygenation index measured by near-infrared spectroscopy and venous jugular bulb saturation in children. Intensive Care Med 2005;31:846–850.

25. Dullenkopf A, Kolarova A, Schulz G, Frey B, Baenziger O, Weiss M. Reproducibility of cerebral oxygenation measurement in neonates and infants in the clinical setting using the NIRO 300 oximeter. Pediatr Crit Care Med 2005;6:344–347.

26. Sorensen LC, Greisen G. Precision of measurement of cerebral tissue oxygenation index using near infrared spectroscopy in term and preterm infants. J Biomed Op 2006;11:05400.

27. Tanner SF, Cornette L, Ramenghi LA, Miall LS, Ridgway JP, Smith MA, Levene MI. Cerebral perfusion in infants and neonates: preliminary results obtained using dynamic susceptibility contrast enhanced magnetic resonance imaging. Arch Dis Child 2003;88:525–530.

28. Wang J, Licht DJ, Jahng GH, et al. Pediatric perfusion imaging using arterial spin labelling. J Magn Res Imag 2003;18:404–413.

29. Licht DJ, Wang J, Silvestre DW, et al. Preoperative cerebral blood flow is diminished in neonates with severe congenital heart defects. J Thorac Cardiovasc Surg 2004;128:841–849.

30. Sharples PM, Stuart AG, Aynsley-Green A, et al. A practical method of serial bedside measurement of cerebral blood flow and metabolism during neurointensive care. Arch Dis Child 1991;66:1326–1332.

31. Garfunkel JM, Baird HW, Siegler J. The relationship of oxygen consumption to cerebral functional activity. J Pediatr 1954;44:64–72.

32. Frewen TC, Kissoon N, Kronick J, Fox M, Lee R, Bradwin N, Chance G. Cerebral blood flow, cross-brain oxygen extraction, and fontanelle pressure after hypoxic–ischemic injury in newborn infants. J Pediatr 1991;118:265–271.

33. Greisen G, Pryds. Intravenous 133Xe clearance in preterm neonates with respiratory distress. Internal validation of CBF-infinity as a measure of global cerebral blood flow. Scand J Clin Lab Invest 1988;48:673–678.

34. Greisen G, Trojaborg W. Cerebral blood flow, PaCO2 changes, and visual evoked potentials in mechanically ventilated, preterm infants. Acta Paediatr Scand 1987;76:394–400.

35. Rubinstein M, Denays R, Ham HR, et al. Functional imaging of brain maturation in humans using iodine 123I-iodoamphetamine and SPECT. J Nucl Med 1989;30:1982–1985.

36. Denays R, Ham H, Tondear M, Piepsz A, Noël P. Detection of bilateral and symmetrical anomalies in technecium-99 HMPAO brain SPECT studies. J Nucl Med 1992;33:485–490.

37. Chiron C, Raynaud C, Maziere B, et al. Changes in regional cerebral blood flow during brain maturation in children and adolescents. J Nucl Med 1992;33:696–703.

38. Ashwal S, Schneider S, Thompson J. Xenon computed tomography measuring blood flow in the determination of brain death in children. Ann Neurol 1989;25:539–546.

39. Volpe JJ, Herscovitch P, Perlman JM, Raichle ME. Positron emission tomography in the newborn. Extensive impairment of regional cerebral blood flow with intraventricular hemorrhage and hemorrhagic cerebral involvement. Pediatrics 1983;72:589–601.

40. Powers WJ, Raichle ME. Positron emission tomography and its application to the study of cerebrovascular disease in man. Stroke 1985;16:361–376.

41. Chugani HT, Phelps ME, Mazziotta JC. Positron emission tomography study of human brain functional development. Ann Neurol 1987;22:487–497.

42. Altman DI, Perlman JM, Volpe JJ, et al. Cerebral oxygen metabolism in newborns. Pediatrics 1993;92:99–104.

43. Cross KW, Dear PRF, Hathorn MKS, et al. An estimation of intracranial blood flow in the newborn infant. J Physiol 1979;289:329–345.

44. Colditz P, Greisen G, Pryds O. Comparison of electrical impedance and 133Xe clearance for the assesment of cerebral blood flow in the newborn infant. Pediatr Res 1988;24:461–464.

45. Zaramella P, Freato F, Quaresima V, et al. Foot pulse oximeter perfusion index correlates with calf muscle perfusion measured by near-infrared spectroscopy in healthy neonates. J Perinatol 2005;25:417–422.

Chapter 5

Functional Echocardiography in the Neonatal Intensive Care Unit

Nicholas J. Evans, DM, MRCPCH

One major limitation in the intensive care of the newborn infant is the lack of tools with which to monitor cardiovascular and hemodynamic function. In most NICUs, there is the ability to continuously monitor invasive blood pressure and heart rate and that is all. Beyond that, heavy reliance is often placed on unvalidated and probably rather crude measures of hemodynamic wellbeing such as acid-base status, skin capillary refill time, and urine output. In the intensive care of the older subject, there is a range of tools for monitoring cardiac output such as thermodilution, continuous Doppler methodologies, and derivations from blood pressure waveforms (1). None of these are available for the neonate, partly because of the need to miniaturize, partly because of commercial conceptions of the NICU as a limited market, and partly because of the complexities of the transitional circulation.

Doppler echocardiography provides a non-invasive technique from which it is possible to derive estimates of a wide range of hemodynamic parameters. Traditionally, it has been specialists who work predominantly outside the NICU (mainly cardiologists) who have had the skills to derive these measures. This resulted in a predominantly snapshot picture of neonatal hemodynamics. Increasingly, neonatal intensivists are developing echocardiographic skills themselves (2). The fact that they are in the NICU all the time has allowed more systematic serial studies, which, in turn, is allowing the research and clinical monitoring potential of these methodologies to develop further. This chapter will describe the functional Doppler echocardiographic measures that can be used in the assessment of the sick newborn infant and how they can be used in common clinical scenarios. Other chapters in this book will provide more details on findings using some of these methods and how the information derived might be used to guide clinical management.

DOPPLER ULTRASOUND

In the simplest terms, ultrasounds reflect off solid or liquid interfaces of different densities to allow definition of structure. In the heart, this is the interface between muscle, fiber, and blood. Projection of these structures against time allows definition of movement, both of the structures themselves but also relative to other structures. This is the essence of M-mode and two-dimensional (2-D) imaging.

The Doppler principle can be applied to ultrasounds because they change frequency as they reflect off moving objects. The direction of change in frequency depends on the direction of movement of the object. Movement toward the transmission source increases frequency while movement away decreases the frequency. This frequency shift is directly proportional to the velocity of the moving object as long as the direction of movement is within $20°$ of straight toward or straight away from the transmission source. This difference between the direction of the ultrasound beam and the reflecting object is called the "angle of insonation." So when this is applied to blood moving in the heart and blood vessels, the various types of Doppler allow determination of two factors: direction and velocity of blood flow.

Accurate determination of velocity allows two further factors to be derived. Firstly, the pressure gradient can be determined via the modified Bernoulli equation. This describes the relationship between pressure gradient and velocity in a fluid stream (pressure gradient $= 4 \times \text{velocity}^2$). Secondly, because flow of a fluid in streamline is the product of mean velocity and cross-sectional area of the stream, if we can estimate the diameter of a blood vessel and measure the mean velocity of the blood, we can estimate blood flow. In the neonate, these flow measures can really only be made in major vessels, as smaller peripheral vessels are too small to measure accurately.

TWO-DIMENSIONAL IMAGING AND NORMAL CARDIAC STRUCTURE

The prerequisite to developing skills in functional echocardiography is a good understanding of cardiac anatomy and the ability to obtain and understand 2-D images from each of the four main ultrasound windows. A common starting point for people wanting to learn echocardiography has been to look over the shoulder of an experienced operator. Many an ultrasound ambition has fallen fallow in this wasteland of a learning approach. You will never learn this way; your understanding will always be one step behind the operator. As ultrasound is essentially a process of converting a 3-D structure into a series of 2-D cuts, if you understand the anatomy in spatial terms, the 2-D images will explain themselves. If you do not understand the anatomy, the 2-D images will remain a mystery. The heart is more difficult to conceptualize in 3-D space than other organs because it is not symmetrical but with application this understanding is possible.

It is beyond the scope of this chapter to describe normal 2-D imaging in detail and other resources for this are available to the reader (3,4). However, to illustrate the points made above, the reader is taken through one view that is particularly useful for hemodynamic assessment: the low parasternal long axis view of the pulmonary artery. Figure 5-1 has four images, which represent the chambers of

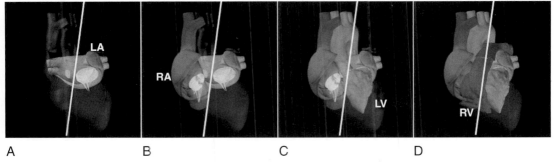

A   B   C   D

FIGURE 5-1 These four frames show the chambers of the heart being progressively added from back to front. The white line shows where the ultrasound beam will transect the heart. (A) The left atrium (LA) at the back of heart with two pulmonary veins coming in each side posteriorly. (B) The right atrium (RA), which is to the right and slightly in front of the LA. (C) The endocardial surface of the left ventricle (LV), which receives blood towards the apex through the mitral valve and ejects it into the ascending aorta, which runs towards the right shoulder in front of the LA. (D) The anterior nature of the right ventricle, which wraps in front of the LV outflow tract before ejecting blood posteriorly into the pulmonary artery. (See color plate.)

the heart being progressively built up from back to front, a fuller explanation of the spatial anatomical relationships is described in the legend to the figure. On each image, the white line represents where the ultrasound beam will cut in the image that is being described. By examining how the line transects each of the structures, you should be able to build up in your own mind how the image will look. This is shown (with more detailed explanation in the legend) for both the heart model and an ultrasound image in Fig. 5-2. The pulmonary artery is particularly good for Doppler studies because its posterior direction takes the blood directly away from the transducer at a minimal angle of insonation. A basic understanding of 2-D imaging can be derived from learning three to four images like this for each of the four ultrasound windows, subcostal, apical, and low and high parasternal.

M-mode ultrasound was the precursor to 2-D imaging and is where ultrasounds down one transmission line are plotted against time (Fig. 5-3). It remains a useful modality for assessing movement of structures and for more accurate measurement of dimensions at defined time points in the cardiac cycle.

TYPES OF DOPPLER

There are three main types of Doppler in common usage: pulsed wave, continuous wave, and color Doppler. Pulsed wave Doppler is most commonly used because it

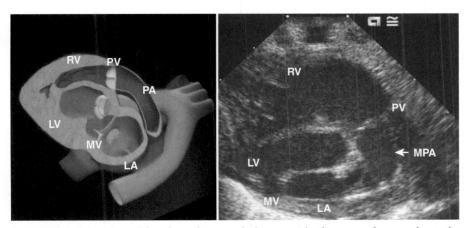

FIGURE 5-2 A heart model and an ultrasound picture cut in the same plane as shown in Fig. 5-1. The RV is seen at the front connecting with the posteriorly directed pulmonary artery. Behind the RV is the LV outflow tract and the LA and mitral valve. (See color plate.)

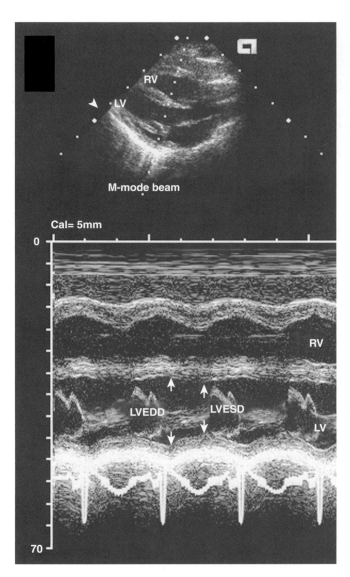

FIGURE 5-3 M-mode plots the ultra-sound signals from the single beam (shown on a 2-D image) against time. This allows movement and dimensions to be more accurately measured. The LV end diastolic diameter (LVEDD) and LV end systolic diameter (LVESD) are shown. (See color plate.)

allows you to focus your velocity assessment at a particular site through an operator guided "range gate" (Fig. 5-4). The limitation of pulsed wave is that it cannot assess velocities over about 2 m/s. Continuous wave Doppler allows assessment of higher velocities but is less focused, receiving signals from the whole line of transmission. Typically both pulsed and continuous wave Doppler are displayed as a velocity time plot, with flow towards the transducer shown as a positive plot and away as a negative plot, Fig. 5-4.

Color Doppler is a development of pulsed wave Doppler where the frequency shift is mapped onto the 2-D image, with flow towards and away from the transducer plotted as different colors. Conventionally, flow away is mapped as blue and towards is mapped as red. Color Doppler has a range of uses but is particularly useful in functional echocardiography to guide pulsed Doppler study and to assess patency of the ductus arteriosus (Fig. 5-4).

WHAT CAN BE MEASURED WITH FUNCTIONAL ECHOCARDIOGRAPHY IN THE NICU?

There is a range of parameters that can be assessed using functional echocardiography, including ductal and atrial shunting (presence, direction, and degree),

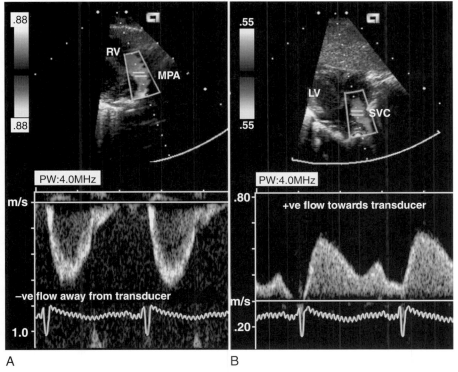

FIGURE 5-4 Pulsed Doppler assesses flow velocity at a defined location (= sign on 2-D image). Flow away from the transducer is negative (A) and towards the transducer positive (B). Color Doppler maps those signals onto the 2-D image with flow away coded blue (A) and towards coded red (B). (See color plate.)

pulmonary artery pressure, flow measures (right and left ventricular output and superior vena cava flow), and myocardial function measures. One factor to emphasize is the close interrelationship of many of these measures. It is a basic rule of fluid mechanics that measurement at a single point in a stream line can be influenced by factors both upstream and downstream of that point. So it is in the heart where, if you take a single measurement, you will often not be able to interpret that measure unless you know what is happening both upstream and downstream from that measure. A commonly encountered example of this in neonatology is a left to right ductal shunt, which will increase the volume load (preload) on the left ventricle and reduce the afterload. So measures of left ventricular input and output in the presence of a significant ductal shunt will be high and measures of function very good, but neither will give you any information about the wellbeing of the systemic circulation. For this reason, studies, whether for research or clinical reasons, need to be as complete as possible.

It also needs to be emphasized that, in common with all non-invasive measures, there are limitations to the accuracy of Doppler ultrasound measurements. Most will have intra-observer variability of about 10% and inter-observer variability of about 20%. The findings need to be interpreted with these limitations to accuracy in mind. These limitations will be minimized if you use more than one method to measure a parameter as a cross-check, take averages from repeated measures, and curtail the number of different observers taking a measurement in the same baby.

We now start by discussing the factors that define the complexity of the transitional circulation relative to the mature circulation, the shunts through the fetal channels, and the potential lability of pulmonary vascular resistance and hence pulmonary arterial pressure.

DUCTAL SHUNTING

Many neonatologists have a conception of the ductus arteriosus as a dichotomous variable, i.e. it is either open or closed. Nothing could be further from the truth and, when looking at the duct with ultrasound, we are struck by the variability of the ductus both in size or degree of constriction and the direction of shunting. The duct can be directly imaged with 2-D ultrasound. Anatomically, it is a continuation of the main pulmonary artery that is slightly offset to the left reflecting the arch it describes into the descending aorta (Fig. 5-5). Thus, with the ultrasound transducer placed at the left upper sternal edge and the beam in a true sagittal plane (straight up and down the body), the duct can be seen leaving the main pulmonary artery close to the junction with the left pulmonary artery and describing an arch into the descending aorta. Patent ducts that are minimally constricted are readily apparent on 2-D imaging (Fig. 5-6), but differentiating a functionally closed from a constricted duct needs color Doppler. Figure 5-7A shows the predominantly blue color Doppler of flow in the main and left pulmonary artery with no flow apparent through the duct. Two-dimensional imaging with color Doppler allows assessment not only of ductal patency but also the degree of ductal constriction. The contrast between the well-constricted duct in Fig. 5-7B and the unconstricted one in Fig. 5-7C is readily apparent. With a well-optimized color Doppler study, it is possible to derive a semi-quantitative assessment of the degree of constriction by measuring the minimum diameter of the shunt within the course of the ductus (5). Color Doppler also allows some assessment of the direction of shunting but accurate assessment of direction of shunting requires pulsed Doppler. The direction of blood flow through the duct is determined by the continuum of the relative pressure at each end. When pulmonary pressures are clearly below systemic the shunt will be left to right (Fig. 5-8A), when they are well above systemic pressures, the shunt will be right to left (Fig. 5-8C). When pulmonary pressures are close to but are not clearly above or below systemic pressures throughout the cardiac cycle, varying degrees of bidirectional shunt are seen (Fig. 5-8B and 5-8C). This range

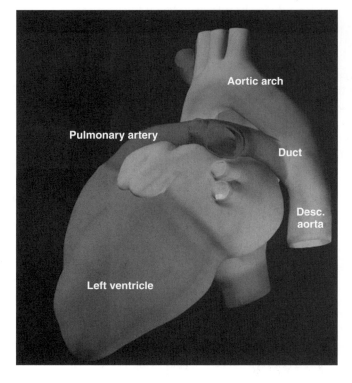

FIGURE 5-5 A model of the heart viewed from the left-hand side. It can be seen that the ductus arteriosus is a continuation of the pulmonary artery and describes an arch into the descending aorta. It is slightly offset to the left reflecting the need to connect with the left-sided descending aorta. (See color plate.)

FIGURE 5-6 A 2-D image of a patent duct adjacent to the root of the left pulmonary artery, which is seen this section as a diverticulum inferior to the duct. The duct describes an arch that is in continuity with the anterior wall of the main pulmonary artery. (See color plate.)

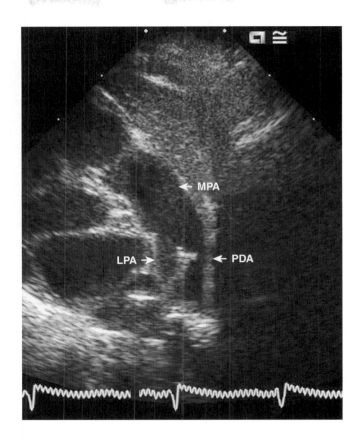

of shunt pattern allows assessment of pulmonary artery pressure in a way that will be described in more detail below.

Echocardiographic determination of patency and shunt direction is relatively straightforward; more controversial are the criteria that should be applied to determine hemodynamic significance. In cardiology, the size of a left to right shunt is often expressed as the ratio of pulmonary to systemic blood flow (Qp:Qs); this, in turn, can be derived by measuring both ventricular outputs with Doppler. With a ductal shunt, the left ventricular output measures the pulmonary blood flow and the right ventricular output, the systemic blood flow. Unfortunately, you cannot use this routinely in the transitional circulation because of the atrial shunts, discussed below, which confound right ventricular output as a measure of systemic blood flow (6). We were able to measure Qp:Qs in a cohort of preterm babies with a PDA in whom there was minimal atrial shunting and compare it to a variety of suggested criteria of ductus arteriosus hemodynamic significance (7). The criteria that had the closest correlation with Qp:Qs was the diameter as measured from the color Doppler as shown in Fig. 5-7. In babies <1500 g during the postnatal week, if the ductal diameter was <1.5 mm, the shunt was usually insignificant and, if >1.5 mm, the shunt was usually significant. If the diameter was over 2 mm, the Qp:Qs was usually more than 2:1 (i.e. twice as much pulmonary blood flow as systemic). The other measure that was useful was the pattern of diastolic flow in the postductal descending aorta. Normally this flow is forwards but, in the presence of an increasing shunt back through a duct, this flow direction becomes progressively absent and then retrograde (Fig. 5-9). In the above-cited studies (7), retrograde diastolic flow was associated with a mean Qp:Qs of 1.6 (i.e. pulmonary blood flow is 60% more than systemic). The same phenomenon that reduces diastolic flow in the postductal aorta also increases diastolic flow in the branch pulmonary arteries. So increased diastolic velocities in the left pulmonary artery has been described as a

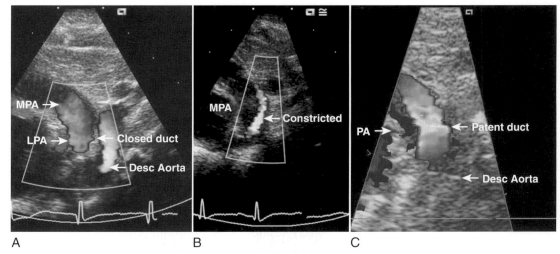

FIGURE 5-7 Three-color Doppler images of the ductal ultrasound cut. (A) Shows a closed duct with the blue streams of the pulmonary artery and descending aorta. The absence of color in the line of the duct shows that it is functionally closed. (B) Shows the red stream of a left to right shunt through a constricted duct, streaming back up the anterior wall of the pulmonary artery. (C) Shows a left to right shunt though an unconstricted duct. (See color plate.)

marker of significance (8). This measure does have the advantage of being technically easier than Doppler in the postductal aorta, just requiring a small adjustment of the Doppler range gate from the ductus into the left pulmonary artery (Fig. 5-10). In clinical practice, we use a combination of the diameter of the duct and the direction of diastolic flow in the descending aorta.

In healthy term babies, the ductus constricts quickly after birth but some shunting is commonly apparent on color Doppler during the first 12 to 24 h (9,10). In term

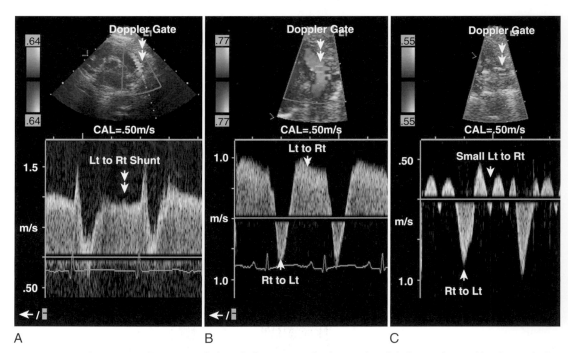

FIGURE 5-8 The range of pattern of ductal shunt on pulsed Doppler. (A) Shows the positive (towards the transducer) trace of a pure left to right shunt. (B) Shows a bidirectional shunt with both left to right (positive) and right to left (negative) components. (C) Shows a predominantly right to left (negative) shunt but with some left to right shunt in diastole. Pure right to left ductal shunts are uncommon. (See color plate.)

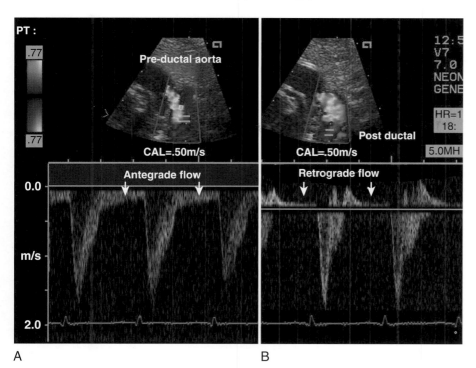

FIGURE 5-9 Compares the normal forward diastolic flow (A), which is also seen with a patent ductus arteriosus (PDA) in the pre-ductal aorta with the retrograde diastolic flow seen in the post ductal aorta in the presence of a significant PDA. (See color plate.)

babies with high oxygen requirements, the ductus also usually constricts quickly, particularly when the problem is primarily in the pulmonary parenchyma. A minority of such babies will have a patent ductus after postnatal day 1 (11). In term babies with primary persistent pulmonary hypertension of the newborn (PPHN), the ductus is more likely to remain patent but is still often well constricted (11).

In the preterm population, the constriction of the ductus in the early hours after birth varies widely from those where the constriction would be equivalent to a term baby to those where there is no constriction (12,13). Contrary to popular belief, even at this early time, the dominant direction of shunting is left to right. In those babies where constriction fails, large systemic to pulmonary shunts can result. So the hemodynamic impact of a ductal shunt in reducing systemic blood flow and increasing pulmonary blood flow can be present from very early after birth (13). These shunts are invariably clinically silent in the first two days, so will only be detected if looked for echocardiographically (14,15). The degree of early ductal constriction also predicts persisting patency, so early echocardiography may offer a way of targeting early treatment of the duct (5,12,13,16).

ATRIAL SHUNTING

The foramen ovale is commonly considered as a site for right to left shunting but not for the much more common phenomenon of left to right shunting through an incompetent foramen ovale (Fig. 5-11) (6,7). The atrial septum is best imaged from the subcostal four chamber view. From this window, it can be imaged in its full length with the foramen ovale easily distinguishable as the loose foraminal flap tissue moves both ways during the cardiac cycle. Some assessment of the relative pressures in the two atria can be derived from this movement but assessment of shunting needs color Doppler. The color Doppler needs to be optimized for the usual low velocity of inter-atrial shunts and, when placed over the foramen ovale,

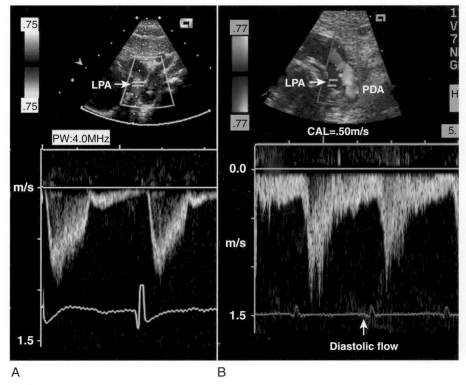

FIGURE 5-10 Compares the diastolic velocity seen in the left pulmonary artery with a closed duct with the increased diastolic velocity (in this case 0.5 m/s) seen with a significant PDA. (See color plate.)

the stream of any shunt should be apparent (Fig. 5-11). Some assessment of the degree of atrial shunting can be derived from the size of the color stream and the ease with which it is imaged (6,7). Like in the ductus, color Doppler gives a good impression of shunt direction but accurate assessment requires pulsed Doppler. The shunt patterns between the atria are complex reflecting a complex pressure relationship. Some shunting through the foramen ovale is commonly apparent even in normal healthy babies and although the dominant direction of shunting is left to right, it is very common to detect a short right to left component in diastole (Fig. 5-12). Thus some degree of bidirectional shunting is a normal finding in the newborn. Indeed, Hiraishi et al. (17) demonstrated that right to left atrial shunting for up to 30% of the cardiac cycle was normal in the neonate. As right heart pressures rise, the duration of right to left shunting within the cardiac cycle will increase. A pure right to left atrial shunt is surprisingly uncommon in babies with pulmonary hypertension although you do see it in extreme cases. A pure right to left atrial shunt should always raise the possibility of congenital heart disease such as total anomalous pulmonary venous drainage.

In the term baby, left to right atrial shunting is usually trivial and transient but, in the preterm baby, it can be both significant and quite persistent (6). The foramen ovale becomes smaller relative to the rest of the heart during the last trimester, so some of this may relate to structural immaturity. However, it is also related to ductal shunting, which will volume load the left atrium increasing the pressure and driving the left to right atrial shunt. It is not uncommon in babies with quite significant ductal shunts to find there is even more blood moving left to right at the atrial level than at the ductal level, and thus both shunts will contribute to a high pulmonary blood flow (6,7).

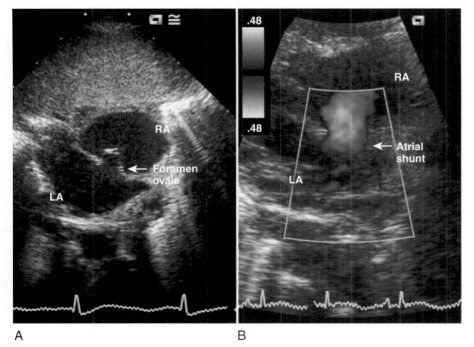

FIGURE 5-11 (A) The 2-D appearance of the atrial septum and foramen ovale in the subcostal four chamber view. (B) The color Doppler of a left to right shunt through an incompetent foramen ovale. (See color plate.)

Ductal and atrial shunts may not necessarily be in the same direction. This reflects the fact that atrial shunting is determined predominantly by filling (or diastolic pressures) while ductal shunting is determined by pressure throughout the cardiac cycle. Thus, it is not uncommon to have a predominantly right to left but bidirectional ductal shunt together with a predominantly left to right atrial shunt.

PULMONARY ARTERY PRESSURE

There are three main methods for estimating pulmonary artery pressure, each of which has strengths and weaknesses. The best methods, because they give you a number, involve application of the modified Bernoulli equation to a ductal shunt or a tricuspid incompetence jet.

Pulmonary Artery Pressure from a Ductal Shunt

The modified Bernoulli equation states that the pressure gradient down which a fluid stream is traveling will be $4 \times \text{velocity}^2$. Thus, if we know the pressure in the systemic circulation and we know velocity of a ductal shunt, we can calculate the pressure gradient across the ductus and so derive the pulmonary artery pressure. For example, if a baby has a left to right ductal shunt with a maximum velocity of 2 m/s then the pulmonary artery pressure must be $4 \times 2^2 = 16$ mm Hg less than the systemic pressure. If the shunt were right to left at 2 m/s then the pulmonary artery pressure must be 16 mm Hg more than systemic pressure.

This is not so straightforward with the common bidirectional ductal shunt pattern that appears as pulmonary pressures start to rise. This bidirectional pattern results from the fact that the pressure wave at each end of the duct is not synchronous (Fig. 5-13). The pressure wave from the right heart arrives before that from

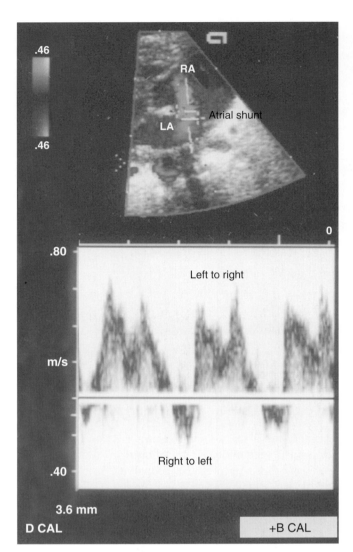

FIGURE 5-12 Pulsed Doppler of a normal bidirectional atrial shunt with a short period of right to left shunting followed by left to right shunting. (See color plate.)

the left. This means that you start to see some right to left shunting in early systole well before pulmonary pressures exceed systemic. It can be seen from Fig. 5-13 that, as pulmonary artery pressure rises relative to systemic, so the velocity and duration of right to left shunting will increase. Musewe et al. (18) estimated that, when the duration of right to left shunt was more than about 30% of the cardiac cycle, pulmonary artery pressure was usually supra-systemic. Less than 30% of the cardiac cycle suggests pulmonary artery pressure is less than systemic. So our approach with bidirectional shunting is to measure the duration of right to left shunting then, if it is more than 30%, use the right to left velocity to estimate the pulmonary artery pressure (PAP). On the other hand, if it is less than 30%, we use the left to right velocity. Apart from this complication, the ductal shunt is very useful for estimating PAP. The main limitation is obviously that the duct is often not patent, particularly in more mature babies.

Pulmonary Artery Pressure from Tricuspid Incompetence

Incompetence of the tricuspid valve in systole is common in the neonate during the transitional period. It is also more likely to be present with pulmonary hypertension, probably because of the tendency for a dilated right ventricle to dilate the tricuspid

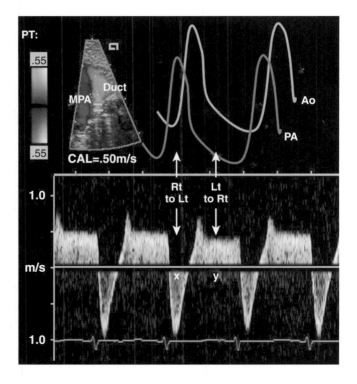

FIGURE 5-13 The two waveforms represent the simultaneous pressure wave at the pulmonary (blue) and aortic (red) end of the duct. The pressure wave at the pulmonary end rises before that at the aortic end. As pulmonary pressure rises (but remains sub-systemic) some right-to-left shunting occurs in early systole. As pulmonary pressure rises further so the duration of this right to left shunt (x) increases. When the duration of right to left shunt is more than about 30% of the cardiac cycle, pulmonary pressure is usually suprasystemic. (See color plate.)

valve ring. The velocity of this incompetent jet can be measured with Doppler and, again using the modified Bernoulli equation, the pressure gradient across the tricuspid valve between the right ventricle and right atrium can be assessed. Because we know that right atrial pressure is usually low (5 to 10 mm Hg), this gradient will approximate to the right ventricular systolic pressure. As long as the pulmonary valve is normal, right ventricular systolic pressure will be the same as pulmonary artery pressure. So if the maximum velocity of a tricuspid incompetence jet is 3 m/s, then the pressure gradient is $(4 \times 3^2 = 36$ mm Hg. Conventionally, 5 mm Hg is added to this gradient to reflect right atrial pressure. So the estimated systolic pulmonary artery pressure in this case would be 41 mm Hg (Fig. 5-14).

The accuracy of this method is dependent on minimizing the angle of insonation. Tricuspid incompetence jets can vary in direction, so this is an important potential source of error. When present, this is probably the most accurate of the indirect methods (19,20). However, the main limitation is that many babies in whom you want to measure pulmonary artery pressure will not have a tricuspid incompetence jet. It was present in only 50% of a cohort of term babies with high oxygen requirements that we studied. Further when pulmonary artery pressure drops, the tricuspid incompetence often disappears, so it is not a very good method for serially monitoring change in pulmonary artery pressure.

Pulmonary Artery Doppler Time to Peak Velocity

This method relies on the observation that as the pulmonary artery pressure rises so the time taken for systolic blood flow to reach its peak velocity in the main pulmonary artery will get shorter (21). This time to peak velocity can be measured and is usually expressed as a ratio to the total right ventricular ejection time. This method has important limitations to its accuracy and is vulnerable to a range of confounders such as right ventricular dysfunction or position of the Doppler range gate. It has also been shown to be of limited accuracy when PAP is raised due to left

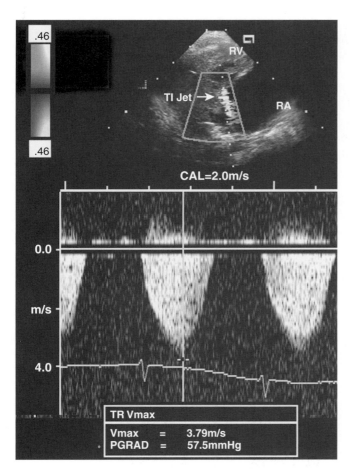

FIGURE 5-14 An example of tricuspid incompetence. The maximum velocity (Vmax) is 3.79 m/s. This means that the pressure gradient (PGRAD) across the valve is $4 \times 3.79^2 = 57.5$ mm Hg. Adding 5 mm Hg for right atrial pressure, this means that the RV systolic pressure is about 63 mm Hg; this will be the same as pulmonary artery systolic pressure. (See color plate.)

to right shunting (22). Pressure is the product of flow and resistance and may be raised if either or both are raised. Considering the physics of this phenomenon, it is probably more a measure of resistance or compliance of the pulmonary circulation. Hence it may be more accurate when pressure is high due to high resistance rather than high flow. It is probably best regarded as a "ballpark" measure when neither of the other two methods discussed above are available. Using this approximation approach, TPV:RVET ratios above 0.3 are normal, 0.2 to 0.3 suggest moderately raised pulmonary artery pressure and less than 0.2 suggests significantly raised pulmonary artery pressure (23,24).

MEASUREMENT OF BLOOD FLOW AND CARDIAC OUTPUT

Blood flow within a vessel is the product of the mean velocity of flow and the cross-sectional area of that vessel. With Doppler, it is possible to measure velocity assuming a minimal angle of insonation and, with the major vessels around the heart, it is possible to derive cross-sectional area, either directly or by estimating from a measured diameter. These two measures have different methodological requirements, in that velocity measurement requires the blood to be flowing at 0° or 180° to the direction of the ultrasound beam and the best measurement of edges with ultrasound is achieved when the ultrasound beam hits the vessel at 90°. These issues mean that there is a significant intrinsic error associated with these measurements. This is particularly true when cross-sectional area is derived from diameter where the conversion will magnify the error. Notwithstanding these problems, we do not have any better method for measuring blood flow in major vessels around the heart in neonatology. The most commonly used measures of blood flow in the heart have been the ventricular outputs, particularly left ventricular output.

Left Ventricular Output

Left ventricular (LV) output is derived by measuring blood flow in the ascending aorta. The ascending aorta leaves the heart heading in the direction of the right shoulder. This direction makes it a great vessel for measuring diameter but an awkward vessel for minimizing angle of insonation to measure velocity. Diameter is usually derived by imaging the ascending aorta in the long axis from the low parasternal window (Fig. 5-15). There is some argument in the literature about the best site for diameter measurement. We have always used in the end-systolic internal diameter just beyond the coronary sinus (Fig. 5-15). Others argue that the diameter of the aortic valve ring or of systolic leaflet separation is more accurate. Probably, where you measure is less important than measuring at a consistent site, in a consistent way and at a consistent time in the cardiac cycle. Cross-sectional area is derived from πr^2. Velocity is best measured from the apical or the suprasternal window but from either view it is difficult to minimize the angle of insonation. Our preference is the apical long axis view because it is better tolerated by the babies (25). The Doppler range gate is placed just beyond the aortic valve and the velocity time trace is recorded. Mean velocity is usually measured as the area under the systolic envelope called the velocity time integral (VTI) and we would usually average this from five cardiac cycles. Using these measures:

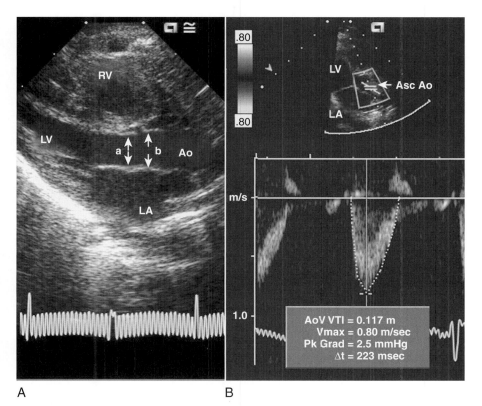

A   B

FIGURE 5-15 (A) Shows the site of measurement of aortic diameter. Some authors recommend measurement of valve ring or leaflet separation (a); we usually use the internal diameter beyond the coronary sinus (b). (B) Shows pulsed Doppler assessment of ascending aortic velocity from the apical long axis view. Velocity time integral (VTI) is derived by tracing around the systolic spectral envelope (VTI = 0.117 m in this case). (See color plate.)

$$\text{stroke volume} = \text{VTI} \times \text{cross-sectional area (mL)}$$

and

$$\text{cardiac output} = \text{stroke volume} \times \text{heart rate (mL/min)}$$

usually also divided by body weight to give mL/kg/min.

This method of measuring LV output has been validated against other more invasive methods (26,27). In general, the correlation against a range of "gold standards" is good although there is significant inter- and intra-observer variability. Intra-observer variability is estimated at about 10% and inter-observer at about 20%, so ideally serial studies should be made by the same person (28). The main problem with LV output as a measure of systemic blood flow in the neonate, particularly the premature neonate, is the extent to which it is confounded by a left to right ductal shunt. If you consider Fig. 5-16, you can see that, in the presence of a ductal shunt, LV output is the sum of systemic blood flow and the shunt across the duct and so it will overestimate systemic blood flow. In fact within this hemodynamic situation, LV output is actually measuring pulmonary blood flow and it is the right ventricular (RV) output that is measuring systemic blood flow. For this reason, RV output is a better measure of systemic blood flow than LV output.

Right Ventricular Output

This is derived by measuring blood flow in the main pulmonary artery. The main pulmonary artery (MPA) heads in a predominantly posterior direction before bifurcating into the two main branches. This direction makes the MPA a great vessel on which to perform Doppler from the low parasternal window with a minimal angle of insonation but not such a good vessel in which to derive diameter. The pulmonary artery is imaged in the long axis as described under the section on "Two-dimensional imaging and normal cardiac structure" earlier in this chapter. We measure diameter from the 2-D image at the insertion of the pulmonary valve leaflets, advancing frame by frame until end-systole, just before the valve closes (Fig. 5-17). The anterior wall is often the most difficult to get a clear view of and there is often a need to experiment with different transducer positions. Doppler is performed from the same window with the range gate just beyond the valve leaflets (Fig. 5-17). This minimizes any disturbance to the flow pattern from ductal shunting. The measures are then used to calculate RV output in the same way as

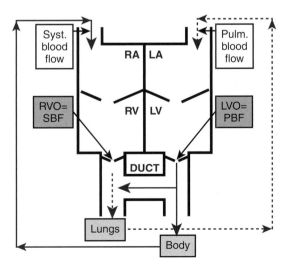

FIGURE 5-16 This schematic diagram of the heart highlights how, in the presence of a left to right ductal shunt, LV output (LVO) is measuring the sum of systemic blood flow and the ductal shunt. This is actually pulmonary blood flow and it is RV output (RVO) that is measuring systemic blood flow.

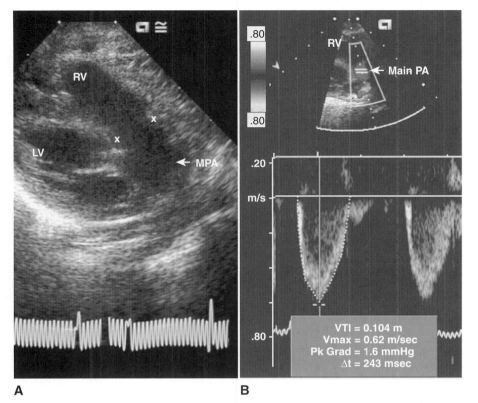

FIGURE 5-17 (A) Shows the site of measurement of pulmonary artery diameter, in end-systole at the valve hinge points. (B) Shows pulsed Doppler assessment of main pulmonary artery velocity with the range gate just beyond the valve. Velocity time integral (VTI) is derived by tracing around the systolic spectral envelope (VTI = 0.104 m in this case). (See color plate.)

described for the LV output. Normal values for both right and left ventricular output would be in the range of 150 to 300 mL/kg/min.

There has been no direct validation of RV output measured in this way. In a group of babies with no atrial or ductal shunting, we found a close correlation between RV output and the directly validated LV output (7). Just as LV output can be confounded by a left to right ductal shunt, RV output can be confounded by a left to right atrial shunt (6,7). While large ductal shunts can develop quite quickly after birth, atrial shunts often take longer to develop, so RV output is a reasonably accurate means of assessing systemic blood flow during the first 24 postnatal hours. However, this variable and unpredictable confounding of both ventricular outputs as measures of systemic blood flow limits their use for studying the natural history of systemic blood flow in babies. Because of this, we developed the concept of measuring cardiac input rather than output, specifically measuring flow returning to the heart via the superior vena cava (SVC).

SUPERIOR VENA CAVA FLOW

Any pump within a closed fluid circuit can only pump out what returns to it and will only return to it what it pumps out. So input to the pump has to be the same as the output, so it is with the heart. The SVC is a good vessel for Doppler as the angle of insonation on flow is small from the low subcostal window and good images for diameter can be obtained from the parasternal window. From a physiologic point of view, SVC flow is not confounded by shunts through the fetal channels and it represents the portion of systemic blood flow that we are most interested in, that from the upper body and brain (14,29). It is difficult to find firm data in the literature as to what proportion of upper body blood flow is cerebral blood flow (CBF), although estimates of 70 to 80% have been suggested for the neonate (30).

Doppler velocity in the SVC is measured from the subcostal window with the transducer as low as possible to minimize the angle of insonation (29). The range gate is placed in the mouth of the SVC just as it enters the right atrium. The velocity traces in the SVC can be quite pleomorphic particularly in babies that are breathing spontaneously and there is often some retrograde flow associated with atrial systole. So we would usually average from 10 cardiac cycles and would include any negative trace (Fig. 5-18). For diameter measurement, the SVC is imaged in the long axis from a low to mid-parasternal position and the SVC can be seen entering the right atrium, often deviating anteriorly just before entry (29). This can be technically the most challenging part of this technique as, with postnatal age, the right lung often inflates over the window. The SVC also varies more in size than the great arteries during the cardiac cycle. To allow for this, we average a maximum and minimum diameter. Whether this is the physiologically correct way to compensate for the variation in diameter is open to question but we adopted this approach because it is simple and easy to apply. These maximum and minimum diameter measurements are much easier from an M-mode trace (Fig. 5-18). However, as with all M-mode diameter measurement it is important to make sure the ultrasound beam is transecting the vessel at right angles. The calculation for SVC flow is then the same as for LV output. Mean SVC flows

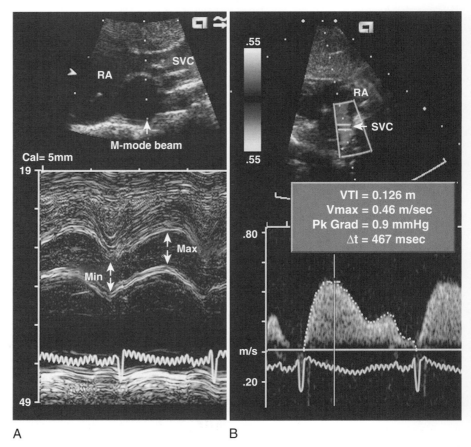

A   B

FIGURE 5-18 (A) Measurement of superior vena cava (SVC) diameter from a mid-parasternal sagittal view. The M-mode beam is dropped through the SVC at the point that is starts to funnel out into the RA. Diameter is averaged from a maximum (max) and minimum (min) diameter. (B) Pulsed Doppler assessment of SVC velocity from a low subcostal view. Velocity time integral (VTI) is derived by tracing around the systolic spectral envelope including any negative trace if present (VTI = 0.126 m in this case). (See color plate.)

increase over the first 48 postnatal hours from about 70 mL/kg/min at 5 h of age to 90 mL/kg/min at 48 h. The normal range during the time frame would be between 40 and 120 mL/kg/min and, in babies with minimal shunting, SVC flow is usually between 30 and 50% of total ventricular output (14,29).

Like RV output, SVC flow has not been directly validated against invasive measures but has been validated against Doppler measured LV output in babies with no shunts (29). It is a more difficult technique to master than the ventricular outputs and is similarly vulnerable to error, probably more so when the SVC is difficult to image for diameter measurement. Its role is probably more as a research tool than a routine clinical tool and it has given us a consistent means with which to study the natural systemic blood flow in the very premature baby. The findings of these studies are touched on below but they will be covered in much more detail in Section III, Chapter 8 and in Section IV.

MYOCARDIAL FUNCTION MEASURES

Neonatologists often place great importance on the traditional LV myocardial function measures of ejection fraction and fractional shortening, possibly because these can be the only hemodynamic measures given in routine echocardiography reports. My view would be that they are not very useful measures in the study of neonatal hemodynamics unless the myocardial dysfunction is severe, in which case you do not need to measure anything to know there is a myocardial problem.

Ejection fraction and fractional shortening are essentially derivations of the same measures, which is the difference between the diastolic and systolic dimensions of the left ventricle. They are most commonly derived from an M-mode study of the left ventricle with the M-mode beam transecting the left ventricle at the tips of the mitral valve (Fig. 5-3). The antero-posterior diameter of the left ventricle is measured in end-systole (LVESD) and end-diastole (LVEDD; Fig. 5-3). The fractional shortening (%) is derived as $[(LVEDD - LVESD)/LVEDD] \times 100$. The ejection fraction is really the same measure but cubes the diameter measurements to convert to an assumed ventricular volume, so is derived as $[(LVEDD^3 - LVESD^3)/LVEDD^3] \times 100$. There are several problems with these measures in the neonate, most importantly M-mode only reflects the movement of the anterior and posterior wall of the left ventricle. In preterm babies because of the complexities of the transitional circulation, the anterior wall of the neonatal LV moves relatively little during contraction compared to the posterior and lateral walls, so A–P M-mode derivations of these measures underestimate LV function. In light of this observation, Lee et al. (31) proposed a method of deriving circumferential shortening by imaging the LV in short axis and tracing the LV endocardial circumference in end-diastole and end-systole and converting to circumferential shortening using the same equation as fractional shortening. The advantage of this method is that it reflects the movement of the entire circumference of the left ventricle not just two walls. The velocity of fractional (or circumferential) fiber shortening (VCF) is another way to derive a function measure from both these measures by using the LV ejection time (LVET). VCF is derived from following equation $VCF = (LVEDD - LVESD)/(LVEDD)(LVET)$. As VCF is also influenced by the heart rate, some investigators recommend to correct for the heart rate using the following equation: $VCF_C = VCF/\sqrt{RR}$ interval where VCF_C is the velocity of circumferential fiber shortening corrected for heart rate.

In essence, VCF measures how fast the myocardium is contracting rather than how far. Mean fractional shortening in healthy newborns is about 35% with a range from 26 to 40% (3), although values lower than this were found by Lee et al. (31) in healthy preterm babies for the reasons cited above. Normal velocity of VCF in a group of preterm babies ranged from 0.8 circ/s (±0.15) shortly after birth to

1.0 circ/s (± 0.18) on postnatal day 5. In term babies, the average was 0.9 circ/s (±0.15) at both times (32).

The overriding problem of all these measures in the neonate is the extent to which they are affected by the load conditions on the left ventricle. Myocardial contractility has three major determinants, the health of the myocardium (which is what we want to assess), the preload on the ventricle (more will improve contractility up to a certain point) and the afterload (more will eventually reduce contractility as the myocardium goes off the top of the Starling curve). So anything that will affect the load conditions will affect these contractility measures. Again ductal shunting is the biggest confounder here, because it increases the preload and reduces the afterload on the left ventricle and so results in excellent measures of contractility in a situation where hemodynamic health may not be good. Other important confounders include hypovolemia, which will reduce contractility, and very high pulmonary vascular resistance in PPHN. The latter can have interesting effects on myocardial function because the high resistance may compromise RV function but the resulting low pulmonary blood flow will also cause low LV preload and hence apparently poor LV function. None of this is possible to work out if you only have a single measure of LV function and do not know what is happening in the rest of the heart.

The above scenario highlights that RV function is probably just as important as LV but the shape of the RV does not lend itself as well to reproducible function measures. However, some investigators have started to look at this by deriving normal values for right ventricular volume measures (33), although it is probably too early to say whether these will develop into clinically useful measures.

One development of the above measures, which is supposed to be more load independent, is the relationship between VCF and LV wall stress (WS). WS is essentially a calculation of afterload and is derived from an equation that included measures of end-systolic blood pressure (ESP), end-systolic LV posterior wall thickness (h) and end systolic diameter (D_{es}). The latter is calculated by dividing the end-systolic circumference by π to reduce error from irregularity of the LV shape. The formula is:

$$\text{VWS} = 0.34(D_{es})(\text{ESP})/h\,[1 + (h/D_{es})]$$

Generally, as LV WS increases so VCFs will slow down, so a plot of the two will produce a negative correlation slope. The steepness of this slope reflects myocardial function; in other words, the more VCF slows in response to an increase in afterload, the worse the myocardial function. The need to derive a slope means that this needs repeated measures at different wall stress. This limits its use in an individual but it may give useful information in cross sectional data in populations of babies. Figure 5-19 compares the VCF versus WS slopes at 3 h of age in preterm infants who did and did not develop low systemic blood flow. The steeper slope in the babies with low systemic blood flow is apparent (34).

MYOCARDIAL FUNCTION: FUTURE DEVELOPMENTS

Data are beginning to emerge in the newborn on two further methodologies for assessing myocardial function, namely measures of diastolic function and tissue Doppler measures. At the moment these data are predominantly limited to normative values, so the role of these methods in clinical or research assessment of hemodynamic pathophysiology is not yet clear. I will describe both briefly here.

Diastolic Function

Diastolic relaxation is an active process in the heart and a compromise of this relaxation can have just as marked effects on cardiac output as compromised systolic

FIGURE 5-19 The relationship between mean velocity of circumferential shortening (mVCF) and LV wall stress in babies who maintained normal systemic blood flow (SBF) and those who developed low SBF. The low SBF babies have a steeper slope suggesting more limited myocardial response to increased LV wall stress.

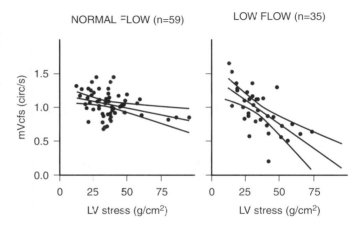

function. In essence, these measures are all derived from the Doppler waveform of the ventricular inflow (Fig. 5-20). This flow pattern reflects the two phases of diastole with an early peak in flow velocity reflecting early ventricular filling (the E wave) with ventricular relaxation and a later peak reflecting active filling as a result of atrial systole (the A wave). A variety of measures of diastolic function can be derived from this flow pattern, most of which are reflections of either velocities of the two phases (maximum, mean, and relative E and A wave ratios) or the acceleration and deceleration times of the two phases. The latter measures need correcting for heart rate

FIGURE 5-20 Shows the normal neonatal pulsed Doppler velocity trace of mitral valve flow that is used to measure diastolic function. The E-wave represents early filling due to active ventricular relaxation while the A-wave represents filling due to atrial systole. Act E-wave shows the acceleration time of early diastolic filling. (See color plate.)

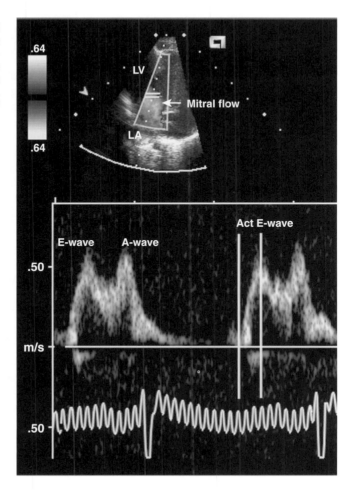

and, at faster heart rates in the newborn, the A wave can be difficult to distinguish from the E wave. Velocity measures taken in isolation will also be as much a reflection of the load conditions as the diastolic function, again the duct will be a big confounder especially in neonates during the immediate postnatal transition.

In the mature healthy heart, 80% of filling occurs in early diastole, so relative dominance of the A wave is a marker of impaired diastolic function. However, in healthy term and preterm neonates, the mean ratio is 1.1:1 and 1:1, respectively, suggesting that reduced diastolic function is normal in the neonate (3). In both term and preterm babies, diastolic function measures improve over the first few months after birth (35). Like most myocardial function measures, there are more data available for the left than right side of the heart. While these measures give interesting physiological insight into the precarious state of the preterm circulation, their relationship to clinical outcome and their role in the assessment of an individual infant have not been clarified.

Tissue Doppler

This methodology uses the low Doppler shift frequencies of high energy generated by the ventricular wall motion, frequencies that are purposely filtered out in standard Doppler blood flow studies (36). There are essentially three variables in ventricular wall motion; velocity, acceleration and displacement. Further, ventricular function depends on contraction of longitudinally and circumferentially orientated fibers. The M-mode myocardial function measures discussed above will give information on displacement and circumferential contraction but tissue Doppler allows much better assessment of velocity, acceleration, and longitudinal contraction. Longitudinal contraction is mainly due to contraction of sub-endocardial fibers and there is evidence from older subjects that abnormalities of wall motion may initially appear in the longitudinal axis. Because the apex of the heart stays relatively stationary during the cardiac cycle, longitudinal motion is assessed best from a four chamber apical view with the Doppler range gate at the base of the heart (Fig. 5-21). From this view, motion of ventricular septal base and tricuspid and mitral annulus can be assessed. The velocity spectral trace has waves that reflect wall velocity in systole and the two phases of diastole.

In older subjects, where much of the tissue Doppler research has been done, there is some evidence that this methodology has significant advantages over more traditional measures of myocardial function (36). Mori et al. (37) have established some normal data in term newborns in comparison to older children but there is little other published work to date. Like diastolic function measures, the clinical usefulness of these measures in the assessment of an individual infant remains to be established.

FUNCTIONAL ECHOCARDIOGRAPHY IN THE NICU IN SPECIFIC CLINICAL SITUATIONS

Although at present there is no evidence that the use of functional echocardiography improves neonatal outcomes, it can provide useful hemodynamic information in almost any sick baby. Because the functional echocardiographer in a NICU will mainly examine structurally normal hearts, the ability to recognize the abnormal patterns of congenital heart disease (CHD) comes quite early in the learning process. Indeed some training in recognizing common congenital heart abnormalities should be part of that learning process. However, this should not be relied on to exclude CHD. In any situation where the primary question is "Does this baby have a structurally normal heart?" it is *vital* that an echocardiogram is performed early in the clinical course by someone skilled in establishing structural normality, usually a

FIGURE 5-21 Shows the tissue Doppler velocity spectrum of longitudinal wall motion at the base of the ventricular septum. Sw shows peak systolic motion velocity, Ew is peak early diastolic filling motion velocity and Aw is peak atrial systolic motion velocity. (See color plate.)

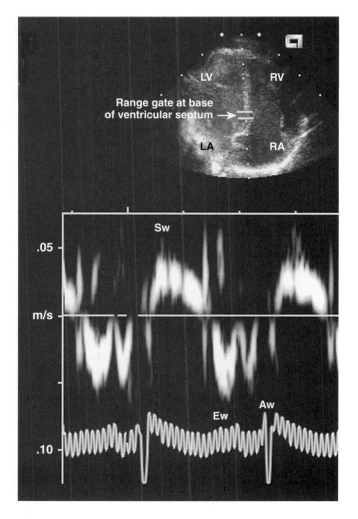

pediatric cardiologist. In most babies where the primary question is "What are the hemodynamics in this sick baby?" the heart will be structurally normal. But there are babies in whom both questions must be answered. Hence, if a neonatologist is going to undertake functional echocardiography, I cannot emphasize strongly enough the importance of working in close collaboration with a pediatric cardiologist.

There are four common scenarios where functional echocardiography plays an important role: (1) the very preterm baby during the transitional period; (2) the baby with suspected PDA; (3) the baby with clinically suspected circulatory compromise (usually hypotensive); and (4) the baby with suspected persistent pulmonary hypertension of the neonate (PPHN). In all these situations, the echocardiogram should be as complete as possible but below I will outline measures that are particularly important in each situation.

The Very Preterm Baby During the Transitional Period

The hemodynamic pathology of the first 12 h of life of the very preterm infant is described in more detail in Section III, Chapter 8. It is a period of exquisite vulnerability to low systemic blood flow and, in our studies, this low systemic blood flow has been associated with a range of adverse preterm outcomes (13,38). We try to perform an echocardiogram between 3 and 9 h of age in all babies born before 28 weeks and babies born after 27 weeks with significant respiratory compromise. This echocardiogram includes a measure of systemic blood flow and an assessment of early ductal constriction and shunt direction

Measurement of Systemic Blood Flow

We recommend measuring both RV output and SVC flow as a cross-check against each other. SVC flow will usually be between 30 and 50% of total systemic blood flow (SBF). For clinical purposes, RV output is a reasonably accurate marker of low SBF because atrial shunts are not usually large early after birth (see above). Full flow measures are time-consuming to derive and, because velocity in the MPA is the dominant determinant of RV output, measuring the maximum velocity in the MPA (PA V_{max}) provides a simple way to screen for low SBF (Fig. 5-22). In our studies, if the PA V_{max} is over 0.45 m/s, low SBF is unlikely and, if the PA V_{max} is less than 0.35 m/s, most babies have low SBF. Between 0.35 and 0.45 m/s is a gray zone where discriminatory accuracy is less good. In practice, I would recommend screening with PA V_{max} and then doing full RV output and/or SVC flow measures in those with a PA V_{max} less than 0.45 m/s (39).

Assessment of Early Ductal Constriction and Shunt Direction

We would assess the degree of ductal constriction by measuring minimum diameter from the color Doppler and the pattern of shunting. The latter is usually predominantly left to right but often has a bidirectional component at this stage. We do this because it has been shown that constriction at this stage predicts subsequent persisting patency (5,12,13,16).

The Preterm Infant with Suspected PDA

This will usually be a baby beyond the first 24 h with signs and/or symptoms suggestive of a PDA. In our hands, an echocardiogram on such a baby includes:

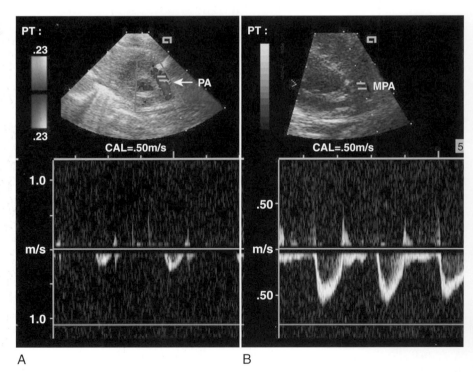

A   B

FIGURE 5-22 Doppler velocity in the pulmonary artery in two babies. (A) The low V_{max} of about 0.2 m/s in a baby with low systemic blood flow (SBF) compared with (B) with a normal V_{max} of about 0.6 m/s. (See color plate.)

- Color Doppler confirmation of patency and minimum diameter from the color Doppler, as a means of assessing likely significance.
- Pulsed Doppler assessment of shunt direction.
- Pulsed Doppler assessment of direction of diastolic flow in the post-ductal descending aorta.
- Pulsed Doppler assessment of velocity of diastolic flow in the left pulmonary artery.

In babies born before 30 weeks with a PDA with a predominantly left to right shunt, a minimum diameter between 1.5 and 2 mm will usually mark a significant shunt and, when over 2 mm, the shunt will almost always be significant. Retrograde diastolic flow in the post-ductal descending aorta and increase velocity diastolic flow in the LPA support the observation that the shunt is likely to be significant.

The Baby with Clinically Suspected Circulatory Compromise

The approach here will vary depending on the presentation. The term baby presenting at birth with low Apgar scores and persisting pallor will usually be due to post-hypoxic acidosis. But an acute fetal bleed with hypovolemia can present this way and the characteristic poorly filled ventricles seen on echocardiography can be helpful in making this diagnosis quickly. In an acute postnatal circulatory collapse in a term baby, then, the need to exclude a ductal dependent systemic circulation is paramount. In the preterm baby undergoing intensive care, such acute collapses will usually have a respiratory origin but it may be cardiac, e.g. cardiac tamponade from a long line extravasating into the pericardium or a ductal dependent systemic circulation. In such situations, prompt diagnosis with echocardiography will be life-saving. The commoner situation for the neonatologist will be the preterm baby with persisting hypotension. These babies usually have a structurally normal heart and functional echocardiography in our practice includes the following:

- A full assessment of ductal patency and significance. PDA causes a global reduction in systolic and diastolic blood pressure during the first postnatal week (40).
- A measure of systemic blood flow, RV output, and/or SVC flow. As the baby grows older, more caution is needed in using pulmonary artery velocities to screen for low flow because significant atrial shunts become more common. In fact, low systemic blood flow is quite uncommon after the first 24 h. Most hypotensive babies after day 1 will have normal or sometimes high systemic blood flow suggesting loss of vascular tone is more important than low cardiac output after the transitional period (13,41,42).
- A visual assessment of myocardial contractility is important in these babies. If it looks poor, I would measure LV fractional shortening.

The Baby with Suspected PPHN

This is usually the term or near-term baby with high oxygen and ventilator requirements. Congenital heart disease can present this way, so these babies must have this possibility excluded early on in their course. Once structural abnormality has been excluded, functional echocardiography in our practice includes the following.

- An assessment of pulmonary artery pressure, ideally from a tricuspid incompetence jet or a ductal shunt. Measure both, if they are present, as a cross-check against each other. Pulmonary artery pressure is surprisingly difficult to predict from a baby's clinical condition (11). The highest pulmonary pressure is found in babies with primary idiopathic PPHN (who may not have very high Fi,o_2 requirements) and babies with severe lung disease.
- An assessment of systemic blood flow, RV output and or SVC flow. These measured are commonly low in such babies, particularly in the first 24 h (11).
- An assessment of ductal constriction and direction of shunting. The ductus usually constricts early and closes in these babies; often well before the oxygen requirement falls (11).
- An assessment of degree and direction of atrial shunting.

CONCLUSION

There is a wealth of hemodynamic information that can be derived by functional echocardiography in the sick neonate. A common theme to many of our research findings in this area is how different actual hemodynamic findings are from what one might expect from conventional thinking in particular clinical scenarios. Further, it is striking how variable hemodynamics are between individual babies and also within the same baby with time. Without echocardiography, you will be guessing the hemodynamics and much of our data would suggest that you will be wrong a fair amount of the time. For functional echocardiography to fulfill its clinical potential, it needs to be available at any time and at short notice in the NICU. Some NICUs will have external diagnostic services that can provide this sort of service but many do not have this sort of access. In these situations, there is much to be said for the neonatologists themselves developing echocardiographic skills in close collaboration with their cardiologists.

REFERENCES

1. Hoffman GM, Ghanayem NS, Tweddell JS. Noninvasive assessment of cardiac output. Semin Thoracic Cardiovas Surg: Ped Cardiac Surg Annual 2005:12–21.
2. Evans N. Echocardiography on neonatal intensive care units in Australia and New Zealand. J Paediat Child Health 2000;36:169–171.
3. Skinner J, Hunter S, Alverson D, eds. Echocardiography for the Neonatologist. London, Churchill Livingstone. 2000.
4. Evans N, Malcolm G. Practical Echocardiography for the Neonatologist. Two multimedia CD-ROMs, Royal Prince Alfred Hospital, 2000 and 2002. www.cs.nsw.gov.au/rpa/neonatal.
5. Evans N, Malcolm G, Osborn DA, Kluckow M. Diagnosis of patent ductus arteriosus in preterm infants. Neoreviews 2004;5:e86–97.
6. Evans N, Iyer P. Incompetence of the foramen ovale in preterm infants requiring ventilation. J Pediatr 1994;125:786–792.
7. Evans N, Iyer P. Assessment of ductus arteriosus shunting in preterm infants requiring ventilation: effect of inter-atrial shunting. J Pediatr 1994;125:778–785.
8. Suzumura H, Nitta A, Tanaka G, Arisaka O. Diastolic flow velocity of the left pulmonary artery of patent ductus arteriosus in preterm infants. Pediatr Int 2001;43:146–151.
9. Evans N, Archer LNJ. Postnatal circulatory adaptation in term and healthy preterm neonates. Arch Dis Child 1990;65:24–26.
10. Lim MK, Hanretty K, Houston AB, Lilley S, Murtagh EP. Intermittent ductal patency in healthy newborn infants: demonstration by colour Doppler flow mapping. Arch Dis Child 1992;67:1217–1218.
11. Evans N, Kluckow M, Currie A. The range of echocardiographic findings in term and near term babies with high oxygen requirements. Arch Dis Child 1998;78:105–111.
12. Kluckow M, Evans N. High pulmonary blood flow, the duct, and pulmonary hemorrhage. J Pediatr 2000;137:68–72.
13. Kluckow M, Evans N. Low superior vena cava flow and intraventricular haemorrhage in preterm infants. Arch Dis Child 2000;82:F188–F194.

14. Skelton R, Evans N, Smythe J. A blinded comparison of clinical and echocardiographic evaluation of the preterm infant for patent ductus arteriosus. J Paediat Child Health 1994;30:406–411.

15. Davis P, Turner-Gomes S, Cunningham K, Way C, Roberts R, Schmidt B. Precision and accuracy of clinical and radiological signs in premature infants at risk of patent ductus arteriosus. Arch Pediatr Adolesc Med 1995;149:1136–1141.

16. Kluckow M, Evans N. Early echocardiographic prediction of symptomatic patent ductus arteriosus in preterm infants undergoing mechanical ventilation. J Pediatr 1995;127:774–779.

17. Hiraishi S, Agata Y, Saito K, et al. Interatrial shunt flow profiles in newborn infants: a colour flow and pulsed Doppler echocardiographic study. Br Heart J 1991;65:41–45.

18. Musewe NN, Poppe D, Smallhorn JF, Hellman J, Whyte H, Smith B, Freedom RM. Doppler echocardiographic measurement of pulmonary artery pressure from ductal Doppler velocities in the newborn. JACC 1990:15:446–456.

19. Yock PG, Popp RL. Non invasive estimation of right ventricular systolic pressure by Doppler ultrasound in patients with tricuspid regurgitation. Circulation 1984;70:657–662.

20. Chan KL, Currie PJ, Seward JB, Hagler DJ, Mair DD, Tajik AJ. Comparison of three Doppler ultrasound methods in the prediction of pulmonary artery pressure. JACC 1987;9:549–554.

21. Kosturakis D, Goldberg SJ, Allen HD, Loeber C. Doppler echocardiographic prediction of pulmonary arterial hypertension in congenital heart disease. Am J Cardiol 1984;53:1110–1115.

22. Matsuda M, Sekiguchi T, Sugishita Y, Kuwako K, Ito I. Reliability of non-invasive estimates of pulmonary hypertension by pulsed Doppler echocardiography. Br Heart J 1986;56:158–164.

23. Evans N, Archer LNJ. Postnatal circulatory adaptation in term and healthy preterm newborns. Arch Dis Child 1990;65:24–26.

24. Evans N, Archer LNJ. Doppler assessment of pulmonary artery pressure and extrapulmonary shunting in the acute phase of hyaline membrane disease. Arch Dis Child 1991;66:6–11.

25. Mandelbaum-Isken VH, Linderkamp O. Cardiac output by pulsed Doppler in neonates using the apical window. Pediatr Cardiol 1991;12:13–16.

26. Alverson DC, Eldridge M, Dillon T, Yabek SM, Merman W. Non invasive pulsed Doppler determination of cardiac output in neonates and children. J Pediatr 1982;101:46–50.

27. Mellander M, Sabel KG, Caidahl K, Solymar L, Eriksson B. Doppler determination of cardiac output in infants and children: comparison with simultaneous thermodilution. Pediatr Cardiol 1987;8:241–246.

28. Hudson I, Houston A, Aitchison T, Holland B, Turner T. Reproducibility of measurements of cardiac output in newborn infants by Doppler ultrasound. Arch Dis Child 1990;65:15–19.

29. Kluckow M, Evans N. Superior vena cava flow. A novel marker of systemic blood flow. Arch Dis Child 2000;82:F182–F187.

30. Drayton MR, Skidmore R. Vasoactivity of the major intracranial arteries in newborn infants. Arch Dis Child 1987;62:236–240.

31. Lee LA, Kimball TR, Daniels SR, Khoury P, Meyer RA. Left ventricular mechanics in the preterm infant and their effect on measurement of cardiac performance. J Pediatr 1992;120:114–119.

32. Takahashi Y, Harada K, Kishkumo S, Arai M, Ishida A, Takada G. Postnatal left ventricular contractility in very low birth weight infants. Pediatrc Cardiology 1997;18:112–117.

33. Clark SJ, Yoxall CW, Subhedar NV. Measurement of right ventricular volume in healthy term and preterm neonates. Arch Dis Child, Fetal Neonatal Ed 2002;87:F89–F93.

34. Osborn D, Evans N, Kluckow M. Left ventricular contractility and wall stress in very preterm infants in the first day of life. Pediatr Res 2007;61:335–340.

35. Schmitz L, Stiller B, Pees C, Koch H, Xanthopoulos A, Lange P. Doppler-derived parameters of diastolic left ventricular function in preterm infants with a birth weight <1500 g: reference values and differences to term infants. Early Human Develop 2004;76:101–114.

36. Isaaz K. Tissue Doppler imaging for the assessment of left ventricular systolic and diastolic function. Curr Opin Cardiol 2002;17:431–442.

37. Mori K, Nakagawa R, Nii M, Edagawa T, Takehara Y, Inoue M, Kuruda Y. Pulsed wave Doppler tissue echocardiography assessment of the long axis function of the right and left ventricles during the neonatal period. Heart 2004;90:175–180.

38. Osborn DA, Evans N, Kluckow M. Hemodynamic and antecedent risk factors of early and late periventricular/intraventricular hemorrhage in premature infants. Pediatrics 2003;112:33–39.

39. Evans N. Which inotrope in which baby? Arch Dis Child 2006;91:F213–220.

40. Evans N, Moorcraft J. Effect of patency of the ductus arteriosus on blood pressure in very preterm infants. Arch Dis Child 1992;67:1169–1173.

41. Noori S, Friedlich P, Wong P, Ebrahimi M, Siassi B, Seri I. Haemodynamic changes after low-dosage hydrocortisone administration in vasopressor-treated preterm and term neonates. Pediatrics 2006;118(4):1456–1466.

42. Lopez SL, Leighton JO, Walther FJ. Supranormal cardiac output ion the dopamine and dobutamine dependent preterm infant. Pediatr Cardiol 1997;18:292–296.

Chapter 6

Near-Infrared Spectroscopy and its Use for the Assessment of Tissue Perfusion in the Neonate

Suresh Victor, MRCPCH, PhD • Michael Weindling, MA, MD, BSC, FRCP, FRCPCH, HON FRCA

Principles of Near-Infrared Spectroscopy
Near-Infrared Spectrophotometers
Measurements of Physiological Variables
Physiological Observations Using NIR spectroscopy
References

Light-based approaches to the assessment of a tissue's oxygen status are attractive to the clinician because they provide the possibility of continuous non-invasive measurements. For example, pulse oximetry, which relies on emission and absorption of light in red and infrared frequencies (660 and 940 nm, respectively), has become widely used in clinical practice. However, this technology only measures hemoglobin oxygen saturation, which is variably related to the partial pressure of oxygen in arterial blood and not oxygen delivery. The arterial oxygen saturation is estimated by measuring the transmission of light through the pulsatile tissue bed; the microprocessor analyses the changes in light absorption due to pulsatile arterial flow and ignores the component of the signal which is non-pulsatile and which results from blood in the veins and tissues. Near-infrared (NIR) spectroscopy technology takes this further and utilizes light in the near-infrared range (700 to 1000 nm).

Using one NIR spectroscopy technique (the continuous wave method with partial venous occlusion, described in more detail below), venous oxygen saturation can be determined, and, from this, oxygen delivery and consumption can be measured. Blood flow can also be measured by continuous wave NIR spectroscopy and the Fick approach, either with a bolus of oxygen or with dye (1,2). However, these methods only allow for intermittent measurements and, more recently, another NIR spectroscopy technique (the time-of-flight method, also described in more detail below) has been used to measure an index of tissue oxygenation continuously (3). Cytochrome activity can also be assessed (4,5), but this has not been achieved in any regular clinical or even research application.

NIR spectroscopy instrumentation consists of fiber-optic bundles or optodes placed either on opposite sides of the tissue being interrogated (usually a limb or the head of a young baby) to measure transmitted light, or close together to measure reflected light. Light enters through one optode and a fraction of the photons are captured by a second optode and conveyed to a measuring device. Multiple light emitters and detectors can also be placed in a headband to provide tomographic imaging of the brain.

In this chapter, we will review the principles of NIR spectroscopy, quantification of physiological variables, and finally some clinically relevant observations that have been made using this technology.

PRINCIPLES OF NEAR-INFRARED SPECTROSCOPY

Near-infrared spectrophotometers are applied in the food industry, geological surveys, and in laboratory analysis. Jöbsis first introduced its use for human tissue in 1977 (6). Since 1985, near-infrared spectrophotometers have been used in newborn infants.

NIR spectroscopy relies on three important phenomena:

- Human tissue is relatively transparent to light in the near-infrared region of the spectrum
- Pigmented compounds known as chromophores absorb light as it passes through biological tissue
- In tissue, there are compounds whose absorption differs depending on their oxygenation status

Human tissues contain a variety of substances whose absorption spectra at near-infrared wavelengths are well defined. They are present in sufficient quantities to contribute significant attenuation to measurements of transmitted light. The concentration of some absorbers such as water, melanin, and bilirubin remain virtually constant with time. However, the concentrations of some absorbing compounds, such as oxygenated hemoglobin (HbO_2), deoxyhemoglobin (HbR), and oxidized cytochrome oxidase (Cyt aa3) vary with tissue oxygenation and metabolism. Therefore changes in light absorption can be related to changes in the concentrations of these compounds.

Dominant absorption by water at longer wavelengths limits spectroscopic studies to less than about 1000 nm. The lower limit on wavelength is dictated by the overwhelming absorption of HbR below 650 nm. However, between 650 and 1000 nm, it is possible with sensitive instrumentation to detect light that has traversed 8 cm of tissue (7).

The absorption properties of hemoglobin alter when it changes from its oxygenated to its deoxygenated form. In the near-infrared region of the spectrum, the absorption of the hemoglobin chromophores (HbR and HbO_2) decreases significantly compared to that observed in the visible region. However, the absorption spectra remain significantly different in this region. This allows spectroscopic separation of the compounds using only a few sample wavelengths. HbO_2 has its greatest absorbency at 850 nm. Absorption by HbR is maximum at 775 nm, so measurement at this wavelength enables any shift in hemoglobin oxygenation to be monitored. The isobestic points (the wavelength at which two substances absorb light to the same extent) for HbR and HbO_2 occur at 590 and 805 nm, respectively. These points may be used as reference points where light absorption is independent of the degree of saturation.

The major part of the NIR spectroscopy signal is derived from hemoglobin (8), but other hemoglobin compounds, such as carboxyhemoglobin, also absorb light in the near-infrared region. However, the combined error due to ignoring these compounds in the measurement of the total hemoglobin signal is probably less than 1% in normal blood. Nevertheless, when monitoring skeletal muscle using NIR spectroscopy, myoglobin and oxymyoglobin must be considered because their near infrared absorbance characteristics are similar to hemoglobin.

NEAR-INFRARED SPECTROPHOTOMETERS

Three different methods of using near-infrared light for monitoring tissue oxygenation are currently used:

- Continuous wave method (9–11)
- Time-of-flight method (also known as time-domain or time-resolved) (12)
- Frequency domain method (11)

The continuous wave method has a very fast response but registers relative change only and it is therefore not possible to make absolute measurements using this technique. Nevertheless, these instruments have been widely used for research studies (1,2,5,13–25). The time-of-flight method needs extensive data processing but provides more accurate measurements. It enables one to explore different information provided by the measured signals and has the potential to become a valuable tool in research and clinical environments. The third approach, which uses frequency domain or phase modulation technology, has a lower resolution than that of the time-of-flight method but has the potential to provide estimates of oxygen delivery sufficiently quickly for clinical purposes. This frequency domain or phase modulation technology is potentially the best candidate for the neonatal intensive care setting and for bedside usage. The principles used in the three methods are described below.

Continuous Wave Instruments

In continuous wave spectroscopy (9), changes in tissue chromophore concentrations from the baseline value can be obtained from the modified Beer–Lambert law. The original Beer–Lambert law describes the absorption of light in a non-scattering medium and states that, for an absorbing compound dissolved in a non-absorbing medium, the attenuation is proportional to the concentration of the compound in the solution and the optical pathlength. Therefore, $A = E \times C \times P$, where A = absorbance (no units), E = extinction coefficient or molar absorbtivity (measured in L/mol/cm), P = pathlength of the sample (measured in cm), and C = concentration of the compound (measured in mol/L). Wray et al. (26) characterized the extinction coefficient of hemoglobin and oxygenated hemoglobin between the wavelengths of 650 and 1000 nm. The extinction coefficients determined by them at four specific wavelengths are as shown in Table 6-1. Mendelson et al. showed that the absorption coefficients of fetal and adult hemoglobin are virtually identical (27).

However, the application of the Beer–Lambert law in its original form has limitations. Its linearity is limited by:

- Deviation in the absorption coefficient at high concentrations (>0.01 M) due to electrostatic interaction between molecules in close proximity; fortunately such concentrations are not met in biological media

Table 6-1	Extinction Coefficients of HbO$_2$ and Hb and Different Wavelengths		
Wavelength (nm)		HbO$_2$	Hb
772		0.71	1.36
824		0.983	0.779
844		1.07	0.778
907		1.2520	0.892

- Scattering of light due to particulate matter in the sample
- Ambient light

When light passes through tissue, it is scattered because of differences in the refractive indices of various tissue components. The effect of scattering is to increase the pathlength traveled by photons and the absorption of light within the tissue. Cell membranes are the most important source of scattering. In neonates, skin and bone tissue become important when the optodes are placed less than 2.5 cm apart (28).

Thus, for light passing through a highly scattering medium, the Beer–Lambert law has been modified to include an additive term, K, due to scattering losses, and a multiplier to account for the increased optical pathlength due to scattering.

Where the true optical distance is known as the differential pathlength (DP), P is the pathlength of the sample, and the scaling factor is the differential pathlength factor (L): thus, $DP = P \times L$. The modified Beer–Lambert law, which incorporates these two additions, is then expressed as $A = P \times L \times E \times C + K$, where A is absorbance, P is the pathlength, E is the extinction coefficient, C is the concentration of the compound, and K is a constant. Unfortunately, K is unknown and is dependent on the measurement geometry and the scattering coefficient of the tissue investigated. Hence this equation cannot be solved to provide a measure of the absolute concentration of the chromophore in the medium. However, if K is constant during the measurement period, it is possible to determine a change in concentration (ΔC) of the chromophore from a measured change in attenuation (ΔA). Therefore, $\Delta A = P \times L \times E \times \Delta C$, or

$$\Delta C = \frac{\Delta A}{P \times L \times E}$$

The differential pathlength factor describes the actual distance traveled by light. As it is dependent on the amount of scattering in the medium, its measurement is not straightforward. The differential pathlength factor has been calculated on human subjects of different ages and in various tissues. Van der Zee et al. (28) and Duncan et al. (29) conducted optical pathlength measurements on human tissue and their results are as shown in Table 6-2.

There is a small change in optical pathlength with gestation, but this is negligible and a constant relationship is assumed (30). Despite gross changes in oxygenation and perfusion before and after death in experimental animals, the optical pathlength at near-infrared wavelengths was found to be nearly constant (maximum difference <9%) (31).

A compound that absorbs light in the spectral region of interest is known as a chromophore. In a medium containing several chromophores (C_1, C_2, and C_3) the overall absorbance is simply the sum of the contributions of each chromophore. Therefore,

$$A = (E_1 C_1 + E_2 C_2 + E_3 C_3)P \times L$$

Table 6-2 Differential Pathlength Factors as Determined by Van Der Zee et al. (28) and Duncan et al. (29)

	Van der Zee	Duncan
Preterm head	3.8 ± 0.57	–
Term head	–	4.99 ± 0.45
Adult forearm	3.59 ± 0.78	4.16 ± 0.78

Table 6-3	Inverse Matrix Coefficients for Hb, HbO$_2$, and Cytochrome aa3 at Different Wavelengths			
	774 nm	825 nm	843 nm	908 nm
Hb	1.363	−0.9298	−0.7538	0.6747
HbO$_2$	−0.7501	−0.5183	−0.0002	1.8881
Cyt aa3	−0.1136	0.7975	0.4691	−1.0945

For a medium containing several chromophores C_1, C_2, C_3

$$\Delta C_1 = Q_1 \Delta A_1 + R_1 \Delta A_2 + S_1 \Delta A_3 + T_1 \Delta A_4$$

$$\Delta C_2 = Q_2 \Delta A_1 + R_2 \Delta A_2 + S_2 \Delta A_3 + T_2 \Delta A_4$$

$$\Delta C_3 = Q_3 \Delta A_1 + R_3 \Delta A_2 + S_3 \Delta A_3 + T_3 \Delta A_4$$

where ΔA_1, ΔA_2, ΔA_3, and ΔA_4 represent changes in absorption at wavelengths such as 774 nm, 825 nm, 843 nm, and 908 nm. ΔC_1, ΔC_2, and ΔC_3 represent changes in the concentrations of C_1, C_2, and C_3 (such as HbR, HbO$_2$, and Cyt aa3). The 12 values of Q, R, S, and T are functions of the absorption coefficients of HbR, HbO$_2$, and Cyt aa3. They are termed near-infrared coefficients. Since the pathlength is wavelength dependent (32), a modification of these inverse matrix coefficients has been made in Table 6-3.

Examples of instruments using continuous wave technology are the NIRO 500 and NIRO 100, made by Hamamatsu Photonic, Japan.

Spatially Resolved Spectroscopy

The continuous wave method, which measures only the intensity of light, is very reliable, but allows only relative or trend measurements due to the lack of information available about pathlength (9). To address this problem using current continuous wave instruments, multiple optodes operating simultaneously are placed around the head. This allows for a pathlength correction, but only when the tissue being interrogated is assumed to be homogeneous. This modification is called spatially resolved spectroscopy. It has reasonable signal to noise ratio and the depth of brain tissue, which can be measured from the surface, varies typically between 1 and 3 cm.

Spatially resolved spectroscopy is a method that measures hemoglobin oxygen saturation. In contrast to standard continuous wave NIR spectroscopy, this technique gives absolute values. A light detector measures tissue oxygenation index with three sensors at different distances from the light source. Scatter and absorption attenuate light passing into tissue. If the distance between the light source and the sensor is large enough (more than 3 cm), the isotropy of scatter distribution becomes so homogeneous that the loss due to scatter is the same at the three sensors. Tissue oxygenation index (TOI) is calculated according to the diffusion equation as follows:

$$TOI(\%) = \frac{K_{HbO_2}}{K_{HbO_2} + K_{HbR}}$$

where K is the constant scattering contribution.

The NIRO 300 (Hamamatsu Inc., Hamamatsu, Japan) was used to determine the cerebral TOI in 15 preterm infants between 26 and 29 weeks, gestation during the first three days after birth. The median TOI increased progressively during the days after birth. It was 57% (95% CI, 54 to 65.7%) on the first day, 66.1% on the second day (95% CI, 61.9 to 82.3%) and 76.1% on the third day (95% CI, 67.8 to 80.1%) (33). In a group of eight preterm infants with hypothermia (body temperature < 35°C), the TOI was found to increase on warming four infants with perinatal asphyxia (34). Naulaers and colleagues have suggested that by using TOI as a measure of venous oxygen saturation, it is possible to measure an equivalent of the fractional extraction of oxygen continuously (34). Recently, Dullenkopf and associates recently examined the reproducibility of cerebral TOI (35). Sensor-exchange experiments (removing the sensor and re-applying another sensor at the same position) and simultaneous left to right forehead measurements revealed only small mean differences (<5%) and no significant differences between corresponding values (35). The same group also showed that much of the variability of cerebral TOI was due to cerebral venous oxygen saturation (36).

Quaresima et al. concluded that TOI reflected mainly the saturation of the intracranial venous compartment of circulation (37). There has been variability in the results of studies aimed at correlating TOI with jugular venous bulb oximetry, possibly because of assumptions made about the distribution of cerebral blood between the arterial and venous compartments; several studies used a fixed ratio of 25:75 (38–40), but Watzman et al. described an arterial-to-venous ratio of 16:84 in normoxia, hypoxia and hypocapnia and also observed considerable biological individual variability (41).

Time-of-flight Instruments

This time-resolved technique consists of emitting a very short laser pulse into an absorbing tissue and recording the temporal response (time of flight) of the photons at some distance from the laser source (12). This method uses a mathematical approximation that is based on diffusion theory to allow for the separation of effects due to light absorbance from those due to light scattering. Thus, the time-of-flight method permits differentiation of one tissue from another. In addition, the scattering component provides further useful information, which may be used for imaging. Functional imaging is an exciting application of the time-of-flight method because, in conjunction with hemoglobin status, scattering changes, which can be mapped optically, may provide information about the electrical and vascular interaction, which determines the functional status of the brain. Disadvantages of this technique, which still need to be addressed, are the large amount of data, which means that data are collected and analyzed relatively slowly (minutes), and information obtained at bedside is not displayed instantaneously but rather a few minutes later.

There have only been a few reports on the use of time of flight instruments in neonates (3). Measurements in neonates at the bedside have not been possible because of the size and the cost of typical laboratory equipment needed for these measurements. However, a new portable TRS device (TRS-10, Hamamatsu Photonics K.K., Hamamatsu, Japan), which has a high data acquisition rate, was recently used clinically. This TRS system can be used (1) for continuous absolute quantification of hemodynamic variables, and (2) for better estimation of light-scattering properties by measurement of differential pathlength factors.

Frequency Domain Instruments

The frequency domain method is based on the modulation of a laser light at given frequencies (11). The frequency domain instrument determines the absorption coefficient and reduces scattering coefficient of the tissue by measuring the AC, DC, and phase change as functions of distance through the tissue. This method allows for correction of the detected signal for the different scattering effects of the fluid and tissue components of the brain using data processing algorithms. Moreover, the phase and amplitude shifts can be used for localization of the signal. Since pathlength is measured directly, the hemoglobin saturation can be measured to ±5% *in vitro* models and ±10% in piglets. Problems include noise and leakage associated with the high frequency signal, but the devices are very compact and appropriate for bedside/incubator use. Further refinement of the technology will be needed to improve accuracy in the clinical setting.

Examples of instruments using this frequency domain technology are manufactured by ISS, Inc., Champaign, IL.

MEASUREMENTS OF PHYSIOLOGICAL VARIABLES

As previously stated, continuous wave NIR spectroscopy does not result in absolute quantitative measurements. In order to derive quantitative values for physiological variables, it is necessary to produce changes in the concentrations of the measured chromophore. This has been done by changing the volume of the cerebral venous compartment, either by tilting the subject head-down (42) or, as we have done, by partial venous occlusion (20), or by using changes in cerebral blood volume induced by ventilation (43). By observing the ratio of the changes in chromophores or the change in chromophore concentration in comparison to another measured variable, it is possible to calculate different physiological variables.

Some assumptions are made. It is assumed that the receiving and transmitting fiber optodes do not move in position and that the distance between the optodes and the scattering characteristics of the tissue remain constant during a measurement. Also, for cerebral measurements it is assumed that there is no contribution to the NIR spectroscopy signal from extra-cerebral hemoglobin (44).

Continuous wave NIR spectroscopy has been used in a number of ways to make measurements relevant to neonatal cerebral and peripheral hemodynamics. The technique has been used to measure peripheral and cerebral venous oxygen saturation, and cerebral and peripheral blood flow.

Venous Oxygen Saturation

Intermittent measurements of both cerebral and peripheral venous oxygen saturation (Sv_{O_2}) have been made using this technology (16,20,42,43,45). The assumption is made that in a steady state, arterial, and venous blood flows are equal. The approach for measuring both cerebral and peripheral Sv_{O_2} is similar, namely to induce a brief increase in the venous compartment (and hence in the concentration of venous hemoglobin) and then to measure that change.

Cerebral Venous Oxygen Saturation

Three techniques have been described for the measurement of cerebral Sv_{O_2} using NIRS (20,42,43). Each involves the calculation of cerebral Sv_{O_2} from the relative changes in HbO_2 and total hemoglobin (the sum of oxygenated and deoxygenated hemoglobin or HbT) that occur when there is an increase in the venous blood volume of the brain. As mentioned earlier, this is achieved either by gravity using a tilt technique (42), or by partial jugular venous occlusion (20) or by using changes in cerebral blood volume induced by ventilation (43).

The partial jugular venous occlusion technique for the measurement of cerebral Sv_{O_2} was developed by our group in Liverpool, UK, and validated by Yoxall et al. (20). In this technique, the monitoring optodes were positioned on the infant's head in the temporal or frontal regions of the same side. The optodes were held firmly in place without any movement using a Velcro band (Ohmeda). A minimum inter-optode distance of 2.5 cm was ensured. In order to establish a baseline, the NIRS data were monitored for a short period when no changes were made. Then a brief jugular venous occlusion was made using gentle pressure on the side of the neck over the jugular vein. The compression lasted for about 5 to 10 s, after which the pressure was released. The brief compression of the jugular vein led to an increase in the blood volume in the head. Since there was no arterial occlusion and because the occlusion was brief, all the increase in hemoglobin concentration monitored using NIR spectroscopy may be assumed to be due to venous blood within the head. The relative changes in HbO_2 concentration and HbT concentration monitored could then be used to calculate the saturation of venous blood within the tissue studied.

Data were recorded every 0.5 s on to a laptop computer using the Onmain program developed at University College London. The differential pathlength factor was set according to Table 6-2. The inter-optode spacing was measured accurately using calipers.

Using a spreadsheet, the HbR and HbO_2 data were visually inspected to determine the point at which both started to rise. The 10 data points (5 s) preceding this were averaged to give a baseline (Fig. 6-1). The increase from this baseline was calculated at each point for the next 5 s (10 data points). The venous saturation every 0.5 s for 5 s following the occlusion was calculated from the change in the concentration of HbO_2 (ΔHbO_2) as a proportion of the change in total hemoglobin concentration (ΔHbT). Therefore,

$$\text{cerebral } Svo_2 = \frac{\Delta HbO_2}{\Delta HbT}$$

The Svo_2 was then calculated as the mean of the 10 values thus obtained. Before calculating the value of cerebral Svo_2, the data obtained during each occlusion were observed to check for a steady baseline and a smooth increase after the occlusion.

Five consecutive occlusions were made over a period of approximately 1 to 2 min and the value of cerebral Svo_2 was obtained from the mean of these five occlusions. Using this technique, cerebral Svo_2 was measured non-invasively with minimal disturbance of the subject and repeated measurements could be made.

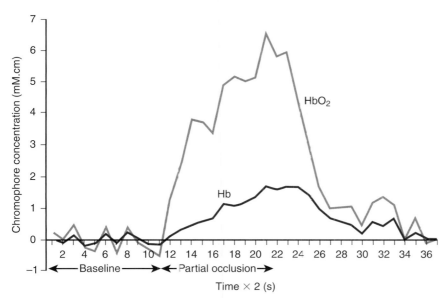

FIGURE 6-1 **Changes in hemoglobin (Hb) and oxygenated hemoglobin (HbO₂) following a partial jugular venous occlusion.** A 5 s baseline is initially recorded. The partial occlusion lasts for 5 to 10 s. Data are acquired by the NIRO every 0.5 s.

This partial jugular venous occlusion technique was validated by comparison with Svo_2 measured by co-oximetry from blood obtained from the jugular bulb during cardiac catheterization (20). Fifteen children were studied, aged three months to 14 years (median, two years) (20). Cerebral Svo_2 by co-oximetry ranged from 36 to 80% (median, 60%) (20). The mean difference (co-oximeter − NIR spectroscopy) was 1.5% (20). Limits of agreement were −12.8% to 15.9% (20). Using partial jugular venous occlusion, measurements were possible in almost all the children studied, including those who were awake and not ventilated and those who were sick and unstable. By contrast, measurements were only possible in 10 of 15 patients studied using the technique described by Wolf et al. (43) and results were only obtained in nine of the 22 patients studied using the tilt technique (42). However, the values obtained using the different techniques are reasonably comparable, considering the different populations studied.

Peripheral Venous Oxygen Saturation

Peripheral Svo_2 can be measured by two methods using NIRS (16,46). One approach, which is described in more detail below, involves measuring changes following venous occlusion. It is similar to that used for cerebral Svo_2 and was developed by Wardle et al. (16) for preterm infants by adapting a method described and validated by De Blasi et al. in adult patients (47). Another approach is a method involving the use of oxygen as an intravascular tracer and it can be used in the same way that measurements of cerebral blood flow are made (see below) (46).

In the venous occlusion method, the optodes were positioned on the upper arm and the interoptode distance was measured using calipers. The optodes were held in place using a small Velcro band (Ohmeda). A brief venous occlusion with a blood pressure cuff around the upper arm was achieved by manually inflating the cuff to 30 mm Hg for approximately 5 to 10 s. This compression of the arm resulted in a rise in the blood volume within the forearm. Since the venous occlusion was brief and there was no arterial occlusion, all the measured increase in hemoglobin within the tissues monitored could assumed to be attributed to an increase in the venous blood. During the initial part of a venous occlusion, hemoglobin accumulated in the tissues owing to cessation of venous flow and the rate of hemoglobin flow was equal to the rate of tissue hemoglobin accumulation during the initial part of the occlusion.

The changes in HbR and HbO_2 concentration were used to calculate the saturation of venous blood within the forearm tissues.

Data were recorded and analyzed as for NIRS measurements of cerebral Svo_2 using partial jugular venous occlusion.

$$\text{Peripheral } Svo_2 = \frac{\Delta HbO_2}{\Delta HbT}$$

NIR spectroscopy measures ΔHbT every 0.5 s (Fig. 6-2). Using a similar approach to that for cerebral venous saturation, the HbT data were visually inspected to determine the point at which it started to rise, the ten data points (5 s) preceding this were averaged to give a baseline and the increase from this baseline was calculated at each point for the next 2 s (four data points). As with cerebral Svo_2 measurements, before calculating the value of the peripheral Svo_2 the data from each occlusion were observed to check for a steady baseline and a smooth increase following the occlusion. Five consecutive occlusions over a period of approximately 1 to 2 min were made and the value of peripheral Svo_2 was obtained from the mean of these five occlusions.

The Svo_2 measurements using the venous occlusion technique made both from the forearms of adults and babies have been compared with co-oximetry measurements. The agreement between the methods was close (21,22). In 19 adult

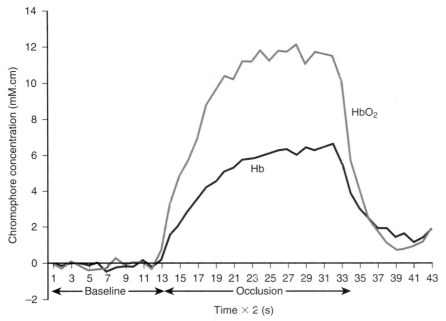

FIGURE 6-2 Changes in hemoglobin (Hb) and oxygenated hemoglobin (HbO₂) following a forearm venous occlusion. A 5 s baseline is initially recorded. The partial occlusion lasts for 5 to 10 s. Data are acquired by the NIRO every 0.5 s.

volunteers, there was a significant correlation between forearm Svo_2 measured by NIR spectroscopy and Svo_2 of superficial venous blood measured by co-oximetry ($r = 0.7$, $P < 0.0001$) (22). When the study was repeated in 16 newborn infants there was again a significant correlation between the two measurements ($r = 0.85$, $P < 0.0001$) (21). The mean difference between the two techniques was 6% and the limits of agreement were -5.1% to 17.1% (21).

Once venous saturation (using partial venous occlusion and continuous wave NIR spectroscopy) and arterial saturation (using pulse oximetry) are known, fractional oxygen extraction can be measured (see below).

Blood Flow

NIR spectroscopy has also been used as a research tool for measuring cerebral and peripheral blood flow. The methods are described below.

From the measurements made using partial venous occlusion, hemoglobin flow (Hb flow) can also be calculated from the slope of a line through the ΔHbT values during the first 2 s of an occlusion using a least squares method, i.e. the rate of increase of HbT within the forearm is used to calculate Hb flow. Hence,

$$\text{Hb flow} = \int \Delta \text{HbT } dt$$

as shown in Fig. 6-3; and,

$$\text{blood flow} = \frac{\text{Hb flow}}{[\text{Hb}]}$$

where [Hb] is hemoglobin concentration.

Blood flow (mL/100 mL/min) is calculated by dividing Hb flow (μmol/100 mL/min) by venous [Hb] in μmol/mL. Since the molecular weight of hemoglobin is 64,500 g/mol, blood flow is:

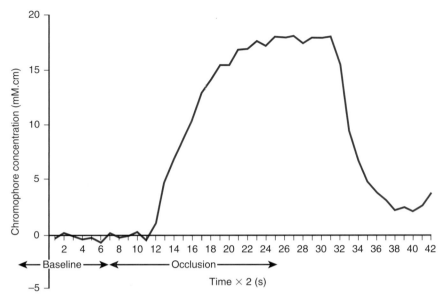

FIGURE 6-3 **Changes in total hemoglobin following a forearm venous occlusion.** A 5 s baseline is initially recorded. The partial occlusion lasts for 5 to 10 s. Data are acquired by the NIRO every 0.5 s.

$$\frac{\text{Hb flow} \times 6.45}{[\text{Hb}]}$$

where blood flow is in mL/100 mL/min, Hb flow is in μmol/100 mL/min, and [Hb] is in g/dL.

An alternative approach to measure flow by NIR spectroscopy is to use a bolus of oxidized hemoglobin as a non-diffusible intravascular tracer (1,2,25). In this technique, the monitoring optodes were positioned on the infant's head in the temporal or frontal regions of the same side. The optodes were held firmly in place without any movement using a Velcro band (Ohmeda). A minimum inter-optode distance of 2.5 cm was used. In order to establish a baseline, the NIR spectroscopy data were monitored for a short period where no changes were made. The measurement is based on the Fick principle, which states that the amount of a non-diffusible intravascular tracer accumulated in a tissue over a time t is equal to the amount delivered in the arterial blood minus the amount removed in the venous blood. If the blood transit time for the brain (t) is less than 6 s, then the amount removed by venous flow will be zero and so increase in tissue tracer content is equal to the amount of tracer delivered by arterial blood flow. Hence, the amount of HbO_2 delivered by arterial flow is [arterial Hb flow $\times$ $\int_0^t \Delta Sa_{O_2}$], where $\int_0^t \Delta Sa_{O_2}$ is the rate of increase in arterial oxygen saturation (Sa_{O_2}) and is measured by pulse oximetry. The equation can be rearranged as

$$\text{Hb flow} = \frac{\Delta HbO_2}{\int_0^t \Delta Sa_{O_2}\ \mathrm{d}t}$$

Total hemoglobin content [HbT] must remain constant through the measurement. The rise in HbO_2 must therefore be accompanied by an equal fall in HbR. To increase the signal to noise ratio ΔHbO_2 is substituted by $\Delta HbD/2$ where $HbD = HbO_2 - HbR$. The equation now reads:

$$\text{hemoglobin flow} = \frac{\Delta HbD}{2\int_0^t \Delta Sa_{O_2}\ \mathrm{d}t}$$

where the hemoglobin flow is in µmol/L/min. The Sa_{O_2} is increased by about 5% over less than 6 s. As Sa_{O_2} is measured peripherally and the HbD is measured on the forehead, there may be an interval of not more than 2 s between the rises of each.

Since the molecular weight of hemoglobin is 64,500 g/mol and the tissue density of the brain is 1.05, cerebral blood flow (mL/100 g/min) is

$$\frac{Hb \times 6.14}{[Hb]}$$

where Hb flow is in µmol/L/min and [Hb] is in g/dL.

The oxygen tracer technique has a major drawback in that it self-selects infants within a range of oxygen requirement. Infants who are saturating close to 100% in room air or in small amounts of oxygen cannot increase their oxygen saturations any further with an oxygen bolus. In addition, infants who are on or close to 100% oxygen cannot be given an oxygen bolus.

PHYSIOLOGICAL OBSERVATIONS USING NIRS

Oxygen Delivery

Oxygen delivery (D_{O_2}) is the total amount of oxygen delivered to the tissue per minute (48). Cerebral oxygen delivery is usually measured as mL of oxygen per 100 g of brain tissue per minute (mL/100g/min) (23).

Oxygen delivery can be calculated from the formula (23):

$$D_{O_2} = cardiac\ output \times arterial\ oxygen\ content$$

$$= cardiac\ output \times (oxygen\ bound\ to\ hemoglobin + dissolved\ oxygen)$$

$$= cardiac\ output \times [([Hb] \times Sa_{O_2} \times 1.39) + (dissolved\ oxygen)]$$

where 1.39 is the oxygen-carrying capacity of hemoglobin. As dissolved oxygen is negligible, D_{O_2} = cardiac output × ([Hb] × Sa_{O_2} × 1.39). While the above formula gives the oxygen delivery to the entire body, oxygen delivery to the brain = cerebral blood flow × ([Hb] × Sa_{O_2} × 1.39). Similarly, oxygen delivery to the peripheral tissue = peripheral blood flow × ([Hb] × Sa_{O_2} × 1.39).

Factors Determining Oxygen Delivery

From the equation D_{O_2} = cardiac output × ([Hb] × Sa_{O_2} × 1.39) it can be seen that the factors affecting oxygen delivery to the brain are blood flow, hemoglobin concentration, and arterial oxygen saturation. Any one of these measurements alone does not adequately describe oxygen delivery. For example, D_{O_2} to an organ may be inadequate due to decreased cerebral blood flow despite the presence of normal oxygen saturation and hemoglobin levels.

Effect of Anemia

Despite the importance of hemoglobin in oxygen transport, total hemoglobin concentration is a relatively poor indicator of the adequacy of the provision of oxygen to the tissues and may not accurately reflect tissue oxygen availability (45). This has been demonstrated in various studies using NIR spectroscopy and is summarized below.

Only a weak but statistically significant negative correlation was demonstrated between blood hemoglobin concentration and cerebral fractional oxygen extraction (FOE) in 91 preterm infants and between blood hemoglobin concentration and peripheral FOE ($n = 94$, $r = -0.21$, $P = 0.04$; Fig. 6-4) (16,18). The authors also

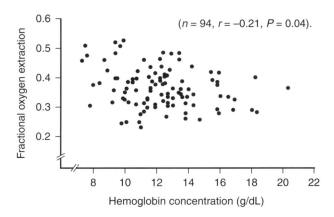

FIGURE 6-4 Correlation between Hb and peripheral fractional oxygen extraction. *Reproduced with permission from Wardle et al. Pediatr Res 1998;44:125.*

compared the cerebral FOE of anemic and non-anemic preterm infants with a relatively small difference in blood hemoglobin concentration between the two groups. There was no significant difference between the cerebral FOE of anemic compared with non-anemic preterm infants (18). However, cerebral FOE decreased immediately after blood transfusion, suggesting that acute changes may produce an effect (18).

Peripheral D_{O_2} increased while peripheral oxygen consumption remained constant after blood transfusion in asymptomatic but not in symptomatic anemic infants (45). In contrast, observations from animals and adult humans have shown little change in cerebral S_{VO_2} during anemic hypoxia (49,50).

Cerebral Oxygen Delivery

Cerebral D_{O_2} has been calculated using the measurements of cerebral blood flow in preterm infants (23). The median cerebral D_{O_2} in infants between 24 and 41 weeks gestation was 83.2 μmol/100 g/min (range, 33.2 to 172.3) (23). Cerebral D_{O_2} overall increases with gestational age ($n = 20$, $\rho = 0.56$, $P < 0.012$) (23) and particularly during the first three days after birth (Fig. 6-5) (51).

Cerebral Blood Flow

Mean global CBF is extremely low in preterm infants and increases with postnatal and gestational age (47). Using NIR spectroscopy, the median of CBF in preterm infants was 9.3 mL/100 g/min (range, 4.5 to 28.3) (23). Similar ranges have been reported by others using the same technique (1,25,42). The finding of extremely low CBF in preterm infants using NIR spectroscopy is consistent with measurements of CBF using the xenon clearance technique (53) and using positron emission tomography (54). Cerebral blood flow values of less than 5.0 mL/100 g/min in the normal or near normal brain of the preterm infant are considerably less than the value of 10 mL/100 g/min that is considered to be the threshold for viability in the adult human brain (55). The very low values of blood flow in the cerebral white matter in the human preterm infant also suggest that there is a small margin of safety between normal and critical cerebral ischemia (55).

Using the oxygen tracer technique and NIR spectroscopy, CBF was found to increase over the first three days after birth in infants between 24 and 31 weeks' gestation (1). In infants between 24 and 34 weeks' gestation, CBF was independent of mean arterial blood pressure and decreased with decrease in transcutaneous carbon dioxide levels (25).

NIR spectroscopy was used to investigate the effects of intravenously administered indomethacin (0.1 to 0.2 mg/kg) on cerebral hemodynamics and D_{O_2} in 13 very preterm infants treated for patent ductus arteriosus (51). Seven infants

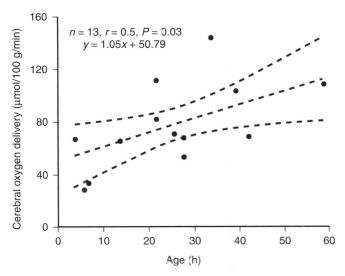

$n = 13$, $r = 0.5$, $P = 0.03$
$y = 1.05x + 50.79$

FIGURE 6-5 Plot of cerebral oxygen delivery against time from birth in hours. There is a significant increase in cerebral oxygen delivery during the measurement, demonstrated by using weighted Pearson correlation coefficient. *Reproduced with permission from Kissack CM et al. J Cereb Blood Flow Metab 2005;25:545.*

received indomethacin by rapid injection (30 s) and six by slow infusion (20 to 30 min) (56). In all infants CBF, Do_2, blood volume, and the reactivity of blood volume to changes in arterial carbon dioxide tension fell sharply after indomethacin (51). There were no differences in the effects of rapid and slow infusion (56).

Peripheral Blood Flow

As described earlier, NIR spectroscopy measures forearm blood flow from the data acquired by the venous occlusion technique (17,46,47). Using this technique De Blasi et al. found that the forearm blood flow in adults at rest was 1.9 ± 0.8 mL/100 mL/min, increasing after exercise to 8.2 ± 2.9 mL/100 mL/min (47). These values correlated well with those made using forearm plethysmography (47).

The partial venous occlusion technique was used to study peripheral oxygen delivery in hypotensive preterm infants between 26 and 29 weeks' gestation (16). In preterm infants, a significant correlation was determined between mean blood pressure and peripheral blood flow (Fig. 6-6) (16,57). Preterm infants with low mean arterial blood pressure of 25 mm Hg (range, 23 to 27) had median peripheral blood flow of 4.6 mL/100 mL/min (range, 3 to 5.97). This was significantly lower than the median peripheral blood flow of 8.3 mL/100 mL/min (range, 6.6 to 10.9) in infants with higher mean arterial blood pressure of 39 mm Hg (range, 30 to 47) (16).

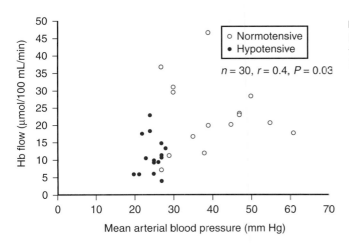

○ Normotensive
● Hypotensive

$n = 30$, $r = 0.4$, $P = 0.03$

FIGURE 6-6 Relationship between mean blood pressure and peripheral hemoglobin flow. *Reproduced with permission from Wardle et al. Pediatr Res 1999;45:343.*

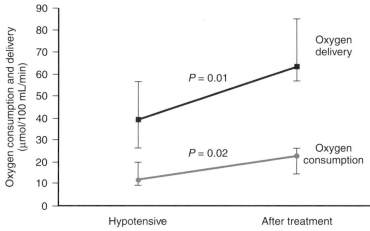

FIGURE 6-7 Changes in forearm oxygen delivery and oxygen consumption after treatment for hypotension. *Reproduced with permission from Wardle et al. Pediatr Res 1999;45:343.*

After treatment of hypotension, the median (interquartile range) forearm oxygen delivery increased significantly ($P = 0.01$) from 37.8 μmol/100 mL/min (25.7 to 59.5) to 64.2 μmol/100 mL/min (57.1 to 83.4) (Fig. 6-7) (16). The median (interquartile range) forearm oxygen consumption increased significantly ($P = 0.02$) from 11.0 μmol/100 mL/min (9.3 to 2.1.4) to 21.7 μmol/100 mL/min (15.9–26.1) (Fig. 6-7) (16).

In a study investigating peripheral oxygen delivery and anemia, forearm blood flow did not correlate with the HbF fraction or the red cell volume (45). Forearm blood flow did not change significantly after transfusion in symptomatic and asymptomatic anemic preterm infants (45). However, in the same study, there was a significant positive correlation between forearm blood flow and postnatal age (45).

Oxygen Consumption

Oxygen consumption (V_{O_2}) is defined as the total amount of oxygen consumed by the tissue per minute (48). The amount of oxygen required by a tissue depends on the functional state of the component cells. Some tissues like the brain, the liver, and the renal cortex have persistently high oxygen demands, while tissues like the spleen have low oxygen demands. Other tissues like the skeletal muscle have variable oxygen demands.

The units for cerebral V_{O_2} are mL of oxygen per 100 g of brain tissue per min (23). V_{O_2} can be calculated from the formula (23):

$$V_{O_2} = \text{cardiac output} \times (\text{arterial oxygen content} - \text{venous oxygen content})$$
$$= \text{cardiac output} \times \begin{bmatrix} ([Hb] \times S_{aO_2} \times 1.39) + (\text{dissolved O}_2) \\ -([Hb] \times S_{vO_2} \times 1.39) + (\text{dissolved O}_2) \end{bmatrix}$$

where 1.39 is the oxygen-carrying capacity of hemoglobin. Since $V_{O_2} =$ cardiac output $\times$ [Hb] $\times (S_{aO_2} - S_{vO_2}) \times 1.39$, cerebral or peripheral $V_{O_2} =$ cerebral or peripheral blood low $\times$ [Hb] $\times (S_{aO_2} - S_{vO_2}) \times 1.39$.

Cerebral Venous Oxygen Saturation and Consumption

By combining measurement of CBF using ^{133}Xe clearance and estimation of cerebral S_{vO_2} using NIRS and head tilt, cerebral V_{O_2} was calculated as 1.0 mL/100 g/min in nine preterm infants and 1.4 mL/100 g/min in 10 asphyxiated term infants (42).

We used NIR spectroscopy with partial jugular venous occlusion to determine cerebral SvO_2 and an oxygen bolus to measure CBF in 20 infants (median gestation, 27 weeks; range, 24 to 41 weeks) (23). The median cerebral VO_2 was 0.52 mL/100 g/min (range, 0.19 to 1.76) and it increased with maturity in line with cerebral DO_2 (see below) and, presumably, increasing cerebral metabolism (23).

Peripheral Venous Oxygen Saturation and Consumption

NIR spectroscopy has been used to study SvO_2 and VO_2 in the forearm of preterm infants. Peripheral SvO_2 when measured by co-oximetry was generally slightly higher than that measured by NIR spectroscopy, and this difference was more pronounced at higher levels of SvO_2 (21). This relationship was significant ($r = 0.528$, $P < 0.05$, $n = 16$).

In a study comparing forearm VO_2 in anemic preterm infants before and after blood transfusion, no differences were found (45). This was irrespective of whether infants were symptomatic or asymptomatic prior to transfusion (45).

Peripheral VO_2 increased significantly after treatment of hypotensive preterm infants (16). In that study, the treatment of hypotension consisted mainly of treatment with dopamine, which is known to stimulate metabolic activity particularly within muscle tissue (16).

The relationship between the use of dopamine and VO_2 has also been studied using NIR spectroscopy. In a study examining peripheral oxygenation in hypotensive preterm babies, treatment of hypotension using volume and/or dopamine increased forearm DO_2 and VO_2 but did not affect FOE (16). Low dose dopamine infusion in young rabbits did not alter cerebral hemodynamics and oxygenation (58).

Fractional Oxygen Extraction

Fractional oxygen extraction (FOE) is the amount of oxygen consumed as fraction of oxygen delivery (48). It has also been called "oxygen extraction ratio" (48), "oxygen extraction" (52), and "oxygen extraction fraction" (59). It is calculated as (18,48):

$$FOE = \frac{V_{O_2}}{D_{O_2}}$$

Since $VO_2 = $ cardiac output $\times [(Hb \times 1.39) \times (SaO_2 - SvO_2)]$ and $DO_2 = $ cardiac output $\times (Hb \times 1.39) \times SaO_2$, then by simplifying the equation,

$$FOE = \frac{Sa_{O_2} - Sv_{O_2}}{Sa_{O_2}}$$

Therefore FOE can be calculated if the SaO_2 and SvO_2 are known. SvO_2 is measured using the methods described above and peripheral SaO_2 is measured by pulse oximetry. The amount of oxygen dissolved in blood is considered to be negligible.

FOE varies from organ to organ and with levels of activity (15). Measurements of FOE for the whole body produce a range of approximately 0.15 to 0.33 (15). That is, the body consumes 15 to 33% of oxygen transported. The heart and brain are likely to have consistently high values of FOE during active states (15).

Cerebral FOE can be calculated using the formula (18):

$$cerebral\ FOE = \frac{cerebral\ V_{O_2}}{cerebral\ D_{O_2}}$$

$$= \frac{CBF \times [Hb] \times (Sa_{O_2} - Sv_{O_2}) \times 1.39}{CBF \times [Hb] \times Sa_{O_2} \times 1.39}$$

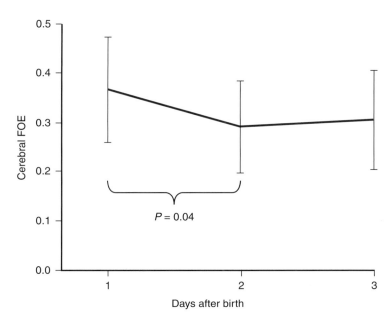

FIGURE 6-8 Changes in cerebral fractional oxygen extraction during the first three days after birth in sick extremely preterm infants. Data are plotted as means with standard deviations. There is a significant decrease in cerebral fractional oxygen extraction between days 1 and 2. *Reproduced with permission from Kissack CM et al. J Cereb Blood Flow Metab 2005;25:545.*

$$= \frac{Sa_{O_2} - Sv_{O_2}}{Sa_{O_2}}$$

Cerebral Sa_{O_2} is assumed to be equal to peripheral Sa_{O_2} as measured by pulse oximetry. The amount of oxygen dissolved in blood is considered to be negligible.

Using NIR spectroscopy and partial jugular venous occlusion in 41 preterm infants (median gestation, 29 weeks; range, 27 to 31 weeks), the mean cerebral FOE was 0.292 (SD = 0.06) (18). In that study, there appeared to be no relationship between cerebral FOE and gestational age or postnatal age (median, 9 days; range, 6 to 19 days) (18). However, when cerebral FOE was measured over the first three days after birth there was a significant decrease in cerebral FOE between days one and two suggesting an increase in CBF and cerebral oxygen delivery (Fig. 6-8) (14,51,57).

A major determinant of cerebral FOE is arterial carbon dioxide (18). A negative correlation between arterial carbon dioxide levels and cerebral FOE has been observed in studies on preterm neonates (18,60). The effect of arterial carbon dioxide on cerebral FOE is related to its effect on cerebral blood flow. The average increase in cerebral FOE with decrease in arterial carbon dioxide was 10.8%/kPa (range, 3.5 to 29) (Fig. 6-9) (18). This is considerably lesser than the reported decrease of 67% (range, 13 to 146) in CBF per kPa decrease in arterial carbon

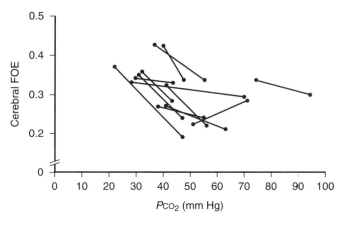

FIGURE 6-9 Relationship between cerebral fractional oxygen extraction (FOE) and P_{CO_2} within individuals. Measurements within individuals are linked by a line. *Reproduced with permission from Wardle et al. J Cereb Blood Flow Metab 2000;20:272.*

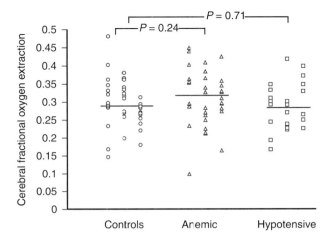

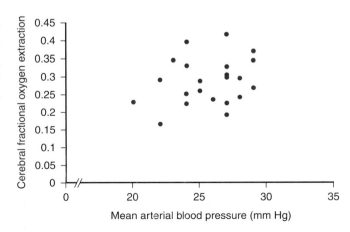

FIGURE 6-10 Cerebral fractional oxygen extraction was compared between three groups of preterm infants. The bar represents the mean value for each group. *Reproduced with permission from Wardle et al. J Cereb Blood Flow Metab 2000;20:272.*

dioxide using ^{133}Xe clearance (61). One possible reason for this may be that cerebral oxygen consumption does not remain constant (62,63), but decreases as a protective response to decreased cerebral oxygen delivery induced by hypocarbia.

Cerebral FOE was not increased in neonates who were considered "hypotensive" when compared with control subjects, and there was no change in cerebral FOE when the blood pressure returned to the normal range after treatment (Figs 6-10 and 6-11) (18). In that study, the median blood pressure was 25 mm Hg (range, 24 to 27 mm Hg) (18). This was confirmed by other studies examining the relationship between mean blood pressure and cerebral FOE at mean blood pressure levels above 20 mm Hg on the first three days after birth (14,57).

The critical level of blood pressure at which cerebral perfusion becomes compromised has not been clearly determined. A study relating CBF to mean blood pressure suggested that the critical level of mean blood pressure was below 23.7 mm Hg and that CBF at mean blood pressure levels above 23.7 mm Hg was independent of mean blood pressure (25). Since all three studies were not conducted at extremely low levels of mean blood pressure, the exact nature of the relationships between measures of cerebral oxygenation and mean blood pressure is still unknown.

Left ventricular output was found to have a weak but significant correlation with cerebral FOE (14). However, much of the relationship was due to two infants with high cerebral FOE. Of the 18 infants with low left ventricular output, cerebral FOE was elevated in only seven. Interestingly, these seven infants were simultaneously hypocarbic (14). This suggests that left ventricular output, which may be reduced by myocardial hypoxic ischemia as well as hypovolemia, is not an

FIGURE 6-11 Relationship between cerebral fractional oxygen extraction and mean arterial blood pressure in hypotensive group. *Reproduced with permission from Wardle et al. J Cereb Blood Flow Metab 2000; 20:272.*

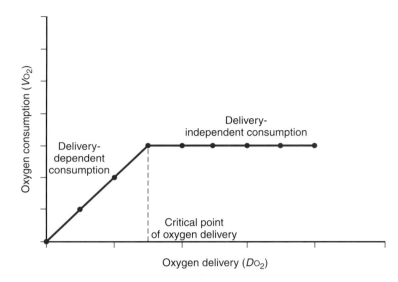

FIGURE 6-12 Biphasic model for oxygen delivery and oxygen consumption.

independent determinant of cerebral FOE. Rather, it seems probable that cerebral FOE is only elevated when left ventricular output is low in the presence of hypocarbia. None of these babies developed cerebral white matter injury. Nevertheless, the observation supports other evidence that hypocarbia is a potentially important cause of brain damage. It also adds weight to the proposition that the mechanism of damage when there is hypocarbia is through cerebral vasoconstriction and cerebral hypoperfusion.

Oxygen Delivery–Consumption Coupling

The relationship between cerebral Do_2 and Vo_2 has been described using the biphasic model (Fig. 6-12). This model was first described by Cain from animal work using dogs (64) and has subsequently been demonstrated in several other animal models (65) and in critically ill adults (66,67) and not in preterm babies. During the phase B–C, as metabolic demand increases or delivery decreases, FOE (Fig. 6-13) rises to maintain aerobic metabolism and consumption remains

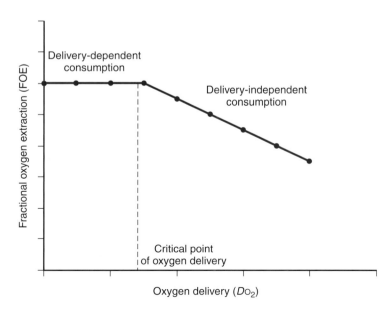

FIGURE 6-13 Biphasic model showing the relationship between oxygen delivery and fractional oxygen extraction.

independent of delivery (48). However at point B–called critical D_{O_2}–the maximum FOE is reached (48). In phase A–B, when V_{O_2} is delivery-dependent, any further increase in V_{O_2} or decline in delivery must lead to tissue hypoxia (48).

The clinical implication of this model is that, tissues, organs, or individuals may be expected to accommodate quite large changes in D_{O_2} without changes in function or critical damage unless D_{O_2} is severely curtailed. One mechanism by which the tissues appear to compensate is by increasing FOE. The exact mechanism by which this occurs is unknown. Since oxygen diffusion to the cell is entirely a passive process, it has been suggested that increased oxygen extraction occurs through capillary dilatation and recruitment (59). However, studies examining this have demonstrated little or no capillary dilatation (68–70). A theoretical model suggests that alterations in membrane diffusability may be responsible for increasing oxygen extraction (59). Another possible mechanism is through changing oxygen–hemoglobin dissociation. As arterial oxygen tension decreases, the affinity of oxygen to hemoglobin decreases dramatically due to the sigmoid shaped relationship. Furthermore, the position of the oxygen–hemoglobin dissociation changes with changing pH, as may occur if there is local hypoxia and consequent acidosis.

The biphasic model is based on the assumption that V_{O_2} remains constant during phase B–C. However, the situation *in vivo* is likely to be different and more complex. V_{O_2} regulates D_{O_2} under normal physiological conditions and D_{O_2} is likely to vary to ensure balance between delivery and consumption, at least till critical D_{O_2} is reached. At this time, further decreases in D_{O_2} result in falling V_{O_2} with diminished metabolism, although not initially hypoxic tissue damage.

Early Postnatal Adaptation

Serial measurements using NIR spectroscopy have been useful in determining postnatal adaptation in premature infants. There is evidence that cerebral D_{O_2} increases during the days after birth: cerebral FOE decreases (14) and there are increases in cardiac output (71), systemic blood pressure (72), and CBF (1). TOI increases during the first three days after birth (73). These observations suggest that the infant is particularly vulnerable to decreased cerebral D_{O_2} on the first day after birth and emphasize the importance of careful resuscitation and the need to maintaining physiologic stability during the hours after birth.

REFERENCES

1. Meek JH, Tyszczuk L, Elwell CE, Wyatt JS. Cerebral blood flow increases over the first three days of life in extremely preterm neonates. Arch Dis Child, Fetal Neonatal Ed 1998;78:F33–F37.
2. Meek JH, Tyszczuk L, Elwell CE, Wyatt JS. Low cerebral blood flow is a risk factor for severe intraventricular haemorrhage. Arch Dis Child, Fetal Neonatal Ed 1999;81:F15–F18.
3. Ijichi S, Kusaka T, Isobe K, et al. Developmental changes of optical properties in neonates determined by near-infrared time resolved spectroscopy. Pediatr Res 2005;58:568–573.
4. Dani C, Bertini G, Reali MF, et al. Brain hemodynamic changes in preterm infants after maintenance dose caffeine and aminophylline treatment. Biol Neonate 2000;78:27–32.
5. Urlesberger B, Pichler G, Gradnitzer E, et al. Changes in cerebral blood volume and cerebral oxygenation during periodic breathing in term infants. Neuropediatrics 2000;31:75–81.
6. Jöbsis FF, Keizer JH, LaManna JC, Rosenthal M. Reflectance spectrophotometry of cytochrome aa3 in vivo. J Appl Physiol 1977;43:858–872.
7. Irwin MS, Thorniley MS, Dore CJ, Green CJ. Near infra-red spectroscopy: a non-invasive monitor of perfusion and oxygenation within the microcirculation of limbs and flaps. Br J Plast Surg 1995;48:14–22.
8. Mancini DM, Bolinger L, Li H, Kendrick K, Chance B, Wilson JR. Validation of near-infrared spectroscopy in humans. J Appl Physiol 1994;77:2740–2747.
9. Stankovic MR, Maulik D, Rosenfeld W, et al. Role of frequency domain optical spectroscopy in the detection of neonatal brain hemorrhage – a newborn piglet study. J Matern Fetal Med 2000;9:142–149.

10. Tsuji M, duPlessis A, Taylor G, et al. Near infrared spectroscopy detects cerebral ischemia during hypotension in piglets. Pediatr Res 1998;44:591–595.

11. Fantini S, Hueber D, Franceschini MA, et al. Non-invasive optical monitoring of the newborn piglet brain using continuous-wave and frequency-domain spectroscopy. Phys Med Biol 1999;44:1543–1563.

12. Alfano RR, Demos SG, Galland P, et al. Time-resolved and nonlinear optical imaging for medical applications. Ann NY Acad Sci 1998;838:14–28.

13. Kissack CM, Garr M, Wardle SP, Weindling AM. Postnatal changes in cerebral oxygen extraction in the preterm infant are associated with intraventricular haemorrhage and haemorrhagic parenchymal infarction but not periventricular leukomalacia. Pediatr Res 2004;56:111–116.

14. Kissack CM, Garr R, Wardle SP, Weindling AM. Cerebral fractional oxygen extraction in very low birth weight infants is high when there is low left ventricular output and hypocarbia but is unaffected by hypotension. Pediatr Res 2004;55:400–405.

15. Wardle SP, Yoxall CW, Weindling AM. Cerebral oxygenation during cardiopulmonary bypass. Arch Dis Child 1998;78:26–32.

16. Wardle SP, Yoxall CW, Weindling AM. Peripheral oxygenation in hypotensive preterm babies. Pediatr Res 1999;45:343–349.

17. Wardle SP, Weindling AM. Peripheral oxygenation in preterm infants. Clin Perinatol 1999;26:947–966.

18. Wardle SP, Yoxall CW, Weindling AM. Determinants of cerebral fractional oxygen extraction using near infrared spectroscopy in preterm neonates. J Cereb Blood Flow Metab 2000;20:272–279.

19. Wardle SP, Weindling AM. Peripheral fractional oxygen extraction and other measures of tissue oxygenation to guide blood transfusions in preterm infants. Semin Perinatol 2001;25:60–64.

20. Yoxall CW, Weindling AM, Dawani NH, Peart I. Measurement of cerebral venous oxyhemoglobin saturation in children by near-infrared spectroscopy and partial jugular venous occlusion. Pediatr Res 1995;38:319–323.

21. Yoxall CW, Weindling AM. The measurement of peripheral venous oxyhemoglobin saturation in newborn infants by near infrared spectroscopy with venous occlusion. Pediatr Res 1996;39:1103–1106.

22. Yoxall CW, Weindling AM. Measurement of venous oxyhaemoglobin saturation in the adult human forearm by near infrared spectroscopy with venous occlusion. Med Biol Eng Comput 1997;35:331–336.

23. Yoxall CW, Weindling AM. Measurement of cerebral oxygen consumption in the human neonate using near infrared spectroscopy: cerebral oxygen consumption increases with advancing gestational age. Pediatr Res 1998;44:283–290.

24. Meek JH, Elwell CE, McCormick DC, et al. Abnormal cerebral haemodynamics in perinatally asphyxiated neonates related to outcome. Arch Dis Child, Fetal Neonatal Ed 1999;81:F110–F115.

25. Tyszczuk L, Meek J, Elwell C, Wyatt JS. Cerebral blood flow is independent of mean arterial blood pressure in preterm infants undergoing intensive care. Pediatrics 1998;102(2, Pt 1):337–341.

26. Wray S, Cope M, Delpy DT, Wyatt JS, Reynolds EO. Characterization of the near infrared absorption spectra of cytochrome aa3 and haemoglobin for the non-invasive monitoring of cerebral oxygenation. Bioch Biophys Acta 1988;933:184–192.

27. Mendelson Y, Kent JC, Mendelson Y, Kent JC. Variations in optical absorption spectra of adult and fetal hemoglobins and its effect on pulse oximetry. IEEE Trans Biomed Eng 1989;36:844–848.

28. van der ZP, Cope M, Arridge SR, et al. Experimentally measured optical pathlengths for the adult head, calf and forearm and the head of the newborn infant as a function of inter optode spacing. Adv Exp Med Biol 1992;316:143–153.

29. Duncan A, Meek JH, Clemence M, et al. Optical pathlength measurements on adult head, calf and forearm and the head of the newborn infant using phase resolved optical spectroscopy. Phys Med Biol 1995;40:295–304.

30. Duncan A, Meek JH, Clemence M, et al. Measurement of cranial optical pathlength as a function of age using phase resolved near infrared spectroscopy. Pediatr Res 1996;39:889–894.

31. Delpy DT, Arridge SR, Cope M, et al. Quantitation of pathlength in optical spectroscopy. Adv Exp Med Biol 1989;248:41–46.

32. Essenpreis M, Cope M, Elwell CE, Arridge SR, van der ZP, Delpy DT. Wavelength dependence of the differential pathlength factor and the log slope in time-resolved tissue spectroscopy. Adv Exp Med Biol 1993;333:9–20.

33. Naulaers G, Morren G, Van Huffel S, et al. Measurement of tissue oxygenation index during the first three days in premature born infants. Adv Exp Med Biol 2003;510:379–383.

34. Naulaers G, Cossey V, Morren G, et al. Continuous measurement of cerebral blood volume and oxygenation during rewarming of neonates. Acta Paediatr 2004;93:1540–1542.

35. Dullenkopf A, Kolarova A, Schulz G, Frey B, Baenziger O, Weiss M. Reproducibility of cerebral oxygenation measurement in neonates and infants in the clinical setting using the NIRO 300 oximeter. Pediatr Crit Care Med 2005;6:378–379.

36. Weiss M, Dullenkopf A, Kolarova A, Schulz G, Frey B, Baenziger O. Near-infrared spectroscopic cerebral oxygenation reading in neonates and infants is asiocated with central venous oxygen saturation. Paediatr Anaesth 2005;15:102–109.

37. Quaresima V, Sacco S, Totaro R, Ferrari M. Noninvasive measurement of cerebral hemoglobin oxygen saturation using two near infrared spectroscopy approaches. J Biomed Opt 2000;5:201–205.

38. Henson LC, Calalang C, Temp JA, Ward DS. Accuracy of a cerebral oximeter in healthy volunteers under conditions of isocapnic hypoxia. Anesthesiology 1998;88:58–65.

39. Kurth CD, Levy WJ, McCann J. Near-infrared spectroscopy cerebral oxygen saturation thresholds for hypoxia–ischemia in piglets. J Cereb Blood Flow Metab 2002;22:335–341.

40. Pollard V, Prough DS, DeMelo AE, Deyo DJ, Uchida T, Stoddart HF. Validation in volunteers of a near-infrared spectroscope for monitoring brain oxygenation in vivo. Anesth Analg 1996;82:269–277.

41. Watzman HM, Kurth CD, Montenegro LM, Rome J, Steven JM, Nicolson SC. Arterial and venous contributions to near-infrared cerebral oximetry. Anesthesiology 2000;93:947–953.

42. Skov L, Pryds O, Greisen G, Lou H. Estimation of cerebral venous saturation in newborn infants by near infrared spectroscopy. Pediatr Res 1993;33:52–55.

43. Wolf M, Duc G, Keel M, Niederer P, von Siebenthal K, Bucher HU. Continuous noninvasive measurement of cerebral arterial and venous oxygen saturation at the bedside in mechanically ventilated neonates. Crit Care Med 1997;25:1579–1582.

44. Owen-Reece H, Smith M, Elwell CE, Goldstone JC. Near infrared spectroscopy. Br J Anaesth 1999;82:418–426.

45. Wardle SP, Yoxall CW, Crawley E, Weindling AM. Peripheral oxygenation and anemia in preterm babies. Pediatr Res 1998;44:125–131.

46. Edwards AD, Richardson C, van der ZP, et al. Measurement of hemoglobin flow and blood flow by near-infrared spectroscopy. J Appl Physiol 1993;75:1884–1889.

47. De Blasi RA, Ferrari M, Natali A, Conti G, Mega A, Gasparetto A. Noninvasive measurement of forearm blood flow and oxygen consumption by near-infrared spectroscopy. J Appl Physiol 1994;76:1388–1393.

48. Leach RM, Treacher DF. The pulmonary physician in critical care * 2: oxygen delivery and consumption in the critically ill. Thorax 2002;57:170–177.

49. Borgstrom L, Johannsson H, Siesjo BK. The influence of acute normovolemic anemia on cerebral blood flow and oxygen consumption of anesthetized rats. Acta Physiol Scand 1975;93:505–514.

50. Paulson OB, Parving HH, Olesen J, Skinhoj E. Influence of carbon monoxide and of hemodilution on cerebral blood flow and blood gases in man. J Appl Physiol 1973;35:111–116.

51. Kissack CM, Garr R, Wardle SP, et al. Cerebral fractional oxygen extraction is inversely correlated with oxygen delivery in the sick, newborn, preterm infant. J Cereb Blood Flow Metab 2005;25:545–553.

52. Greisen G. Cerebral blood flow and energy metabolism in the newborn. Clin Perinatol 1997;24:531–546.

53. Pryds O, Greisen G, Skov LL, Friis-Hansen B. Carbon dioxide-related changes in cerebral blood volume and cerebral blood flow in mechanically ventilated preterm neonates: comparison of near infrared spectrophotometry and [133]xenon clearance. Pediatr Res 1990;27:445–449.

54. Altman DI, Powers WJ, Perlman JM, Herscovitch P, Volpe SL, Volpe JJ. Cerebral blood flow requirement for brain viability in newborn infants is lower than in adults. Ann Neurol 1988;24:218–226.

55. Volpe JJ. Neurobiology of periventricular leukomalacia in the premature infant. Pediatr Res 2001;50:553–562.

56. Edwards AD, Wyatt JS, Richardson C, et al. Effects of indomethacin on cerebral haemodynamics in very preterm infants. Lancet 1990;335:1491–1495.

57. Victor S, Weindling AM, Appleton RE, Beirne M, Marson AG. Relationship between blood pressure, electroencephalograms, cerebral fractional oxygen extraction and peripheral blood flow in very low birth weight newborn infants. Pediatr Res 2006;59:314–319.

58. Koyama K, Mito T, Takashima S, Suzuki S. Effects of phenylephrine and dopamine on cerebral blood flow, blood volume, and oxygenation in young rabbits. Pediatr Neurol 1990;6:87–90.

59. Hayashi T, Watabe H, Kudomi N, et al. A theoretical model of oxygen delivery and metabolism for physiologic interpretation of quantitative cerebral blood flow and metabolic rate of oxygen. J Cereb Blood Flow Metab 2003;23:1314–1323.

60. Victor S, Appleton RE, Beirne M, Marson AG, Weindling AM. Effect of carbon dioxide on background cerebral electrical activity and fractional oxygen extraction in very low birth weight infants just after birth. Pediatr Res 2005;58:579–585.

61. Greisen G, Trojaborg W. Cerebral blood flow, PaCO2 changes, and visual evoked potentials in mechanically ventilated, preterm infants. Acta Paediatr Scand 1987;76:394–400.

62. Rosenberg AA. Response of the cerebral circulation to profound hypocarbia in neonatal lambs. Stroke 1988;19:1365–1370.

63. Rosenberg AA. Response of the cerebral circulation to hypocarbia in postasphyxia newborn lambs. Pediatr Res 1992;32:537–541.

64. Cain SM. Oxygen supply dependency in the critically ill – a continuing conundrum. Adv Exp Med Biol 1992;317:35–45.

65. Adams RP, Dieleman LA, Cain SM. A critical value for O_2 transport in the rat. J Appl Physiol 1982;53:660–664.

66. Mohsenifar Z, Goldbach P, Tashkin DP, Campisi DJ. Relationship between O_2 delivery and O_2 consumption in the adult respiratory distress syndrome. Chest 1983;84:267–271.

67. Astiz ME, Rackow EC, Falk JL, Kaufman BS, Weil MH. Oxygen delivery and consumption in patients with hyperdynamic septic shock. Crit Care Med 1987;15:26–28.

68. Bereczki D, Wei L, Otsuka T, et al. Hypoxia increases velocity of blood flow through parenchymal microvascular systems in rat brain. J Cereb Blood Flow Metab 1993;13:475–486.

69. Pinard E, Engrand N, Seylaz J. Dynamic cerebral microcirculatory changes in transient forebrain ischemia in rats: involvement of type I nitric oxide synthase. J Cereb Blood Flow Metab 2000;20:1648–1658.

70. Seylaz J, Charbonne R, Nanri K, et al. Dynamic in vivo measurement of erythrocyte velocity and flow in capillaries and of microvessel diameter in the rat brain by confocal laser microscopy. J Cereb Blood Flow Metab 1999;19:863–870.
71. Evans N, Kluckow M. Early determinants of right and left ventricular output in ventilated preterm infants. Arch Dis Child, Fetal Neonatal Ed 1996;74:F88–F94.
72. Cunningham S, Symon AG, Elton RA, Zhu C, McIntosh N. Intra-arterial blood pressure reference ranges, death and morbidity in very low birthweight infants during the first seven days of life. Early Hum Dev 1999;56:151–165.
73. Naulaers G, Morren G, Van Huffel S, Casaer P, Devlieger H. Cerebral tissue oxygenation index in very premature infants. Arch Dis Child, Fetal Neonatal Ed 2002;87:F189–F192.

Chapter 7

Advanced Magnetic Resonance Neuroimaging Techniques in the Neonate with a Focus on Hemodynamic-related Brain Injury

Ashok Panigrahy, MD • Stefan Blüml, PhD

This chapter discusses the recent advances in magnetic resonance imaging (MRI) with a special focus on assessing hemodynamics and hypoxic ischemic lesions in the neonatal brain in an environment specifically adapted to meet the needs of critically ill preterm and term neonates when undergoing MRI studies. Specifically, MR diffusion imaging (both diffusion weighted imaging and diffusion tensor imaging) and MR spectroscopy are both used clinically to evaluate acute hypoxic ischemic injury to the neonatal brain. MR neonatal perfusion imaging and functional MR (fMR) are new emerging fields showing promise in directly and non-invasively evaluating cerebral blood flow (CBF) and the development of brain function, respectively. Each section will provide a brief description of the technique and briefly discuss the role of each technique in the evaluation of different pattern of brain injury in the neonate secondary to hypotension or cardiovascular arrest.

MAGNETIC RESONANCE-COMPATIBLE NEONATAL INCUBATOR AND NEONATAL HEAD COIL

MRI studies of critically ill preterm and term neonates are difficult because of the need to provide consistent, reliable and effective monitoring and support for respiratory and cardiovascular functions and fluid–electrolyte and thermoregulatory homeostasis throughout the examination. Thus, one needs to bring either the MRI suite to the neonatal intensive care unit (NICU) or the NICU to the MRI suite. Our approach has been to bring the NICU to the MRI suite, i.e. to develop the ability to provide uninterrupted intensive care including monitoring and full clinical support for critically ill preterm and term neonates while undergoing MRI studies. We have accomplished this by the use of an FDA-approved MR-compatible incubator (Lammers Medical Technology, Lübeck, Germany) and monitoring system (1).

In addition, manufacturers of MRI systems usually provide only general "one fits all" coils, i.e. a head coil designed for use in adults. However, this approach results in inferior image quality in children and, especially, newborns. Coils appropriately tailored to the body size of the neonate indeed offer superior signal-to-noise ratio (SNR) and image contrast for the neonatal patient population. Improvements in SNR, in turn, can be used to reduce scan time, improve image resolution, or do both.

By utilizing the MR-compatible incubator with air flow, humidity, and temperature regulation, monitoring and respiratory devices and specialized integrated radiofrequency head and body coils (Advanced Imaging Research Inc., Cleveland, Ohio, USA), we have recently demonstrated that this MR-compatible incubator provides a safe and controlled environment for critically ill preterm and term newborns (Fig. 7-1). In addition, we showed that the use of the integrated radiofrequency head and body coils optimized for newborns improves the quality of MRI (1).

DIFFUSION-WEIGHTED IMAGING AND DIFFUSION TENSOR IMAGING IN THE NEONATAL BRAIN

Diffusion-weighted MRI is based on the microscopic movement of water molecules in brain tissue (2). There are two basic imaging sequences that are being used to obtain quantitative information about water diffusion and the two images can be combined to calculate the apparent diffusion coefficient (ADC) map. The ADC map is an instrument- and MR sequence-independent parameter.

The second method is termed diffusion tensor imaging (DTI) (3–5), which uses a set of diffusion-weighted images to obtain a more complete picture of the water diffusion including quantitative parameters. These quantitative parameters correlate with sequences of myelination in the developing brain (5,6). DTI can be used for the evaluation of a neonate with hypoxic–ischemic brain injury and periventricular white matter injury. It can also be used to map white matter tracts because water movement across fibers is hindered by white matter elements (7,8) and to generate tractography data to evaluate selected tracts (i.e. optic radiations) in the neonate (Fig. 7-2).

QUANTITATIVE PROTON MRS OF THE NEONATAL BRAIN

The signal used by MRI to create anatomical maps is generated primarily by the hydrogen nuclei, also known as protons (^{1}H), of water molecules (H_2O). In contrast, ^{1}H MRS analyzes signal of protons attached to other molecules.

In neonates with hypotensive ischemic brain injury, early acute injury can be detected by MRS when both diffusion imaging and conventional imaging are negative (9–15). Within the first 24 h of injury, MRS can detect elevated levels of lactate in the cerebral cortex or basal ganglia depending on the pattern of injury. Reduced levels of N-acetyl-aspartate (NAA) and elevated glutamate/glutamine are then usually detected after 24 h (Fig. 7-3). The role of MRS in evaluating perinatal white matter injury is similar in the acute phase of injury, where initially lactate is elevated, then NAA is reduced and glutamate/glutamine is elevated. Knowledge of the normal developmental changes in MRS metabolites across development is necessary when interpreting pathologic cases (9–15).

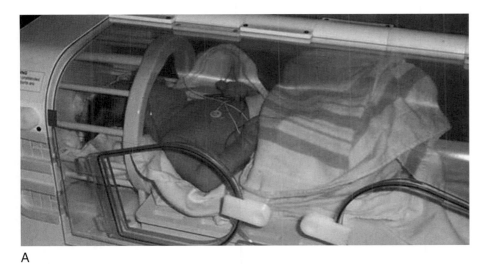

A

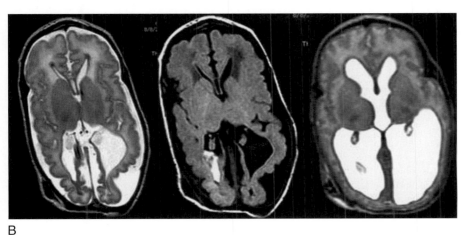

B

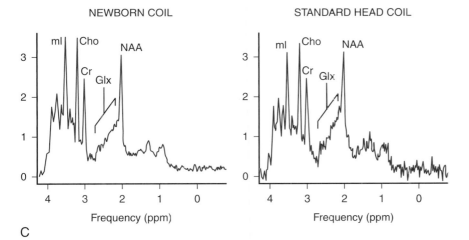

C

FIGURE 7-1 (A) MR-compatible incubator with a patient set-up for a MR examination. Physiological monitoring is performed using MR-compatible equipment. Note, that the specialized newborn head coil is already in place. (B) T2-weighted FSE MRI (left), FLAIR MRI (middle), and single-shot FSE image (right). (C) The improvement in signal-to-noise is demonstrated by two MR spectra acquired from two-months old babies with the newborn coil (left) and the standard head coil (right). The random noise signal at 0 ppm is approximately three times higher when the standard head coil was used.

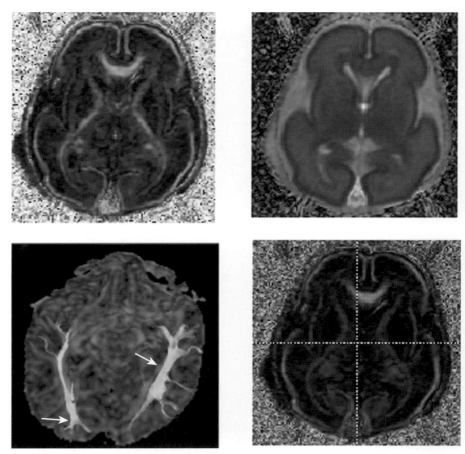

FIGURE 7-2 Diffusion tensor imaging of a preterm neonate (25 weeks' gestation, one week old) with fractional anisotropy map (top left), mean diffusivity map (top right), color direction specific (blue: cranial caudal; green: transverse; and red: anterior posterior) fractional anisotropy map (bottom right) and tractography of the optic radiations (bottom left). (See color plate.)

"Abnormal" peaks can also be observed after the ingestion of alcohol, using specialized diets (ketone bodies such as acetone after ketogenic diet (16)) or following the administration of large amounts of medications such as mannitol or propylene glycol solvent for drugs) (Fig. 7-4).

PERFUSION MAGNETIC RESONANCE IMAGING OF NEONATAL BRAIN INJURY

There are three major classes of MRI techniques that can measure perfusion in the brain. The first class is based upon the use of intravascular contrast agents, which can change the magnetic susceptibility of blood causing a change in the magnetic resonance signal. The second class of techniques is arterial spin-labeling (ASL), in which arterial blood is tagged magnetically before it enters the brain tissue being measured and then the amount delivered to the tissue is measured (17–19). The third class is based on the blood oxygenation level dependent (BOLD) effect, in which changes in blood oxygenation results in change in the magnetic resonance signal. Each technique is sensitive to specific perfusion states with the contrast method providing the best measurement of cerebral blood volume, the ASL technique is most useful in the measurement of CBF, and the BOLD technique is the most sensitive to the change in local oxygenation fraction. The BOLD technique is used for fMR discussed in the last section of this chapter.

In dynamic contrast to magnetic resonance perfusion techniques, gadolinium, a paramagnetic substance that does not cross the normally intact

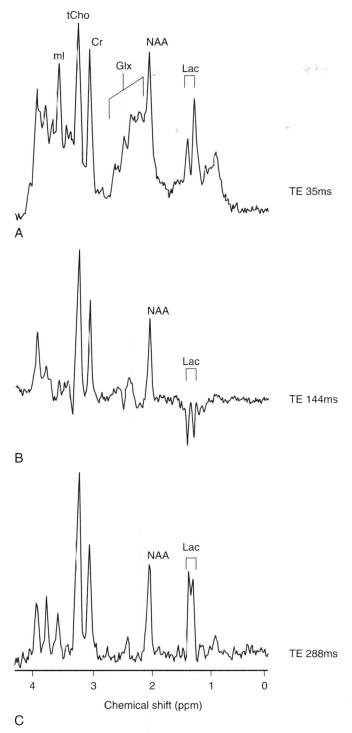

FIGURE 7-3 Single-voxel proton magnetic resonance spectroscopy (MRS) of the basal ganglia of a term infant with hypoxic–ischemic injury. The top figure (A) is a spectrum acquired using short echo time (35 ms), which shows a myoinositol peak (left side of the spectrum), elevated glutamate/glutamine peak next to a reduced NAA peak (middle spectrum), and an elevated lactate doublet next to a lipid peak (right side of the spectrum). The middle figure (B) is a spectrum acquired using long echo time (144 ms) showing a lactate doublet peak inverted and reduced NAA but with non-visualization of myoinositol, glutamate, and lipids. The bottom figure (C) is a spectrum acquired using even longer echo time (244 ms) and it is similar to Fig. 7-3B except that the lactate doublet has reverted.

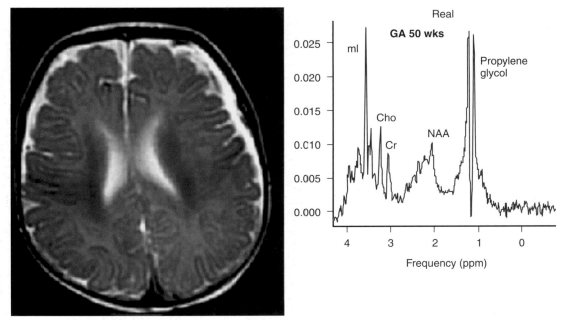

FIGURE 7-4 Short-echo proton magnetic resonance spectroscopy of occipital gray matter in a full-term neonate showing a propylene glycol (right) peak from a solvent used in medication being administered to the patient.

blood–brain barrier, is injected intravenously T2 or susceptibility weighted magnetic resonance images are then obtained (Fig. 7-5). As the contrast passes through the brain tissue, a magnetic field difference is created between the blood vessel filled with contrast and the surrounding brain tissue. The perfusion imaging dataset is used to create a signal intensity/time activity curve, and this curve is then used to calculate relative cerebral blood volume, relative CBF, and mean transit time. One study using dynamic susceptibility contrast-enhanced MRI demonstrated that maps of relative CBF could be acquired especially in more mature neonates (19). These authors found that relative CBF was greater in gray matter structures compared to white matter structures, which has also been our experience. Indeed, we have found that, depending on the timing of perfusion imaging performed relative to the acute hypoxic injury, there may be a relatively increased flow in region of acute infarction, which is probably related to luxury perfusion or increased metabolism (Fig. 7-6).

Pulsed (PASL) or continuous (CASL) arterial spin-labeling (ASL) (20–22) allows quantitative cerebral perfusion imaging without the use of exogenous contrast agents (Fig. 7-6). When pulsed ASL is used a quantitative perfusion map is calculated by mathematical formulas to account for the difference in magnetization/signal intensity between labeling and unlabeling images and relate the difference to regional CBF. Continuous ASL sequences use the same type of sequences except that the blood is contiguously tagged for a longer period of time on a thinner slab of tissue.

In one study, the PASL technique was used to quantify preoperative CBF in 25 infants with congenital heart disease (23). The mean CBF value for the cohort was 19.7 ± 9.1 mL/100 g/min. This value is less compared to that found in another study in healthy term infants (50 ± 3.4 mL/100 g/min), which calculated CBF using ^{133}Xe clearance methodology (24). In the study on neonates with congenital heart disease (23), periventricular leukomalacia (PVL) occurred in 28% of the cases (7/25) and was associated with decreased baseline CBF values. Recently, ASL has been performed with a 3 T magnet in neonates for evaluation of regional cerebral perfusion (25). Interestingly, this study found that perfusion in the basal

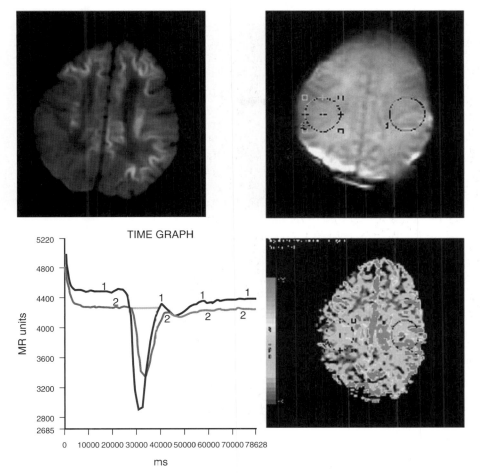

FIGURE 7-5 Dynamic contrast susceptibility perfusion magnetic resonance imaging (MRI) of hypoxic–ischemic injury in the neonatal brain. Top left: Diffusion map showing abnormal restricted diffusion in the bilateral cerebral cortex, left greater then right, with a "peripheral" pattern of injury. Top right: Gradient echo–echo planar magnetic resonance perfusion raw image obtained at the same level with placement of two ROIs. Bottom left: Time–activity curve showing the signal change over time of the contrast bolus through the region of interest. Bottom right: The generated cerebral blood volume map shows a relatively increased blood flow in the cortex relative to white matter and increased cerebral blood volume in the regions of acute infarction likely representing luxury compensatory reactive perfusion. (See color plate.)

ganglia (30–39 mL/100 g/min) was higher than in cortical gray matter (16–19 mL/100 g/min) or white matter (10–15 mL/100 g/min).

Of note, with reference to neonates suffering ischemia-related brain injury, we have found a large incidence of focal white matter necrosis in MRI studies in both preterm and term infants with congenital heart disease (26). In analyzing the neuropathology of 38 infants dying after cardiac surgery, we tested a set of questions related to the severity and patterns of brain injury, cardiopulmonary bypass (CPB), deep hypothermic circulatory arrest (DHCA), and age of the infants at the time of surgery. In all infants dying after cardiac surgery, irrespective of the modality, cerebral white matter damage (PVL or diffuse white matter gliosis) was the most significant lesion in terms of severity and incidence, followed by a spectrum of gray matter lesions. The patterns of brain injury were not age-related in the limited time-frame analyzed, except that infants who developed acute PVL after both closed and DHCA/CPB surgery (14/38 infants, 34%) were significantly younger at the time of death (median age 13.0 days) compared to unaffected infants (median age at death

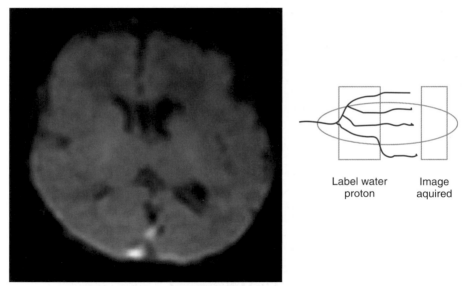

FIGURE 7-6 Left panel: Raw unprocessed arterial spin-labeled images acquired using FAIR (flow-sensitive alternating inversion recovery) technique in a full-term newborn signal with a focal area of cavitation seen near the left frontal horn. Note the high signal seen in the straight and the sagittal sinus near the level of the torcula. Also note that the signal intensity of the periventricular and deep white matter in decreased relative to the cortex. Right panel: A diagram showing how the arterial blood is tagged by a radio-frequency pulse. The arterial blood then flows into the imaging slice, where its magnetization results in change in signal intensity.

42.5 days) ($P = 0.031$). This observation suggests that the brain in the neonatal period (= 28 postnatal days) but not later is at risk for acute PVL even in term neonates, and likely reflects the vulnerability of immature (premyelinating) white matter to hypoxia–ischemia.

FUNCTIONAL MAGNETIC RESONANCE IMAGING IN THE NEWBORN PERIOD

The functional magnetic resonance imaging (fMRI) technique was introduced in 1992 by Ogawa et al. (27) and Kwong et al. (28) using repetitive MRI. Using rapid MRI acquisition they were able to observe transient changes in the magnetic resonance signal caused by hemodynamic changes. These changes occur when increased blood flow supplies more oxygen to the tissue than can be extracted by the cells. The oxygen content in the venous blood is increased, which reduces the magnetic susceptibility gradient between the capillary component and the surrounding parenchyma. As a result of this effect, known as the blood oxygen level dependent (BOLD) effect, the magnetic resonance signal of the effected brain region is increased by decreased $T2^*$ spin de-phasing. Since then, BOLD imaging has been widely adopted as an effective non-invasive method to detect blood flow changes associated with regional brain activation. The BOLD magnetic nesonance signal change can be observed about one second after the onset of a task, e.g. a hand movement, and reaches its maximum after about four seconds and remains at this maximum level during task performance. BOLD changes the magnetic resonance signal by 3 to 7% depending on the magnetic field strength of the magnetic resonance system and the brain region. In order to use the BOLD effect to image brain activation, one needs a $T2^*$ sensitive MRI sequence and the subject needs to alternate between activation and rest states (present and absent BOLD signal, respectively). Repetitive BOLD sensitive acquisition used while a participant is performing an alternating task/rest condition, e.g. finger tapping, results in a series of brain volumes which contain the BOLD magnetic resonance signal changes. These changes can be depicted by image processing and the statistical analysis of each voxel time-series of the brain volume. The result is a functional brain activation map, which shows 3D areas with or without BOLD changes during the specific task performed. Common practice is to visualize these brain maps laid on top of high-resolution anatomical images, because of the low spatial resolution of rapid functional BOLD imaging. The magnetic susceptibility of blood is altered depending on the blood concentration of deoxyhemoglobin.

Functional MRI is an established technique in the adult to measure brain activation from passive or active tasks performed during imaging. There have been studies of newborn fMRI as well, predominately of the visual system, although the auditory and sensory-motor systems have also been investigated (29). Because of their small head size, the use of the standard magnetic resonance head coils results in suboptimal picture quality in the neonate (30) affecting the ability to obtain high-quality fMRI studies. As mentioned earlier, to overcome these difficulties, we have utilized a magnetic resonance compatible incubator with a built-in radio-frequency head coil optimized for the neonatal brain volume (30). In this study we have demonstrated that fMRI and high-resolution structural MRI of the newborn brain can be achieved with this novel design. Since the onset and early postnatal development of hemispheric lateralization in the human brain are unknown, we also studied cortical activation induced by passive extension and flexion of the hand in neonates using fMRI (31). In contrast to that seen in older age groups, somatosensory areas in the pre- and postcentral gyri of the neonate showed no significant hemispheric lateralization at term. Rather, our findings from independent left- and right-hand experiments suggest the presence of an

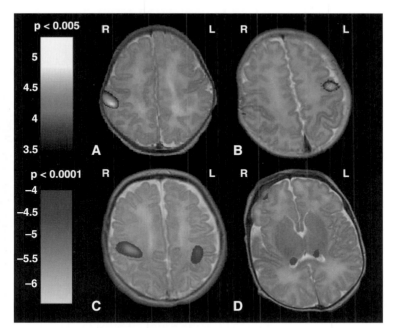

FIGURE 7-7 BOLD changes in sensorimotor areas and thalamus from passive extension and flexion stimulation. (A) Contralateral activation from left-hand stimulation of a 40-week gestation female (at 42-week postmenstrual age) newborn. (B) Right-hand stimulation of a 26-week gestation female (at 39-week postmenstrual age) newborn. Findings are comparable to adult results for sensorimotor activation. (C) Bi-hemispheric BOLD changes (36.4% during left-hand task and 31.3% during right hand of the population), which are unique for the newborn. Bilateral deactivation in a 40-week gestational age male (at 43 weeks postmenstrual age) newborn from left-hand stimulation. Additional significant BOLD changes have been found in frontal lobe and thalamus (41.7% of the population). (D) Thalamic deactivation in both hemispheres in a 39-week gestational age male (at 42 weeks postmenstrual age) newborn from left-hand stimulation. (See color plate.)

emerging trend of contralateral lateralization of the somatosensory system at around term gestation (Fig. 7-7). The slight although statistically insignificant advantage of contralateral dominance (9.1% left hand and 12.5% right hand) found in this study suggests a trend toward the lateralization we know in the mature human brain. Findings in infants confirm rapid maturation of lateralization and suggest the presence of a developmental step between birth and about two to six months of age. In addition, the symmetry between left- and right-hand findings confirms establishment of unilateral sensorimotor function and validates the methodological approach. In this context, a comprehensive fMRI study of somatosensory genesis in younger premature newborns (24 to 32 weeks' gestation) and somatosensory pruning in older infants (two to six months) reported for emerging language lateralization (32) would be intriguing. Taken these findings together, it appears that the somatosensory system is not specialized between midgestation and early postnatal life and appears to develop later through postnatal pruning (32).

In summary, recent advances in MRI technology have enabled us to investigate changes in total and regional CBF even in preterm neonates. However, much more data need to be collected within the framework of well-designed clinical studies to gain a deeper insight in the normal development of total and regional CBF regulation and the impact of brain injury and pathological processes on the regulation of CBF and oxygen delivery in the brain of the immature human neonate.

ACKNOWLEDGMENTS

The authors thank Hari Keshava (quantitative diffusion tensor measurements); Stephan Erberich PhD (neonatal fMRI); Marvin D. Nelson MD, Istvan Seri MD, PhD, and Floyd Gilles MD for support and advice; the staff of the Newborn and Infant Critical Care Unit and MRI program at CHLA. Grant support: Radiological Society of North American and Rudi Schulte Research Institute and NIH pediatric research loan repayment grant.

REFERENCES

1. Bluml S, Friedlich P, Erberich S, Wood JC, Seri I, Nelson MD. MR imaging of newborns by using an MR-compatible incubator with integrated radiofrequency coils: initial experience. Radiology 2002;231:594–601.
2. Beaulieu C. The basis of anisotropic water diffusion in the nervous system – a technical review. NMR Biomed 2002;15:435–455.
3. Le Behan D, Mangin JF, Poupon C, et al. Diffusion tensor imaging: concepts and applications. J Magn Reson Imaging 2001;13:534–546.
4. Basser PJ, Jones DK. Diffusion-tensor MRI: theory, experimental design and data analysis – a technical review. NMR Biomed 2002;5:456–467.
5. Wimberger DM, Roberts TP, Barkovich AJ, et al. Identification of "premyelination" by diffusion-weighted MRI. J Comput Assist Tomogr 1995;19:23–33.
6. Evans AC, for the Brain Development Cooperative Group. The NIH MRI study of normal brain development. Neuroimage 2006;30:184–202.
7. Mori S, Crain BJ, Chacko VP, et al. Three-dimensional tracking of axonal projections in the brain by magnetic resonance imaging. Ann Neurol 1999;45:265–269.
8. Basser PJ, Pajevic S, Pierpaoli C, et al. In vivo fiber tractography using DT–MRI data. Magn Reson Med 2000;44:625–632.
9. Kreis R, Hofmann L, Kuhlmann B, Boesch C, Bossi E, Hueppi PS. Brain metabolite composition during early human brain development as measured by quantitative in vivo 1H magnetic resonance spectroscopy. Magn Reson Med 2002;48:949–958.
10. Ernst T, Kreis R, Ross BD. Absolute quantitation of water and metabolites in the human brain. I. Compartments and water. J Magn Reson 1993;102:1–8.
11. Shu SK, Ashwal S, Hosouser BA, et al. Prognostic value of 1-H MRS in perinatal CNS insults. Pediatr Neurol 1997;17:309–318.
12. Hanrahan JD, Sargentoni J, Azzopardi D, et al. Cerebral metabolism within 18 hours of birth asphyxia: a proton magnetic resonance spectroscopy study. Pediatr Res 1996;39:584–590.
13. Holshouser BA, Ashwahl S, Luh GY, et al. Proton MR spectroscopy after acute central nervous system injury: outcome prediction in neonates, infants, and children. Radiology 1997;202:487–496.

14. Huppi PS, Posse S, Lazeyras F, et al. Magnetic resonance in preterm and term newborns: H-1 spectroscopy in developing brain. Pediatr Res 1991;30:574–578.
15. Vigneron DB, Barkovich AJ, Noworolski SM, et al. Three-dimensional proton MR spectroscopic imaging of premature and term neonates. Am J Neuroradiol 2001;22:1424–1433.
16. Seymour KJ, Bluml S, Sutherling J, Sutherling W, Ross BD. Identification of cerebral acetone by 1H-MRS in patients with epilepsy controlled by ketogenic diet. Magma 1999;8:33–42.
17. Ball Jr WS, Holland SK. Pefusion imaging in the pediatric patient. Magn Reson Imaging Clin N Am 2001;9:207–230.
18. Huisman TA, Sorenson AG. Perfusion-weighted magnetic resonance imaging of the brain: techniques and application in children. Eur Radiol 2004;14:59–72.
19. Tanner SF, Cornette L, Ramenghi LA, Miall, LS, Ridgway JP, Smith MA, Levene MI. Cerebral perfusion in infants and neonates: preliminary results obtained using dynamic susceptibility contrast enhanced magnetic resonance imaging. Arch Dis Child, Fetal Neonatal Ed 2003;88:F525–F530.
20. Detre JA, Leigh JS, Williams DS, Koretsky AP. Perfusion imaging. Magn Reson Med 1992;23:37–45.
21. Buxton RB, Frank LR, Wong EC, Siewert B, Warach S, Edelman RR. A general kinetic model for quatitative perfusion imaging with arterial spin labeling. Magn Reson Med 1998;40:383–396.
22. Detre JA, Aslop DC. Perfusion fMRI with are terial spin labeling based perfusion imaging techniques for MRI. In Functional MRI. Moonen CTW, Bandetti PA, eds. Heidelberg, Springer-Verlag, 1999:47–62.
23. Licht DJ, Wang J, Silvestre DW, et al. Preoperative cerebral blood flow is diminished in neonates with severe congenital heart defects. J Thorac Cadiovasc Surg 2004;128:841–849.
24. Greisen G, Borch K White matter injury in the preterm neonate: the role of perfusion. Dev Neurosci 2001;23:209–212.
25. Miranda MJ, Olofsson K, Sidaros K. Noninvasive measurements of regional cerebral perfusion in preterm and term neonates by magnetic resonance arterial spin labeling. Pediatr Res 2006;60:359–363.
26. Kinney HC, Panigrahy A, Newberger J, Jonas R, Sleeper LA. Hypoxic–ischemic brain injury in infants with congenital heart disease dying after cardiopulmonary bypass surgery. Acta Neuropathol (Berlin) 2005;110:563–578.
27. Ogawa S, Tank DW, Menon R, Ellermann JM, Kim SG, Merkle H, Ugurbil K. Intrinsic signal changes accompanying sensory stimulation: functional brain mapping with magnetic resonance imaging. Proc Natl Acad Sci USA 1992;89:5951–5955.
28. Kwong KK, Belliveau JW, Chesler DA, et al. Dynamic magnetic resonance imaging of human brain activity during primary sensory stimulation. Proc Natl Acad Sci USA 1992;89:5675–5679.
29. Seghier ML, Lazeyras F, Huppi PS. Functional MRI of the newborn. Semin Fetal Neonatal Med 2006;11:479–488.
30. Erberich SG, Friedlich P, Seri I, Nelson Jr MD, Bluml S. Functional MRI in neonates using neonatal head coil and MR compatible incubator. Neuroimage 2003;20:683–692.
31. Erberich GS, Panigrahy A, Friedlich P, Seri I, Nelson MD, Gilles F. Somatosensory lateralization in the newborn brain. Neuroimage 2006;29:155–161.
32. Dehaene-Lambertz G, Dehaene S, Hertz-Pannier L. Functional neuroimaging of speech perception in the infants. Science 2002;298:2013–2015.

Clinical Presentations of Neonatal Shock

Chapter 8

Clinical Presentations of Neonatal Shock: The VLBW Infant during the First Postnatal Day

Martin Kluckow, MBBS, PhD • Istvan Seri, MD, PhD

The birth of a very low birth weight (VLBW) infant creates a unique set of circumstances that can adversely affect the cardiovascular system resulting in cardiovascular compromise. The cardiovascular system of the fetus is adapted to an *in utero* environment that is constant and stable. The determinants of cardiac output, such as preload and afterload, are maintained in equilibrium without interference from the external factors that may affect a neonate born prematurely. Postnatal factors that can affect the cardiovascular function of the VLBW infant include perinatal asphyxia, positive pressure respiratory support, which may alter preload, and changes in afterload occurring with the rapid transition from the fetal circulation characterized by low systemic vascular resistance to the neonatal circulation with higher peripheral vascular resistance in the immediate transitional period. These changes of the transitional circulation combined with predominantly systemic to pulmonary shunts at the atrial and ductal level through persisting fetal channels, can further reduce potential systemic blood flow (Fig. 8-1).

The situation is further complicated by the difficulty in assessing the adequacy of the cardiovascular system in the VLBW infant. The small size of the infant and the frequent presence of shunting at both ductal and atrial level precludes the use of many of the routine cardiovascular assessment techniques used in children and adults to determine cardiac output. As a result clinicians are forced to fall back on more easily measured parameters such as the blood pressure. However, blood

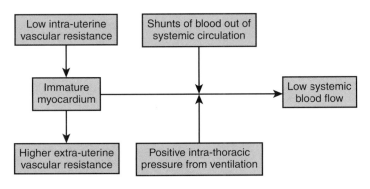

FIGURE 8-1 Suggested model of how the various external and internal influences on the cardiovascular system of the VLBW infant can result in low systemic blood flow.

pressure is but one measure of the cardiovascular system and changes in the blood pressure do not necessarily reflect changes in the cardiac output and subsequent changes in organ blood flow and tissue oxygen delivery (see Section I, Chapter 1 and Chapter 2).

Hypotension occurs in up to 30% of VLBW infants with between 16 and 52% of these infants receiving treatment with volume expansion and up to 39% receiving vasopressors (1). Similarly, low systemic blood flow in the first 24 h is seen in up to 35% of VLBW infants, but not all of these infants will have hypotension (2). There is a wide variation in the assessment and management of cardiovascular compromise both among institutions and individual clinicians (1). As with many other areas in medicine where there is variation in practice with multiple treatment options, the lack of good evidence for both when to treat cardiovascular compromise and whether treatment benefits the long-term outcome of infants, underlies this uncertainty. This chapter explores the importance of the unique changes involved in the transitional circulation during the first postnatal day and how they impact upon the presentation, assessment, and management of neonatal shock.

DEFINITION OF HYPOTENSION AND ITS RELATIONSHIP TO LOW SYSTEMIC PERFUSION

Hypotension can be defined as the blood pressure value where vital organ blood flow autoregulation is lost. If effective treatment is not initiated at this point, blood pressure may further decrease and reach the "functional threshold" and then the "ischemic threshold" resulting in neuronal dysfunction and tissue ischemia with permanent organ damage, respectively. The blood pressure causing loss of autoregulation or function, or the critical blood pressure resulting in direct tissue damage has not been clearly defined for the VLBW neonate in the immediate postnatal period (3). The distinction between the three levels of hypotension is important because, although loss of autoregulation and cellular function may predispose to brain injury, reaching the ischemic threshold of hypotension by definition is associated with direct tissue damage. Finally, these thresholds may be affected by several factors including gestational- and postmenstrual age, the duration of hypotension, and the presence of acidosis and/or infection.

In addition to the level of maturity and postnatal age, factors such as the pathogenesis of shock and illness severity may also influence the relationship between blood pressure, organ blood flow autoregulation and tissue ischemia. Although the normal autoregulatory blood pressure range is not known, in clinical practice there are generally two definitions of early hypotension in widespread use:

- Mean blood pressure less than 30 mm Hg in any gestation infant in the first postnatal days. This definition is based on pathophysiological associations between cerebral injury (white matter damage or intraventricular hemor-rhage) and mean blood pressure < 30 mm Hg (4,5) and to a lesser degree on more recent data looking at maintenance of cerebral blood flow (CBF) measured by near infra-red (NIR) spectroscopy over a range of blood pressures suggesting a reduction in CBF when a particular mean blood pressure threshold is reached (6,7). It is important to note that, although the 10th centile for infants of all gestational ages is at or above 30 mm Hg by the third postnatal day, in more immature infants the normal mean blood pressure is lower than 30 mm Hg during the first three days (8). Therefore, it is too simplistic to use a single cut-off value for blood pressure across a range of gestation and postnatal ages.

- Mean blood pressure less than the gestational age in weeks during the first postnatal days, which roughly correlates with the 10th centile for age in tables of normative data (4,9). This definition has also been supported by professional body guidelines such as the Joint Working Group of the British Association of Perinatal Medicine (10). Again this rule of thumb applies mainly in the first 24 to 48 h of extrauterine life – after this time there is a gradual increase in the mean blood pressure so that most premature infants have a mean blood pressure above 30 mm Hg by day 3 (9).

The current definitions are not related to physiologic endpoints such as maintenance of organ blood flow or tissue oxygen delivery. However, most (7,11,12) but not all (13) studies using ^{133}Xe clearance or NIR spectroscopy to assess changes in CBF found that the lower limit of the autoregulatory blood pressure range may be around 30 mm Hg even in the one-day-old extremely low birth weight (ELBW) neonate. Indeed, preterm neonates with a mean blood pressure at or above 30 mm Hg appear to have an intact static autoregulation of their CBF during the first postnatal day (14). It is reasonable to assume that, although the gestational age-equivalent blood pressure value is below the CBF autoregulatory range, this value is still higher than the suspected ischemic blood pressure threshold for the VLBW patient population (13).

A confounding finding to the straightforward-appearing blood pressure–CBF relationship has been provided by a series of studies using superior vena cava (SVC) flow measurements to indirectly assess brain perfusion in the VLBW neonate with a focus on the ELBW infant in the immediate postnatal period (2,15). The findings of these studies suggest that, in the ELBW neonate, blood pressure in the normal range may not always guarantee normal vital organ (brain) blood flow. In the compensated phase of shock, by redistributing blood flow from non-vital organs (muscle, skin, kidneys, intestine, etc.), neuroendocrine compensatory mechanisms ensure that blood pressure and organ blood flow to vital organs (brain, heart, adrenals) are maintained within the normal range. With progression of the condition, shock enters an uncompensated phase and blood pressure and vital organ perfusion decrease. Since the immature myocardium of the ELBW neonate may not be able to compensate for the sudden increase in peripheral vascular resistance immediately following delivery, cardiac output may fall (15,16). Yet, despite the decrease in cardiac output, many ELBW neonates maintain their blood pressure in the normal range by redistributing blood flow to the organs that are vital at that particular developmental stage. It is conceivable that the rapidly developing cerebral cortex and white matter of the ELBW neonate is not yet among the vital organs with appropriately developed autoregulatory capacity (12,15,16). However, by the second postnatal day, normal blood pressure is highly likely to be associated with normal brain and systemic blood flow (15,16). Thus, the vasculature of the cerebral cortex and white matter of the ELBW neonate may mature rapidly and become a "high-priority" vascular bed soon after delivery (16,17).

THE TRANSITIONAL CIRCULATION IN THE VLBW INFANT

The traditional understanding of the changes occurring in the transitional circulation of the preterm infant suggests that atrial and ductal shunts in the first postnatal hours are of little significance and are bidirectional or primarily right to left in direction as a result of the higher pulmonary vascular resistance expected in the newborn premature infant (18). In contrast to this understanding, longitudinal studies using bedside non-invasive echocardiography show significant variability in the time taken for the preterm infant to transition from the *in utero* right-ventricle dominant, low resistance circulation to the bi-ventricular higher resistance postnatal circulation. Shortly after delivery, the severing of the umbilical vessels, the inflation of the lungs with air, and the associated changes in oxygenation lead to a sudden increase in the resistance in the systemic circulation and a lowering of resistance in the pulmonary circulation. Cardiac output now passes in a parallel fashion through the pulmonary and the systemic circulation except for the blood flow shunting through the closing fetal channels.

In normal full-term infants the ductus arteriosus is functionally closed by the second postnatal day and the right ventricular pressure usually falls to adult levels by about two to three days after birth (19,20). This constriction and functional closure of the ductus arteriosus is then followed by anatomical closure over the next two to three weeks. In contrast, in the VLBW infant there is frequently a failure of complete closure of both the foramen ovale and the ductus arteriosus in the expected time frame, probably due to immaturity of the mechanisms involved (21,22). The persistence of the fetal channels leads to blood flowing preferentially from the aorta to pulmonary artery resulting in a relative loss of blood from the systemic circulation and excessive blood being passed through the pulmonary circulation. Contrary to traditional understanding, this systemic to pulmonary shunting can occur as early as the first postnatal hours, with recirculation of 50% or more of the normal cardiac output back into the lungs (23). The myocardium subsequently attempts to compensate by increasing the total cardiac output. There can be up to a twofold increase in the left ventricular (LV) output by one hour of age, resulting primarily from an increased stroke volume, rather than increased heart rate (24). A significant proportion of this increased blood flow is likely to be passing through the ductus arteriosus (25). There is a wide range of early ductal constriction, with some infants able to effectively close or minimize the size of the ductus arteriosus within a few hours of birth whilst others achieve an initial constriction followed by an increase in size of the ductus and yet another group having a persistent large ductus arteriosus with no evidence of early constriction and subsequent limitation of shunt size (26). In this early postnatal period both ductal and atrial shunts are frequently large in size and the direction of shunting is predominantly left to right, i.e. systemic to pulmonary. This results in an increase in the pulmonary blood flow relative to the systemic blood flow and movement of blood flow away from the systemic circulation. Again, contrary to traditional beliefs, pulmonary blood flow can be more than twice the systemic blood flow as early as the first few postnatal hours (26). This amount of pulmonary blood flow may be enough to cause clinical effects, such as reduced systemic blood pressure and blood flow, increases in ventilatory requirements or even pulmonary hemorrhagic edema.

In utero, the fetal communications of the foramen ovale and ductus arteriosus result in a lack of separation between the left and right ventricular outputs, making it difficult to quantitate their individual contributions. In addition to heart rate, the ventricular systolic function is determined by the physiological principles of preload (distension of the ventricle by blood prior to contraction), contractility (the intrinsic ability of the myocardial fibers to contract), and afterload (the combined resistance of the blood, the ventricular walls, and the vascular beds). The myocardium of the VLBW infant is less mature than that of a term infant with fewer mitochondria and less energy stores. This results in a limitation in the ability to respond to changes in the determinants of the cardiac output, in particular the afterload (27). Consequently the myocardium of the VLBW infant, just like the fetal myocardium, is likely to be less able to respond to stresses that occur in the postnatal period such as increased peripheral vascular resistance with the resultant increase in afterload. There is a significant difference in the influence of determinants of cardiac output in the newborn premature infant with a dramatically increased afterload and changes in the preload caused by the inflation of the lungs. Furthermore, the effect of lung inflation on preload is different when lung inflation occurs by positive pressure ventilation rather than by the negative intrathoracic pressures generated by spontaneous breathing. The newborn ventricle is more sensitive to changes in the afterload, such that small changes can have large effects especially if the preload and contractility are not optimized (27).

Failure of the normal transitional changes to occur in a timely manner can result in impairment of cardiac function leading to low cardiac output states and hypotension in the VLBW infant. As oxygen delivery is primarily related to both the oxygen content of the blood and to the volume of blood flow to the organ (28), delivery of oxygen to vital organs may be impaired where there is cardiovascular impairment. Therefore, the timely identification and appropriate management of early low cardiac output states and hypotension is of vital importance in the overall care of the VLBW infant.

Physiological Determinants of the Blood Pressure in the VLBW Infant

The product of cardiac output and peripheral vascular resistance determines arterial blood pressure. The main influences on the cardiac output are the preload or blood volume and myocardial contractility. The peripheral vascular resistance is determined by the vascular tone, which in the presence of an unconstricted ductus arteriosus may not only be the systemic peripheral vascular resistance, but is also contributed to by the pulmonary vascular resistance. Myocardial contractility is difficult to assess in the newborn as the accepted measures of contractility in the adult, such as the echocardiographic measure of fractional shortening, are adversely influenced by the asymmetry of the ventricles caused by the *in utero* right ventricular dominance. In this regard, use of load independent measures of cardiac contractility, such as mean velocity of fractional shortening or LV wall stress indices, may provide more useful information (29); see also Section II, Chapter 5 (Fig. 8-2). Some studies have found a relationship between myocardial

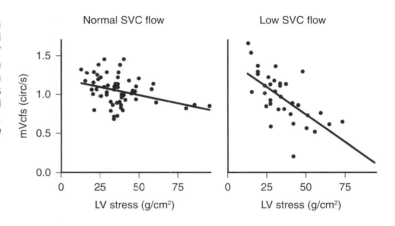

FIGURE 8-2 Relationship between mean velocity of circumferential fiber shortening (mVCFs) and LV wall stress at 3 h in infants with low and normal superior vena cava (SVC) flows in the first 24 h. Infants who developed low SVC flow had reduced LV contractility ($P=0.02$). *Reproduced with permission from Osborn et al. (29).*

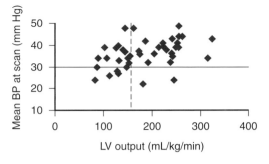

FIGURE 8-3 **The weak relationship between mean systemic blood pressure and simultaneously measured left ventricular (LV) output.** Some infants with a mean blood presure (BP) greater than 30 mm Hg have critically low cardiac output (<150 mL/kg/min) and conversely some infants with normal LV output have low mean blood pressure. *Reproduced with permission from Kluckow and Evans (31).*

dysfunction and hypotension in the preterm infant (30) whilst others have not (31), even though a similar measurement method was used. Similarly, blood volume correlates poorly with blood pressure in hypotensive neonates (32,33). Due to the unique characteristics of the newborn cardiovascular system discussed earlier, systemic blood pressure is closely related to changes in the systemic vascular resistance. As systemic vascular resistance cannot be measured directly, the measurement of cardiac output or systemic blood flow becomes an essential element in understanding the changes occurring in the cardiovascular system of the VLBW infant.

In the absence of measurement of cardiac output and systemic vascular resistance, clinicians have tended to rely on blood pressure as the sole assessment of circulatory compromise. However, in the VLBW neonate with a closed ductus arteriosus during the first 24 to 48 h, there is only a weak relationship between mean blood pressure and cardiac output (31) (Fig. 8-3). Relying on measurements of blood pressure alone can lead the clinician to make assumptions about the underlying physiology of the cardiovascular system that may not be correct especially during the period of early transition with the fetal channels open. Indeed, many hypotensive preterm infants potentially have a normal or high left ventricular output (31,34,35). One of the reasons for this apparent paradox relates to the presence of a hemodynamically significant ductus arteriosus, which causes an increase in left ventricular output whilst also causing a reduction in the overall systemic vascular resistance. Variations in the peripheral vascular resistance may cause a change in the underlying cardiac output that does not affect the blood pressure. This phenomenon makes it possible for two infants with the same blood pressure to have markedly different cardiac outputs. Thus, the physiologic determinants of blood pressure may affect the blood pressure in multiple ways – acting via an effect on cardiac performance and thus cardiac output, altering the vascular resistance or sometimes altering both.

Clinical Determinants of Blood Pressure in the VLBW Infant

Gestational Age and Postnatal Age

Both gestational age and postnatal age are major determinants of the systemic blood pressure as can be seen by examining nomograms and tables of normal blood pressure data (see Section I, Chapter 3). Generally blood pressure is higher in more mature infants and progressively increases with advancing postnatal age. The reasons why blood pressure increases with postnatal age are unclear but are probably related to changes in the underlying vascular tone mediated by various humoral regulators and possibly upregulation of receptors involved in myocardial responses. Simultaneously, there are temporal physical changes in the transitional circulation such as closure of the ductus arteriosus, which will affect both blood pressure and blood flow.

Use of Antenatal Glucocorticoid Therapy

There is evidence that a significant number of sick VLBW infants have relative adrenal insufficiency and that this condition may be one of the underlying causes of cardiovascular dysfunction and the propensity to inflammation in these patients contributing to the pathogenesis of clinical conditions such as bronchopulmonary dysplasia (36–38). Low cortisol levels have been documented in hypotensive infants requiring inotropic support (39). The use of antenatal glucocorticoids to assist in fetal lung maturation may therefore have an additional effect of improving neonatal blood pressure. Likely mechanisms for this effect include the acceleration of cardiovascular adrenergic receptor expression and maturation of myocardial structure and function. The enhanced adrenergic receptor expression also increases the sensitivity of the myocardium and peripheral vasculature to endogenous catecholamines (40). Randomized controlled trials of the use of antenatal glucocorticoids have shown variable effects on the neonatal blood pressure. In some, there was an increase in the mean blood pressure of VLBW infants in the treated group with a decreased need for vasopressor/inotropic support (41,42), whilst others have shown little difference between the mean blood pressures of infants whose mothers did or did not receive antenatal steroids (43,44).

Blood Loss

Acute blood loss in the VLBW infant can result from prenatal events such as fetomaternal hemorrhage, antepartum hemorrhage or twin–twin transfusion syndrome, intrapartum events such as a tight nuchal cord resulting in an imbalance between blood flow to and from the fetus, or postnatally from a large subgaleal hematoma or hemorrhage into an organ such as the liver or brain. Acute blood loss can result in significant hypotension but due to the immediate compensatory mechanisms of the cardiovascular system this effect may be delayed. Similarly, a drop in the infant's hemoglobin level can also be delayed following significant hemorrhage.

Positive Pressure Ventilation

Many VLBW infants are exposed to positive pressure respiratory support in the first postnatal days. Positive end expiratory pressure (PEEP) or nasal continuous positive airway pressure (CPAP) is often utilized to reduce the atelectasis resulting from collapse of unstable alveoli when surfactant is lacking, particularly in more immature infants. Although surfactant deficiency is the main reason for provision of positive pressure support, there is also a contribution from sepsis and immaturity of the lungs without surfactant deficiency. The use of high ventilation pressures in the premature infant who has a relatively small chest can result in secondary interference with cardiac function. Function can be impaired by a reduction in the preload from reduced systemic or pulmonary venous return, or direct compression of cardiac chambers resulting in a reduced stroke volume or an increase in afterload. This latter scenario is particularly concerning for the right ventricle (RV) and may reduce cardiac output. As the right and left sides of the heart are connected in series, a reduction in the RV output will also result in a reduction in the LV cardiac output.

Studies in VLBW infants have shown a fall off in the systemic oxygen delivery if the PEEP was greater than 6 cm of water and a reduction in the cardiac output at a PEEP level of 9 cm water (45) in mechanically ventilated infants. A study of VLBW infants (mean gestational age 29 weeks) before and during treatment with mechanical ventilation for severe respiratory distress syndrome demonstrated a reduction in left ventricular dimensions and filling rate with a resultant decrease in the cardiac output by about 40% compared to control values. The addition of a packed cell blood transfusion prevented the decrease in ventricular size and reduction in cardiac output (46). The blood pressure did not change significantly in the group where cardiac output dropped. In longitudinal clinical studies of blood pressure and blood flow, mean airway pressure has a consistently negative influence on both mean blood pressure (31,47) and systemic blood flow (15,48).

Patent Ductus Arteriosus

A patent ductus arteriosus may not be recognized clinically in the first days after delivery as the flow through it is generally not turbulent and therefore no murmur is audible (49). Despite this, the flow is almost always left to right or bidirectional with a predominantly left to right pattern (23). A patent ductus arteriosus is usually thought to be associated with a low diastolic blood pressure (BP) but some data suggest that it can be associated with both low diastolic and systolic BP, making a patent ductus arteriosus one of the possible causes of systemic hypotension (50). As clinical detection of a patent ductus arteriosus in the first postnatal days is difficult (49), an echocardiogram is required for early diagnosis. The classical clinical signs of a murmur, bounding pulses and a hyperdynamic precordium, usually become evident only after the third postnatal day making clinical detection much more accurate at that time (49).

Systemic Vascular Resistance

There is a reciprocal relationship between the systemic vascular resistance and cardiac output in the healthy term, preterm, and sick ventilated infant (51). This relationship is particularly important when considering the use of vasopressor-inotropes such as dopamine in preterm infants where an increase in the peripheral vascular resistance can increase the blood pressure but have no impact on, or even decrease, the cardiac output (52). The peripheral resistance varies markedly in the preterm infant and can be affected by numerous factors, including environmental temperature, carbon dioxide level (51), the maturity of the sympathoadrenal system (53), patency of the ductus arteriosus (26), presence of vasoactive substances such as catecholamines, prostacyclin, and nitric oxide, and sepsis. It is important to remember that, in patients with a patent ductus arteriosus, the left ventricle is exposed to the combined pulmonary and systemic vascular resistance. The potential variability of the peripheral resistance in VLBW infants means that significant changes in cardiac output or blood flow cannot be identified by measurement of the systemic blood pressure alone.

ASSESSMENT OF CARDIOVASCULAR COMPROMISE IN THE SHOCKED VLBW INFANT

Because of the wide variation in blood pressure levels at varying gestations and postnatal ages, some authors have cautioned against the simplicity of just treating low BP alone but suggest that the clinician should look for some other evidence of hypoperfusion such as increased capillary return, oliguria, or metabolic acidosis (54). The assessment of the cardiovascular adequacy in the VLBW infant is more of a challenge than in infants and adults. Measures of cardiovascular function used in these groups, such as pulmonary wedge pressure, central venous pressure, and cardiac output measured via thermodilution, are impractical in the preterm infant due to their size and fragility and the frequent presence of cardiac shunting. Assessment usually consists of a mainly clinical appraisal of the perfusion via capillary refill time (CRT) and urine output and the documentation of the pulse rate and blood pressure. The acid base balance and evidence of lactic acidosis are a further adjunct to this assessment but, unless serum lactate levels are serially monitored, monitoring changes in pH and base deficit may be misleading due to the increased bicarbonate losses through the immature kidneys. Indeed, the use of all of these parameters have limitations in the newborn and particularly in the VLBW infant.

Capillary Refill Time

Although CRT is a widely utilized proxy of both cardiac output and peripheral resistance in neonates, normal values have only recently been documented for this group of infants (55). A number of confounding factors lead to the CRT being potentially inaccurate and these include the different techniques used (sites tested and pressing time), inter-observer variability, ambient temperature (56), medications, and maturity of skin blood flow control mechanisms. In addition, even in older children receiving intensive care, there is only a weak relationship between the CRT and other hemodynamic measures such as the stroke volume index (57). A recent study investigating the relationship between a measure of systemic blood flow (superior vena cava (SVC) flow) and CRT in VLBW infants showed that a CRT of 3 s had only 55% sensitivity and 81% specificity for predicting low systemic blood flow. However, a markedly increased CRT of 4 s or more was more closely correlated with low blood flow states (58).

Urine Output

Following urine output is useful in the assessment of cardiovascular wellbeing in the adult; however, the immature renal tubule in VLBW infants is inefficient at concentrating the urine and therefore may be unable to appropriately reduce urine flow in the face of high serum osmolality (59). As a result, even if the glomerular filtration rate is decreased markedly, there can be little or no change in urine output. In addition, accurate measurement of urine output is not easy in VLBW infants, generally requiring collection via a urinary catheter or via a collection bag, both techniques being invasive with significant potential complications.

Pulse Rate

A rising pulse rate is usually indicative of hypovolemia in the adult. The mechanism relies on a mature autonomic nervous system, with detection of reduced blood volume and then blood pressure via baroreceptors and subsequent increase in the heart rate in an attempt to sustain appropriate cardiac output. Neonates, especially preterm infants, have a faster baseline heart rate and immature myocardium and autonomic nervous system, potentially affecting the cardiovascular response to hypovolemia. There are many other influences on the heart rate in the immediate postnatal period so it cannot be relied upon as an accurate assessment of cardiovascular status.

Metabolic Acidosis/Lactic Acidosis

Tissue hypoxia, due to low arterial oxygen tension, inadequate blood flow, or a combination of these two factors, results in a switch to anaerobic metabolism at the cellular level. Reduced systemic blood flow may therefore result in an increase in the serum lactate. Serum lactate levels have been correlated with illness severity and mortality in critically ill adults (60–64) and in ventilated neonates with respiratory distress syndrome (62,65–67). The normal lactate level in this group of infants is less than 2.5 mmol/L (65,66) and there is an association with mortality as the serum lactate level increases above this threshold.

compensate for the decreased oxygen delivery any more. In addition, the documented increase in the cardiac output (or systemic blood flow) in some VLBW infants with hypotension may be an additional compensatory mechanism preserving oxygen delivery to the brain.

Several studies have suggested that autoregulation is intact in many preterm babies but appears to be compromised in a subgroup who seem to be at particularly high risk of peri/intraventricular hemorrhage (PIVH) (80,81). It has been suggested that infants suffering severe PIVH are more likely to have blood pressure passive changes in cerebral blood flow (4–7,82) and oxygenation in the first postnatal days.

Peri/Intraventricular Hemorrhage

A number of studies have described associations between low mean blood pressure and subsequent PIVH and neurological injury (4,5,83–86). It was these observations of an association between systemic blood pressure and cerebral injury that led to current recommendations for treatment of blood pressure. Despite these statistical associations, a large population based study has not found systemic hypotension to be an independent risk factor for PIVH in VLBW infants (87). Furthermore, there is no evidence from appropriately designed, prospective, controlled clinical trials that treatment of hypotension decreases the incidence of PIVH and neurological injury.

Periventricular Leukomalacia

The potential relationship between low cerebral blood flow and white matter injury due to the specific vulnerability of the periventricular white matter in the preterm infant has led to concerns that hypotension may be a precursor of white matter injury. Observational data again have shown a relationship between hypotension (often mean arterial blood pressure below 30 mm Hg) and adverse cranial ultrasound findings (5). However, as with P/IVH, larger population-based studies have failed to identify systemic hypotension as an independent risk factor for white matter injury (88,89). It is conceivable that the pathogenesis of periventricular leukomalacia (PVL) just like that of PIVH, is multifactorial and, in addition to changes in cerebral perfusion pressure, factors such as specific or nonspecific inflammation and oxidant injury play a significant role in its development.

Long-term Neurodevelopmental Outcome

Hypotension in VLBW infants has been correlated with longer term adverse neurodevelopmental outcome (85,86,90,91). A study of systemic blood flow in VLBW infants demonstrated an independent relationship between low systemic blood flow (particularly the duration of the insult) and adverse neurodevelopmental outcome at three years of age (92).

TREATMENT OPTIONS IN THE MANAGEMENT OF CARDIOVASCULAR COMPROMISE/SHOCK IN THE VLBW INFANT

The appropriate management of shock in the VLBW infant will vary according to the underlying physiology. The clinician must take into account a number of possible factors, including the infant's gestational age, postnatal age, measures of cardiovascular adequacy such as cardiac output or systemic blood flow if available, and associated pathological conditions. An early echocardiogram can assist greatly in the diagnostic process by providing information about the presence, size, and direction of the ductus arteriosus shunt, presence of pulmonary hypertension, assessment of cardiac contractility, adequacy of venous filling, and measurement of cardiac output or systemic blood flow.

Prior to instituting specific treatment for hypotension potentially reversible causes such as a measurement error (transducer height in comparison to patient's right atrium, calibration of the transducer, air bubble, or blood, clot in the measurement catheter), patent ductus arteriosus, hypovolemia from blood or fluid loss, pneumothorax, use of excessive mean airway pressure, sepsis, and adrenocortical insufficiency should be considered and managed appropriately. Therapeutic options that have a physiologic basis for efficacy and have been subjected to clinical trial include volume loading (with crystalloid or colloid), vasopressor/inotropes and inotropic agents, and hydrocortisone and other glucocorticoids. Table 8-1 suggests an approach to the use of these therapies according to the likely underlying mechanism of cardiovascular compromise and Table 8-2 summarizes the data regarding each individual intervention.

Closing the Ductus Arteriosus

A large and unconstricted ductus arteriosus has been associated with hypotension on the first postnatal day (50). Early assessment of the ductus arteriosus in infants who are hypotensive for no obvious reason may demonstrate a large PDA that could be closed using a cyclooxygenase inhibitor such as indomethacin or ibuprofen. There are no trials of the use of cyclooxygenase inhibitors being used primarily to treat hypotension, however, there is some evidence that they assist in maintenance of normal systemic blood flow (93). The trials of prophylactic indomethacin have shown a reduced incidence of PIVH – stabilization of the transitional circulation may be one mechanism for this effect. This effect, however, must be weighed against the potential of these agents to reduce cerebral blood flow (94). The hemodynamic effect of a large unconstricted PDA (> 1.5 mm on color Doppler measurement) (95) on the transitional circulation of the preterm infant can be significant and sometimes results in other complications such as the development of pulmonary hemorrhagic edema (96). Consequently it appears to be prudent to treat an unconstricted PDA during the first postnatal days with an initial dose of 0.2 mg/kg of indomethacin, followed by further doses according to response.

Volume Expansion

Hypotension on the first postnatal day in the VLBW infant is rarely associated with absolute hypovolemia unless there has been significant perinatal blood loss. Hypovolemia should be suspected where there is pallor associated with tachycardia, especially in the setting of peripartum blood loss or a very tight nuchal cord. Infants with sepsis, particularly of later onset, can have significant absolute hypovolemia due to leakage of fluid into tissue spaces and may benefit from volume expansion. Other clinical scenarios associated with absolute hypovolemia include infants with subgaleal hematomas or other intracavity hemorrhage. Studies of the relationship between the blood volume and blood pressure in premature infants show a poor correlation suggesting that low blood volume is not synonymous with low blood pressure (32,33,97). Similarly, other groups have found that infants with hypotension and associated acidosis have reduced left ventricular output and impaired cardiac contractility (30). The usefulness of volume expansion in this setting is questionable as it may lead to a worsening of cardiac function and cardiogenic failure. Routine use of volume expansion in preterm infants on the first day to improve outcome is not supported by the evidence (98).

Table 8-1   Treatment Options According to Underlying Mechanism of Cardiovascular Compromise on the First Postnatal Day

Patient Group	Clinical Issues	Cardiovascular Parameters	Suggested Management
Extreme preterm infant during transitional period	Early low systemic blood flow	Normal or low BP Low blood flow/cardiac output Large ductus arteriosus Higher systemic vascular resistance (unless born with chorioamnionitis) Poor myocardial contractility	Saline 10–20 mL/kg Dobutamine 5–20 μg/kg/min – adjust to blood flow Second line: Add dopamine 5 μg/kg/min titrate carefully to BP
VLBW infant with PDA	Low BP PDA signs	Low BP Large PDA, Left to right shunt	Indomethacin first, then treatment of flow/pressure if required
VLBW infant with asphyxia	Myocardial damage Low systemic blood flow	Normal or low BP Poor myocardial contractility	Saline 10–20 mL/kg (care if myocardial function is affected) Dobutamine 5–20 μg/kg/min – adjust to blood flow Second line: Add dopamine 5 μg/kg/min titrate to BP (or low-dose epinephrine)
VLBW infant with suspected sepsis or chorioamnionitis – **high output**	High output cardiac failure secondary to sepsis	Normal or low BP High systemic blood flow Low systemic vascular resistance/capillary leak	Volume replacement – may require more than 20 mL/kg Dopamine 5 μg/kg/min titrated to BP Second line: Epinephrine 0.05 μg/kg/min titrated to BP
VLBW infant with suspected sepsis or chorionamnionitis – **low output**	Sepsis and poor myocardial function	Normal or low BP Normal or low systemic blood flow High systemic vascular resistance	Saline 10–20 mL/kg Dobutamine 15–20 μg/kg/min – adjust to blood flow Second line: (low blood flow) Epinephrine 0.05 μg/kg/min Second line: (hypotension) Dopamine 5 μg/kg/min titrate to BP (or epinephrine)
VLBW infant with acute fluid loss (intraventricular/pulmonary hemorrhage)	Acute hypovolemia	Normal or low blood pressure Poor venous filling pressures	Volume replacement – may require more than 20 mL/kg, including blood transfusion Dopamine 5 μg/kg/min titrated to BP Second line: Epinephrine 0.05 μg/kg/min titrated to BP

There appears to be little difference in efficacy between crystalloid and colloid solutions in the treatment of systemic hypotension (99,100). There have been concerns over the use of 5% albumin in older children and adults in intensive care settings and an association with increased morbidity (101). Colloid solutions are more expensive than normal saline and are derived from donated blood with the associated risk of

Table 8-2 Cardiovascular Interventions Used in Preterm Infants on the First Day

Intervention	Dose	Receptors/Effects	Indications	Considerations	Evidence
Volume (normal saline or colloid)	10–20 mL/kg	*Short term ↑SBF	Hypovolemia suspected – perinatal blood loss, infant pale with ↑HR	No evidence of improved outcome. Excess fluid associated with increased mortality, PDA, and CLD	Cohort (104) SR of RCTs (151)
Dobutamine	5–20 μg/kg/min	β: ↑contractility, ↓PVR/SVR → ↑SBF	First line for low SBF Pulmonary hypertension Asphyxia	Corrects hypotension in 60%. Tachycardia if no volume expansion	SR of RCTs (104,117)
Dopamine	2–10 μg/kg/min	**Dopamine:** ↑renal blood flow. β: ↑contractility, ↓PVR/SVRα: ↑SVR net effect: ↑BP, Ø, or ↑ SBF (CBF)	Hypotension; consider second line for low SBF	In hypotensive infants may increase CBF	SR of RCT (104,117) RCT (106)
	>10 μg/kg/min	α >> β → ↑↑SVR ↑↑PVR net effect: ↑↑ BP, Ø, or ↓ SBF	Refractory hypotension Septic shock	May substantially reduce SBF	SR of RCT (104,117)
Epinephrine	0.05–0.375 μg/kg/min	β > α: ↑BP, ↑SBF (CBF)↑SVR>PVR	Hypotension; consider second line for low SBF	In hypotensive infants may increase CBF	RCT (106)
	>0.375 μg/kg/min	α > β: ↑↑BP, ↑SVR > PVR net effect: ?↓SBF	Refractory hypotension Septic shock	May substantially reduce SBF	None in preterm
Hydrocortisone*	2–10 mg/kg/day in 2–4 divided doses	↑SVR, ↑BP, Ø, or ↑ SBF^	Refractory hypotension Adrenal insufficiency	Early steroids associated with intestinal perforation. High dose steroids ↑BSL	RCT (107)^ Prospective Observational (140)
Dexamethasone**	0.25 mg/kg single dose	↑SVR, ↑BP, unknown effect on SBF	Refractory hypotension Adrenal insufficiency	Early steroids associated with intestinal perforation. High dose steroids ↑BSL	RCT (137)
Milrinone	0.75 μg/kg/min × 3 h, then 0.2 μg/kg/min	**Type III phosphodiesterase inhibitor:** unknown effects on contractility; ↓SVR, ↓PVR →↑SBF	Low SBF	May cause hypotension	Pilot study (126)

The table is adapted from Osborn (150).

Abbreviations: ↑ = increase; ↓ = decrease; → = leads to; Ø = no change; BP = blood pressure; BSL = Blood sugar level; CBF = cerebral blood flow; CLD = chronic lung disease; HR = heart rate; PDA = patent ductus arteriosus; PVR = pulmonary vascular resistance; RCT = randomized controlled trial; SBF = systemic blood flow; SR = systematic review; SVR = Systemic vascular resistance.   *Recommended doses for low-dose hydrocortisone administration in VLBW neonates are 1 mg/kg/dose Q12 hours.   **Dexamethasone administration (even at low doses) to the VLBW neonates during the first postnatal week is NOT recommended.

blood-borne infection. In the VLBW infant the increased capillary permeability may contribute to leakage of albumin into the extravascular compartment, increasing tissue oncotic pressure and resulting in tissue fluid retention, impaired gas exchange in the lungs, and potentially causing injury to the brain. Randomized trials have shown improvement in blood pressure in hypotensive infants given volume but no change in short-or long-term outcomes. In infants who have had an identified fluid loss such as a hemorrhage at the time of delivery or excessive transepidermal water loss with excessive weight loss from use of radiant heat, replacement with the type of fluid lost is appropriate. Volume expansion probably increases LV output, but it is less effective than inotropes at increasing the blood pressure. One trial showed dopamine to be more effective than plasma in improving the blood pressure in hypotensive preterm infants (102). Observational studies have shown a short-term improvement in systemic blood flow after volume expansion (58).

As the accurate diagnosis of absolute or relative hypovolemia is difficult in the neonate, and hypovolemia results in reduced efficacy of vasopressor inotropes, it is reasonable to initially treat hypotension with 10 to 20 mL/kg of normal saline solution over 30 to 60 min. Trials that have used a volume load prior to giving an inotrope (i.e. dobutamine) reported no reflex tachycardia in response to the inotrope suggesting that volume load may lessen the reduction in preload that occurs with vasodilation potentially associated with the use of dobutamine. In an infant requiring positive pressure respiratory support, even if the infant is not hypovolemic, a volume load may increase the central venous pressure sufficiently to improve venous return to the heart. As there is an association between excess fluid administration in premature infants and adverse outcomes, including increased incidence of patent ductus arteriosus, necrotizing enterocolitis, chronic lung disease (103), and mortality, excessive and inappropriate administration of volume should be avoided. If normalization of the blood pressure is not achieved with a single dose of volume replacement, then early initiation of a vasopressor-inotrope or an inotrope should be the next step considered.

Vasopressor-inotropes, Inotropes, and Lusitropes

These agents have been used in neonates for many years in the treatment of hypotension. Vasopressor-inotropes, such as dopamine and epinephrine, increase both myocardial contractility and SVR; inotropes, such as dobutamine, increase myocardial contractility and exert a variable vasodilatory action on the periphery; and lusitropes, such as milrinone, work primarily as peripheral vasodilators with a variable degree of inotropy or no inotropic effect. They were introduced without randomized and blinded trials and there is still no evidence that use of these treatments improves important neonatal outcomes such as death and disability. Studies of vasopressor-inotropes and inotropes have focused on the effect on blood pressure and only recently have the effects of these medications on cardiac output, the main determinant of oxygen delivery to tissues, been taken into account (52,104). The mechanisms of action of these vasoactive agents are complex and affected by the developmental maturation of the cardiovascular and autonomic nervous systems. Consequently these agents can alter the relationship between the systemic blood pressure and systemic blood flow and, if only the blood pressure is monitored a change in the blood flow may not be appreciated during treatment.

Dopamine

Dopamine is the most commonly used sympathomimetic amine for the treatment of hypotension in the VLBW infant. Dopamine is a precursor to both epinephrine and norepinephrine, but is also a naturally occurring catecholamine. The drug stimulates the cardiovascular alpha- and beta-adrenergic and dopaminergic

DOSE-DEPENDENT EFFECTS OF DOPAMINE IN NEONATES*

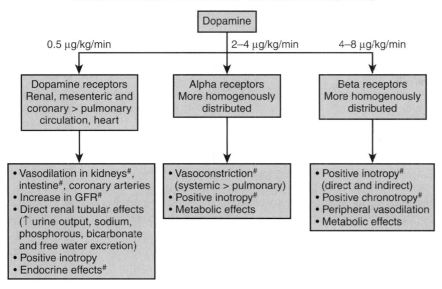

* Without adrenoreceptor downregulation
# Demonstrated effects in preterm neonates

FIGURE 8-5 In the preterm neonate, low doses of dopamine stimulate the dopaminergic receptors. At low-to-medium doses, effects of alpha-adrenergic receptor stimulation also appear. At medium-to-high doses (> 8 to 10 µg/kg/min), effects of both beta- and alpha-receptor stimulation dominate the hemodynamic response to the drug. However, this response is influenced by several factors (state of cardiovascular adrenergic receptor expression, etc.) regulated by the level of maturity and disease severity (3). See text for details. *Reprinted with permission from Seri (148).*

receptors in a dose-dependent manner (105). Manifestation of the hemodynamic actions of dopamine (and the other sympathomimetic amines) is affected by several factors. These include the level of expression of the adrenergic receptors and intracellular signaling systems, adrenal function, developmentally regulated maturity of the myocardium, and the dysregulated release of local vasodilators such as endogenous nitric oxide and vasodilatory prostaglandins (3). Figure 8-5 illustrates the dose-dependent cardiovascular and renal actions of dopamine.

Potential cardiovascular and renal side effects of dopamine administration include tachycardia, hypertension and/or decreased systemic perfusion (at high doses) and increased urinary sodium, phosphorus, free water, and bicarbonate losses, respectively (105). Dopamine also plays a role in the short-term physiological regulation of sodium–potassium–ATPase activity and exerts certain endocrine and paracrine actions (105). These effects include but are not limited to the temporary inhibition of prolactin, TSH, growth hormone, and gonadotropin release from the pituitary and increased renin-angiotensin activity. Additionally, dopamine plays a role in the peripheral regulation of breathing and influences certain aspects of leukocyte function (105). It is unclear whether these transient endocrine and paracrine dopaminergic actions have short- or long-term clinical significance in the preterm neonate.

As mentioned earlier, dopamine administered exogenously acts via dopaminergic and adrenergic receptors, with varying effects at different doses. At lower doses it acts via increasing myocardial contractility in a dose-dependent fashion, but at higher doses (> 10 µg/kg/min), peripheral vasoconstriction and increased afterload play an increasing role in its effect on blood pressure. It is this increase in the afterload that may also affect cardiac function, particularly in the very preterm infant where the immature ventricle may not be as able to maintain cardiac output with increasing peripheral vascular resistance. Accordingly, lower doses of

CARDIOVASCULAR EFFECTS OF EPINEPHRINE IN NEONATES*

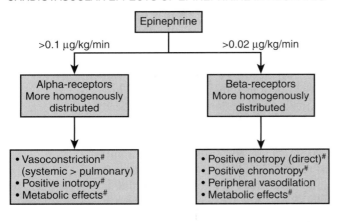

* Without adrenoreceptor downregulation
# Demonstrated effects in preterm neonates

FIGURE 8-7 In the preterm neonate, at low to medium doses of epinephrine, effects of beta- and then alpha-adrenergic receptor stimulation become apparent. The cardiovascular response is influenced by several factors (state of cardiovascular adrenergic receptor expression, etc.) regulated by the level of maturity and disease severity (3). See text for details. *Reprinted with permission from Seri (148).*

low-dose epinephrine in hypotensive very preterm infants in the first day similar increases were reported in cerebral blood flow and oxygenation as measured by NIR spectroscopy. Both vasopressor-inotropes were equally efficacious at increasing blood pressure. No other clinical benefits to either medication were reported (106). As epinephrine at higher doses has a peripheral vasoconstrictive effect it may be of particular use in infants with pathological peripheral vasodilation due to septic shock. The dose range used in neonates ranges from 0.05 to 2.6 µg/kg/min (118) or beyond.

Milrinone

Milrinone is a phosphodiesterase-3 inhibitor and therefore it increases intracellular cyclic adenosine monophosphate (cAMP) concentrations. In the adult it has both a positive inotropic effect (particularly improving myocardial diastolic function) and a peripheral vasodilatory effect. Although this combination of actions is potentially very efficacious in preterm infants in the first postnatal hours, where the immature myocardium is struggling against the increased afterload of the postnatal circulation, it is not known if milrinone acts as a true inotrope in the neonate. Indeed, findings of studies in immature animal models show that class III phosphodiesterase inhibitors such as amrinone have minimal (119), no, or even negative (120,121) inotropic effects. It has been suggested that the developmentally regulated variation in the effect of phosphodiesterase inhibitors on myocardial contractility is a consequence of the developmental imbalance between class III and IV phosphodiesterases in the sarcoplasmic reticulum of the immature myocardium (122). However, these negative inotropic effects exhibited in neonatal puppies become positive within a few days after birth (121). Indeed, milrinone has been shown to be effective in treatment of low cardiac output syndrome (LCOS) in infants after cardiac surgery by increasing cardiac output. LCOS in this patient population is associated with a rise in both systemic and pulmonary resistance (123,124). The ability of the myocardium to adapt to an increased afterload is compromised by the effects of cardiac bypass, similar to the myocardium of the preterm infant in transition, which may be compromised by the postnatal changes in afterload. In a multicenter randomized trial, there was a dose-dependent reduction of incidence of LCOS when milrinone was used preventatively in infants after cardiac surgery (125). A single pilot study of the use of milrinone in preterm infants using a modified dosing regimen to prevent low blood flow demonstrated that the potential side effect of significant hypotension was not seen and all infants maintained adequate cardiac output when compared to historical controls (126).

Treatment of VLBW Neonates with Vasopressor-resistant Shock

More than 50% of hypotensive VLBW infants requiring dopamine at doses > 10 μg/kg/min during the immediate postnatal period cannot be weaned off the drug for well over three to four days and many develop vasopressor-resistant hypotension (3,36,127,128). These VLBW neonates with vasopressor dependence or with vasopressor-resistant hypotension often respond to relatively low doses of hydrocortisone with an improvement in blood pressure and urine output and frequently wean off vasopressor support within 24 to 72 h (3,36,127–130). Several factors may explain the corticosteroid responsiveness of vasopressor-resistant hypotension in neonates especially in those born before 30 weeks' gestation. These factors include the downregulation of the adrenergic receptors in critical illness (131) and a relative or absolute adrenal insufficiency of the VLBW neonate (36,37,127).

The attenuated cardiovascular responsiveness to catecholamines in critical illness is, at least in part, caused by the downregulation of the cardiovascular adrenergic receptors and their intracellular signaling systems (131). Findings that reversal of receptor downregulation requires new protein synthesis and that the expression of the adrenergic receptors and type-1 angiotensin 2 receptors in the cardiovascular system is inducible by glucocorticoids (132,133) explain why steroid administration reverses adrenergic receptor downregulation. Moreover, corticosteroids inhibit prostacyclin production and the induction of nitric oxide synthase (134), limiting the pathological vasodilation associated with the non-specific or specific inflammatory response in the critically ill neonate. These genomic effects of steroids result in synthesis and membrane-assembly of new receptor proteins and require several hours to take place. In addition to their genomic effects, steroids exert certain non-genomic actions (135,136) resulting in a rapid increase in the sensitivity of the cardiovascular system to catecholamines. These effects include the direct inhibition of catecholamine metabolism, the decrease in norepinephrine reuptake into the sympathetic nerve endings, the increase in cytosolic calcium availability in myocardial and vascular smooth muscle cells, and the improvement in capillary integrity (130,133). The result of these complex actions is an improvement in blood pressure and cardiovascular status occurring within hours after the initiation of hydrocortisone administration in the neonate (130).

Relative adrenal insufficiency, especially in the VLBW neonate, is the other factor thought to contribute both to the increased incidence of vasopressor resistance and the enhanced responsiveness to hydrocortisone in this patient population (37). Several lines of indirect evidence suggest that the VLBW neonate has a developmentally regulated limited adrenal reserve. Thus, in these patients, relative adrenal insufficiency contributes to the disruption of the balance between adrenergic receptor destruction and synthesis resulting in decreased sensitivity of the cardiovascular system to endogenous and exogenous catecholamines. Therefore, steroid administration especially in the hypotensive ELBW neonate may also be considered as a hormone replacement therapy (130).

Although the effects of low-dose hydrocortisone on blood pressure, urine output and vasopressor requirement have been more extensively studied (36,127,129,130), only preliminary data are available on the other aspects of the hemodynamic response to low-dose hydrocortisone. Two clinical trials have assessed the usefulness of corticosteroids in hypotensive preterm infants. The first was a randomized controlled trial (RCT) of dopamine and hydrocortisone which found that 81% of hypotensive infants had a response to hydrocortisone at a dose of 2 to 10 mg/kg/day (107). In another RCT, a single dose of dexamethasone (0.25 mg/kg) allowed weaning of the epinephrine infusion compared with placebo (137). Several case series have also reported positive responses to hydrocortisone or dexamethasone in infants with refractory hypotension (129,130,138,139). The hydrocortisone administration-associated changes in cardiac output, systemic vascular resistance, and organ blood flow are extremely important because hydrocortisone, at least in theory, may increase blood pressure at the expense of systemic perfusion if it would primarily enhance the peripheral vasoconstrictive effects of vasopressors. However, recent findings indicate that hydrocortisone improves all aspects of cardiovascular function, including cardiac output and organ blood flows (140).

Potential side effects of hydrocortisone administration are numerous but the increase in gastrointestinal perforations when it is concomitantly administered with indomethacin is the most important acute side effect. This severe complication limits the use of hydrocortisone to VLBW neonates not receiving indomethacin. It is important to note that hydrocortisone administration without indomethacin treatment does not increase the incidence of isolated gastrointestinal perforations. Finally, although low-dose hydrocortisone exposure during the first postnatal week and high-dose, prolonged hydrocortisone exposure after the first postnatal week do not appear to affect long-term neurodevelopment (141,142), more data are needed to ensure that hydrocortisone administration to VLBW neonates during and after neonate transition does not adversely affect neurodevelopment in this vulnerable patient population. Therefore, hydrocortisone should be used with caution in the VLBW neonate and its use, at least at present, should be restricted to cases with vasopressor resistance.

PRESENTATION AND MANAGEMENT OF CARDIOVASCULAR COMPROMISE IN THE VLBW INFANT ON THE FIRST POSTNATAL DAY

There are several different potential mechanisms that result in hypotension and/or decreased systemic blood flow on the first postnatal day. Each of these mechanisms needs to be considered individually when planning appropriate assessment and treatment:

- Delay in the adaptation of the immature myocardium to the sudden increase in systemic vascular resistance occurring at birth (transient myocardial dysfunction)
- Peripheral vasodilation and hyperdynamic myocardial function primarily in VLBW neonates born to mothers with chorioamnionitis
- Perinatal depression with secondary myocardial dysfunction and/or abnormal peripheral vasoregulation

Some insight into the appropriate combination of therapies can be obtained by looking beyond just the measurement of blood pressure and beginning to assess other parameters that impact upon the cardiovascular adequacy. The underlying cause for cardiovascular compromise should be sought from the history, the physical examination and by utilizing other available information such as that obtained from functional echocardiography.

Transient Myocardial Dysfunction

During the first postnatal day, VLBW neonates may present with shock because of the inability of the immature myocardium to pump against the increased peripheral vascular resistance occurring in the immediate period after delivery (144). While attempting to maintain adequate perfusion pressure, the immature neonate's vasoconstrictive vasoregulatory response to decreased systemic perfusion may include cerebral vasoconstriction in addition to vasoconstriction in the vascular beds of the non-vital organs. The more immature the neonate the higher the likelihood that systemic (and cerebral) hypoperfusion will occur during the first postnatal day (2,15). Although a significant number of these patients will also be hypotensive, in others blood pressure may remain within the normal range. Thus, despite having "normal" blood pressure, some of these neonates may have a temporarily compromised CBF. Recognition of this presentation requires the ability to assess cerebral blood flow at the bedside using SVC flow measurements and functional echocardiography (2,104) and/or NIR spectroscopy (6,13,16).

Management of this presentation of circulatory compromise is difficult and findings in the literature are somewhat contradictory. In a series of studies using SVC blood flow as a surrogate measure of CBF in VLBW neonates during the first postnatal day, Evans et al. described the hemodynamics of systemic and cerebral hypoperfusion (2,15), the relationship between recovery from hypoperfusion and the development of PIVH, the weak relationship between SVC blood flow and systemic blood pressure (31), and the association between neurodevelopmental outcome at three years of age and low SVC blood flow during the first 24 postnatal hours (92). In addition, this group performed a randomized blinded clinical trial with a crossover design to compare the effects of dopamine and dobutamine at 10 and 20 µg/kg/min on SVC flow and blood pressure in VLBW neonates during the first postnatal day (104). They found that dopamine improved systemic blood pressure more effectively in this group of infants, while dobutamine was better at increasing SVC flow at the two doses tested. Since pharmacodynamics rather than pharmacokinetics determine the cardiovascular response to these sympathomimetic amines, the limitation of this study was the lack of stepwise titration of the drugs in search for the optimal hemodynamic response. Indeed, a recent study using continuous NIR spectroscopy monitoring to assess the relative changes in CBF demonstrated that, by stepwise titration of dopamine or epinephrine, both drugs are equally effective in the low-to-moderate dose range at improving blood pressure and CBF in VLBW neonates during the first postnatal day (106). It is of note that, although the use of continuous NIR spectroscopy monitoring to assess cerebral intravascular oxygenation and cerebral blood volume allows for data collection for a longer period of time (hours) and provides reliable information for the relative changes in these parameters, the absolute values are not known when one uses the continuous NIR spectroscopy measurements rather than intermittently checking for absolute CBF values with NIR spectroscopy.

Finally, recent findings using multiple (not continuous) measurements of CBF by NIR spectroscopy to assess the response of CBF and blood pressure to dopamine in ELBW neonates during the first two postnatal days suggest that these patients respond to moderate-to-high doses of dopamine with an increase in both the blood pressure and CBF (7). However, although CBF returns to the presumed normal range as blood pressure normalizes, its autoregulation remains impaired. The authors also calculated the lower elbow of the autoregulatory curve in their patients and found that it is around 29 mm Hg. One of the limitations of the findings is that the bilinear regression analysis used in this study combines two small patient populations predefined by treatment criteria. The findings of this study also suggest that, once CBF autoregulation is lost in preterm neonates, it does not recover immediately after the normalization of the blood pressure with dopamine. Indeed, findings of an earlier study support this notion and indicate that, in sick preterm neonates, it may take up to 30–40 min or more for CBF autoregulation to recover after blood pressure has been normalized (53). Another approach to the treatment of poor systemic perfusion in the one-day-old VLBW neonate is currently being investigated in an ongoing double blind randomized clinical trial using prophylactic milrinone shortly after delivery in an attempt to prevent systemic hypoperfusion (126). The results are not available as yet.

In summary, treatment of the hypotensive one-day-old VLBW neonate remains complex even if systemic perfusion can be assessed by functional echocardiography.

The use and stepwise titration of low-to-moderate dose dopamine (17,53,105,106) or epinephrine (106) to achieve blood pressure values somewhat higher than the gestational age of the patient is a preferred approach during the first postnatal day by most neonatologists especially if systemic perfusion can only be assessed by the less than reliable indirect signs of systemic hemodynamics such as urine output and CRT. Whether using milrinone to prevent systemic hypoperfusion following delivery in the VLBW neonate will result in improved short- and long-term outcomes is not known at present. If there is evidence of myocardial dysfunction, dobutamine is the first line medication and low-dose dopamine may be added if blood pressure decreases upon initiation of dobutamine administration. However, one must bear in mind that systemic vascular resistance should only be increased very carefully by dopamine as it may induce further decreases in the cardiac output secondary to myocardial dysfunction. If assessment of systemic perfusion (SVC flow) is available (2), the systemic hemodynamic effects of the careful titration of a vasopressor-inotrope (dopamine or epinephrine) or an inotrope (dobutamine) can be followed. Finally, it is important to note that it is not known whether the use of dopamine or dobutamine as the first-line vasoactive agent in the treatment of hypotension in the one-day old VLBW neonate has a more favorable impact on mortality and short- or long-term morbidity.

Vasodilation and Hyperdynamic Myocardial Function

Recent data indicate that VLBW neonates born after chorioamnionitis, especially if they also present with funisitis, develop hypotension and increased cardiac output within a few hours after delivery (145). The presentation of hypotension with increased cardiac output suggests that systemic vascular resistance is lower in VLBW neonates born after chorioamnionitis. These alterations in the cardiovascular function correlate with cord blood interleukin-6 levels (145). In addition, the presence of maternal fever or a neonatal immature-to-total (I/T) white blood cell ratio over 0.4 is associated with decreased left ventricular fractional shortening. In summary, these findings indicate that, in VLBW neonates born after chorioamnionitis, hypotension is primarily caused by vasodilation although a variable degree of myocardial dysfunction may also contribute to the hemodynamic disturbance especially in neonates with an increased I/T ratio.

Based on these findings, treatment of hypotension in the one-day-old VLBW neonate born after chorioamnionitis should be tailored to address both components of the cardiovascular compromise (vasodilation and potential myocardial dysfunction). In these cases, dobutamine administration alone may lead to further decreases in systemic vascular resistance especially in patients with increased cardiac output and little or no myocardial compromise. Therefore, carefully titrated low-to-moderate doses of dopamine (or epinephrine) will likely be effective in these patients. However, one should bear in mind that dopamine or epinephrine at higher doses my increase systemic vascular resistance to levels where cardiac output may be compromised and, despite improving blood pressures, systemic blood flow may decrease. Thus, if functional echocardiography is not available, the indirect measures of tissue perfusion (urine output, CRT, base deficit and/or serum lactate levels) should be carefully followed to monitor for the state of blood flow to the organs and vasopressor support needs to be adjusted accordingly.

Perinatal Depression with Secondary Myocardial Dysfunction And/or Abnormal Peripheral Vasoregulation

Perinatal asphyxia with secondary myocardial dysfunction occurs in both term and VLBW infants (145). Administration of volume in this setting is common as the

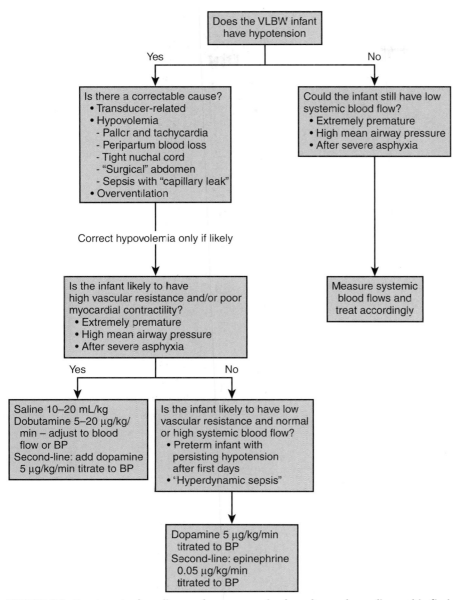

FIGURE 8-8 Treatment of cardiovascular compromise based on echocardiographic findings. *Adapted from Subhedar (150), Obsorn (151), and Obsorn and Evans (152).*

infant is often thought to be poorly perfused and hypotensive. There is, however, little evidence that this group of infants is hypovolemic (147) unless there has been specific blood loss or a tight nuchal cord as discussed earlier. The perfusion will usually improve with adequate resuscitation and respiratory support. Preterm infants with evidence of perinatal asphyxia and multiorgan dysfunction require careful management of fluid balance to prevent volume overload and subsequent cardiac failure – in this group inotropes such as dobutamine (and maybe milrinone) are probably of most use. Administration of excessive volume in the setting of asphyxia, with the added risk of an underlying myocardial injury being present, may result in fluid overload and cardiogenic heart failure. In this situation, the judicious use of a vasopressor-inotrope such as dopamine or an inotrope such as dobutamine is preferable (110,148). There is some suggestion that a hypoxic ischemic insult may also impair proper peripheral vasoregulation resulting in an infant who is unable to adjust blood pressure in response to physiological changes.

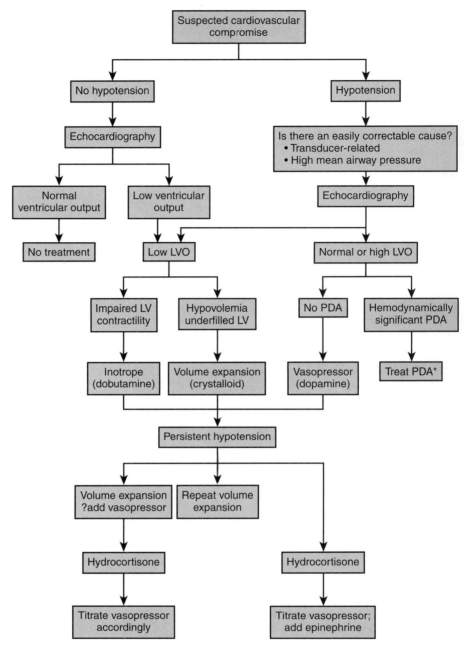

*Treat PDA and allow pulmonary vascular resistance to increase to combate left-to-right shunting (keep Paco$_2$ at 45–55 mm Hg, arterial pH at 7.25–7.35, and O$_2$ saturation 82–90%.

FIGURE 8-9 Treatment of cardiovascular compromise based on clinical findings. *Adapted from Obsorn (151), and Obsorn and Evans (152).*

However, direct evidence for this notion is lacking due to the difficulties in appropriately assessing peripheral vascular resistance.

CONCLUSION

The appropriate assessment and treatment of the VLBW infant with cardiovascular impairment or full-blown shock requires the clinician to obtain adequate information about the etiology and underlying physiologic determinants of the condition. An understanding of the actions of the therapeutic options available and the specific effects of these treatments on the circulation of the VLBW infant is also important (Table 8-2). Figure 8-8 shows an approach to the management of hypotension in the VLBW infant based on clinical information. The addition of a functional echocardiogram to the assessment process provides information about the size and shunt direction of the ductus arteriosus, the function of the myocardium and its filling as well as about the cardiac output and calculated peripheral vascular resistance. Figure 8-9 summarizes the approach to management of hypotension in the VLBW infant using the additional information provided by the functional echocardiogram.

REFERENCES

1. Al Aweel I, Pursley DM, Rubin LP, et al. Variations in prevalence of hypotension, hypertension, and vasopressor use in NICUs. J Perinatol 2001;21:272–278.
2. Kluckow M, Evans N. Superior vena cava flow in preterm infants: a novel marker of systemic blood flow. Arch Dis Child, Fetal Neonatal Ed 2000;82:182–187.
3. Seri I. Circulatory support of the sick preterm infant. Semin Neonatol 2001;6:85–95.
4. Watkins AM, West CR, Cooke RW. Blood pressure and cerebral haemorrhage and ischaemia in very low birthweight infants. Early Hum Dev 1989;19:103–110.
5. Miall-Allen VM, de Vries LS, Whitelaw AG. Mean arterial blood pressure and neonatal cerebral lesions. Arch Dis Child 1987;62:1068–1069.
6. Tsuji M, Saul JP, du PA, et al. Cerebral intravascular oxygenation correlates with mean arterial pressure in critically ill premature infants. Pediatrics 2000;106:625–632.
7. Munro MJ, Walker AM, Barfield CP. Hypotensive extremely low birth weight infants have reduced cerebral blood flow. Pediatrics 2004;114:1591–1596.
8. Nuntnarumit P, Yang W, Bada-Ellzey HS. Blood pressure measurements in the newborn. Clin Perinatol 1999;26:981–996.
9. Hegyi T, Carbone MT, Anwar M, et al. Blood pressure ranges in premature infants. i. the first hours of life. J Pediatr 1994;124:627–633.
10. Development of audit measures and guidelines for good practice in the management of neonatal respiratory distress syndrome. Report of a joint working group of the British Association of Perinatal Medicine and the research unit of the Royal College of Physicians. Arch Dis Child 1992;67:1221–1227.
11. Greisen G, Borch K. White matter injury in the preterm neonate: the role of perfusion. Develop Neurosci 2001;23:209–212.
12. Greisen G. Autoregulation of cerebral blood flow in newborn babies. Early Hum Dev 2005;81:423–428.
13. Tyszczuk L, Meek J, Elwell C, et al. Cerebral blood flow is independent of mean arterial blood pressure in preterm infants undergoing intensive care. Pediatrics 1998;102:337–341.
14. Seri I, Abbasi S, Wood DC, et al. Regional hemodynamic effects of dopamine in the sick preterm neonate. J Pediatr 1998;133:728–734.
15. Kluckow M, Evans N. Low superior vena cava flow and intraventricular haemorrhage in preterm infants. Arch Dis Child, Fetal Neonatal Ed 2000;82:188–194.
16. Kissack CM, Garr R, Wardle SP, et al. Cerebral fractional oxygen extraction in very low birth weight infants is high when there is low left ventricular output and hypocarbia but is unaffected by hypotension. Pediatr Res 2004;55:400–405.
17. Seri I. Hemodynamics during the first two postnatal days and neurodevelopment in preterm neonates. J Pediatr 2004;145:573–575.
18. Friedman AH, Fahey JT. The transition from fetal to neonatal circulation: normal responses and implications for infants with heart disease. Semin Perinatol 1993;17:106–121.
19. Mahoney LT, Coryell KG, Lauer RM. The newborn transitional circulation: a two-dimensional Doppler echocardiographic study. J Am Coll Cardiol 1985;6:623–629.
20. Gentile R, Stevenson G, Dooley T, et al. Pulsed Doppler echocardiographic determination of time of ductal closure in normal newborn infants. J Pediatr 1981;98:443–448.
21. Evans N, Iyer P. Longitudinal changes in the diameter of the ductus arteriosus in ventilated preterm infants: correlation with respiratory outcomes. Arch Dis Child, Fetal Neonatal Ed 1995;72:F156–F161.
22. Seidner SR, Chen YQ, Oprysko PR, et al. Combined prostaglandin and nitric oxide inhibition produces anatomic remodeling and closure of the ductus arteriosus in the premature newborn baboon. Pediatr Res 2001;50:365–373.
23. Evans N, Iyer P. Assessment of ductus arteriosus shunt in preterm infants supported by mechanical ventilation: effects of interatrial shunting. J Pediatr 1994;125:778–785.
24. Agata Y, Hiraishi S, Oguchi K, et al. Changes in left ventricular output from fetal to early neonatal life. J Pediatr 1991;119:441–445.
25. Drayton MR, Skidmore R. Ductus arteriosus blood flow during first 48 hours of life. Arch Dis Child 1987;62:1030–1034.
26. Kluckow M, Evans N. Low systemic blood flow in the preterm infant. Semin Neonatol 2001;6:75–84.

27. Teitel DF. Physiologic development of the cardiovascular system in the fetus. In Fetal and Neonatal Physiology. Polin RA, Fox WW, eds. Philadelphia, WB Saunders, 1998:827–836.

28. Weindling AM, Kissack CM. Blood pressure and tissue oxygenation in the newborn baby at risk of brain damage. Biol Neonate 2001;79:241–245.

29. Osborn D, Evans N, Kluckow M. Diagnosis and treatment of low systemic blood flow in preterm infants. NeoReviews 2004;5:e109–e121.

30. Gill AB, Weindling AM. Echocardiographic assessment of cardiac function in shocked very low birthweight infants. Arch Dis Child 1993;68:17–21.

31. Kluckow M, Evans N. Relationship between blood pressure and cardiac output in preterm infants requiring mechanical ventilation. J Pediatr 1996;129:506–512.

32. Bauer K, Linderkamp O, Versmold HT. Systolic blood pressure and blood volume in preterm infants. Arch Dis Child 1993;69:521–522.

33. Barr PA, Bailey PE, Sumners J, et al. Relation between arterial blood pressure and blood volume and effect of infused albumin in sick preterm infants. Pediatrics 1977;60:282–289.

34. Lopez SL, Leighton JO, Walther FJ. Supranormal cardiac output in the dopamine- and dobutamine-dependent preterm infant. Pediatr Cardiol 1997;18:292–296.

35. Pladys P, Wodey E, Beuchee A, et al. Left ventricle output and mean arterial blood pressure in preterm infants during the 1st day of life. Eur J Pediatr 1999;158:817–824.

36. Ng PC, Lam CW, Fok TF, et al. Refractory hypotension in preterm infants with adrenocortical insufficiency. Arch Dis Child, Fetal Neonatal Ed 2001;84:F122–F124.

37. Watterberg KL. Adrenal insufficiency and cardiac dysfunction in the preterm infant. Pediatr Res 2002;51:422–424.

38. Hanna CE, Jett PL, Laird MR, et al. Corticosteroid binding globulin, total serum cortisol, and stress in extremely low-birth-weight infants. Am J Perinatol 1997;14:201–204.

39. Scott SM, Watterberg KL. Effect of gestational age, postnatal age, and illness on plasma cortisol concentrations in premature infants. Pediatr Res 1995;37:112–116.

40. Sasidharan P. Role of corticosteroids in neonatal blood pressure homeostasis. Clin Perinatol 1998;25:723–740.

41. Moise AA, Wearden ME, Kozinetz CA, et al. Antenatal steroids are associated with less need for blood pressure support in extremely premature infants. Pediatrics 1995;95:845–850.

42. Demarini S, Dollberg S, Hoath SB, et al. Effects of antenatal corticosteroids on blood pressure in very low birth weight infants during the first 24 hours of life. J Perinatol 1999;19:419–425.

43. LeFlore JL, Engle WD, Rosenfeld CR. Determinants of blood pressure in very low birth weight neonates: lack of effect of antenatal steroids. Early Hum Dev 2000;59:37–50.

44. Leviton A, Kuban KC, Pagano M, et al. Antenatal corticosteroids appear to reduce the risk of postnatal germinal matrix hemorrhage in intubated low birth weight newborns. Pediatrics 1993;91:1083–1088.

45. Trang TT, Tibballs J, Mercier JC, et al. Optimization of oxygen transport in mechanically ventilated newborns using oximetry and pulsed Doppler-derived cardiac output. Crit Care Med 1988;16:1094–1097.

46. Maayan C, Eyal F, Mandelberg A, et al. Effect of mechanical ventilation and volume loading on left ventricular performance in premature infants with respiratory distress syndrome. Crit Care Med 1986;14:858–860.

47. Skinner JR, Boys RJ, Hunter S, et al. Pulmonary and systemic arterial pressure in hyaline membrane disease. Arch Dis Child 1992;67:366–373.

48. Evans N, Kluckow M. Early determinants of right and left ventricular output in ventilated preterm infants. Arch Dis Child, Fetal Neonatal Ed 1996;74:F88–F94.

49. Skelton R, Evans N, Smythe J. A blinded comparison of clinical and echocardiographic evaluation of the preterm infant for patent ductus arteriosus. J Paediatr Child Health 1994;30:406–411.

50. Evans N, Moorcraft J. Effect of patency of the ductus arteriosus on blood pressure in very preterm infants. Arch Dis Child 1992;67:1169–1173.

51. Fenton AC, Woods KL, Leanage R, et al. Cardiovascular effects of carbon dioxide in ventilated preterm infants. Acta Paediatr 1992;81:498–503.

52. Roze JC, Tohier C, Maingueneau C, et al. Response to dobutamine and dopamine in the hypotensive very preterm infant. Arch Dis Child 1993;69:59–63.

53. Seri I, Rudas G, Bors Z, et al. Effects of low-dose dopamine infusion on cardiovascular and renal functions, cerebral blood flow, and plasma catecholamine levels in sick preterm neonates. Pediatr Res 1993;34:742–749.

54. Versmold HT, Kitterman JA, Phibbs RH, et al. Aortic blood pressure during the first 12 hours of life in infants with birth weight 610 to 4,220 grams. Pediatrics 1981;67:607–613.

55. Strozik KS, Pieper CH, Roller J. Capillary refilling time in newborn babies: normal values. Arch Dis Child, Fetal Neonatal Ed 1997;76:F193–F196.

56. Schriger DL, Baraff L. Defining normal capillary refill:variation with age, sex, and temperature. Ann Emerg Med 1988;17:932–935.

57. Tibby SM, Hatherill M, Murdoch IA. Capillary refill and core–peripheral temperature gap as indicators of haemodynamic status in paediatric intensive care patients. Arch Dis Child 1999;80:163–166.

58. Osborn DA, Evans N, Kluckow M. Clinical detection of low upper body blood flow in very premature infants using blood pressure, capillary refill time, and central–peripheral temperature difference. Arch Dis Child, Fetal Neonatal Ed 2004;89:F168–F173.

59. Linshaw MA. Concentration of the urine. In Fetal and Neonatal Physiology. Polin RA, Fox WW, eds. Philadelphia WB Saunders, 1998:1634–1653.

60. Cady LDJ, Weil MH, Afifi AA, et al. Quantitation of severity of critical illness with special reference to blood lactate. Crit Care Med 1973;1:75–80.

61. Peretz DI, Scott HM, Duff J, et al. The significance of lacticacidemia in the shock syndrome. Ann NY Acad Sci 1965;119:1133–1141.

62. Rashkin MC, Bosken C, Baughman RP. Oxygen delivery in critically ill patients. Relationship to blood lactate and survival. Chest 1985;87:580–584.

63. Vincent JL, Dufaye P, Berre J, et al. Serial lactate determinations during circulatory shock. Crit Care Med 1983;11:449–451.

64. Weil MH, Afifi AA. Experimental and clinical studies on lactate and pyruvate as indicators of the severity of acute circulatory failure (shock). Circulation 1970;41:989–1001.

65. Beca JP, Scopes JW. Serial determinations of blood lactate in respiratory distress syndrome. Arch Dis Child 1972;47:550–557.

66. Deshpande SA, Platt MP. Association between blood lactate and acid–base status and mortality in ventilated babies. Arch Dis Child, Fetal Neonatal Ed 1997;76:F15–F20.

67. Graven SN, Criscuolo D, Holcomb TM. Blood lactate in the respiratory distress syndrome: significance in prognosis. Am J Dis Child 1965;110:614–617.

68. Butt WW, Whyte HW. Blood pressure monitoring in neonates: comparison of umbilical and peripheral artery measurements. J Pediatr 1984;105:630–632.

69. Colan SD, Fujii A, Borow KM, et al. Noninvasive determination of systolic, diastolic and end-systolic blood pressure in neonates, infants and young children: comparison with central aortic pressure measurements. Am J Cardiol 1983;52:867–870.

70. Emery EF, Greenough A. Non-invasive blood pressure monitoring in preterm infants receiving intensive care. Eur J Pediatr 1992;151:136–139.

71. Kimble KJ, Darnall Jr RA, Yelderman M, et al. An automated oscillometric technique for estimating mean arterial pressure in critically ill newborns. Anesthesiology 1981;54:423–425.

72. Lui K, Doyle PE, Buchanan N. Oscillometric and intra-arterial blood pressure measurements in the neonate: a comparison of methods. Australian Paediatric Journal 1982;18:32–34.

73. Park MK, Menard SM. Accuracy of blood pressure measurement by the Dinamap monitor in infants and children. Pediatrics 1987;79:907–914.

74. Dannevig I, Dale HC, Liestol K, et al. Blood pressure in the neonate: three non-invasive oscillometric pressure monitors compared with invasively measured blood pressure. Acta Paediatr 2005;94:191–196.

75. Alverson DC, Eldridge M, Dillon T, et al. Noninvasive pulsed Doppler determination of cardiac output in neonates and children. J Pediatr 1982;101:46–50.

76. Walther FJ, Siassi B, Ramadan NA, et al. Pulsed Doppler determinations of cardiac output in neonates: normal standards for clinical use. Pediatrics 1985;76:829–833.

77. Lou HC, Lassen NA, Friis-Hansen B. Impaired autoregulation of cerebral blood flow in the distressed newborn infant. J Pediatr 1979;94:118–121.

78. Victor S, Marson AG, Appleton RE, et al. Relationship between blood pressure, cerebral electrical activity, cerebral fractional oxygen extraction, and peripheral blood flow in very low birth weight newborn infants. Pediatr Res 2006;59:314–319.

79. Wardle SP, Yoxall CW, Weindling AM. Peripheral oxygenation in hypotensive preterm babies. Pediatr Res 1999;45:343–349.

80. Perlman JM, McMenamin JB, Volpe JJ. Fluctuating cerebral blood-flow velocity in respiratory-distress syndrome. Relation to the development of intraventricular hemorrhage. N Engl J Med 1983;309:204–209.

81. Pryds O, Greisen G, Lou H, et al. Heterogeneity of cerebral vasoreactivity in preterm infants supported by mechanical ventilation. J Pediatr 1989;115:638–645.

82. Pryds O, Greisen G, Lou H, et al. Heterogeneity of cerebral vasoreactivity in preterm infants supported by mechanical ventilation. J Pediatr 1989;115:638–645.

83. Bada HS, Korones SB, Perry EH, et al. Mean arterial blood pressure changes in premature infants and those at risk for intraventricular hemorrhage. J Pediatr 1990;117:607–614.

84. Cunningham S, Symon AG, Elton RA, et al. Intra-arterial blood pressure reference ranges, death and morbidity in very low birthweight infants during the first seven days of life. Early Hum Dev 1999;56:151–165.

85. Grether JK, Nelson KB, Emery ES, et al. Prenatal and perinatal factors and cerebral palsy in very low birth weight infants. J Pediatr 1996;128:407–411.

86. Fanaroff JM, Wilson-Costello DE, Newman NS, et al. Treated hypotension is associated with neonatal morbidity and hearing loss in extremely low birth weight infants. Pediatrics 2006;117:1131–1135.

87. Heuchan AM, Evans N, Henderson Smart DJ, et al. Perinatal risk factors for major intraventricular haemorrhage in the Australian and New Zealand Neonatal Network 1995–97. Arch Dis Child, Fetal Neonatal Ed 2002;86:F86–F90.

88. de Vries LS, Regev R, Dubowitz LM, et al. Perinatal risk factors for the development of extensive cystic leukomalacia. Am J Dis Child 1988;142:732–735.

89. Perlman JM, Risser R, Broyles RS. Bilateral cystic periventricular leukomalacia in the premature infant: associated risk factors. Pediatrics 1996;97:822–827.

90. Goldstein RF, Thompson RJ, Jr., Oehler JM, et al. Influence of acidosis, hypoxemia, and hypotension on neurodevelopmental outcome in very low birth weight infants. Pediatrics 1995;95:238–243.

91. Low JA, Froese AB, Galbraith RS, et al. The association between preterm newborn hypotension and hypoxemia and outcome during the first year. Acta Paediatr 1993;82:433–437.

92. Hunt RW, Evans N, Rieger I, et al. Low superior vena cava flow and neurodevelopment at 3 years in very preterm infants. J Pediatr 2004;145:588–592.

93. Osborn DA, Evans N, Kluckow M. Effect of early targeted indomethacin on the ductus arteriosus and blood flow to the upper body and brain in the preterm infant. Arch Dis Child, Fetal Neonatal Ed 2003;88:F477–F482.

94. Patel J, Roberts I, Azzopardi D, et al. Randomized double-blind controlled trial comparing the effects of ibuprofen with indomethacin on cerebral hemodynamics in preterm infants with patent ductus arteriosus. Pediatr Res 2000;47:36–42.

95. Kluckow M, Evans N. Early echocardiographic prediction of symptomatic patent ductus arteriosus in preterm infants undergoing mechanical ventilation. J Pediatr 1995;127:774–779.

96. Kluckow M, Evans N. Ductal shunting, high pulmonary blood flow, and pulmonary hemorrhage. J Pediatr 2000;137:68–72.

97. Wright IM, Goodall SR. Blood pressure and blood volume in preterm infants. Arch Dis Child, Fetal Neonatal Ed 1994;70:F230–F231.

98. Randomised trial of prophylactic early fresh-frozen plasma or gelatin or glucose in preterm babies: outcome at 2 years. Northern Neonatal Nursing Initiative Trial Group [see comments]. Lancet 1996;348:229–232.

99. Emery EF, Greenough A, Gamsu HR. Randomised controlled trial of colloid infusions in hypotensive preterm infants. Arch Dis Child 1992;67:1185–1188.

100. So KW, Fok TF, Ng PC, et al. Randomised controlled trial of colloid or crystalloid in hypotensive preterm infants. Arch Dis Child, Fetal Neonatal Ed 1997;76:F43–F46.

101. Nadel S, De Munter C, Britto J, et al. Albumin: saint or sinner? Arch Dis Child 1998;79:384–385.

102. Gill AB, Weindling AM. Randomised controlled trial of plasma protein fraction versus dopamine in hypotensive very low birthweight infants. Arch Dis Child 1993;69:284–287.

103. Van Marter LJ, Leviton A, Allred EN, et al. Hydration during the first days of life and the risk of bronchopulmonary dysplasia in low birth weight infants. J Pediatr 1990;116:942–949.

104. Osborn D, Evans N, Kluckow M. Randomized trial of dobutamine versus dopamine in preterm infants with low systemic blood flow. J Pediatr 2002;140:183–191.

105. Seri I. Cardiovascular, renal and endocrine actions of dopamine in neonates and children. J Pediatr 1995;126:333–344.

106. Pellicer A, Valverde E, Elorza MD, et al. Cardiovascular support for low birth weight infants and cerebral hemodynamics: a randomized, blinded, clinical trial. Pediatrics 2005;115:1501–1512.

107. Bourchier D, Weston PJ. Randomised trial of dopamine compared with hydrocortisone for the treatment of hypotensive very low birthweight infants. Arch Dis Child, Fetal Neonatal Ed 1997;76:F174–F178.

108. Klarr JM, Faix RG, Pryce CJ, et al. Randomized, blind trial of dopamine versus dobutamine for treatment of hypotension in preterm infants with respiratory distress syndrome. J Pediatr 1994;125:117–122.

109. Seri I, Tulassay T, Kiszel J, et al. Cardiovascular response to dopamine in hypotensive preterm neonates with severe hyaline membrane disease. Eur J Pediatr 1984;142:3–9.

110. DiSessa TG, Leitner M, Ti CC, et al. The cardiovascular effects of dopamine in the severely asphyxiated neonate. J Pediatr 1981;99:772–776.

111. Perez CA, Reimer JM, Schreiber MD, et al. Effect of high-dose dopamine on urine output in newborn infants. Crit Care Med 1986;14:1045–1049.

112. Seri I, Evans J. Addition of epinepherine to dopamine increases blood pressure and urine output in critically ill extremely low birth weight infants with uncompensated shock. Pediatr Res 1998;43:194A.

113. Ruffolo RR, Jr. The pharmacology of dobutamine. American Journal of the Medical Sciences 1987;294:244–248.

114. Noori S, Friedlich P, Seri I. Cardiovascular and renal effects of dobutamine in the neonate. NeoReviews 2004;5:E22–E26.

115. Martinez AM, Padbury JF, Thio S. Dobutamine pharmacokinetics and cardiovascular responses in critically ill neonates. Pediatrics 1992;89:47–51.

116. Stopfkuchen H, Queisser-Luft A, Vogel K. Cardiovascular responses to dobutamine determined by systolic time intervals in preterm infants. Crit Care Med 1990;18:722–724.

117. Subhedar NV, Shaw NJ. Dopamine versus dobutamine for hypotensive preterm infants. Cochrane Database of Systematic Reviews 2003;CD001242.

118. Heckmann M, Trotter A, Pohlandt F, et al. Epinephrine treatment of hypotension in very low birthweight infants. Acta Paediatr 2002;91:566–570.

119. Artman M, Kithas PA, Wike JS, et al. Inotropic responses change during postnatal maturation in rabbit. Am J Physiol 1988;255(Part 2):H335–H342.

120. Klitzner TS, Shapir Y, Ravin R, et al. The biphasic effect of amrinone on tension development in newborn mammalian myocardium. Pediatr Res 1990;27.

121. Binah O, Legato MJ. Developmental changes in the cardiac effects of amrinone in the dog. Circ Res 1983;52:747–752.

122. Akita T, Joyner RW, Lu C, et al. Developmental changes in modulation of calcium currents of rabbit ventricular cells by phosphodiesterase inhibitors. Circulation 1994;90:469–478.

123. Wernovsky G, Wypij D, Jonas RA, et al. Postoperative course and hemodynamic profile after the arterial switch operation in neonates and infants. A comparison of low-flow cardiopulmonary bypass and circulatory arrest. Circulation 1995;92:2226–2235.

124. Chang AC, Atz AM, Wernovsky G, et al. Milrinone: systemic and pulmonary hemodynamic effects in neonates after cardiac surgery. Crit Care Med 1995;23:1907–1914.

125. Hoffman TM, Wernovsky G, Atz AM, et al. Efficacy and safety of milrinone in preventing low cardiac output syndrome in infants and children after corrective surgery for congenital heart disease. Circulation 2003;107:996–1002.

126. Paradisis M, Evans N, Kluckow M, et al. Pilot study of milrinone for low systemic blood flow in very preterm infants. J Pediatr 2006;148:306–313.

127. Ng PC, Lee CH, Lam CW, et al. Transient adrenocortical insufficiency of prematurity and systemic hypotension in very low birthweight infants. Arch Dis Child, Fetal Neonatal Ed 2004;89:F119–F126.

128. Seri I, Noori S. Diagnosis and treatment of neonatal hypotension outside the transitional period. Early Hum Dev 2005;81:405–411.

129. Helbock HJ, Insoft RM, Conte FA. Glucocorticoid-responsive hypotension in extremely low birth weight newborns. Pediatrics 1993;92:715–717.

130. Seri I, Tan R, Evans J. Cardiovascular effects of hydrocortisone in preterm infants with pressor-resistant hypotension. Pediatrics 2001;107:1070–1074.

131. Hausdorff WP, Caron MG, Lefkowitz RJ. Turning off the signal: desensitization of beta-adrenergic receptor function. FASEB Journal 1990;4:2881–2889.

132. Hadcock JR, Malbon CC. Regulation of beta-adrenergic receptors by "permissive" hormones: glucocorticoids increase steady-state levels of receptor mRNA. Proc Natl Acad Sci USA 1988;85:8415–8419.

133. Segar JL, Bedell K, Page WV, et al. Effect of cortisol on gene expression of the renin–angiotensin system in fetal sheep. Pediatr Res 1995;37:741–746.

134. Knowles RG, Salter M, Brooks S, et al. Glucocorticoids inhibit the expression of an inducible, but not the constitutive, nitric oxide synthase in vascular endothelial cells. Proc Natl Acad Sci USA 1990;87:10043–10047.

135. Seri I, Evans J. Controversies in the diagnosis and management of hypotension in the newborn infant. Current Opinion in Pediatrics 2001;13:116–123.

136. Wehling M. Specific, nongenomic actions of steroid hormones. Annu Rev Physiol 1997;59:365–393.

137. Gaissmaier RE, Pohlandt F. Single-dose dexamethasone treatment of hypotension in preterm infants. J Pediatr 1999;134:701–705.

138. Fauser A, Pohlandt F, Bartmann P, et al. Rapid increase of blood pressure in extremely low birth weight infants after a single dose of dexamethasone. Eur J Pediatr 1993;152:354–356.

139. Kopelman AE, Moise AA, Holbert D, et al. A single very early dexamethasone dose improves respiratory and cardiovascular adaptation in preterm infants. J Pediatr 1999;135:345–350.

140. Noori S, Friedlich P, Ebrahimi M, Wong P, Siassi B, Seri I. Hemodynamic changes following low-dose hydrocortisone administration in vasopressor-treated preterm and term neonates. [In Press] Pediatrics 2006;.

141. Heide-Jalving M, Kamphuis PJ, van der Laan MJ, et al. Short- and long-term effects of neonatal glucocorticoid therapy: is hydrocortisone an alternative to dexamethasone? Acta Paediatr 2003;92:827–835.

142. Lodygensky GA, Rademaker K, Zimine S, et al. Structural and functional brain development after hydrocortisone treatment for neonatal chronic lung disease. Pediatrics 2005;116:1–7.

143. Watterberg KL, Shaffer ML, Mishefske MJ, et al. Growth and neurodevelopmental outcomes after early low-dose hydrocortisone treatment in extremely low birth weight infants. Pediatrics 2007;120:40–48.

144. Evans N, Seri I. Cardiovascular compromise in the newborn infant. In Avery's Diseases of the Newborn. Taeusch HW, Ballard RA, Gleason CA, eds. Philadelphia WB Saunders, 2004:398–409.

145. Yanowitz TD, Jordan JA, Gilmour CH, et al. Hemodynamic disturbances in premature infants born after chorioamnionitis: association with cord blood cytokine concentrations. Pediatr Res 2002;51:310–316.

146. Cabal LA, Devaskar U, Siassi B, et al. Cardiogenic shock associated with perinatal asphyxia in preterm infants. J Pediatr 1980;96:705–710.

147. Yao AC, Lind J. Blood volume in the asphyxiated term neonate. Biol Neonate 1972;21:199–209.

148. Walther FJ, Siassi B, Ramadan NA, et al. Cardiac output in newborn infants with transient myocardial dysfunction. J Pediatr 1985;107:781–785.

149. Seri I. Management of hypotension and low systemic blood flow in the very low birth weight neonate during the first postnatal week. J Perinatol 2006;26:S8–S13.

150. Subhedar NV. Treatment of hypotension in newborns. Seminars in Neonatology 2003;8:413–423.

151. Osborn DA. Diagnosis and treatment of preterm transitional circulatory compromise. Early Hum Dev 2005;81:413–422.

152. Osborn DA, Evans N. Early volume expansion for prevention of morbidity and mortality in very preterm infants. Cochrane Database of Systematic Reviews 2004;CD002055.

Chapter 9

The Very Low Birth Weight Neonate with a Hemodynamically Significant Ductus Arteriosus during the First Postnatal Week

Shahab Noori, MD • Istvan Seri, MD, PhD

Signs and Symptoms of PDA

Cardiovascular Adaptation to PDA

Effects of Hemodynamically Significant PDA on Blood Pressure

Effects of Hemodynamically Significant PDA on Organ Perfusion

Changes in Cardiac Function Following PDA Ligation

Summary

References

During fetal life increased pulmonary vascular resistance results in a diversion of the blood from the pulmonary to the systemic circulation through the wide-open ductus arteriosus (DA). As a consequence, the right ventricle contributes significantly to the systemic blood flow and its output is about twice that of the left ventricle (1). In addition, pulmonary blood flow is normally low *in utero*. This is important as increased pulmonary blood flow associated with ductal constriction or closure *in utero* results in alterations in the pulmonary vascular bed and the development of pulmonary hypertension after birth. Clinical and laboratory observations have shown hypertrophy and increased reactivity of the muscular layer of the pulmonary vasculature in the event of closure or constriction of the DA *in utero* (2–4). Thus, the DA acts as a pop-off valve to decrease right ventricular afterload, which, as mentioned above, is inherently high due to elevated pulmonary vascular resistance present in fetal life. The physiologically elevated pulmonary vascular resistance and the role of the DA in ensuring the contribution of the right ventricular output to systemic blood flow in the fetus explain why premature closure of the DA results in right ventricular failure and decreased systemic blood flow leading to hydrops and eventually to fetal demise.

With the first breath after birth, the pulmonary vascular resistance drops significantly and the ensuing increase in oxygen tension further reduces pulmonary vascular resistance. Since the direction of flow in the patent ductus arteriosus (PDA) depends on the relative resistances in the systemic and pulmonary circulation, the postnatal decrease in pulmonary resistance results in changes in the pattern of ductal flow from purely right-to-left *in utero* to bidirectional during the transitional period and to purely left-to-right thereafter. The transition in the flow pattern of the PDA appears to be rather short. In one study of preterm infants of less than 30 weeks' gestation, 52% of the neonates had pure left-to-right ductal shunts at 5 hours of postnatal life while 43% exhibited predominantly left-to-right shunts and only 2% had pure right-to-left shunts at this time (5). In term infants, in the absence of any pathology adversely affecting the normal postnatal reduction of the pulmonary vascular resistance, postnatal transition is short and ends with functional closure of the DA within the first 48 hours after birth. The functional closure of the DA depends, at least in part, on the thickness of the muscular layer determining its intrinsic tone and on the balance between local vasodilators and vasoconstrictors. In preterm infants, the balance of vasoconstrictors and vasodilators favors patency of the DA and the poor intrinsic tone prevents effective ductal constriction, a step crucial in ductal closure (6,7). The incidence of PDA is inversely related to gestational age, and underlying pathology such as respiratory distress syndrome (RDS) may delay the process of postnatal circulatory transition especially in premature infants of <30 weeks' gestation (8).

After functional closure, the DA undergoes significant changes and its anatomical closure prevents reopening of the vessel. Unlike in term neonates, in preterm infants, especially in those that are extremely premature, the DA frequently reopens after it has functionally closed (9–11). Induction of muscle media hypoxia is a prerequisite for anatomical closure of the DA (12). Oxygen supply to the muscle media in the late preterm and term neonate is provided directly from the oxygenated blood in the vessel lumen as well as from the adventitia through the vasa vasorum. With constriction of the DA, the vasa vasorum obliterate, resulting in the development of hypoxia within the muscle media. However, oxygen supply in the thin-walled DA of the extremely premature infant only depends on the luminal flow because of the ability of the oxygen to diffuse through the entire vessel wall and there is no or only minimal vasa vasorum present in the adventitia. Therefore, constriction of the immature DA does not lead to the development of tissue hypoxia (13) resulting in incomplete anatomical closure or reopening of DA in the extremely premature neonate.

The increased mortality and morbidity associated with the presence of a PDA stems from a combination of pulmonary overcirculation and a decrease in blood flow to the systemic circulation. The increased pulmonary blood flow, the resulting damage to the capillary bed, and pulmonary edema result in increased requirement for ventilatory support and may explain the higher incidence of associated bronchopulmonary dysplasia (BPD) in immature neonates with a PDA. Furthermore, the systemic hypoperfusion explains, at least in part, the increased incidence of intraventricular hemorrhage (IVH), periventricular leukomalacia (PVL) and necrotizing enterocolitis (NEC) in preterm neonates with a PDA. However, it is important to note that this is only an association and the cause and effect relationship of PDA with these morbidities has recently been questioned (14,15).

This chapter will discuss the effects of PDA on the cardiovascular system and systemic, pulmonary, and organ blood flows, with a special emphasis on how the premature heart copes with the increased preload and decreased peripheral vascular resistance associated with the significant left-to-right shunting across the PDA.

SIGNS AND SYMPTOMS OF PDA

The development of cardiovascular compromise and the degree of the symptomatology of the PDA depend on the size and direction of the shunt, duration of ductal patency, extent of the "steal phenomenon," and adequacy of the compensatory mechanisms of the premature myocardium and other organs.

The pattern of the ductal shunt depends on the size of the DA and relative resistance in the pulmonary and systemic circulation (5). In uncomplicated situations, the shunt pattern changes from bidirectional to left-to-right before complete closure of the DA. In the majority of preterm infants, the DA is open in the first few days of postnatal life. During this stage, the pulmonary and systemic hemodynamic effects of PDA appear to be well compensated. This explains why the specificity and sensitivity of the clinical diagnosis of PDA are low during the first few postnatal days (16–18). With time, however, the classic signs and symptoms of PDA appear, including the presence of a hyperactive left ventricular impulse, increased pulse pressure, systolic murmur, and the increased need for ventilatory support (19). In most cases, the clinically silent PDA during the first few days goes undetected unless an echocardiogram is performed. Although color Doppler is very sensitive in diagnosing a PDA, the mere presence of a ductal flow is a poor indicator of the hemodynamic disturbances that might be caused by the PDA. Although not well defined, a hemodynamically significant PDA (hsPDA) usually refers to a state where the left-to-right shunt across the PDA has created a significant volume overload of the heart and it is often associated with exhaustion of the compensatory mechanisms resulting in pulmonary edema and systemic hypoperfusion. Using echocardiographic measures, the left atrial to aortic root diameter ratio (LA:AO) (20,21), the size of the DA, and/or estimation of the ductal flow (22,23) have been used to define an hsPDA. The LA:AO ratio estimates the significance of PDA by assessing the degree of volume overload of the left side of the heart. Presuming a normal mitral valve and left ventricle function, the size of the left atrium is indicative of the left ventricular preload. However, this index does not necessarily reflect the degree of pulmonary overcirculation, as the presence of a stretched patent foramen ovale (PFO) or atrial septal defect (ASD) reduces the left atrial diameter and therefore the LA:AO ratio. In addition, a presumably normal LA:AO ratio does not say anything about the degree of steal phenomenon from the systemic circulation. In the presence of a non-restricting PFO/ASD, a small left atrial diameter (lower preload) may, at least theoretically, interfere with the compensatory increase in LV output to offset the systemic steal phenomenon. Defining the size of the PDA by color Doppler is another more objective way to assess the hemodynamic significance of ductal patency. A PDA size of 1.6 or 2 mm has been used as an indicator of a hemodynamically significant PDA. Kluckow and Evans showed that a ductal diameter of >1.6 mm at 5 hours of postnatal life predicts occurrence of hsPDA in preterm infants of <30 weeks' gestation (5,22). Unfortunately, estimation of the ductal flow by measuring the ductal diameter and the flow velocity is also less than perfect because of the problems associated with the accurate determination of the ductal diameter and the frequent presence of a turbulent flow, respectively. Despite these shortcomings, determination of the LA:AO ratio and the size of and the flow through the PDA is useful as these indices appear to correlate with clinical symptomatology. More recently, diastolic flow velocity of the left pulmonary artery (24), transductal velocity ratio (25), and ratio of the left ventricular output to superior vena cava (SVC) flow (26) have been used in an attempt to quantify the hemodynamic significance of the PDA. Finally, serum levels of B-type natriuretic peptide (BNP) have been suggested as a possible indicator of an hsPDA (27–29). Although BNP serum levels correlate well with echocardiographic markers of an hsPDA (29), the large variability in the proposed cutoff value defining an hsPDA among the different studies and the low specificity of this test render it less than optimal for routine clinical use.

CARDIOVASCULAR ADAPTATION TO PDA

Cardiac output is the result of the interactions among preload, afterload, myocardial contractility, and heart rate. Under normal conditions and in the absence of a PDA, the left cardiac output of a neonate is in the range of 150–300 mL/kg per min. Since blood flow to the lungs is increased in the presence of a left-to-right shunt through the DA, venous return from the pulmonary circulation to the left atrium is also increased resulting in an increase in the preload of the left ventricle. Studies have consistently shown a higher left ventricle end-diastolic volume (preload) when the DA is open with a predominantly left-to-right shunting pattern. According to the Starling curve, the increase in myocardial muscle fiber stretch from higher preload augments stroke volume. Indeed, most but not all (30,31) studies have demonstrated a significantly increased left ventricular output in the presence of a PDA with predominantly left-to-right shunting (32–39). In a lamb model where DA was infiltrated with formalin and ductal patency was regulated by a mechanical occluder, Clyman et al. studied the effect of increasing degree of shunting through the PDA (35). Compared to when the DA was closed, stroke volume increased by 33%, 66%, and 97% as the ductal shunt increased by 31%, 50%, and 67% of the baseline left ventricular stroke volume, respectively. However, in the clinical setting, the presence of a PFO significantly alters the effect of PDA on stroke volume as it decompresses the left atrium. In fact, it has been shown that in the presence of a significant PFO flow, the right ventricular output may even be higher than the left ventricular output despite the presence of the significant left-to-right shunt through the PDA (40).

It appears that, despite the significant volume overload in the presence of a PDA, the left ventricle is quite capable of handling the additional volume. Preterm lambs with an open DA are able to increase their stroke volume when challenged with a fluid bolus, even though the degree of the increase is less than when the DA is closed (34). The decrease in the total peripheral vascular resistance associated with the presence of a PDA results in a reduction of the left ventricle afterload. The reduction in the afterload may in turn enhance the ability of the myocardiums to increase the stroke volume.

There are significant differences in both the structure and function of the myocardium between preterm and term neonates and older children and adults. These differences put the immature myocardium at a disadvantage as far as contractility is concerned (41). Furthermore, since perfusion to the myocardium primarily takes place during diastole, it is expected that myocardial performance would be adversely affected in patients with an hsPDA when diastolic blood pressure is low. However, although the findings of some studies suggest the presence of myocardial ischemia (42,43) and a deterioration of myocardial performance, most of the published data indicate that myocardial perfusion and function are maintained. Moreover, since the higher preload is associated with a greater stretch of the myocardial fibers in the presence of a PDA, myocardial contractility should actually increase. Therefore, some authors have stated that the mere maintenance of myocardial contractility in preterm neonates with a PDA in fact suggests deterioration of myocardial function. However, using a load-independent measure of myocardial contractility, Barlow et al. showed that hsPDA had no effect on contractility (44). Similarly, contractility, assessed by a load-independent index, has been reported to remain unchanged after ligation of the DA (45). In addition, a recent study showed that cardiac troponin T, a marker of myocardial cell injury, is not elevated in preterm infants with a PDA during the first postnatal week (46). However, as in this small study the PDA was treated prior to becoming hemodynamically significant, caution should be exercised with the interpretation of the findings.

As the heart rate remains unchanged whether the DA is open or closed, the increase in cardiac output is solely result of the increase in the stroke volume. The increase in cardiac output, at least initially, may offset the systemic hemodynamic effects of the PDA. However, in a significant number of very low birth weight (VLBW) infants, this compensatory mechanism will eventually fail and systemic perfusion becomes inadequate. At this stage, signs and symptoms of organ and tissue hypoperfusion initially present in the form of poor peripheral perfusion and decreased urine output while later hypotension and lactic acidosis develop.

EFFECTS OF HEMODYNAMICALLY SIGNIFICANT PDA ON BLOOD PRESSURE

Hypotension commonly occurs in the presence of an hsPDA (47–49). Even as early as the first postnatal day, PDA is clearly associated with hypotension (49). Blood pressure is the product of the interaction between cardiac output and peripheral vascular resistance. In general, systolic blood pressure is primarily affected by the changes in stroke volume while diastolic blood pressure is mainly reflective of changes in peripheral vascular resistance. Traditionally, low diastolic blood pressure has been considered the hallmark of an hsPDA and many studies have supported this notion (39,44). However, studies that looked more specifically at the relationship between blood pressure and PDA have shown a similar decrease in both systolic and diastolic blood pressure, at least in the first postnatal week (47,48). Ratner et al. examined the association between blood pressure and PDA in a group of preterm infants weighing <1200 g during the first postnatal week (47). None of the babies were treated with indomethacin or cardiotropic medications. By the second postnatal day, there was a significant decrease in both systolic and diastolic blood pressure in patients with an hsPDA. In addition, they reported no significant differences in the pulse pressure between patients with and without a PDA (Fig. 9-1). Evans and Moorcraft studied the effects of hsPDA on blood pressure during the first postnatal week (48). The presence of an hsPDA was assessed by daily echocardiography and blood pressure was continuously monitored using an umbilical catheter. In infants with a birth weight between 1000 and 1500 g, there was a slight but nonsignificant difference in systolic, diastolic, and mean blood pressure between patients with and without an hsPDA. In contrast, in infants with a birth weight <1000 g, the systolic, diastolic, and mean blood pressures were significantly lower in the hsPDA group (Figs 9-2 and 9-3). As in the previous study (47), pulse pressure was not increased in patients with an hsPDA during the first postnatal week (48). As discussed earlier, since stroke volume increases and vascular resistance decreases in the presence of an hsPDA, it is expected for the systolic blood pressure to be maintained or slightly decrease while diastolic blood pressure is to disproportionately decrease. Since the cardiac output, ductal shunt volume, and

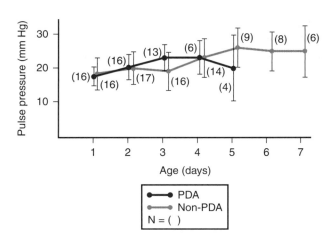

FIGURE 9-1 Similar pulse pressure in PDA and non-PDA preterm infants in the first week of life (47).

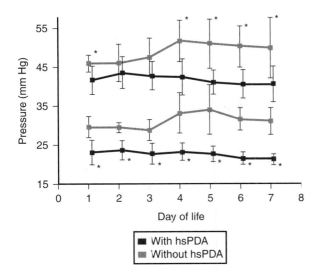

FIGURE 9-2 Changes in systolic and diastolic BP in infants <1000 g with and without an hsPDA during the first week of life (48).

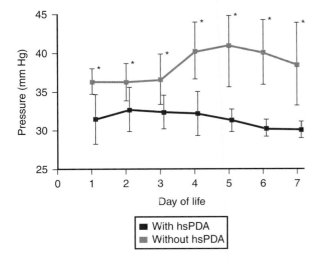

FIGURE 9-3 Changes in mean BP in infants <1000 g with and without an hsPDA during the first week of life (48).

peripheral resistance were not measured in the above studies, the reason for lack of a wide pulse pressure cannot be determined. The authors speculated that failure of a compensatory increase in the cardiac output secondary to myocardial immaturity might be the cause of the more uniform reduction in the systolic and diastolic blood pressure. However, since the severity and duration of the PDA shunt likely determine the extent of the diastolic steal phenomenon and therefore the pattern of hypotension, a definitive conclusion about the interaction between PDA and blood pressure cannot be drawn, at least for the human neonate. According to findings in immature animals, a significant decrease in systolic blood pressure occurs only when the PDA shunt is moderate or large. Yet, a decrease in the diastolic and mean blood pressure occurs even when the shunt is small (35).

EFFECTS OF HEMODYNAMICALLY SIGNIFICANT PDA ON ORGAN PERFUSION

The mechanisms causing organ hypoperfusion in the presence of an hsPDA include the systolic and diastolic steal phenomena leading to a decrease in systemic blood flow and the development of hypotension resulting in a decrease in perfusion pressure.

In addition, treatment strategies used to facilitate closure of the PDA, such as indomethacin administration, may have an effect on organ blood flow independent of the hemodynamic changes associated with the presence of an hsPDA.

The studies on the effects of an hsPDA on organ perfusion have primarily focussed on changes in perfusion of the brain and intestine. Blood flow velocity measured by the Doppler technique has been the primary mode used to assess organ blood flow in the neonate although cerebral blood flow has also been assessed using near infrared (NIR) spectroscopy. In addition, in animal models, the microsphere technique has also been utilized. It is important to note that these techniques have significant limitations and that at present we do not have the ability to continuously measure absolute blood flow to the different organs in the human neonate.

As for using the Doppler technique, the amount of blood flowing through a vessel is a function of the vessel diameter (cross-sectional area) and mean blood flow velocity. Because of the small size of the vessels of interest in the neonate (e.g. anterior or middle cerebral artery), accurate measurement of the diameter is not possible. In addition, it is presumed that the diameter of the vessel remains constant during the cardiac cycle, a notion that has been repeatedly challenged. Despite these limitations, however, Doppler velocity measurements and velocity-derived indices have been shown to have fairly good correlations with more invasive measures of organ blood flow (50–52). The most commonly used indicators of organ blood flow are systolic, diastolic, and mean blood flow velocities, velocity time integral, pulsatility index (PI), and resistive index (RI). As the PI and RI are inversely related to flow and directly related to vascular resistance, an increase in the PI or RI indicates a reduction in organ blood flow.

Cerebral Blood Flow

Although some studies suggested maintenance of cerebral blood flow in the presence of an hsPDA (33,39), the majority of the studies found a disturbance in cerebral hemodynamics. Furthermore, indomethacin, used commonly for the pharmacological closure of the PDA, has a direct albeit transient vasoconstrictive effect in the cerebral circulation (53).

In a group of preterm infants, Perlman et al. evaluated changes in blood flow velocity in the anterior cerebral artery on a daily basis starting from the first postnatal day (54). Using the Doppler technique, they demonstrated a decrease in diastolic blood flow velocity in the presence of an hsPDA.

Several investigators have reported a retrograde diastolic flow and an increase in the PI in the anterior cerebral artery in the presence of PDA; findings suggestive of a decrease in cerebral blood flow (55,56). In contrast, Shortland et al. found no difference in cerebral blood flow velocity between infants with or without a PDA in a cohort of 120 preterm infants (57). However, they reported a higher incidence of PVL in infants with retrograde blood flow in the anterior cerebral artery. Therefore, it is possible that only a subset of patients with a PDA is adversely affected and these include patients with an hsPDA or a diastolic steal phenomenon. A recent study by Jim et al. demonstrated a correlation between an hsPDA assessed by the LA:AO ratio and both end-diastolic velocity and RI in the anterior cerebral artery in VLBW infants (58). Although the correlations were weak, these data suggest that with a more severe left-to-right shunt across the PDA, cerebral blood flow progressively decreases. Interestingly, in preterm lambs (33) and humans (39) cerebral blood flow is maintained in the presence of a PDA when left cardiac output is increased. It is conceivable that the increase in the cardiac output, at least to a certain point, ensures adequate cerebral perfusion in patients with a PDA. Indeed, Baylen et al. have reported a decrease in cerebral blood flow when cardiac output was compromised in preterm lambs (30).

Study	Treatment n/N	Control n/N	Relative risk (fixed) 95% CI	Weight (%)	Relative risk (fixed) 95% CI
Bada 1989	27/71	37/70		7.8	0.72 [0.50, 1.04]
Bandstra 1988	43/99	62/100		12.8	0.70 [0.53, 0.92]
Hanigan 1988	6/56	11/55		2.3	0.54 [0.21, 1.35]
Krueger 1987	4/15	5/17		1.0	0.91 [0.30, 2.77]
Mahony 1985	12/54	17/56		3.5	0.73 [0.39, 1.38]
Ment 1985	6/24	14/24		2.9	0.43 [0.20, 0.93]
Ment 1988	2/19	8/17		1.8	0.22 [0.05, 0.91]
Ment 1994b	25/209	40/222		8.1	0.66 [0.42, 1.05]
Morales-Suarez 1994	20/40	22/40		4.6	0.91 [0.60, 1.38]
Puckett 1985	15/16	10/16		2.1	1.50 [1.01, 2.24]
Rennie 1986a	10/24	9/26		1.8	1.20 [0.59, 2.45]
Supapannachart 1999	5/15	5/15		1.0	1.00 [0.36, 2.75]
TIPP 2001	236/601	234/601		48.7	1.01 [0.88, 1.16]
Vincer 1985	11/15	8/15		1.7	1.38 [0.78, 2.41]
Total (95% CI)	422/1258	482/1274		100.0	0.88 [0.80, 0.98]

Test for heterogeneity chi-square = 27.30 df = 13 p = 0.0113
Test for overall effect = –2.43 p = 0.01

0.1 0.2   1   5 10
Favors treatment   Favors control

FIGURE 9-4 Meta-analysis of randomized controlled study of indomethacin prophylaxis showed reduction in the incidence of IVH in prophylactic indomethacin group compared to the control (59).

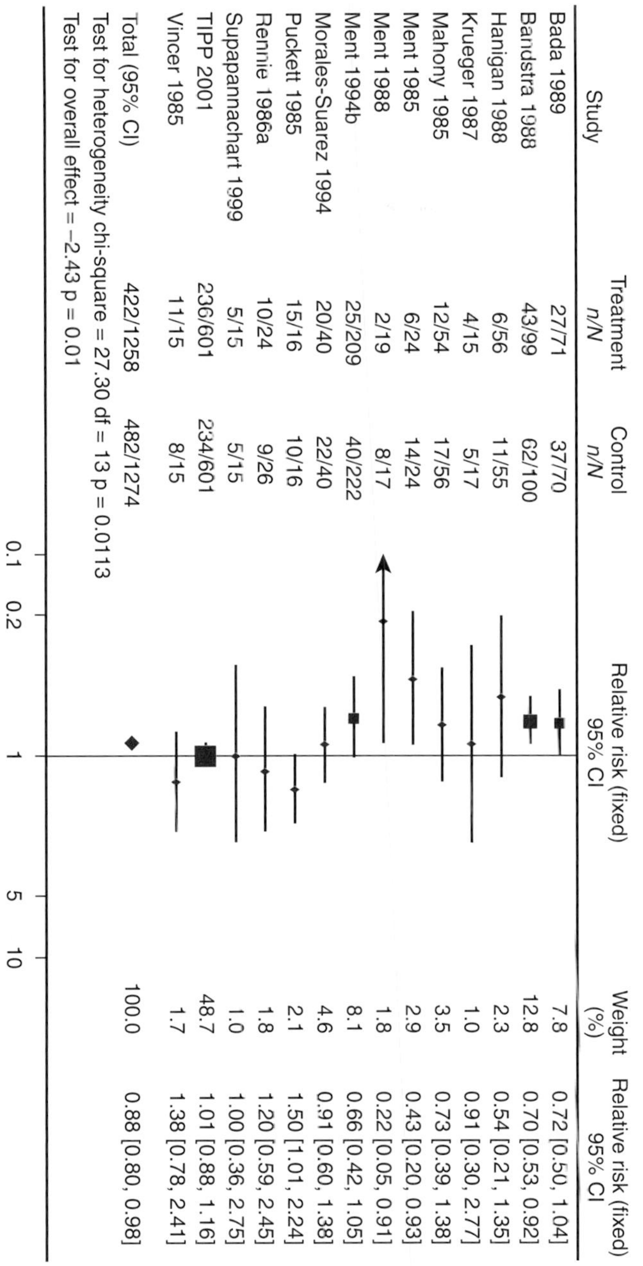

The adverse impact of an hsPDA on the cerebral circulation is strengthened by the findings that prophylactic indomethacin administration significantly decreases the incidence of both IVH and hsPDA (Fig. 9-4). Although the direct cerebral vasoconstrictive effect of indomethacin may contribute to the decreased incidence of IVH in preterm neonates receiving prophylactic indomethacin, surgical closure of the DA has also been reported to decrease the incidence of IVH (60).

Superior Mesenteric and Celiac Artery Blood Flow

Intestinal hypoperfusion is a known risk factor for NEC. Studies evaluating blood flow to the abdominal organs in general and to the superior mesenteric artery (SMA) in particular have uniformly demonstrated a decrease in blood flow in

FIGURE 9-5 Organ blood flow in preterm lambs with and without PDA (35).

| | Ductus left-to-right shunt | | | | | |
| | Small (n = 18) | | Moderate (n = 25) | | Large (n = 20) | |
	Closed	Open	Closed	Open	Closed	Open
Spleen (mL/min/100 g)	178 ± 133	110 ± 92*	216 ± 136	135 ± 100†	259 ± 155	106 ± 55‡
Gastrointestinal (mL/min/100 g)	74 ± 40	59 ± 34§	78 ± 41	54 ± 32‡	80 ± 39	34 ± 16∥
Adrenal (mL/min/100 g)	278 ± 142	218 ± 124§	322 ± 179	202 ± 109∥	300 ± 104	205 ± 208§
Carcass (mL/min/100 g)	9.5 ± 3.8	8.3 ± 2.8	9.2 ± 2.8	6.6 ± 1.8∥	7.7 ± 2.2	4.3 ± 1.5∥
Kidneys (mL/min/100 g)	160 ± 50	139 ± 64§	154 ± 73	113 ± 59‡	140 ± 48	88 ± 45‡
Liver (mL/min/100 g)	23 ± 13	18 ± 10*	28 ± 18	20 ± 12‡	30 ± 20	16 ± 12∥
Brain (mL/min/100 g)	40 ± 20	34 ± 15	37 ± 12	31 ± 10†	39 ± 8	28 ± 6‡
Heart (mL/min/100 g)	96 ± 47	114 ± 61	111 ± 47	123 ± 84	82 ± 36	83 ± 42
LV (mL/min/100 g)	102 ± 52	125 ± 73§	136 ± 61	152 ± 123	93 ± 41	97 ± 41
LV in/LV out	1.13 ± 0.49	1.03 ± 0.46§	1.22 ± 0.48	1.08 ± 0.32*	1.35 ± 0.48	1.09 ± 0.37†

Values represent mean ± SD.
Carcass = skin, skeletal muscle, bone; heart = total heart; LV = LV free wall; LV in/LV out = blood flow to inner third of LV divided by flow to outer two-thirds.
*$P < 0.01$, open vs closed.
†$P < 0.005$
‡$P < 0.0005$
§$P < 0.05$
∥$P < 0.00005$

the presence of an hsPDA. In addition, administration of indomethacin appears to directly also reduce intestinal blood flow.

Clyman et al. studied the effects of small, moderate and large left-to-right PDA shunting on systemic and organ blood flow using the microsphere technique in preterm lambs during the first 10 hours after delivery (35). Shunts were classified as small, moderate, or large if they were less than 40%, 40 to 60%, and greater than 60% of the left ventricular cardiac output, respectively. Even with a small ductal shunt, there were significant reductions in blood flow to abdominal organs (Fig. 9-5). With the increase in shunt size, there was a further decrease in organ blood flow. The compromise in organ blood flow occurred despite significant increases in cardiac output. Furthermore, there was evidence that decreased perfusion pressure and localized vasoconstriction were responsible for the reduction in organ blood flow. Baylen et al. first also documented compromised organ blood flows (including the gastrointestinal tract) in more immature preterm lambs with a PDA during the first few postnatal hours (30), although they could not reproduce these findings in a more recent study (33).

Meyers et al. studied the effects of PDA and indomethacin on intestinal blood flow and oxygen consumption in preterm lambs in the immediate newborn period (38). Blood flow was measured using the microsphere technique. These authors demonstrated that shunting across the PDA or indomethacin administration decreases blood flow in the terminal ileum. However, oxygen consumption in the terminal ileum remained unchanged whether the ductus was open or closed and autoregulation of oxygen consumption was only compromised in presence of indomethacin. As the study involved only slightly premature animals in the first few hours after delivery, it is not known whether autoregulation remains intact in the more premature primate in case of a prolonged ductal patency.

In a group of preterm infants with a large PDA, Martin et al. reported a retrograde diastolic flow in the descending aorta, which resolved after closure of DA (55). Similarly, Deeg et al. demonstrated a decrease in both the systolic and diastolic blood flow velocities in the celiac artery in preterm infants with a PDA; a finding implying that a decrease in the blood flow in the celiac artery has occurred in these patients (56).

Using ultrasound, Shimada et al. assessed left cardiac output and abdominal aortic blood flow in VLBW infants before and after ductal closure and compared the findings to those obtained in patients without a PDA (39). Blood flow in the abdominal aorta was significantly lower in the PDA group before closure of the DA than after ductal closure or in the control group (Fig. 9-6). Furthermore, they demonstrated that abdominal aorta blood flow was compromised despite the presence of a significantly higher left ventricular cardiac output in the PDA group before closure of the DA.

Coombs et al., also using the Doppler technique, studied the effects of symptomatic PDA and indomethacin administration on SMA and celiac artery blood flow in preterm infants (61). PDA was diagnosed based on clinical symptoms. In the presence of a clinically diagnosed PDA, there was an abnormal blood flow pattern (absent or retrograde diastolic blood flow) in both arteries but more so in the SMA. In addition, they showed that indomethacin decreased peak systolic velocity in the SMA especially when given as a bolus.

The findings of decreased systemic and gastrointestinal blood flow in preterm neonates with a PDA and indomethacin administration may, at least in part,

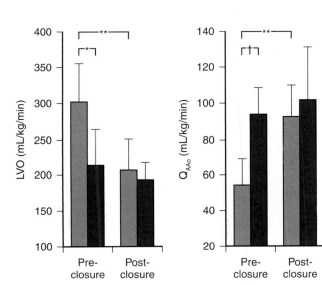

FIGURE 9-6 Left ventricular output (LVO) and blood flow volume of the abdominal aorta (QAAo) before and after closure of ductus arteriosus by mefenamic acid. ▨ values for hsPDA group; ▮ values for group without hsPDA. Values are expressed as mean ± SD. $*P < 0.002$; $**P < 0.001$; $\dagger P < 0.0001$ (37).

explain the increased incidence of NEC and spontaneous intestinal perforations under these clinical scenarios, respectively. However, although early ligation of the PDA decreases the incidence of NEC (60), randomized studies on prophylactic indomethacin treatment have not shown a decrease in the incidence of NEC. A recent metanalysis of 11 randomized controlled studies on prophylactic indomethacin administration to decrease mortality and morbidity in preterm infants revealed no beneficial effects on the incidence of NEC (59) (Fig. 9-7). There are several possible explanations for the lack of effectiveness of prophylactic indomethacin in reducing the incidence of NEC. First, studies on the use of prophylactic indomethacin were not designed to evaluate the impact of PDA closure on the incidence of NEC. Rather, these studies were primarily designed to determine the

FIGURE 9-7 Meta-analysis of randomized controlled study of indomethacin prophylaxis showed no difference in the incidence of NEC in prophylactic indomethacin group compared to the control (59).

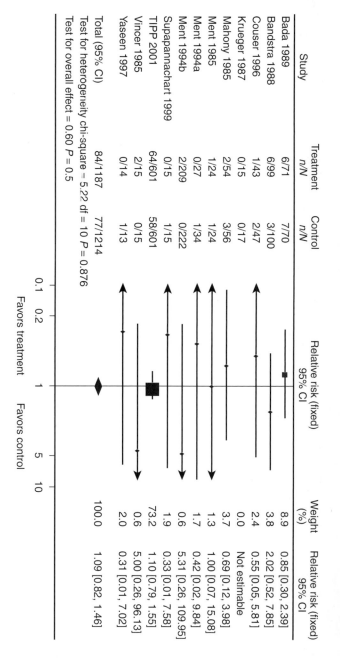

efficacy of early indomethacin in the prevention of IVH or in the prevention of the extension of a pre-existing IVH (62–65) or to examine the effect of prophylactic indomethacin on ductal closure (63,66–68) or neurodevelopmental (69,70) or pulmonary outcome (71,72). In addition, in these studies, the control groups received indomethacin or PDA ligation if the ductus remained open further complicating our ability to critically examine the impact of ductal closure on the incidence of NEC. Second, indomethacin itself has a direct negative impact on intestinal blood flow and autoregulation of oxygen consumption and these actions may counter the potential beneficial hemodynamic effects associated with the pharmacological closure of the DA.

CHANGES IN CARDIAC FUNCTION FOLLOWING PDA LIGATION

Given the detrimental hemodynamic effects of an hsPDA on systemic and pulmonary organ blood flows, one would expect an improvement in the clinical status following removal of ductal shunting by ligation. However, in clinical practice the neonatologist often observes deterioration in the patient's condition immediately after surgical ligation of the DA before seeing an improvement. Indeed, some investigators reported worsening of the cardiovascular status evidenced by an increase in the requirement for vasopressor support in about one-third of the preterm infants immediately following ligation (45,73).

As discussed earlier, the cardiac adaptive processes to a PDA with left-to-right shunt include an increase in left ventricular output (mostly stroke volume) in response to the increased preload and the ductal steal phenomenon. Therefore, if other variables remain unchanged and according to Starling's law the mere removal of ductal shunting with a resultant decrease in the preload would be expected to lead to a reduction in left cardiac output and perhaps a decrease in the force of contraction. These changes may not necessarily indicate deterioration in cardiac function; rather, they represent a return to the normal basal function. However, reduction in preload is not the only change that occurs after surgical closure of the DA. Several other factors such as prolonged exposure of the immature myocardium to volume overload and the sudden change in the SVR following ligation may have an impact on cardiac function in a way that cannot be explained by change in the preload alone.

However, there are only limited data in the literature on the effects of PDA ligation on cardiac function. Most animal studies have evaluated myocardial performance after ductal ligation in the first 24 hours of birth (30,74). Therefore, applying the findings of animal studies to humans is inappropriate since, in the clinical practice, the preterm infant has usually been exposed to the effects of ductal shunting for days or sometimes weeks before surgical ligation takes place. A recent study by McCurnin et al. describes the effects of PDA ligation performed on the 6th day of postnatal life on cardiopulmonary function in the preterm baboon (75). These authors found medium-term beneficial effects of PDA ligation on left and right myocardial performance. However, the study did not examine the changes in cardiac function in the immediate postoperative period.

As for humans, there are only a few studies addressing this issue in preterm infants. Lindner et al. assessed cardiac function by measuring left ventricular output, stroke volume and heart rate two days after PDA ligation and compared the findings to pre-ligation measurements (37). They reported a significant decrease in left ventricular output and stroke volume without a significant change in heart rate. In contrast, Kimball et al. found an increase in systemic vascular resistance and heart rate and no change in the myocardial contractility, left ventricular output, or afterload (76). It is unclear as to why left cardiac output did not decrease as expected with a reduction in the preload, although there was a statistically not significant 20% decrease in left cardiac output in this study enrolling only a small number of patients. In addition to these studies describing the changes in systolic function, we have recently reported our findings on diastolic and global myocardial function after PDA ligation (45). We found a significant reduction in preload and left ventricular output two hours after ligation without further changes at 24 hours post-ligation. The reduction in left ventricular output appears to have been the result of a decrease in stroke volume as the heart rate remained unchanged. Similar to Kimball et al., we found no change in contractility or afterload despite an increase in systemic vascular resistance after ligation. While the afterload is affected by changes in systemic vascular resistance primarily via changes in the blood pressure, the left ventricular diameter and wall thickness are among the other factors that affect afterload. We speculate that, following PDA ligation, the decrease in left ventricular diameter and the increase in wall thickness offset the effects of the increase in systemic vascular resistance on afterload with the net result being no change in the afterload. In addition, we found no change in diastolic function as assessed by indices derived from mitral inflow and tissue Doppler studies. We also assessed the global myocardial function (both systolic and diastolic) using the myocardial performance index (MPI) (77,78). Interestingly, the changes in the MPI indicated deterioration of myocardial function immediately after ligation with a partial recovery by 24 hours post-ligation. The deterioration in myocardial performance may be the result of the acute decrease in the length of myofibrils immediately following the ductal ligation-induced volume unloading. However, myocardial performance improves with time perhaps by resetting the myocyte to the new loading condition. Thus, these findings suggest that the decrease in stroke volume immediately following ligation is caused by both the acute volume unloading of the left ventricle and the deterioration in cardiac function. Furthermore, we found that the size of PDA correlates best with the deterioration in myocardial function after ligation suggesting a direct relation of the severity of volume overload with the post-ligation myocardial performance.

Therefore, apart from a significant reduction in left ventricular output (stroke volume), there are no major changes in systolic and diastolic function after PDA ligation in preterm infants. However, it appears that a subtle deterioration in myocardial performance occurs immediately after ligation, which probably contributes to the decrease in stroke volume. It is still unclear as to why a subset of preterm infants presents with hypotension and increased requirement for vasopressors following PDA ligation. While left ventricular output measured in the aorta proximal to the DA decreases after ligation, the changes in effective left ventricular output (i.e. the portion of the left ventricular output supplying the systemic circulation and not shunting into the pulmonary circulation before ductal ligation) are not known. Therefore, it is unclear whether the hypotension observed in a significant portion of these preterm infants is the result of a decrease in effective left ventricular output due to myocardial dysfunction, a decrease in systemic vascular resistance after the initial rise or a combination of these two cardiovascular changes. In addition, downregulation of cardiovascular adrenergic receptors, relative adrenal insufficiency and anesthesia could also be associated with alterations in vasomotor tone, requiring escalation of vasopressor support to maintain blood pressure in critically ill preterm neonates undergoing surgery (79,80).

SUMMARY

Patent ductus arteriosus is a common problem in preterm infants born at less than 30 weeks' gestational age. Contrary to the common belief, the shunt across the PDA is primarily left-to-right very soon after birth. If the DA remains open, it will result in a progressively increasing pulmonary overcirculation and left-sided cardiac volume overload. Despite the immaturity of myocardium, the heart is capable of increasing the cardiac output even in VLBW neonates. The increase in cardiac output is a result of the increase in the stroke volume, usually without a significant change in heart rate. Because of the diversion of blood from the aorta to the pulmonary artery, the increase in left ventricular output does not usually translate to an increase in or even maintenance of *effective* left cardiac output. While the increase in the left ventricular output and other compensatory mechanisms may initially offset the effects of the ductal shunt on the systemic circulation, with time effective left cardiac output is reduced. Indeed, both animal and human studies show compromised organ blood flows especially to organs supplied by the aorta distal to the PDA. The PDA is also a significant cause of hypotension in preterm infants. The hypotension and systolic and diastolic steal phenomena can lead to organ hypoperfusion and lactic acidosis. Finally, the persistence of an hsPDA will eventually lead to congestive heart failure.

REFERENCES

1. Clyman RI, et al., eds. Maternal–Fetal Medicine. Philadelphia, WB Saunders, 1999:249.
2. Levin DL, Mills LJ, Weinberg AG. Hemodynamic, pulmonary vascular, and myocardial abnormalities secondary to pharmacologic constriction of the fetal ductus arteriosus. A possible mechanism for persistent pulmonary hypertension and transient tricuspid insufficiency in the newborn infant. Circulation 1979;60:360–364.
3. Van Marter LJ, Leviton A, Allred EN, Pagano M, Sullivan KF, Cohen A, Epstein MF. Persistent pulmonary hypertension of the newborn and smoking and aspirin and nonsteroidal antiinflammatory drug consumption during pregnancy. Pediatrics 1996;97:658–663.
4. Alano MA, Ngougmna E, Ostrea EM Jr, Konduri GG. Analysis of nonsteroidal antiinflammatory drugs in meconium and its relation to persistent pulmonary hypertension of the newborn. Pediatrics 2001;107:519–523.
5. Evans N, Malcolm G, Osborn D, Kluckow M. Diagnosis of patent ductus arteriosus in preterm infants. NeoReview 2004;5:e86–97.
6. Clyman RI, Waleh N, Black SM, Riemer RK, Mauray F, Chen YQ. Regulation of ductus arteriosus patency by nitric oxide in fetal lambs: the role of gestation, oxygen tension, and vasa vasorum. Pediatr Res 1998;43:633–644.
7. Kajino H, Chen YQ, Seidner SR, et al. Factors that increase the contractile tone of the ductus arteriosus also regulate its anatomic remodeling. Am J Physiol, Regul Integr Comp Physiol 2001;281:R291–R301.
8. Reller MD, Rice MJ, McDonald RW. Review of studies evaluating ductal patency in the premature infant. J Pediatr 1993;122:S59–S62.
9. Gonzalez A, Sosenko IR, Chandar J, Hummler H, Claure N, Bancalari E. Influence of infection on patent ductus arteriosus and chronic lung disease in premature infants weighing 1000 grams or less. J Pediatr 1996;128:470–478.
10. Narayanan M, Cooper B, Weiss H, Clyman RI. Prophylactic indomethacin: factors determining permanent ductus arteriosus closure. J Pediatr 2000;136:330–337.
11. Keller RL, Clyman RI. Persistent Doppler flow predicts lack of response to multiple courses of indomethacin in premature infants with recurrent patent ductus arteriosus. Pediatrics 2003;112:583–587.
12. Clyman RI, Chan CY, Mauray F, et al. Permanent anatomic closure of the ductus arteriosus in newborn baboons: the roles of postnatal constriction, hypoxia, and gestation. Pediatr Res 1999;45:19–29.
13. Kajino H, Goldbarg S, Roman C, et al. Vasa vasorum hypoperfusion is responsible for medial hypoxia and anatomic remodeling in the newborn lamb ductus arteriosus. Pediatr Res 2002;51:228–235.
14. Laughon MM, Simmons MA, Bose CL. Patency of the ductus arteriosus in the premature infant: is it pathologic? Should it be treated?. Curr Opin Pediatr 2004;16:146–151.
15. Brooks JM, Travadi JN, Patole SK, Doherty DA, Simmer K. Is surgical ligation of patent ductus arteriosus necessary? The Western Australian experience of conservative management. Arch Dis Child, Fetal Neonatal Ed 2005;90:F235–F239.
16. Skelton R, Evans N, Smythe J. A blinded comparison of clinical and echocardiographic evaluation of the preterm infant for patent ductus arteriosus. J Paediatr Child Health 1994;30:406–411.
17. Davis P, Turner-Gomes S, Cunningham K, Way C, Roberts R, Schmidt B. Precision and accuracy of clinical and radiological signs in premature infants at risk of patent ductus arteriosus. Arch Pediatr Adol Med 1995;149:1136–1141.

18. Urquhart DS, Nicholl RM. How good is clinical examination at detecting a significant patent ductus arteriosus in the preterm neonate? Arch Dis Child 2003;88:85–86.

19. Ellison RC, Peckham GJ, Lang P, et al. Evaluation of the preterm infant for patent ductus arteriosus. Pediatrics 1983;71:364–372.

20. Johnson GL, Breart GL, Gewitz MH, Brenner JI, Lang P, Dooley KJ, Ellison RC. Echocardiographic characteristics of premature infants with patent ductus arteriosus. Pediatrics 1983;72:864–871.

21. Iyer P, Evans N. Re-evaluation of the left atrial to aortic root ratio as a marker of patent ductus arteriosus. Arch Dis Child, Fetal Neonatal Ed 1994;70:F112–F117.

22. Kluckow M, Evans N. Early echocardiographic prediction of symptomatic patent ductus arteriosus in preterm infants undergoing mechanical ventilation. J Pediatr 1995;127:774–779.

23. Phillipos EZ, Robertson MA, Byrne PJ. Serial assessment of ductus arteriosus hemodynamics in hyaline membrane disease. Pediatrics 1996;98:1149–1153.

24. Suzumura H, Nitta A, Tanaka G, Arisaka O. Diastolic flow velocity of the left pulmonary artery of patent ductus arteriosus in preterm infants. Pediatr Int 2001;43:146–151.

25. Davies MW, Betheras FR, Swaminathan M. A preliminary study of the application of the transductal velocity ratio for assessing persistent ductus arteriosus. Arch Dis Child, Fetal Neonatal Ed 2000;82:F195–F199.

26. El Hajjar M, Vaksmann G, Rakza T, Kongolo G, Storme L. Severity of the ductal shunt: a comparison of different markers. Arch Dis Child, Fetal Neonatal Ed 2005;90:F419–F422.

27. Choi BM, Lee KH, Eun BL, Yoo KH, Hong YS, Son CS, Lee JW. Utility of rapid B-type natriuretic peptide assay for diagnosis of symptomatic patent ductus arteriosus in preterm infants. Pediatrics 2005;115:e255–e261.

28. Sanjeev S, Pettersen M, Lua J, Thomas R, Shankaran S, L'Ecuyer T. Role of plasma B-type natriuretic peptide in screening for hemodynamically significant patent ductus arteriosus in preterm neonates. J Perinatol 2005;25:709–713.

29. Flynn PA, da Graca RL, Auld PA, Nesin M, Kleinman CS. The use of a bedside assay for plasma B-type natriuretic peptide as a biomarker in the management of patent ductus arteriosus in premature neonates. J Pediatr 2005;147:38–42.

30. Baylen BG, Ogata H, Ikegami M, Jacobs HC, Jobe AH, Emmanouilides GC. Left ventricular performance and regional blood flows before and after ductus arteriosus occlusion in premature lambs treated with surfactant. Circulation 1983;67:837–843.

31. Tamura M, Harada K, Takahashi Y, Ito T, Toyono M, Ishida A, Takada G. Changes in left ventricular diastolic filling patterns before and after the closure of the ductus arteriosus in very-low-birth weight infants. Tohoku J Exp Med 1997;182:337–346.

32. Alverson DC, Eldridge MW, Johnson JD, et al. Effect of patent ductus arteriosus on left ventricular output in premature infants. J Pediatr 1983;102:754–757.

33. Baylen BG, Ogata H, Oguchi K, Ikegami M, Jacobs H, Jobe A, Emmanouilides GC. The contractility and performance of the preterm left ventricle before and after early patent ductus arteriosus occlusion in surfactant-treated lambs. Pediatr Res 1985;19:1053–1058.

34. Clyman RI, Roman C, Heymann MA, Mauray F. How a patent ductus arteriosus affects the premature lamb's ability to handle additional volume loads. Pediatr Res 1987;22:531–535.

35. Clyman RI, Mauray F, Heymann MA, Roman C. Cardiovascular effects of patent ductus arteriosus in preterm lambs with respiratory distress. J Pediatr 1987;111:579–587.

36. Walther FJ, Kim DH, Ebrahimi M, Siassi B. Pulsed Doppler measurement of left ventricular output as early predictor of symptomatic patent ductus arteriosus in very preterm infants. Biol Neonate 1989;56:121–128.

37. Lindner W, Seidel M, Versmold HT, Dohlemann C, Riegel KP. Stroke volume and left ventricular output in preterm infants with patent ductus arteriosus. Pediatr Res 1990;27:278–281.

38. Meyers RL, Alpan G, Lin E, Clyman RI. Patent ductus arteriosus, indomethacin, and intestinal distension: effects on intestinal blood flow and oxygen consumption. Pediatr Res 1991;29:569–574.

39. Shimada S, Kasai T, Konishi M, Fujiwara T. Effects of patent ductus arteriosus on left ventricular output and organ blood flows in preterm infants with respiratory distress syndrome treated with surfactant. J Pediatr 1994;125:270–277.

40. Evans N, Iyer P. Assessment of ductus arteriosus shunt in preterm infants supported by mechanical ventilation: effect of interatrial shunting. J Pediatr 1994;125:778–785.

41. Noori S, Seri I. Pathophysiology of newborn hypotension outside the transitional period. Early Hum Dev 2005;81:399–404.

42. Guller B, Bozic C. Right-to-left shunting through a patent ductus arteriosus in a newborn with myocardial infarction. Cardiology 1972;57:348–357.

43. Way GL, Pierce JR, Wolfe RR, McGrath R, Wiggins J, Merenstein GB. ST depression suggesting subendocardial ischemia in neonates with respiratory distress syndrome and patent ductus arteriosus. J Pediatr 1979;95:609–611.

44. Barlow AJ, Ward C, Webber SA, Sinclair BG, Potts JE, Sandor GG. Myocardial contractility in premature neonates with and without patent ductus arteriosus. Pediatr Cardiol 2004;25:102–107.

45. Noori S, Friedlich P, Seri I, Wong P. Changes in myocardial function and hemodynamics after ligation of the ductus arteriosus in preterm infants. J Pediatr 2007;150:597–602.

46. Trevisanuto D, Zaninotto M, Altinier S, Plebani M, Zanardo V. High serum cardiac troponin T concentrations in preterm infants with respiratory distress syndrome. Acta Paediatr 2000;89:1134–1136.

47. Ratner I, Perelmuter B, Toews W, Whitfield J. Association of low systolic and diastolic blood pressure with significant patent ductus arteriosus in the very low birth weight infant. Crit Care Med 1985;13:497–500.

48. Evans N, Moorcraft J. Effect of patency of the ductus arteriosus on blood pressure in very preterm infants. Arch Dis Child 1992;67:1169–1173.

49. Pladys P, Wodey E, Beuchee A, Branger B, Betremieux P. Left ventricle output and mean arterial blood pressure in preterm infants during the 1st day of life. Eur J Pediatr 1999;158:817–824.

50. Hansen NB, Stonestreet BS, Rosenkrantz TS, Oh W. Validity of Doppler measurements of anterior cerebral artery blood flow velocity: Correlation with brain blood flow in piglets. Pediatrics 1983;72:526–531.

51. Greisen G, Johansen K, Ellison PH, Fredriksen PS, Mali J, Friis-Hansen B. Cerebral blood flow in the newborn: comparison of Doppler ultrasound and 133xenon clearance. J Pediatr 1984;104:411–418.

52. Raju TN. Cerebral Doppler studies in the fetus and the newborn infant. J Pediatr 1991;119:165–174.

53. Lundell BP, Sonesson SE, Cotton RB. Ductus closure in preterm infants. Effects on cerebral hemodynamics. Acta Paediatr Scand (Suppl) 1986;329:140–147.

54. Perlman JM, Hill A, Volpe JJ. The effect of patent ductus arteriosus on flow velocity in the anterior cerebral arteries: ductal steal in the premature newborn infant. J Pediatr 1981;99:767–771.

55. Martin CG, Snider AR, Katz SM, Peabody JL, Brady JP. Abnormal cerebral blood flow patterns in preterm infants with a large patent ductus arteriosus. J Pediatr 1982;101:587–593.

56. Deeg KH, Gerstner R, Brandl U, et al. Doppler sonographic flow parameter of the anterior cerebral artery in patent ductus arteriosus of the newborn infant compared to a healthy control sample. Klin Padiatr 1986;198:463–470.

57. Shortland DB, Gibson NA, Levene MI, Archer LN, Evans DH, Shaw DE. Patent ductus arteriosus and cerebral circulation in preterm infants. Dev Med Child Neurol 1990;32:386–393.

58. Jim WT, Chiu NC, Chen MR, Hung HY, Kao HA, Hsu CH, Chang JH. Cerebral hemodynamic change and intraventricular hemorrhage in very low birth weight infants with patent ductus arteriosus. Ultrasound Med Biol 2005;31:197–202.

59. Fowlie PW, Davis PG. Prophylactic intravenous indomethacin for preventing mortality and morbidity in preterm infants. Cochrane Database Syst Rev 2002;3:CD000174.

60. Cassady G, Crouse DT, Kirklin JW, et al. A randomized, controlled trial of very early prophylactic ligation of the ductus arteriosus in babies who weighed 1000 g or less at birth. N Engl J Med 1989;320:1511–1516.

61. Coombs RC, Morgan ME, Durbin GM, Booth IW, McNeish AS. Gut blood flow velocities in the newborn: effects of patent ductus arteriosus and parenteral indomethacin. Arch Dis Child 1990;65:1067–1071.

62. Bada HS, Green RS, Pourcyrous M, et al. Indomethacin reduces the risks of severe intraventricular hemorrhage. J Pediatr 1989;115:631–637.

63. Bandstra ES, Montalvo BM, Goldberg RN, et al. Prophylactic indomethacin for prevention of intraventricular hemorrhage in premature infants. Pediatrics 1988;82:533–542.

64. Ment LR, Duncan CC, Ehrenkranz RA, et al. Randomized low-dose indomethacin trial for prevention of intraventricular hemorrhage in very low birth weight neonates. J Pediatr 1988;112:948–955.

65. Ment LR, Oh W, Ehrenkranz RA, Phillip AG, et al. Low-dose indomethacin therapy and extension of intraventricular hemorrhage: a multicenter randomized trial. J Pediatr 1994;124:951–955.

66. Couser RJ, Ferrara TB, Wright GB, Cabalka AK, Schilling CG, Hoekstra RE, Payne NR. Prophylactic indomethacin therapy in the first twenty-four hours of life for the prevention of patent ductus arteriosus in preterm infants treated prophylactically with surfactant in the delivery room. J Pediatr 1996;128:631–637.

67. Mahony L, Caldwell RL, Girod DA, Hurwitz RA, Jansen RD, Lemons JA, Schreiner RL. Indomethacin therapy on the first day of life in infants with very low birth weight. J Pediatr 1985;106:801–805.

68. Supapannachart S, Khowsathit P, Patchakapati B. Indomethacin prophylaxis for patent ductus arteriosus (PDA) in infants with a birth weight of less than 1250 grams. J Med Assoc Thai 1999;82:S87–S92.

69. Ment LR, Vohr B, Allan W, et al. Outcome of children in the indomethacin intraventricular hemorrhage prevention trial. Pediatrics 2000;105:485–491.

70. Schmidt B, Davis P, Moddemann D, et al. Trial of Indomethacin Prophylaxis in Preterms Investigators. Long-term effects of indomethacin prophylaxis in extremely-low-birth-weight infants. N Engl J Med 2001;344:1966–1972.

71. Vincer M, Allen A, Evans J, Nwaesei C, Stinson D, Rees E, Fraser A. Early intravenous indomethacin prolongs respiratory support in very low birth weight infants. Acta Paediatr Scand 1987;76:894–897.

72. Yaseen H, al Umran K, Ali H, Rustum M, Darwich M, al-Faraidy A. Effects of early indomethacin administration on oxygenation and surfactant requirement in low birth weight infants. J Trop Pediatr 1997;43:42–46.

73. Moin F, Kennedy KA, Moya FR. Risk factors predicting vasopressor use after patent ductus arteriosus ligation. Am J Perinatol 2003;20:313–320.

74. Taylor AF, Morrow WR, Lally KP, Kinsella JP, Gerstmann DR, deLemos RA. Left ventricular dysfunction following ligation of the ductus arteriosus in the preterm baboon. J Surg Res 1990;48:590–596.

75. McCurnin DC, Yoder BA, Coalson J, et al. Effect of ductus ligation on cardiopulmonary function in premature baboons. Am J Respir Crit Care Med 2005;172:1569–1574.

76. Kimball TR, Ralston MA, Khoury P, Crump RG, Cho FS, Reuter JH. Effect of ligation of patent ductus arteriosus on left ventricular performance and its determinants in premature neonates. J Am Coll Cardiol 1996;27:193–197.
77. Tei C, Ling LH, Hodge DO, et al. New index of combined systolic and diastolic myocardial performance: a simple and reproducible measure of cardiac function – a study in normals and dilated cardiomyopathy. J Cardiol 1995;26:357–366.
78. Tei C, Nishimura RA, Seward JB, Tajiik J. Noninvasive Doppler-derived myocardial performance index: correlation with simultaneous measurement of cardiac catheterization. J Am Soc Echocardiogr 1997;10:1969–1978.
79. Seri I, Evans J. Controversies in the diagnosis and management of hypotension in the newborn infant. Curr Opin Pediatr 2001;13:116–123.
80. Ng PC, Lee CH, Lam CW, et al. Transient adrenocortical insufficiency of prematurity and systemic hypotension in very low birthweight infants. Arch Dis Child, Fetal Neonatal Ed 2004;89:F119–F126.

Chapter 10

The Preterm Neonate with Relative Adrenal Insufficiency and Vasopressor-resistant Hypotension

Cynthia Cole, MD, MPH

Relative Adrenal Insufficiency

Vasopressor-resistant Hypotension

Evidence of Relative Adrenal Insufficiency in Sick Premature Infants

RAI, Cardiovascular Insufficiency, and Vasopressor-resistant Hypotension in
  Sick Premature Infants

Cardiovascular and Stress Effects of Cortocosteroids and Proposed
  Mechanisms

Summary

References

Relative adrenal insufficiency (RAI) and vasopressor-resistant hypotension are closely associated, serious disorders described in severely ill patients, including extremely premature infants. Undoubtedly, RAI and vasopressor-resistant hypotension occur together in many critically ill patients. However, some severely ill patients manifest vasopressor-resistant hypotension and no clear evidence of RAI and, vice versa, some critically sick patients have RAI but no evidence of vasopressor-resistant hypotension. The mechanisms that precipitate and fuel vasopressor-resistant hypotension and RAI are complex, highly interactive, and incompletely understood.

In this chapter, we review RAI and vasopressor-resistant hypotension, including proposed mechanisms for each, and summarize available evidence that RAI and vasopressor-resistant hypotension occur in sick premature infants. We also discuss the effects and proposed mechanisms by which corticosteroid therapy acts to resolve vasopressor-resistant hypotension with or without RAI.

RELATIVE ADRENAL INSUFFICIENCY

In the mid-nineteenth century, Thomas Addison described manifestations of primary adrenal insufficiency as "general languor and debility, remarkable feebleness of the heart's action, irritability of the stomach...occurring in connection with a diseased condition of the suprarenal capsules..." (http://wehner.org/addison.htm). Now, more than 150 years after the original description of Addison's disease, these manifestations of adrenal insufficiency extend to the recently described disorder "relative" adrenal insufficiency (RAI). Since the 1980s, RAI has been diagnosed in

preterm infants (24 to 36 weeks' gestation) with left ventricular output (LVO) ≤180 mL/min/kg had greater mortality (6/14, 64%) during the first postnatal day compared to infants with LVO >180 mL/min/kg (9/71, 13%) (P = 0.001). Mortality was highest in infants <31 weeks' gestation who had lower LVO (9/10, 90%). Scott et al. measured serum cortisol values in 54 of the 85 infants reported by Alverson. Infants with LVO ≤180 mL/min/kg had significantly lower cortisol values than infants with LVO >180 mL/min/kg (16). In addition, infants with low LVO and low cortisol levels did not respond well to surfactant therapy. However, it should be kept in mind that LVO is influenced by left-to-right shunting at the level of the ductus arteriosus and, to a lesser extent, the foramen ovale during the first postnatal day and thus it does not appropriately represent systemic perfusion as long as these fetal channels are open (85,86). In separate reports, Scott and Watterberg described lower cortisol levels in preterm infants who required inotropic support and surfactant therapy than preterm infants not receiving vasopressor therapy (12) and suggested that RAI in premature infants is associated with presence of a PDA (82).

Among publications and abstracts regarding adrenal function and/or hydrocortisone effect on vasopressor hypotension in sick premature infants or baboons, five human reports (1,2,5,10,17,32,39) and one baboon study (40) document low cortisol values and vasopressor-resistant hypotension responsive to corticosteroid treatment, Three studies report a similar presentation without cortisol data (5,10,25). Vasopressor-resistant hypotension responded to corticosteroid therapy in all but two infants (17) among reported neonates. Responding infants weaned from vasopressor support often within two days. Other neonatal reports about the effect of hydrocortisone on blood pressure or other outcomes are not comparable to these nine studies due to different objectives and inclusion criteria that did not limit their study to infants with vasopressor responsive hypotension and/or specific cortisol criteria. Efird et al. reported that prophylactic hydrocortisone therapy for five days (versus placebo) in extremely low birth weight infants reduced the use of vasopressors during the first two postnatal days (88).

The study by Yoder et al. of a very premature baboon model provides the most direct evidence that RAI, cardiovascular insufficiency, and prematurity are related (40). This group of investigators documented in previous studies that the majority of extremely premature baboons, delivered at ~67% of baboon gestation (~26 weeks human gestation), required volume expansion and vasopressor therapy to treat hypotension, oliguria, and acid–base imbalance. Many of the premature baboons also required hydrocortisone to treat vasopressor-resistant hypotension (89). Yoder et al. then demonstrated that decreased urinary free cortisol excretion in the first day of life correlated with decreased left ventricular function. Furthermore, hydrocortisone therapy (0.5 to 1.0 mg/kg/day for one to two days) corrected hypotension and left ventricular dysfunction, reduced vasopressor/ inotrope use and mortality, and increased serum cortisol to levels comparable to cortisol levels seen in baboons with no evidence of adrenal insufficiency or cardiovascular dysfunction through the end of the study at two weeks of extrauterine life (40).

CARDIOVASCULAR AND STRESS EFFECTS OF CORTOCOSTEROIDS AND PROPOSED MECHANISMS

The goal of corticosteroid therapy is to maintain homeostasis during stress and minimize organ dysfunction. The HPA axis and the adrenergic and sympathetic nervous system are the primary mediators of stress response. Under normal conditions, all forms of stress increase ACTH and cortisol production.

Corticosteroid cardiovascular effects maintain myocardial contractility, vascular tone, endothelial integrity, and vascular responsiveness to catecholamines and angiotensin II. Corticosteroids attenuate the pro-inflammatory cytokine response, reduce vascular permeability in the presence of acute inflammation, decrease the dysregulated production of nitrous oxide (NO) and other vasodilators, and modulate free water distribution within the vascular compartment (5,29,30,90–92).

Corticosteroids also modulate the immune response and counteract the inflammatory cascade. Acute exposure to inflammatory cytokines may increase affinity of glucocorticoid receptors. Acute exposure to inflammatory cytokines (e.g. IL-1 IL-6, TNF-alpha) can activate the HPA axis, which decreases inflammatory response, and may increase ligand affinity of glucocorticoid receptors. Cortisol feedback regulates the period for immunosuppressive and catabolic needs during stress. On the other hand, prolonged exposure to cytokines alters the HPA axis response. Low levels of ACTH are documented in patients with severe sepsis. Chronic increase in IL-6 can suppress ACTH production. Prolonged exposure to TNF-alpha may decrease adrenal function, CRH stimulation of ACTH production.

Corticosteroids exert their effects through genomic (slower) and non-genomic mechanisms (faster) (29,90,92). Genomic glucocorticoid effects reverse vasopressor-refractory hypotension by upregulating cardiovascular α- and β-adrenergic receptors through synthesis and membrane-assembly of new receptor proteins, a process that occurs over hours. Other genomic effects include glucocorticoid mediation of the sympathetic nerve activity and maturational changes in Na^+, K^+-ATPase enzyme activity, myosin fibers, and other components of cardiac muscle (29,93,94). However, the rapid response of the cardiovascular system to corticosteroids is thought to occur via non-genomic mechanisms through interaction with putative cell membrane-bound steroid receptors (6). Via their genomic and non-genomic actions, corticosteroids rapidly sensitize the cardiovascular system to catecholamines. This corticosteroid effect occurs by increasing catecholamine levels through increased catecholamine synthesis and inhibition of catecholamine metabolism, by a primarily mineralocorticoid-mediated increase in intracellular calcium, by inhibition of prostacyclin and nitric oxide vasodilation, and by improved capillary integrity.

Response time of sick premature infants to glucocorticoid therapy for vasopressor-resistant hypotension varies among reports. Helbock reported increase in blood pressure as early as 30 min and within 2 h following hydrocortisone therapy (1 mg) in 25- to 26-week gestation infants with vasopressor-resistant hypotension (32). Gaissmaier and Pohlandt noted improvement in vasopressor-resistant hypotension in 4 to 8 h following a single injection of dexamethasone (39). Seri et al. (5) and Noori et al. (25) reported increase in blood pressure within 2 h following hydrocortisone and low-dose dexamethasone (0.1 mg/kg) administration, respectively. Based on their case series, Helbock and Ng speculated that response time for reversal of vasopressor-resistant hypotension may be dose-related (17,32). Bellissant and Annane reported increased vascular responsiveness to phenylephrine 1 h after hydrocortisone administration in 12 adult patients with septic shock (95).

Hydrocortisone therapy at stress doses (34) or low doses (91), compared to placebo, accelerated shock reversal (i.e. reduced duration of vasopressor therapy) in adult patients with septic shock. Oppert et al. also noted that low-dose hydrocortisone reduced cytokine production in patients with early hyperdynamic septic shock regardless of a patient's adrenal response to ACTH. The hydrocortisone-induced hemodynamic effect of accelerating shock reversal was more dramatic in adrenal "non-responders" (RAI) compared to "responders." The findings by Oppert et al. suggest that the hydrocortisone-mediated hemodynamic effect is related, in part, to adrenal reserve status, and the immunomodulatory effect is independent of adrenal reserve (91). Currently, there are insufficient data in neonates to recommend specific glucocorticoid interventions, particularly as related to criteria for treatment, type of glucocorticoid, dosage, and duration. This uncertainty is further fueled by the documented increases in spontaneous ileal perforations in premature neonates co-exposed to either hydrocortisone or dexamethasone and indomethacin as well as by the documented deleterious effects of dexamethasone on neurodevelopment in preterm neonates (64,96). Whether hydrocortisone administered at low doses in the immediate postnatal period affects neurodevelopment in premature neonates is not known at this time (97,98). Finally, there is ongoing debate in other pediatric and adult critical care regarding indications, efficacy, high-dose short course vs. low-dose longer course.

SUMMARY

Adequate HPA axis and adrenal function are vital to postnatal adaptation in extremely premature infants. Clinical, biochemical, and physiological evidence indicate that RAI and vasopressor-resistant hypotension are serious disorders in sick, premature infants, which, respond to corticosteroid therapy with improvements in the cardiovascular status. However, whether this improvement translates to improved mortality and/or morbidity is not known. However, recent research provides important insight into RAI and vasopressor-resistant hypotension and stimulates consideration of mechanisms for RAI and vasopressor-resistant hypotension. Management of the critically ill hypotensive preterm infant remains challenging and requires a better understanding of the pathophysiology of neonatal shock and improvements in our ability to evaluate cardiac output, organ blood flow, and tissue perfusion at the bedside.

However, one major challenge is to improve our understanding of the pathogenesis and epidemiology of RAI and vasopressor-resistant hypotension in terms of determinants, mechanisms, and patterns, and their relationship with acute and long-term morbidity/mortality. Ultimately, we need to provide evidence that our interventions also improve clinically meaningful outcomes. In addition, we need to ask questions such as "What is the temporal interaction of vasopressor-resistant hypotension and RAI?", "Does acute inflammatory response precipitate vasopressor-resistant hypotension with secondary RAI," and "Is RAI due to prematurity the primary precipitating event in sick premature infants?"

Another challenge is to improve diagnostic methods to assess adrenal function and vasopressor-resistant hypotension and criteria for treatment. Which patient needs therapy? Corticosteroid therapy improves vasopressor-resistant hypotension even in patients with no evidence of RAI. What evaluations provide reliable information early in the neonatal course? Are serum cortisol values the optimal measure of adrenal function? Can one improve diagnosis and prognosis by combining responses of different tests (99)? Could serum or urine evaluations of adrenal function refine diagnosis? Will simultaneous measurements of inflammatory mediators improve our understanding and guide therapy? Accurate, timely diagnosis will target higher risk patients for investigational and clinical interventions and avoid unnecessary exposure of lower risk infants to glucocorticoid therapy.

Hydrocortisone is often prescribed for extremely premature neonates with evidence of vasopressor-resistant hypotension. But, many questions regarding therapy are not resolved. What factors influence choice of corticosteroid, dosage, duration, and response to therapy for individual patients (100)? Are different corticosteroid regimens necessary depending upon the severity of illness or the patient's response? What regimens will maximize effectiveness and minimize harm? Scientifically, ethically sound research is necessary to resolve these questions.

REFERENCES

1. Colasurdo MA, Hanna CE, Gilhooly JT, et al. Hydrocortisone replacement in extremely premature infants with cortisol insufficiency. Clin Res 1989;37:180A.
2. Ward RM, Rich-Denson C. Addisonian crisis in extremely premature neonates. Clin Res 1991;39:11A.
3. Hanna CE, et al. Hypothalamic pituitary adrenal function in the extremely low birth weight infant. J Clin Endocrinol Metab 1993;76:384–387.
4. Ho J, et al. Septic shock and sepsis: a comparison of total and free plasma cortisol levels. J Clin Endocrinol Metab 2005.
5. Seri I, Tan R, Evans J. Cardiovascular effects of hydrocortisone in preterm infants with pressor-resistant hypotension. Pediatrics 2001;107:1070–1074.
6. Schneider AJ, Voerman HJ. Abrupt hemodynamic improvement in late septic shock with physiological doses of glucocorticoids. Intensive Care Med 1991;17:436–437.
7. Briegel J, et al. Haemodynamic improvement in refractory septic shock with cortisol replacement therapy. Intensive Care Med 1992;18:318.
8. Caplan RH, et al. Occult hypoadrenalism in critically ill patients. Arch Surg 1994;129:456.
9. Guttentag SH, Rubin LP, Douglas R, Ringer SA, Berg G, Liley H. The glucocorticoid pathway in ill and well extremely low birthweight infants. Pediatric Res 1991;29:77A.
10. Fauser A, Pohlandt F, Bartmann P, Gortner L. Rapid increase of blood pressure in extremely low birth weight infants after a single dose of dexamethasone. Eur J Pediatr 1993;152:354–356.
11. Reynolds JW, Hanna CE. Glucocorticoid-responsive hypotension in extremely low birth weight newborns. Pediatrics 1994;94:135–136.
12. Scott SM, Watterberg KL. Effect of gestational age, postnatal age, and illness on plasma cortisol concentrations in premature infants. Pediatr Res 1995;37:112–116.
13. Watterberg KL, Scott SM. Evidence of early adrenal insufficiency in babies who develop bronchopulmonary dysplasia. Pediatrics 1995;95:120–125.
14. Bouchier D, Weston PJ. Randomised trial of dopamine compared with hydrocortisone for the treatment of hypotensive very low birth weight infants. Arch Dis Child Fetal Neonatal Ed 1997;76:F174–F178.
15. Hanna CE, et al. Corticosteroid binding globulin, total serum cortisol, and stress in extremely low-birth-weight infants. Am J Perinatol 1997;14:201–204.
16. Scott SM, Alverson DC, Backstrom C, Bessman S. Positive effect of cortisol on cardiac output in the preterm infant. Pediatr Res 1995;37:236A.
17. Ng PC, et al. Refractory hypotension in preterm infants with adrenocortical insufficiency. Arch Dis Child Fetal Neonatal Ed 2001;84:F122–F124.
18. Korte C, et al. Adrenocortical function in the very low birth weight infant: improved testing sensitivity and association with neonatal outcome. J Pediatr 1996;128:257–263.
19. Cooper MS, Stewart PM. Corticosteroid insufficiency in acutely ill patients. N Engl J Med 2003;348:727–734.
20. Annane D, et al. Effect of treatment with low doses of hydrocortisone and fludrocortisone on mortality in patients with septic shock. JAMA 2002;238:862–871.
21. Seri I, et al. Cardiovascular response to dopamine in hypotensive preterm neonates with severe hyaline membrane disease. Eur J Pediatr 1984;142:3–9.
22. Seri I. Circulatory support of the sick preterm infant. Semin Neonatol 2001;6:85–95.
23. Roze J, Ch Tohier C, Maingueneau C, Lefevre M, Mouzard A. Response to dobutamine and dopamine in the hypotensive very preterm infant. Arch Dis Child Fetal Neonatal Ed 1993;69:59–63.
24. Rivers EP, et al. Adrenal insufficiency in high-risk surgical ICU patients. Chest 2001;119:889–896.
25. Noori S, et al. Cardiovascular effects of low-dose dexamethasone in very low birth weight neonates with refractory hypotension. Biol Neonate 2005;89:82–87.
26. Noori S, Seri I. Pathophysiology of newborn hypotension outside the transitional period. Early Hum Dev 2005;81:399–404.
27. Ng PC, Fok TF, Lee CH, Ma KC, Chan IHS, Wong E. Refractory hypotension in preterm infants with adrenocortical insufficiency. Arch Dis Child Fetal Neonatal Ed 2001;84:F122–F124.
28. Ng PC, et al. Transient adrenocortical insufficiency of prematurity and systemic hypotension in very low birthweight infants. Arch Dis Child Fetal Neonatal Ed 2004;89:F119–F126.
29. Lamberts SW, Bruining HA, de Jong FH. Corticosteroid therapy in severe illness. N Engl J Med 1997;337:1285–1292.
30. Keh D, et al. Immunologic and hemodynamic effects of 'low-dose" hydrocortisone in septic shock: a double-blind, randomized, placebo-controlled, crossover study. Am J Respir Crit Care Med 2003;167:512–520.
31. Huysman MW, et al. Adrenal function in sick very preterm infants. Pediatr Res 2000;48:629–633.
32. Helbock HJMI, Conte FA. Glucocorticoid-responsive hypotension in extremely low birth weight newborns. Pediatrics 1993;92:715–717.
33. Dimopoulou I, et al. Hypothalamic–pituitary–adrenal axis dysfunction in critically ill patients with traumatic brain injury: incidence, pathophysiology, and relationship to vasopressor dependence and peripheral interleukin-6 levels. Crit Care Med 2004;32:404–408.
34. Briegel J, Gorst H, Haller M, et al. Stress doses of hydrocortisone reverse hyperdynamic septic shock: a prospective, randomized, double blind, single center study. Crit Care Med 1999;27:723–732.
35. Annane D, Briegel J, Sprung CL. Corticosteroid insufficiency in acutely ill patients. N Engl J Med 2003;348:2157–2159.

36. Annane D, et al. Clinical equipoise remains for issues of adrenocorticotropic hormone administration, cortisol testing, and therapeutic use of hydrocortisone. Crit Care Med 2003;31:2250–2251; author reply 2252–2253.

37. Alverson D, Scott SM, Backstrom C, Bessman S. Persistently low cardiac output during the first day of life predicts high mortality in preterm infants with respiratory distress syndrome. Pediatr Res 1995;37:193A.

38. Hoen S, et al. Cortisol response to corticotropin stimulation in trauma patients: influence of hemorrhagic shock. Anesthesiology 2002;97:807–813.

39. Gaissmaier RE, Pohlandt F. Single-dose dexamethasone treatment of hypotension in preterm infants. J Pediatr 1999;134:701–705.

40. Yoder BA, Martin H, McCurnin DC, Coalson JJ. Impaired urinary cortisol excretion and early cardiopulmonary dysfunction in immature baboons. Pediatr Res 2002;51:426–432.

41. Ng PC, et al. Reference ranges and factors affecting the human corticotropin-releasing hormone test in preterm, very low birth weight infants. J Clin Endocrinol Metab 2002;87:4621–4628.

42. Joosten KF, et al. Endocrine and metabolic responses in children with meningoccocal sepsis: striking differences between survivors and nonsurvivors. J Clin Endocrinol Metab 2000;85:3746–3753.

43. Chrousos GP. The hypothalamic–pituitary–adrenal axis and immune mediated inflammation. N Engl J Med 1995;332:1351–1362.

44. Watterberg KL, et al. Effect of dose on response to adrenocorticotropin in extremely low birth weight infants. J Clin Endocrinol Metab 2005;90:6380–6385.

45. Dickstein G, et al. Adrenocorticotropin stimulation test: effects of basal cortisol level, time of day, and suggested new sensitive low dose test. J Clin Endocrinol Metab 1991;72:773–778.

46. Annane D. Time for a consensus definition of corticosteroid insufficiency in critically ill patients. Crit Care Med 2003;31:1868–1869.

47. Arnold J, et al. Longitudinal study of plasma cortisol and 17-hydroxyprogesterone in very-low-birth-weight infants during the first 16 weeks of life. Biol Neonate 1997;72:148–155.

48. Agus M. One step forward: an advance in understanding of adrenal insufficiency in the pediatric critically ill. Crit Care Med 2005;33:911–912.

49. Contreras LN, et al. A new less-invasive and more informative low-dose ACTH test: salivary steroids in response to intramuscular corticotrophin. Clin Endocrinol (Oxf) 2004;61:675–682.

50. Hoen S, et al. Hydrocortisone increases the sensitivity to alpha1-adrenoceptor stimulation in humans following hemorrhagic shock. Crit Care Med 2005;33:2737–2743.

51. Marik PE, Zaloga GP. Adrenal insufficiency during septic shock. Crit Care Med 2003;31:141–145.

52. Williams HW, Bluhy RG. Diseases of the adrenal cortex. In Harrison's Principles of Internal Medicine. Facuci AS, Isselbacher KJ, et al. eds. New York, McGraw-Hill, 1998:2035–2057.

53. Pizarro CF, Damiani D, Carcillo JA. Absolute and relative adrenal insufficiency in children with septic shock. Crit Care Med 2005;33:855–859.

54. Pittinger TP, Sawin RS. Adrenocortical insufficiency in infants with congenital diaphragmatic hernia: a pilot study. J Pediatr Surg 2000;35:223–225; discussion 225–226.

55. Rothwell PM, Udwadia ZF, Lawler PG. Cortisol response to corticotropin and survival in septic shock. Lancet 1991;337:582–583.

56. Briegel J, et al. Immunomodulation in septic shock: hydrocortisone differentially regulates cytokine responses. J Am Soc Nephrol 2001;12(Suppl. 17):S70–S74.

57. Ng PC, Lam CWK, Fok TF, Lee CH, Ma KC, Chan IHS, Wong E. The pituitary–adrenal responses to exogenous human corticotropin-releasing hormone in preterm, very low birth weight infants. J Clin Endocrinol Metab 1997;82:797–799.

58. Bolt RJ, van Weissenbruch MM, Cranendonk A, Lafeber HN, Delemarre-Van De Waal HA. The corticotrophin-releasing hormone test in preterm infants. Clin Endocrinol 2002;56:207–213.

59. Thomas S, et al. Response to ACTH in the newborn. Arch Dis Child 1986;61:57–60.

60. Soliman AT, et al. Circulating adrenocorticotropic hormone (ACTH) and cortisol concentrations in normal, appropriate-for-gestational-age newborns versus those with sepsis and respiratory distress: cortisol response to low-dose and standard-dose ACTH tests. Metabolism 2004;53:209–214.

61. Karlsson R, et al. Timing of peak serum cortisol values in preterm infants in low-dose and the standard ACTH tests. Pediatr Res 1999;45:367–369.

62. Karlsson R, et al. Adrenocorticotropin and corticotropin-releasing hormone tests in preterm infants. J Clin Endocrinol Metab 2000;85:4592–4595.

63. Watterberg KL, et al. Prophylaxis against early adrenal insufficiency to prevent chronic lung disease in premature infants. Pediatrics 1999;104:1258–1263.

64. Watterberg KL, et al. Prophylaxis of early adrenal insufficiency to prevent bronchopulmonary dysplasia: a multicenter trial. Pediatrics 2004;114:1649–1657.

65. Hingre RV, et al. Adrenal steroidogenesis in very low birth weight preterm infants. J Clin Endocrinol Metab 1994;78:266–270.

66. Bolt RJ, et al. Maturity of the adrenal cortex in very preterm infants is related to gestational age. Pediatr Res 2002;52:405–410.

67. Trainer PJ, et al. Urinary free cortisol in the assessment of hydrocortisone replacement therapy. Horm Metab Res 1993;25:117–120.

68. Ng PC, Fok TF, Lee CH, Ma KC, Chan IHS, Wong E. The pituitary–adrenal responses to exogenous human corticotropin-releasing hormone in preterm, very low birth weight infants. J Clin Endocrinol Metab 1997;82:797–799.

69. Jett PL, et al. Variability of plasma cortisol levels in extremely low birth weight infants. J Clin Endocrinol Metab 1997;82:2921–2925.

70. al Saedi S, et al. Reference ranges for serum cortisol and 17-hydroxyprogesterone levels in preterm infants. J Pediatr 1995;126:985–987.

71. Mesiano S, Jaffe RB. Developmental and functional biology of the primate fetal adrenal cortex. Endocr Rev 1997;18:378–403.

72. Tsuneyoshi I, Kanmura Y, Yoshimura N. Nitric oxide as a mediator of reduced arterial responsiveness in septic patients. Crit Care Med 1996;24:1083–1086.

73. Tsuneyoshi I, Kanmura Y, Yoshimura N. Lipoteichoic acid from Staphylococcus aureus depresses contractile function of human arteries in vitro due to the induction of nitric oxide synthase. Anesth Analg 1996;82:948–953.

74. Tsuneyoshi I, Kanmura Y, and. Yoshimura N. Methylprednisolone inhibits endotoxin-induced depression of contractile function in human arteries in vitro. Br J Anaesth 1996;76:251–257.

75. Annane D, Bellissant E, Sebille V, et al. Impaired pressor sensitivity to noradrenaline in septic shock patients with and without impaired adrenal function reserve. Br J Clin Pharm 1998;46:589–597.

76. Lee MM, et al. Serum adrenal steroid concentrations in premature infants. J Clin Endocrinol Metab 1989;69:1133–1136.

77. Heckmann M, et al. Reference range for serum cortisol in well preterm infants. Arch Dis Child Fetal Neonatal Ed 1999;81:F171–F174.

78. Watterberg KL, Gerdes JS, Cook KL. Impaired glucocorticoid synthesis in premature infants developing chronic lung disease. Pediatr Res 2001;50:190–195.

79. Linder N, et al. Longitudinal measurements of 17-alpha-hydroxyprogesterone in premature infants during the first three months of life. Arch Dis Child Fetal Neonatal Ed 1999;81:F175–F178.

80. Ng PC, et al. Early pituitary–adrenal response and respiratory outcomes in preterm infants. Arch Dis Child Fetal Neonatal Ed 2004;89:F127–F130.

81. Scott SM. Evidence for developmental hypopituitarism in ill preterm infants. J Perinatol 2004;24:429–433.

82. Watterberg KL, et al. Links between early adrenal function and respiratory outcome in preterm infants: airway inflammation and patent ductus arteriosus. Pediatrics 2000;105:320–324.

83. Peltoniemi O, et al. Pretreatment cortisol values may predict responses to hydrocortisone administration for the prevention of bronchopulmonary dysplasia in high-risk infants. J Pediatr 2005;146:632–637.

84. Pladys P, et al. Left ventricle output and mean arterial blood pressure in preterm infants during the 1st day of life. Eur J Pediatr 1999;158:817–824.

85. Seri I. Management of hypotension and low systemic blood flow in the very low birth weight neonate during the first postnatal week. J Perinatol 2006;26(Suppl. 1):S8–S13.

86. Noori S, Friedlich P, Wong P, Ebrahimi M, Siassi B, Seri I. Hemodynamic changes following low-dose hydrocortisone administration in vasopressor-treated neonates. Pediatrics 2006;118:1456–1466.

87. Palta M, Gabbert D, Weinstein MR, Peters ME. Multivariate assessment of traditional risk factors for chronic lung disease in very low birth weight neonates. J Pediatr 1991;119:285–292.

88. Efird MM, et al. A randomized-controlled trial of prophylactic hydrocortisone supplementation for the prevention of hypotension in extremely low birth weight infants. J Perinatol 2005;25:119–124.

89. Coalson JJ, et al. Neonatal chronic lung disease in extremely immature baboons. Am J Respir Crit Care Med 1999;160:1333–1346.

90. Seri I, Evans JR. Why do steroids increase blood pressure in preterm infants? J Pediatr 2000;136:420–421.

91. Oppert M, et al. Low-dose hydrocortisone improves shock reversal and reduces cytokine levels in early hyperdynamic septic shock. Crit Care Med 2005;33:2457–2464.

92. Shenker Y, Skatrud JB. Adrenal insufficiency in critically ill patients. Am J Respir Crit Care Med 2001;163:1520–1523.

93. Segar JL, et al. Effect of antenatal glucocorticoids on sympathetic nerve activity at birth in preterm shee. Am J Physiol 1998;274(1 Pt 2):R160–R167.

94. Wang ZM, Celsi G. Glucocorticoids differentially regulate the mRNA for Na^+, K^+-ATPase isoforms in the infant rat heart. Pediatr Res 1993;33:1–4.

95. Bellissant E, Annane D. Effect of hydrocortisone on phenylephrine mean arterial pressure dose–response relationship in septic shock. Clin Pharmacol Ther 2000;68:293–303.

96. Paquette L, Friedlich P, Ramanathan R, Seri I. Cumulative doses of indomethacin and concurrent use of corticosteroids predict spontaneous intestinal perforation in very low birth weight neonates. J Perinatol 2006;26:486–492.

97. Seri I. Hydrocortisone is effective in treatment of vasopressor-resistant hypotension in very low birth weight neonates. J Pediatr 2006;149:422–423.

98. Lodygensky GA, Rademaker K, Zimine S, et al. Structural and functional brain development after hydrocortisone treatment for neonatal chronic lung disease. Pediatrics 2005;116:1–7.

99. Annane D, et al. A 3-level prognostic classification in septic shock based on cortisol levels and cortisol response to corticotropin. JAMA 2000;283:1038–1045.

100. Aucott SW. Hypotension in the newborn: who needs hydrocortisone? J Perinatol 2005;25:77–78.

Chapter 11

Clinical Presentations of Systemic Inflammatory Response in Term and Preterm Infants

Rowena G. Cayabyab, MD • Istvan Seri, MD, PhD

Perinatal Inflammation, Cord Blood Cytokines, and Postnatal
Hemodynamic Variables

Clinical Presentations of Neonatal Shock in Infants with Systemic
Inflammatory Response Syndrome

Pulmonary Hypertension Associated with SIRS

Treatment of the Hypotensive Neonate with SIRS

References

Neonatal infection is one of the major causes of mortality around the world. The incidence of neonatal sepsis ranges from 1/1000 to 23/1000 live births with a mortality rate of 5/1000 to 34/1000 live births (1). Neonatal infection could present as systemic inflammatory response of different severity as temperature instability, tachypnea, tachycardia, and lethargy or as respiratory and circulatory failure rapidly progressing to multiorgan dysfunction (2).

Systemic inflammatory response starts with inflammation as a response to exogenous (microbial, physical, or chemical) agents or endogenous (immunologic or neurologic) factors. The response is initiated when inflammatory cells at the site of inflammation, such as macrophages, are activated and rapidly produce TNF-α and IL-1. These cytokines in turn activate the cytokine cascade resulting in the generation of proinflammatory cytokines, IL-6, and IL-8, as well as other chemokines (3,4). Inflammatory stimuli also trigger the synthesis of anti-inflammatory cytokines and specific cytokine inhibitors to control the extent of the inflammatory response. Anti-inflammatory cytokines such as IL-10, IL-13, IL-4, and IL-11 inhibit the synthesis of proinflammatory cytokines (5,6) while the naturally occurring proinflammatory cytokine inhibitors neutralize proinflammatory cytokine activity by binding to proinflamamtory cytokine receptors, decoy receptor antagonist, and cytokine binding proteins. The interplay among these proinflammatory cytokines, anti-inflammatory cytokines, and naturally occurring cytokine inhibitors determines the inflammatory response and its effectiveness to contain the inflammatory response and bring about resolution of the initiating process (7).

Systemic inflammatory response syndrome (SIRS) develops as a result of an imbalance in the production of proinflammatory and anti-inflammatory cytokines. The main known mediators involved in the evolution of SIRS are cytokines, nitric oxide, platelet activating factor (PAF), and eicosanoids. The systemic response to infection is mediated via macrophage-derived cytokines that target end organ receptors in response to injury or infection. However, production of anti-inflammatory protein and lipid molecules will also take place to attenuate and halt the inflammatory response (5). These mediators initiate overlapping processes that directly influence the endothelium, cardiovascular, hemodynamic, and coagulation mechanisms. If a balance between pro- and anti-inflammatory substances is not established and homeostasis restored, a massive proinflammatory reaction (i.e. SIRS) and multiple organ dysfunction (MODS) may ensue. Thus, after the first proinflammatory mediators are released, the body mounts a compensatory anti-inflammatory reaction to the initial inflammatory response. The anti-inflammatory reaction may be as robust and sometimes even more robust than the proinflammatory response (8). In addition to proinflammatory cytokines, other mediators such as NO, PAF, prostaglandins, and leukotrienes are also produced. These molecules are responsible for activating complement, coagulation, and kinin cascades as well.

Interactions between pro- and anti-inflammatory cytokines play an important role in the clinical manifestations and outcomes of systemic infections and other diseases in preterm and term neonates and children (9–12). Although it has been reported that proinflammatory activity positively correlates with gestational age (13,14), some studies have shown that preterm neonates are also able to mount a potent inflammatory response sometimes even surpassing the adult response (14–18). However, in the presence of a robust proinflammatory response, preterm neonates are unable to mount an appropriate anti-inflammatory response commensurate to the injury. The immaturity of the anti-inflammatory response in preterm infants could be the reason why newborns develop enhanced systemic inflammatory responses to an insult (19,20).

PERINATAL INFLAMMATION, CORD BLOOD CYTOKINES, AND POSTNATAL HEMODYNAMIC VARIABLES

Chorioamnionitis is the most common cause of SIRS in the preterm newborn. Cord blood IL-6 concentration is the most sensitive and specific plasma marker of chorioamnionitis and it is the strongest predictor of blood pressure immediately after delivery (21). IL-6 concentration correlates inversely with systolic, mean, and diastolic blood pressure in the neonate. The findings of decreased blood pressure and increased cardiac output in infants with placental inflammation and fetal vessel inflammation (funisitis) suggest that systemic vascular resistance decreases in infants born after chorioamnionitis. In addition, infants born after chorioamnionitis and presenting with funisitis have higher IL-6 and IL-1β concentrations and right ventricular cardiac output compared to their counterparts without funisitis. Clinically these preterm neonates present with increased heart rate and decreased mean and diastolic blood pressures (22–25). These hypotensive neonates also have an impaired cerebral blood flow (CBF) autoregulation (pressure passive cerebral circulation) (26) predisposing them to decreased CBF while hypotensive potentially contributing to their white matter injury (27,29). With correction of hypotension and improvement of cerebral perfusion these infants may develop periventricular–intraventricular hemorrhage during the reperfusion phase of the hemodynamic compromise. Indeed in this patient population, there is an association between wide blood pressure swings and brain injury (28,29). Finally, chorioamnionitis with fetal inflammatory response has been associated with premature birth and an increased risk for postnatal mortality and morbidity including white matter injury and cerebral palsy, periventricular intraventricular hemorrhage, and chronic lung disease (30–35).

CLINICAL PRESENTATIONS OF NEONATAL SHOCK IN INFANTS WITH SYSTEMIC INFLAMMATORY RESPONSE SYNDROME

In adults and pediatric patients, SIRS is defined as a systemic inflammatory response to a wide variety of insults manifested by two or more of the following conditions: temperature $> 38°C$ or $< 36°C$, heart rate > 90 beats/min, respiratory rate > 20 breaths/min, $Paco_2 < 32$ mm Hg, WBC $>12,000/mm^3$ or < 4000 mm^3 or $> 10\%$ immature forms (8). If left untreated, SIRS can evolve into full-blown shock (most often due to sepsis), multiple organ dysfunction and death. Shock develops when oxygen delivery becomes inadequate to satisfy tissue oxygen demand. The etiology, pathophysiology, and phases of neonatal shock are described in Section I, Chapter 1 in detail.

In this chapter, we will only discuss the major cellular mechanisms of the circulatory compromise specifically associated with SIRS.

Activation of ATP-sensitive Potassium (K_{ATP}) Channels in Vascular Smooth Muscle

Alterations in the membrane potential of smooth muscle cells play a critical role in the modulation of vascular tone (35). Although a variety of ion transporters and channels regulate the membrane potential in vascular smooth muscle cells, potassium channels appear to play a primary role. Of the four types of potassium channels, K_{ATP} channels are the best understood and appear to have a critical role in the pathogenesis of vasodilatory shock. The opening of K_{ATP} channels allows an efflux of potassium leading to hyperpolarization of the cell membranes and prevention of calcium entry into the cell. The resulting impaired ability of the vascular smooth muscle cell to increase its intracellular calcium concentration attenuates catecholamine- and/or angiotensin-induced vasoconstriction. K_{ATP} channels are physiologically activated by decreases in intracellular ATP concentrations and increases in the intracellular concentrations of lactate and hydrogen; mechanisms that link cellular metabolism to vascular tone and blood flow (36,37). Under normal conditions, these channels are closed. However, with increased tissue metabolism or tissue hypoxia, activation of these channels results in vasodilatation and increased blood flow and oxygen delivery provided that perfusion pressure (systemic blood pressure) is maintained in the normal range. Neurohormonal activators of K_{ATP} channels are atrial natriuretic peptide, calcitonin gene-related peptide, and adenosine as well as locally generated nitric oxide (NO) (38–41).

Increased Synthesis of Nitric Oxide

In the pathogenesis of sepsis and septic shock, NO initially exerts beneficial effects. However, with the progression of the condition, the effects of NO become deleterious (42). Nitric oxide has both pro- and anti-inflammatory as well as oxidant and anti-oxidant properties (43). Overproduction of NO and the subsequent formation of peroxynitrite are among the most important mediators for the late phase of hypotension, vasoplegia, cellular suffocation, apoptosis, lactic acidosis, and multiorgan failure in septic shock (44). The toxicity of NO itself may be enhanced by the formation of peroxynitrite resulting in DNA and cell membrane damage (45), and the multiple organ dysfunction that often accompanies severe sepsis may be related, at least in part, to the cellular effects of excess NO or peroxynitrite. The vasodilating action of nitric oxide is mediated through the activation of myosin light chain phosphatase and potassium channels in the plasma membrane of the vascular smooth muscle cell (36). The increased NO release has also been implicated in the diminished response to vasopressors. Accordingly, pharmacologic inhibition of inducible nitric oxide synthase (iNOS) activity or iNOS deficiency is associated with a loss of endotoxin-induced vasodilatation (46). The vascular hyporeactivity to catecholamines and endothelin seen in septic shock or decompensated hemorrhagic shock is also markedly improved by the administration of inhibitors of NO synthesis (47–51). Vasopressin responses to catecholamines during sepsis are greater in knockout mice without the gene for inducible iNOS than in wild type mice (50). Furthermore, NO may exert direct and indirect effects on cardiac function in sepsis. Increases in myocardial iNOS activity have been reported in response to endotoxin or cytokines and are inversely correlated with myocardial performance (52). The negative inotropic effects of NO are probably mediated by cGMP and the impairment in coronary autoregulation and oxygen utilization (53). Plasma NO levels in neonates with septic shock are higher than in neonates with sepsis alone and they correlate with TNF-α levels and illness severity (54).

Deficiency of Vasopressin

Vasopressin is a peptide hormone that has several important physiologic functions. It is released into the circulation upon stimulation by increased plasma osmolality or as a baroreflex response. Vasopressin plays a key role in the regulation of body fluid balance through its antidiuretic action mediated by renal vasopressin V_2 receptors coupled to adenyl cyclase and thus the generation of cAMP. Vasopressin also exerts vascular effects by causing vasoconstriction mediated by the V_1 receptors coupled to phospholipase C and thus increased intracellular Ca^{2+} concentration in the vascular smooth muscle cell (55). Under pathological conditions, endotoxin stimulates vasopressin release directly and independently of baroreceptor activity (56). In addition, proinflammatory cytokines (IL-1β, IL-6, TNF-α) enhance vasopressin production (57–60). Plasma vasopressin levels reveal a biphasic pattern during septic shock both in animals and humans. In the early phase of shock, vasopressin is significantly elevated while in the late phase, vasopressin levels are inappropriately low for the degree of hypotension (60,61). The decrease in vasopressin production contributes to diminished vasoconstriction but does not affect the antidiuretic action of the hormone. The most likely reason for the low vasopressin levels in the late phase of septic shock is impaired vasopressin secretion. Possible mechanisms are the exhaustion of pituitary vasopressin stores in response to baroreceptor-mediated hormone release, autonomic dysfunction, and increased production and release of NO in the posterior pituitary gland. Interestingly, although patients with septic shock have a relative deficiency of vasopressin, the sensitivity of the systemic circulation to exogenous vasopressin is increased. The mechanisms of vasopressin hypersensivity in septic shock include the increased availability of and alterations in V_1 receptor expression, potentiation of the vasoconstrictive effects of catecholamines by the vasopressin-mediated direct inactivation of K_{ATP} channels, vasopressin-induced increases in the synthesis of endothelin-1 and corticosteroids, attenuation of endotoxin- and IL-1β-stimulated NO synthesis, and the presence of autonomic dysfunction (60–65).

PULMONARY HYPERTENSION ASSOCIATED WITH SIRS

Pulmonary hypertension is the single most consistently seen circulatory disturbance in every animal model of sepsis (66–68). In the animal model of group B streptococcal (GBS) disease, pulmonary hypertension may present early or late in the disease process. Early-phase pulmonary hypertension is mediated by thromboxane-A_2 and it can be prevented by pretreatment with indomethacin (69,70). On the other hand, late-phase pulmonary hypertension occurs independent of prostaglandin production, and is associated with pulmonary injury and edema (71,72).

There are several pathophysiological factors contributing to the development of pulmonary hypertension in septic newborns. Inflammation causes endothelial dysfunction resulting in an immediate increase in circulating vasoactive substances such as inflammatory cytokines $TNF\alpha$, $IL-1\beta$, and $IL-6$ (73,74). These polypeptide mediators are released from circulating inflammatory and resident lung cells in response to epithelial and endothelial injury triggering second messenger pathways favoring vasoconstriction and smooth muscle proliferation (75). In addition, as described earlier, inflammatory conditions such as sepsis cause induction of endothelial NO synthesis attenuating catecholamine- and endothelin-mediated vasoconstriction in the systemic circulation. However, in the pulmonary circulation, the synthesis of and responsiveness to the vasoconstrictor prostagland in thromboxane are undiminished (76). This finding may explain the coexistence of pulmonary hypertension and systemic hypotension during septicemia. In neonates, concurrent hypoxic exposure can further amplify the inflammation-mediated pulmonary vasoconstriction. Hypoxia is associated with increased pulmonary thromboxane synthase activity and decreased prostacyclin synthesis suggesting altered production of arachidonic acid metabolites contributing to hypoxic vasoconstriction.

The elevation in pulmonary artery pressure in neonatal sepsis results in right-to-left shunting through the fetal channels (ductus arteriosus and foramen ovale) and causes systemic hypoxemia and tissue oxygen deprivation. Hypoxemia is further aggravated in infants who are hypotensive by enhancing right-to-left shunting. In addition, in the absence of shunting through the fetal channels, pulmonary hypertension leads to decreased left ventricular filling and thus systemic perfusion while long-standing pulmonary hypertension causes impaired right ventricular function potentially affecting systemic perfusion and blood pressure even after the resolution of pulmonary hypertension (75).

TREATMENT OF THE HYPOTENSIVE NEONATE WITH SIRS

In patients with SIRS, the immediate recognition of the condition and initiation of appropriate therapeutic intervention is crucial. If SIRS is secondary to an infectious agent, broad-spectrum antibiotic therapy as well as cardiovascular and respiratory support must be initiated as soon as possible. In neonates with septic shock, decreased peripheral vascular resistance and relative and absolute hypovolemia are the main culprits of the circulatory compromise (77,78). In children and newborns with septic shock, aggressive fluid resuscitation significantly improves outcome (79,80). The use of normal saline and blood products to correct coagulopathy and improve the oxygen carrying capacity of the blood is the recommended approach for volume resuscitation. Early initiation and escalation of vasopressor therapy with dopamine or epinephrine is essential in patients with septic shock (81–83). Some studies have reported the use of low-dose hydrocortisone in septic shock with relative adrenal insufficiency in adults (79) and children (84) to improve survival. In neonates, relative adrenal insufficiency has been recognized as an etiology for volume- and vasopressor-resistant hypotension (85–87) and the use of low-dose hydrocortisone (88,89) facilitates weaning patients off of vasopressor support (see Section III, Chapter 10). Apart from its genomic and non-genomic effects on the cardiovascular system, administration of low-dose hydrocortisone also improves capillary permeability improving intravascular blood volume. Newborns with pulmonary hypertension warrant appropriate ventilatory management and administration of iNO. In addition, patients with refractory hypotension and septic shock may respond to low-dose vasopressin administration. Use of vasopressin may be useful in the treatment of septic shock presenting with high cardiac output and low systemic vascular resistance but could be deleterious if used in a patient with severe left ventricular dysfunction (58–60). In addition, experimental studies raise concern about the use of vasopressin in patients at risk for ischemia in multiple vascular beds (90,91). Finally, the use of functional echocardiography has become an emerging tool to follow changes in systemic and pulmonary circulation in neonates with cardiovascular compromise providing potentially useful information on myocardial function, systemic blood flow (cardiac output), systemic vascular resistance and organ blood flow (92). It is important to emphasize, however, that at present there is no evidence that the use of functional echocardiography improves outcomes in neonates with shock (93).

REFERENCES

1. Vergnano S, Sharland M, Kazembe P, Mwansambo C, Heath PT. Neonatal sepsis. Arch Dis Child, Fetal Neonatal Ed 2005;90:F220–F224.
2. Botwinski C. Systemic inflammatory response syndrome. Neonatal Network 2001;20:21–28.
3. Pruitt JH, et al. Interleukin-1 and interleukin-1 antagonism in sepsis, systemic inflammatory response syndrome and septic shock. Shock 1995;3:235.
4. Moldawer LL. Biology of proinflammatory cytokines and their antagonists. Crit Care Med 1994;22:S3.
5. van der Poll T, van Deventeer SJH. Cytokines and anticytokines in the pathogenesis of sepsis. Infect Dis North Am 1999;13:413.
6. Opal SM, DePalo VA. Anti-inflammatory cytokines. Chest 2000;117:1162.
7. Kilpatrick L, Harris MC. Cytokines and inflammatory response in the fetus and the neonate. In Fetal and Neonatal Physiology 3rd edn. Polin RA, Fox WW, Abman S. Philadelphia PA, WB Saunders Co, 2003:1555–1572.
8. Bone RC, Grodzin C, Balk P. Sepsis. A novel hypothesis for pathogenesis of the disease process. Chest 1997;112:235–243.
9. Jones CA, Cayabyab RG, Kwong KYC, et al. Undetectable interleukin 10 and persistent IL-8 expression early in hyaline membrane disease: a possible developmental basis for the predisposition to chronic lung inflammation in preterm newborns. Pediatr Res 1996;39:966–975.
10. Edelson MB, et al. Circulating pro and counterinflammatory cytokine levels and severity in necrotizing enterocolitis. Pediatrics 1999;103:766.
11. Doughty L, Carcillo JA, Kaplan S, Janosky J. The compensatory anti-inflammatory cytokine interleukin-10 response in pediatric sepsis induced multiple organ failure. Chest 1998;113:1625–1631.
12. Kawada J, Kimura H, Ito Y, et al. Evaluation of systemic inflammatory response in neonates with herpes simplex virus infection. J Infect Dis 2004;190:494.
13. Weatherstone KB, Rich EA. Tumor necrosis factor/cachectin and interleukin 1 secretion by cord blood monocytes from preterm and term neonates. Pediatr Res 1989;25:342–346.
14. Dembiski J, Behrendt D, Martini R, Heep A, Bartmann P. modulation of pro and anti inflammatory cytokine production in very preterm infants. Cytokine 2003;21:200–206.
15. Schultz C, Temming P, Bucsky P, Gopel W, Strunk T, Hartel C. immature anti-inflammatory response in the neonates. Clin Exp Immunol 2004;135:130–136.
16. Schultz C, Rott C, Temming P, Schlenke P, Moller J, Bucsky P. enhanced interleukin-6 and interleukin-8 in term and preterm infants. Pediatr Res 2002;51:317–322.
17. Dammann O, Phillips TM, Alred EN, O'Shea TM, Paneth N. mediators of fetal inflammation in extremely low gestational age newborns. Cytokine 2001;13:234–239.
18. Ng PC, Li K, Wong RPO, Chui K, Wong E, Li G, Fok TF. Proinflammatory and anti-inflammatory cytokine responses in preterm infants with systemic infections. Arch Dis Child, Fetal Neonatal Ed 2003;88:F209–F213.
19. Blahnik M, Ramanathan R, Riley C, Minoo P. lipopolysaccharide induced tumor necrosis factor-α and IL-10 production by lung macrophge from preterm and term neonates. Pediatr Res 2001;50:726–731.
20. Kwong KYC, Jones CA, Cayabyab R, et al. The Effects of IL-10 on proinflammatory cytokine expression (IL-1β and IL-8 in hyaline membrane disease (HMD). Clin Immunol Immunopathol 1998;88:105–113.
21. Yanowitz TD, Jordan AJ, Gilmour CH, et al. Hemodynamic disturbances in preterm infants born after chorioamnionitis: association with cord blood cytokine concentrations. Pediatr Res 2002;51:310–316.
22. Gomez R, Roberto R, Ghezzi F, Yoon BH, Mazor M, Berry SM. The fetal inflammatory response syndrome. Am J Obstet Gynecol 1998;179:194–202.
23. D'Alquen D, Kramer BW, Seidinspinner S, et al. Activation of umbilical cord cells and fetal inflammatory response in preterm infants with chorioamnionitis and funisitis. Pediatr Res 2005;57:263–269.
24. Yanowitz TD, Baker RW, Roberts JM, Brozanski BS. Low blood pressure among very low birth weight infants with fetal vessel inflammation. J Perinatol 2004;24:299–304.

25. Greisen G. Autoregulation of cerebral blood flow in newborn babies. Early Hum Devel 2005;81:423–428.

26. Munro MJ, Walker AM, Barfield C. Hypotensive extremely low birth weight infants have reduced blood flow. Pediatrics 2004;114:1591–1596.

27. Bada H, Korones S, Perry EH, et al. Mean arterial blood pressure changes in premature infants and those at risk for intraventricular hemorrhage. J Pediatr 1990;177:607–614.

28. Tsuji, M Saul PJ, du Plessis A, et al. Cerebral intravascular oxygenation correlates with mean arterial pressure in critically premature infants. Pediatrics 2000;106:615–632.

29. Yoon BH, Romero R, Kim KS, et al. A systemic fetal inflammatory response and the development of bronchopulmonary dysplasia. Am J Obstet Gynecol 1999;181:773–779.

30. Watterberg K, Demers L, Scott S, Murphy S. Chorioamnionitis and early lung in infants in whom bronchopulmonary dyspalsia develops inflammation. Pediatrics 1996;97:210–215.

31. Cayabyab RG, Jones CA, Kwong KYC, Hendershott C, Lecart C, Ramanathan R, Minoo P. Lung expression of IL-1β in premature infants: A marker for maternal chorioamnionitis and predictor of adverse neonatal outcome. J Matern Fetal Neonatal Med 2003;14:205–211.

32. Mittendoerf R, Montag A, Macmillan W, et al. Components of the systemic fetal inflammatory response syndrome as predictors of impaired neurologic outcomes in children. Am J Obstet Gynecol 2003;188:1436–1438.

33. Saliba E, Henrot A. inflammatory mediators and neonatal brain damage. Biol Neonate 2001;79:224–227.

34. duPlessis AJ, Volpe JJ. Perinatal brain injury in the preterm and term newborn. Curr Opin Neurol 2002;15:151–157.

35. Jackson WF. Ion channels and vascular tone. Hypertension 2000;35:173–178.

36. Quayle JM, Nelson MT, Standen NB. ATP sensitive and inwardly rectifying potassium channels in smooth muscle. Physiol Rev 1997;77:1165–1232.

37. Keung EC, Li Q. Lactate activates ATP sensitive potassium channels in guinea pig ventricular myocytes. J Clin Invest 1991;88:1772–1777.

38. Arnalich F, Hernanz A, Jimenez M, et al. Relationship between circulating levels of calcitonin gene related peptide, nitric oxide metabolites and hemodynamic changes in human septic shock. Regul Peptides 1996;65:115–121.

39. Martin C, Leone M, Viviand X, Ayem ML, Guieu ??. High adenosine plasma concentration as a prognostic index for outcome in patients with septic shock. Crit Care Med 2000;28:3198–3202.

40. Frajewicki V, Kahana L, Yechiele H, Brod V, Kohan R, Bitterman H. effects of severe hemorrhage on plasma ANP and glomerular ANP receptors. Am J Physiol 1997;273:R1623–R1630.

41. Murphy ME, Brayden JE. Nitric oxide hyperpolarizes rabbit mesenteric arteries via ATP sensitive potassium channels. J Physiol 1995;486:47–58.

42. Groenveld AB, Sipkema P. Interaction of oxyradicals, antioxidants and nitric oxide during sepsis. Crit Care Med 2000;28:2161.

43. Wink DA, Miranda KM, Espey MG. Mechanisms of the antioxidant effect of nitric oxide. Antioxid Reox Signal 2001;3:203–213.

44. Szabo C. Role of poly(ADP-ribose) synthetase activation in the suppression of cellular energetics in response to nitric oxide and peroxynitrite. Biochem Soc Trans 1997;25:924–929.

45. Burney S, Caulfield JL, Niles JC, et al. The chemistry of DNA damage from nitric oxide and peroxynitrate. Mutat Res 1999;42:37–49.

46. Hauser B, Bracht H, Matejovic M, Radermacher P, Venkatesh B. nitric oxide synthase inhibition in sepsis? Lessons learned from animal studies. Anest Anal 2005;101:488–498.

47. Thiemermann C, Szabo C, Mitchell JA, Vane JR. Vascular hyporeactivity to vasoconstrictor agents and hemodynamic decompensation in hemorrahgic shock is mediated by nitric oxide. Proc Natl Acad Sci USA 2003;90:271–376.

48. Hollenberg SM, Cunnion RE, Zimmenerg J. Nitric oxide synthase inhibition reverses arteriolar hyporesponsiveness to catecholamines in septic rats. Am J Physiol 1993;264:H660–H663.

49. Hollenberg SM, Piotrowski MJ, Parrillo JE. Nitric oxide synthase inhibition reverses arteriolar responsiveness to endothelin-1 in septic rats. Am J Phyisol 1997;272:R969–R974.

50. Hollenberg SM, Broussard M, Osman J, Parrillo JE. Increased microvascular reactivity and improve mortality in septic mice lacking inducible nitric oxide synthase. Circ Res 2000;86:774–778.

51. Kilbourn R. Nitric oxide synthase inhibitors – a mechanism based treatment in septic shock. Crit Care Med 1999;27:2019–2022.

52. Liu S, Adcock IM, Old RW, Barnes PJ, Evans TW. Lipopolysaccharide treatment in vivo induces widespread tissue expression of inducible nitric oxide synthase mRNA. Biochem Biophys Res Commun 1993;196:1208–1213.

53. Taylor BS, Geller DA. Molecular generation of the human inducible nitric oxide synthase (iNOS) gene shock 2000;13:413–424.

54. Shi Y, Li H, Shen C, A et al. Plasma nitric oxide levels in newborn infants with sepsis. J Pediatr 1993;123:435–438.

55. Brackett DJ, Schaefer CF, Tompkins P, et al. Evaluation of cardiac output, total peripheral vascular resistance and plasma concentration of vasopressin in the conscious, unrestrained rat during endotoxemia. Circ Shock 1985;17:273–284.

56. Kasting NW, Mazurek MF, Martin JB. Endotoxin increases vasopressin release independently of known physiological stimuli. Am J Physiol 1985;248:E420–424.

57. Mastorakos G, Weber JS, Magiakou MA, Gunn H, Churosus GP. Hypothalamic–pituitary–adrenal axis activation and stimulation of systemic vasopressin secretion by recombinant interleukin-6 in

humans: Potential implications for the syndrome of inappropriate vasopressin secretion. J Clin Endocrinol Metab 1994;79:934–939.

58. Chikanza IC, Petrou P, Chrousos G. Perturbations of arginine vasopressin secretion during inflammatory stress. Pathophysiologic implications. Ann NY Acad Sci 2000;917:825–834.

59. Zelawski P, Patchev VK, Zelazowska EB, Chrousos GP, Gold PW. Release of hypothalamic corticotropin releasing hormone and arginine vasopressin by interleukin1 β and α MSH: studies in rats with different susceptibility to inflammatory disease. Brain Res 1993;631:22–26.

60. Sharshar T, Blanchard A, Paillard M, Raphael JC, Gajdos P, Annane D. Circulating vasopressin levels in septic shock. Circulation 1997;95:1122–1125.

61. Landry DW, Levin HR, Gallant EM, et al. Vasopressin deficiency contributes to the vasodilatation of septic shock. Circulation 1997;95:1122–1125.

62. Landry DW, Levin HR, Gallant EM, et al. Vasopressin pressor hypersensitivity in vasodilatory septic shock. Crit Care Med 1997;25:1279–1282.

63. Obstrich Md, Bestul DJ, Jung R, Fish DN, Mclaren R. The role of vasopressin in vasodilatory septic shock. Pharmacotherapy 2004;24:1050–1063.

64. Malay MB, Ashton R, Landry D, Townsend R. Low dose vasopressin in the treatment of vasodilatory septic shock. J Trauma 1999;47:699–710.

65. Mutlu GM, Factor P. Role of vasopressin in the management of septic shock. Intensive Care Med 2004;30:1276–1291.

66. Peevey KJ, Chartrand SA, Wiseman HJ, Boerth RC, Olson RD. Myocardial dysfunction in group B streptococcal shock. Pediatr Res 1985;19:511–513.

67. Peevey KJ, Reed T, Chartrand SA, Olson RD, Boerth R. the comparison of myocardial dysfunction in three forms of experimental septic shock. Pediatr Res 1986;20:1240–1242.

68. Meadow Wl, Meus JP. Early and late hemodynamic consequences of group B streptococcal sepsis in piglets: effects on systemic, pulmonary and mesenteric circulations. Circ Shock 1986;19:347–356.

69. Hammerman C, Komar K, Meadow W, et al. Selective inhibition of thromboxane synthase reduces group B β-hemolytic streptococci induced pulmonary hypertension in piglets. Dev Pharmacol Ther 1988;11:306–312.

70. Runkle B, Goldberg RN, Streitfeld MM. cardiovascular changes in group B streptococcal sepsis in the piglet: Response to indomethacin and relationship to prostacyclin and thromboxane A2. Pediatr Res 1984;18:874–878.

71. Fike CD, Kaplowitz MR, Pfister SL. Arachidonic acid metabolites and an early stage of pulmonary hypertension in the chronically hypoxic newborn pigs. Am J Physiol Lung Cell Mol Physiol 2003;284:316–323.

72. Meadow W, Rudinsky B. Inflammatory mediators and neonatal sepsis. Clin Perinatol 1995;22:519–536.

73. Lei Y, Zhen J, Ming XL, Jian HX. Induction of higher expression of IL-1β and TNF α lower expression of IL-10 and cyclic guanosine monophosphate by pulmonary arterial hypertension following cardiopulmonary bypass. Asian J Surg 2002;25:203–208.

74. Saetre T, Hoiby EA, Aspelin T, Lenmark G, Lyberg T. Acute serogroup A streptococcal shock: a porcine model. J Infect Dis 2000;182:133–141.

75. Dashinamurti S. pathophysiologic mechanism of persistent pulmonary hypertension of the newborn. Pediatr Pulmonol 2005;39:492–503.

76. Ermert M, Merkele, M Mootz R, et al. Endotoxin priming of the cyclooxygenase-2 thromboxane axis in isolated rat lungs. Am J Physiol Lung Cell Mol Physiol 2000;278:1195–1203.

77. Noori S, Friedlich P, Seri, I. Pathophysiology of shock in the fetus and the neonate. In Fetal and Neonatal Physiology 3rd edn. Polin RA, Fox WW, Abman S. Philadelphia PA, WB Saunders Co, 2003:772–781.

78. Seri I, Noori S. diagnosis and treatment of neonatal hypotension outside of the transitional period. Early Hum Develop 2005;82:405–411.

79. Carcillo JA, Fields AI. American College of Critical Care Medicine Task Force Committee Members: Clinical practice parameters for hemodynamic support of pediatric and neonatal patients in septic shock. Crit Care Med 2002;30:1365–1378.

80. Han YY, Carcillo J, Dragotta MA, et al. Early reversal of pediatric–neonatal septic shock by community physicians is associated with improved outcomes. Pediatrics 2003;11:793–799.

81. Seri I, Abbasi S, Wood DC, Gerdes JS. Regional hemodynamic effects of dopamine in sick preterm neonate. J Pediatr 1998;133:728–734.

82. Seri I. cardiovascular, renal and endocrine actions of dopamine in neonates and children. J Pediatr 1995;126:333–344.

83. Seri I, Rudas G, Bors Z, Kanyicsa B, Tulassay T. effects of low dose dopamine infusion on cardiovascular and renal functions, cerebral blood flow, and plasma catecholamine levels in preterm infants. Pediatr Res 1993;34:742–749.

84. Annane D, Sebille V, Charpentier C, et al. Effect of treatment with low doses of hydrocortisone and fludrocortisone on the mortality in patients with septic shock. JAMA 2002;288:862–871.

85. Ng PC, Lam CWK, Fok TF, et al. Refractory hypotension in preterm infants with adrenocortical insufficiency. Arch Dis Child, Fetal Neonatal Ed 2001;84:F122–F124.

86. Tantivit P, Subramanian N, Garg M, Rangasamy R, Delemos RA. Low serum cortisol levels in term newborns with refractory hypotension. J Perinatol 1999;19:352–357.

87. Watterberg K. Adrenal insufficiency and cardiac dysfunction in the preterm infant. Pediatr Res 2002;51:422–424.

88. Seri I, Tan R, Evans J. Cardiovascular effects of hydrocortisone in preterm infants with pressor resistant hypotension. Pediatrics 2001;107:1070–1074.

89. Noori S, Friedlich P, Wong P, Ebrahimi M, Siassi B, Seri I. Hemodynamic changes following low-dose hydrocortisone administration in vasopressor-treated neonates. Pediatrics 2006;118:1456–1466.

90. Liedel JL, Meadow W, Nachman J, Koogler T, Kahana MD. Use of vasopressin in refractory hypotension in children with vasodilatory shock: Five cases and review of the literature. Pediatr Crit Care Med 2002;3:15–18.

91. Tsuneyoshi I, Yamada H, Kakihana Y, et al. Hemodynamic and metabolic effects of low dose vasopressin infusions in vasodilatory septic shock. Crit Care Med 2001;29:487–493.

92. Osborn D. Diagnosis and treatment of preterm transitional circulatory compromise. Early Hum Develop 2005;81:413–422.

93. Kluckow M, Seri I, Evans N. Functional echocardiography – an emerging clinical tool for the neonatologist: medical progress article. J Pediatr 2007;150:125–130.

Chapter 12

Shock in the Surgical Neonate

Philippe Friedlich, MD, MS Epi, MBA • Cathy Shin, MD, FACS, FAAP • Caterina Tiozzo, MD • Istvan Seri, MD, PhD

A significant number of neonates are born with problems that require surgery or develop such problems after birth. This chapter highlights the issues that are specific to the cardiovascular compromise of neonates requiring surgery. The discussion focusses on a review of the general pathophysiological principles involved in the clinical management of shock in these patients and on the most frequently encountered surgical conditions that require urgent or emergency cardiovascular attention.

DEFINITION AND PHASES OF NEONATAL SHOCK

The etiology, clinical presentations, phases, and pathophysiology of neonatal shock are discussed in detail in Section I, Chapter 1. Here, we briefly review the most important features of neonatal shock with a special attention to their relevance to the surgical neonate.

Shock develops when O_2 delivery to the tissues is inadequate to satisfy cellular metabolic demand. Independent of the etiology, there are three phases of shock with each being characterized by unique pathophysiological changes. In the compensated phase, vital organ function is maintained by intrinsic neurohormonal compensatory mechanisms resulting in distribution of organ blood flow primarily to the heart, brain, and adrenal glands, and away from other "non-vital" organs. Several hormones and local factors affecting myocardial function, organ blood flow distribution, capillary integrity, systemic and pulmonary vascular resistance, and cellular metabolism play a central role in the regulation of these specific hemodynamic changes. Stroke volume, central venous pressure, and urine output all decrease. However, blood pressure remains within normal limits because the increase in myocardial contractility and heart rate maintains cardiac output close to the normal range. It is important to note that, since blood pressure is the function of blood flow and systemic vascular resistance, blood pressure by definition does not appropriately reflect the status of organ blood flow in the non-vital organs. This notion is especially important in the non-acidotic extremely low birth weight

(ELBW) preterm neonate with immature myocardium and compensated shock during the first postnatal day (1–3). If the circulatory compromise advances, neonatal shock enters its uncompensated phase where failure of the neurohormonal compensatory mechanisms result in decreased myocardial contractility, stroke volume, and blood pressure with ensuing significant decreases in organ blood flow and tissue perfusion and the development of lactic acidosis. If treatment is delayed and/or the condition rapidly deteriorates in cases with fulminant sepsis, myocarditis, or asphyxia with multiorgan failure, neonatal shock enters its irreversible phase where complete organ failure dominates the clinical picture and death invariably occurs.

PATHOGENESIS OF NEONATAL SHOCK

The clinical presentation, pathophysiology, and treatment of neonatal shock are significantly affected by the primary etiology of the condition. As discussed in detail in Chapter 1, hypovolemia, myocardial dysfunction, and abnormal regulation of peripheral vascular tone are the primary etiological factors leading to shock in the neonate. In addition, in the critically ill neonate, more than one of these factors may be involved. For example, in a newborn with septic shock, the capillary leak-induced relative hypovolemia, direct myocardial injury, and abnormal regulation of vascular tone may all contribute to the development of the circulatory compromise.

DIAGNOSIS OF CIRCULATORY COMPROMISE AND SHOCK

There is no universally accepted agreement on what the gold standard for the diagnosis of circulatory compromise in the neonate should be. Conventionally, blood pressure has been used as the gold standard. The major reason for this is that, in addition to heart rate, blood pressure is the only meaningful hemodynamic parameter that can be continuously monitored in absolute numbers. The other hemodynamic parameters important in the assessment of tissue perfusion, such as cardiac output (systemic blood flow) and blood flow to organs (such as cerebral, renal, intestinal, or pulmonary blood flow), can only be assessed in absolute numbers at one point at a time or, when measured continuously, only relative changes in these parameters can be monitored. In addition, the available monitoring techniques allowing for assessment of the hemodynamic parameters in the neonate (echocardiography, near infrared (NIR) spectroscopy, magnetic resonance imaging (MRI) and so on) all have significant limitations (see Section II) and there are no data linking hemodynamic compromise and its treatment to changes in neonatal outcomes. Accordingly, the gestational- and postnatal age-dependent blood pressure range that "warrants intervention" is not known (see Section I, Chapter 3). Finally, even if we knew the normal blood pressure range, relying solely on blood pressure carries the inherent risk of overlooking the compensated phase of shock. The indirect and commonly used clinical signs of circulatory compromise, such as increased heart rate, slow skin capillary refill time, increased core peripheral temperature difference, low urine output, and acidosis, either have limitations in aiding the prompt diagnosis of circulatory compromise or, as in the very preterm neonate in the immediate postnatal period, are simply of limited clinical value (see Section III, Chapter 8). Despite the limitations of these indirect measures of cardiovascular compromise, their combined use and/or the changes in these measure occurring over time are predictive for adverse outcome. For example, when blood pressure and capillary refill time are being assessed together (4) or when there is evidence for worsening lactic acidosis, outcome becomes more predictable (5).

Respiratory Disorders

Congenital Diaphragmatic Hernia

Congenital diaphragmatic hernia (CDH) is a defect of the diaphragm thought to be due to an early failure of the pleuroperitoneal canal closure in early gestation resulting in a spectrum of pulmonary hypoplasia (6). The incidence of CDH has been estimated between 1/3000 and 1/5000 live births (7).

The defect allows the abdominal organs, such as the stomach and bowel, and occasionally the liver and spleen, to enter the thoracic cavity. These organs displace the heart and lung compromising lung and cardiac development *in utero* and result in decreases in respiratory gas exchange and cardiac output and function after delivery. A major cause of hypoxemia associated with CDH is right-to-left shunting through the foramen ovale (FO) and/or patent ductus arteriosus (PDA) caused by the associated pulmonary hypertension. Persistent pulmonary hypertension in infants with CDH has many etiologies and significantly affects the outcome of these neonates.

Prenatal factors affecting the development of postnatal pulmonary hypertension in patients with CDH have been partly explained by the impact of the mediastinal shift and the malposition of the heart on fetal circulation and cardiac development (8,9).

The neonatal heart is normally positioned on the left side of the thoracic cavity with the interventricular septum at a 45° angle to the midline sagittal plane. Indeed, Baumgart et al. have shown that cardiac malposition is common in neonates with CDH who require extracorporeal membrane oxygenation (ECMO) perioperatively (9). The malposition of the heart is caused by herniation of the abdominal viscera into the thorax also resulting in a mediastinal shift, and pulmonary hypoplasia. Interestingly, the return of the heart to a more normal position after surgical repair of the diaphragm predicts a better outcome, whereas failure to return to a more normal axis after diaphragmatic repair has been associated with poor outcomes (9).

In addition to causing malposition of the heart, CDH may affect the development of the heart itself. Indeed, an adequate left ventricular mass favors survival, whereas neonates with CDH and significant left ventricle hypoplasia are less likely to survive (10). A redistribution of fetal cardiac output away from the left ventricle toward the right side was proposed to occur in infants with CDH based on the finding of a markedly increased pulmonary valve to aortic valve flow ratio compared with healthy fetuses (11). This redistribution also seems to be associated with development of low left ventricular mass (11).

Several mechanisms may contribute to cardiovascular compromise in patients with severe CDH. For example, lung hypoplasia may diminish pulmonary blood flow returning to the left atrium during fetal life. By the mid- to late-third trimester, 22% of combined cardiac output normally circulates through the pulmonary vasculature *in utero*. However, this pulmonary blood flow may be reduced by as much as half with severe lung hypoplasia in patients with CDH (12). There is also evidence that normal fetal pulmonary artery blood flow is necessary for normal pulmonary vascular and airway development and that diminished cardiac mass with severe CDH *in utero* may be used as an indicator of the severity of pulmonary hypoplasia (13,14). Since a diminished left ventricle size in the fetus with CDH has been documented, it has been suggested that a decreased left ventricular mass is an intrinsic part of this anomaly (14). In addition, the extent of left ventricle hypoplasia may be a predictor of poor outcomes, as infants with the smallest left ventricular mass more frequently require preoperative ECMO support and often experience poor outcomes (14). Furthermore, CDH patients often experience cardiac stun while receiving ECMO support (15). This phenomenon may be due to the inability of a relatively small left ventricle to adapt to the increased afterload effect of the aortic cannula (15,16). Furthermore, the malposition of the cardiac angle within the thorax in the fetus may impede venous return to the right side of the heart from the umbilical circulation. Since umbilical flow returning from the placenta is normally directed by the ductus venosus across the foreman ovale into the left atrium, such flow contributes to left ventricular output (17). As the shift in cardiac position in patients with CDH may redirect the venous return into the right atrium, it could result in an imbalance between pulmonary and aortic flows (10). Lastly, the redistribution of cardiac output away from the left heart may be further enhanced by the poor function of the underdeveloped left ventricle, resulting in poor outcome (18).

In view of the complex pulmonary and cardiovascular problems facing the neonate with CDH, patients with prenatal diagnoses should be delivered at centers with a multidisciplinary team available at all times and with the ability to deliver advanced modalities of respiratory and cardiovascular therapies, including ECMO. After delivery, prenatally diagnosed infants, or as soon as the diagnosis of CDH is suspected, infants must not be ventilated by bag and mask and should be immediately intubated and ventilated using a low peak inspiratory pressure not exceeding 24 cm of water to minimize the potential for the development of an air leak syndrome (19). With a significant increase in the risk of air leak secondary to lung hypoplasia, the use of neuromuscular blockade and sedation has been recommended to minimize both barotrauma and the possibility of bowel distention, and to enhance decompression of the hollow abdominal organs displaced into the intrathoracic cavity (20). Once the airway has been stabilized, appropriate arterial and central venous access established, and the patient has been transferred to the neonatal intensive care unit (NICU), right-to-left shunting is usually monitored by the use of pre- and postductal pulse oximetry. Blood pressure support is usually also instituted with the judicious use of volume administration and, if appropriate, the continuous infusion of vasopressors or inotropes. An echocardiogram is essential in the assessment of the cardiac structure and function immediately following the stabilization of the patient. Repeat functional echocardiograms may also assist in the management of cardiovascular status. According to general practice but without much supporting evidence, preductal arterial oxygen saturation is maintained close to 90%. The utility of conventional versus high frequency oscillatory ventilation has been extensively debated and remains unclear (20,21). If hypoxemia resulting from pulmonary hypertension does not respond to the initial mechanical ventilatory methodologies, a trial of inhaled nitric oxide (iNO) is warranted (22). Finally, if all else fails the infant with CDH is managed by use of ECMO (20).

The intraoperative and postoperative care of patients with congenital diaphragmatic hernia often includes the use of volume support in the form of colloids and/or crystalloids and vasoactive agents. There is very little and only anecdotal evidence of how much and what kind of volume and vasopressor or inotrope therapy to use. Ideally, with the reduction of the defect and a return of abdominal contents into the peritoneum, improved venous return and cardiac output will result in improvement of systemic and pulmonary blood flow. Some neonates with more severe pulmonary hypoplasia will experience a potentially fatal rebound pulmonary hypertensive crisis following ECMO and surgery, with some responding to iNO while some of the non-responders may respond to the addition of sildenafil to iNO (23). Finally, it is uncertain if the recent improvement in survival rates of neonates with CDH translates into better long-term outcomes (24).

Cystic Congenital Adenomatoid Malformation

The term congenital cystic adenomatoid malformation (CCAM) reflects the histopathological features of the presentation (25). It is believed that CCAM results from a cessation of bronchopulmonary maturation and concomitant overgrowth of mesenchymal elements at about the 5th to 6th weeks of gestation and produces the adenomatoid appearances of the anomaly (26). There are two major classifications of CCAM. One classification divides the presentation into three types on the basis of their histopathological characteristics while the other uses the size of the cysts within the mass to separate the macrocystic presentation (single or multiple cysts with diameters > 5 mm) from the microcystic type with very small cysts and echodense homogeneous lungs (26). As for the clinical presentation in the immediate postnatal period, many patients with CCAM are asymptomatic at birth (26). However, since a small bronchial communication often exists within the CCAM, infections and overinflation of the cystic lesions will frequently lead to respiratory pathology during infancy.

Antenatal ultrasound has increased the detection of CCAM and it provides a chance to also identify fetuses who will remain asymptomatic after birth (27,28). In general, the majority of CCAM lessions does not lead to significant abnormalities of lung or heart development in the fetus and regression and/or lack of growth of these lesions occur frequently (27,28).

A very small proportion of these malformations behave in a more aggressive fashion, forming a rapidly expanding space-occupying lesion. This may lead to the development of hydrops fetalis due to the elevated central venous pressure caused by cardiac compression and altered hemodynamics (29). In the hydropic fetus, Doppler study of the inferior vena cava can demonstrate a significantly greater degree of flow reversal with atrial contractions as compared to normal fetuses (29).

When faced with cardiopulmonary complications and when a large single cyst is involved, *in utero* drainage by thoracocentesis or a thoracoamniotic shunt has had varying success for fetal salvage (30). Similarly, *in utero* fetal surgery via maternal hysterotomy and fetal thoracotomy and lobectomy has been attempted and for now should be restricted to specialized fetal therapy centers (30,31).

In the immediate postnatal period, the asymptomatic lesions can be safely followed with computerized tomography (CT) scanning or MRI. The timing of the surgical management in asymptomatic cases is dictated by the potential development of recurrent infection (32). In symptomatic lesions, respiratory distress is usually an acute postnatal event. Lobectomy remains the procedure of choice to prevent residual disease and recurrence in the remaining lobe (32).

Vascular Tumors

Hepatic Vascular Tumors

The most common hepatic vascular anomalies in infancy are hepatic hemangioma and arterio-venous malformations (AVMs). These two disorders are biologically different yet exhibit similarities in their pathophysiology, including fast flow hemodynamics. These lesions often manifest themselves in the neonatal period with hepatomegaly, congestive heart failure, and anemia (33). Although liver hemangiomas often regress spontaneously, complications associated with liver hemangiomas still result in a mortality rate of up to 30% (34). Unlike hemangiomas, AVMs are unlikely to regress spontaneously and have a higher, albeit not well-documented, mortality rate (35).

Most cases of infantile hepatic hemangioma are benign vascular tumors and are the second most common liver tumor in infants after hepatoblastomas (36). Infants with hepatic hemangioma, especially with its capillary form (hemangioendothelioma), typically develop congenital hepatomegaly, congestive heart failure, and significant anemia.

The prenatal imaging techniques, including ultrasound, color Doppler imaging, and ultrafast MRI, are providing critical information for early diagnosis and successful management of such conditions. Typical color Doppler flow patterns of hemangioma demonstrate enlarged vessels with high flow velocity associated with corresponding abrupt changes in the vessel caliber and arterio-venous shunts.

Fetal hepatic hemangioma can result in non-immune hydrops fetalis and high-output cardiac failure due to the arterio-venous shunting associated volume overload. More than 55% of hepatic hemangioma diagnosed in the fetus has been associated with hydrops fetalis and a mortality rate over 55%. In the absence of hydrops fetalis, the mortality rates are lower and estimated at less than 30% (36). Neither the size, the total enlargement, the side of the affected liver lobe, nor gestational age is a significant variable predicting the likelihood of the development of hydrops (36). The optimal pre- and perinatal management strategies include the use of serial ultrasound and/or MRI monitoring of the fetus for signs of hydrops fetalis. Postnatally, the diagnosis is confirmed or established by ultrasound, CT scan, and/or MRI, with MRI being the preferred investigative modality as it can accurately define the extent and nature of the vascular lesion, alleviating the need for diagnostic arteriography.

Infantile hepatic hemangioendothelioma rarely presents with asymptomatic hepatomegaly. The classical manifestations are prominent massive hepatomegaly, out of proportion to the associated high-output cardiac failure resulting from the arterio-venous communications (37). Over 50% of the cardiac output may be diverted to the hepatic hemangioendothelioma resulting in severe cardiovascular compromise (38) and patients with significant congestive heart failure have a mortality rate approaching 70 and 90% (39,40). The younger the age at presentation, the more severe are the cardiovascular symptoms (41). Treatment of infantile hepatic hemangioendothelioma initially consists of supportive medical management and depends on the degree of shunting through intrahepatic arterio-venous fistulae along with the severity of the resultant congestive heart failure (42,43). Progression of symptoms despite medical therapy is an indication for hepatic arteriography and embolization (42,44). Neonates not responding to medical management have a poor prognosis for long-term survival.

Sacrococcygeal Teratoma

Sacrococcygeal teratoma is one of the most common tumors in newborns with an estimated incidence of 1/20,000 to 1/40,000 births (45). Sacrococcygeal teratoma is defined as a neoplasm composed of tissue from either all three germ layers or multiple foreign tissues lacking organ specificity (46). The American Academy of Pediatric surgery section classification uses a four-level staging classification based on the location, the ease of resection, and the malignant potential of these tumors.

Prenatal diagnosis of sacrococcygeal teratoma can be done by ultrasonographic imaging (47,48). Large prenatally diagnosed sacrococcygeal teratomas usually are highly vascular and can easily lead to fetal high output cardiac failure, resulting in hepatomegaly, placentomegaly, and non-immune hydrops (47,48). As with liver AVMs, the development of intrauterine fetal high output failure in fetuses with sacrococcygeal teratoma is caused by arterio-venous shunting within the tumor and/or occurs secondarily to hemorrhage within the tumor itself, leading to severe fetal anemia and poor outcomes (49). When hydrops develops in fetuses with sacrococcygeal teratoma, dilatation of the cardiac ventricular chambers and of the inferior vena cava occurs due to the large venous return from the lower body (50). Fetal intervention and resection have been attempted in fetuses whose courses were complicated with significant congestive heart failure and hydrops fetalis (49,51,52).

In the postnatal management of patients with sacrococcygeal teratoma, the clinical presentation of a hyperdynamic cardiovascular state should be anticipated and treated accordingly. Postnatal echocardiography should be obtained to assess cardiac function and frequent reassessment using functional echocardiography may be of benefit.

Finally, the long-term outcomes are variable for patients with sacrococcygeal teratoma and prenatal diagnoses prior to 30 weeks of gestation, especially with large tumors, tend to have worse prognoses (49,51). Recommendations for long-term monitoring include serial serum alpha-fetal protein levels and radiological examination every three months. Consideration for postsurgical chemotherapy regimens will depend on the specific pathological nature of the immature elements (53).

Gastrointestinal Disorders

Several gastrointestinal neonatal surgical conditions may result in cardiovascular collapse or shock. Many of these disorders require prompt attention to initial fluid resuscitation as well as the coordination of care between perinatal, obstetric, and neonatal teams. With improvement in prenatal diagnosis, an increasing number of infants are diagnosed prenatally with correctible surgical malformations allowing forfetal intervention, planned delivery in a tertiary surgical center, and antenatal counseling using a multidisciplinary approach.

Gastroschisis and Omphalocele

Gastroschisis and omphalocele are relatively frequently diagnosed fetal anomalies. The incidence of gastroschisis has been increasing worldwide and this condition primarily affects fetuses whose mothers are less than 20 years of age (54).

The effect of timing and mode of delivery on outcomes of neonates with gastroschisis is unclear. However, the present recommendations for delivery of these patients in a tertiary care facility with close coordination of obstetric, neonatal, and pediatric surgical care are supported by some evidence (55).

The immediate postnatal management of the neonate with gastroschisis is directed toward preventing excessive fluid losses, hypothermia, and trauma to the exteriorized intestines. In these patients, following stabilization and evaluation for anesthesia, the surgeons usually attempt primary closure if the abdominal cavity volume allows closure of the external fascia. Following abdominal closure, excessive abdominal wall tensions can lead to a compartment syndrome, including vena cava compression, compromised respiratory status, and on rare occasions potential bowel ischemia. To avoid this complication, most surgeons estimate the intra-abdominal pressure with the use of a nasogastric or bladder catheter. If the estimated pressure is greater than 20 mm Hg, a silo is used to stage the closure of the abdominal wall. Because the closure and tension associated with compartment syndrome often lead to poor peripheral perfusion, metabolic acidosis, and decreased urine output, the immediate postsurgical management often includes significant fluid resuscitation. Especially in large defects following closure, the increased intra-abdominal pressure often results in some degree of capillary leak, resulting in pulmonary and soft tissue edema. Recent recommendations favor performing the reduction over time to prevent potential complications of the abdominal compartment syndrome and improve tolerance for early feeding and shorter hospital stays (56,57). However, these recommendations are mainly not evidence-based.

Similarly to gastroschisis, the use of routine prenatal screening and fetal ultrasonography has led to significant proportions of omphalocele being detected by the early second trimester. However, contrary to gastroschisis, there is a relatively high incidence of association of genetic syndromes with omphalocele. Therefore, prenatal diagnosis of fetuses with omphalocele includes a very careful evaluation for potential chromosomal anomalies as well as malformations of other organs.

To decrease the chance of an omphalocele rupture, delivery by cesarean section is recommended. Upon delivery, trauma to the lesion needs to be avoided. In general, an omphalocele with ruptured membranes carries the same cardiovascular risks, clinical presentation, and treatment approaches as gastroschisis with most small-to-medium size omphaloceles having good outcomes unless associated with severe cardiac, central nervous system or other malformations. Giant omphaloceles present a challenge for medical and surgical management.

Necrotizing Enterocolitis

Necrotizing enterocolitis (NEC) is one of the most common gastrointestinal medical and/or surgical emergencies often affecting preterm neonates. With a mortality rate often approaching 50% in preterm infants with a birth weight < 1500 g and with the associated respiratory failure, systemic inflammatory response syndrome and cardiovascular collapse, The pathogenesis of NEC is multifactorial and likely includes significant decreases in gastrointestinal perfusion in general and mucosal perfusion in particular. Risk factors for NEC include but are not limited to prematurity, hypoxemic ischemic insult, presence of a patent ductus arteriosus with "diastolic aortic steal," and time to full enteral feeding.

Medical management of infants with NEC should include decompression of the intestines, abstinence from enteral feeding, broad-spectrum antibiotics, fluid resuscitation, and support of the respiratory and cardiovascular compromise. Surgical care may include the placement of a temporary drain or formal laparotomy with intestinal resection as appropriate. During laparotomy, the increased insensible and transmembraneous fluid losses need to be addressed while in the pre- and postoperative period the complex cardiovascular effects of the associated systemic inflammatory response syndrome require constant attention (see Section I, Chapter 1 and Section III, Chapter 11).

REFERENCES

1. Kluckow M, Evans N. Relationship between blood pressure and cardiac output in preterm infants requiring mechanical ventilation. J Pediatr 1996;129:506.
2. Kluckow M, Evans N. Superior vena flow in preterm infants: A novel marker of systemic blood flow. Arch Dis Child 2000;82:F182.
3. Seri I, Evans J. Controversies in the diagnosis and management of hypotension in the newborn infant. Curr Opin Pediatr 2001;13:116.
4. Osborn DA, Kluckow M, Evans N. Blood pressure, capillary refill, and central–peripheral temperature difference. Clinical detection of low upper body blood flow in very premature infants. Arch Dis Child, Fetal Neonatal Ed 2004;89:F168–F173.
5. Deshpande SA, Platt MP. Association between blood lactate and acid–base status and mortality in ventilated babies. Arch Dis Child, Fetal Neonatal Ed 1997;76:F15–F20.
6. Harrison MR, Adzick NS, Flake AW. Correction of congenital diaphragmatic hernia. VI. Hard lessons. J Pediatr Surg 1993;28:1411–1418.
7. Puri P, Gorman F. Lethal nonpulmonary anomalies associated with congenital diaphragmatic hernia: Implications for early intrauterine surgery. J Pediatr Surg 1984;19:29–32.
8. Ryan CA, Perreault T. Johnston-Hodgson A, Finer NN. Extracorporeal membrane oxygenation and cardiac malformation. J Pediatr Surg 1994;29:878.
9. Baumgart S, Paul JJ, Huhta JC. Cardiac malformation, redistribution of fetal cardiac output, and left heart hypoplasia reduce survival in neonates with congenital diaphragmatic hernia requiring extracorporeal membrane oxygenation. J Pediatr Surg 1998;133:57–62.
10. Schwartz SM, Vermilion RP, Hirschl RB. Evaluation of left ventricular mass in children with left sided congenital diaphragmatic hernia. J Pediatr 1994;125:447.
11. Rasanen J, Wood DC, Weiner S, Ludomirski A, Huhta JC. Role of the pulmonary circulation in the distribution of human fetal cardiac output during the second half of pregnancy. Circulation 1996;94:1068–1073.
12. Karamanoukian HL, Glick PL, Wilcox DT, O'Toole SJ, Rossman JE, Aziazkhan RG. Pathophysiology of congenital diaphragmatic hernia. XI: Anatomic and biochemical characterization of the heart in the fetal lamb CDH model. J Pediatr Surg 1995;30:925–929.
13. Karamanoukian HL, O'Toole SJ, Rossman JR, Sharma A, Holm BA. Can cardiac weight predict lung weight in patients with congenital diaphragmatic hernia? J Pediatr Surg 1996;31:823–825.
14. Schwartz SM, Vermillion RP, Hirschl RB. Evaluation of left ventricular mass in children with left-sided diaphragmatic hernia. J Pediatr 1994;125:447–451.
15. Martin GR, Short BL, Abbot C, O'Brian A. Cardiac stun in infants undergoing extracorporeal membrane oxygenation. J Thorac Cardiovasc Surg 1991;101:607–611.
16. Martin GR, Short BL. Doppler echocardiographic evaluation of cardiac performance in infants on prolonged extracorporeal membrane oxygenation. Am J Cardiol 1988;62:929–934.

17. Kiserud T, Eik-Nes SH, Blaas HG, Hellevik LR. Ultrasonographic velocimetry of the fetal ductus venosus. Lancet 1991;338:1412–1414.

18. Sharland GK, Lockhart SM, Heward AJ, Allan LD. Prognosis in fetal diaphragmatic hernia. Am J Obstet Gynecol 1991;166:9–13.

19. Finer NN, Tierney A, Etches PC, et al. Congenital diaphragmatic hernia: developing a protocolized approach. J Pediatr Surg 1998;33:1331.

20. Ford JW. Neonatal ECVMO: Current controversies and trends. ECMO: current controversies and trends. Neonatal Netw 2006;25:229–238.

21. Moya FR, Lally KP. Evidence-based management of infants with congenital diaphragmatic hernia. Semin Perinatol 2005;29:112–117.

22. Kinsella JP, Abnam SH. Inhaled nitric oxide therapy in children. Paediatr Respir Rev 2005;6:190–198.

23. Noori S, Friedlich P, Seri I. Cardiovascular effects of sildenafil in neonates and infants with congenital diaphragmatic hernia. Neonatology 2007;91:92–100.

24. Chiu PP, Sauer C, Mihailovic A, Adatia I, Bohn D, Coates AL, Langer JC. The price of success in the management of congenital diaphragmatic hernia: is improved survival accompanied by and increase in long-term morbidity? J Pediatr Surg 2006;41:888–892.

25. Chin KY, Tang MY. Congenital adenomatoid malformation of one lobe of a lung with general anasarca. Arch Pathol 1949;48:221–229.

26. Bailey PV, Tracey Jr T, Connors RH, deMello D, Lewis JE, Weber TR. Congenital bronchopulmonary malformations. Diagnostic and therapeutic considerations. J Thorac Cardiovasc Surg 1990;99:597–603.

27. Van Leeuwen K, Teitelbaum DH, Hirschi RB, et al. Prenatal diagnosis of congenital cystic adenomatoid malformation and its potential postnatal presentation, surgical indications and natural history. J Paediatr Surg 1999;34:794–798.

28. Marshall KW, Blane CE, Teitelbaum DH, Van Leeuwen K. CCAM: impact of prenatal diagnosis and charging strategies in treatment of asymptomatic patient. AJR, Am J Roentgenol 2000;175:1551–1554.

29. Mahle WT, Rychik J, Tian ZY, et al. Echocardiographic evaluation of the fetus with congenital cystic adenomatoid malformation. Ultrasound Obstet Gynecol 2000;16:620–624.

30. Adzick NS, Harrison MR, Crombleholme TM, Flake AW, Howell LJ. Fetal lung lesions: management and outcome. Am J Obstet Gynecol 1998;179:884–889.

31. Khosa JK, Leong SL, Borzi PA. Congenital cystic adenomatoid malformation of the lung: indications and timing of surgery. Pediatr Surg Int 2004;20 505–508.

32. Keidar S, Ben-Sira L, Weinberg M, Jaffa AJ, Silbiger A, Vinograd I. The postnatal management of CCAM. Isr Med Assoc J 2001;3:258–261.

33. Boon LM, Burrows PE, Paltiel HJ, Lund DP, Ezekowitz RAB, Folkman J, Mulliken JB. Hepatic vascular anomalies in infancy. A twenty-seven years experience. J Pediatr 1996;129:346–354.

34. Cohen RC, Myers NA. Diagnosis and management of massive hepatic hemangiomas in childhood. J Pediatr Surg 1986;21:6–9.

35. Mulliken JB, Young AE. Vascular Birthmarks: Hemangiomas and Malformations. Philadelphia, WB Saunders, 1988.

36. Bartsch EMP, Paek BW, Yoshizawa J, et al. Giant fetal hepatic hemangioma. Fetal Diag Ther 2003;18:59–64.

37. Samuel M, Spitz L. Infantile hepatic hemangioendothelioma: the role of surgery. J Pediatr Surg 1995;30:1425–1429.

38. Rocchini AP, Rosenthal A, Isenberg HJ, Nadas AD. Hepatic hemangioendothelioma: hemodynamic observation and treatment. Pediatrics 1976;57:131–135.

39. Daller JA, Bueno J, Gutierrez J, et al. Hepatic hemangioendothelioma: V. Clinical experience and management strategy. J Ped Surg 1999;34:98–106.

40. Fishman SJ, Mulliken JB. Hemangiomas and vascular malformations of infancy and childhood. Pediatr Clin North Am 1993;40:1177–1200.

41. Davenport M, Hansen L, Heaton ND, Howard ER. Hemangioendothelioma of the liver in infants. J Pediatr Surg 1995;30:44–48.

42. Holcomb GW, O'Neil JA, Mahboubi S, Bishop HC. Experience with hepatic hemangioendothelioma in infancy and childhood. J Pediatr Surg 1988;23:661–666.

43. Fellows KE, Hoffer FA, Karkowitz RI, O'Neil Jr JA. Multiple collaterals to hepatic infantile hemangioendotheliomas and arteriovenous malformations: effects of embolization. Radiology 1991;181:813–818.

44. Iyer CP, Stanley P, Mahour GH. Hepatic hemangiomas in infants and children: a review of 30 cases. Am Surg 1996;62:356–360.

45. Isaacs HJ. Tumors of the Fetus and Newborns. Philadelphia, WB Saunders Company, 1997.

46. Mahour GH, Woolley MM, Trinedi SN. Sacrococcygeal teratoma: a 33 year experience. J Pediatr Surg 1975;10:183–188.

47. Bond SJ, Harrison MR, Schmidt KG. Death due to high output cardiac failure in fetal coccygeal teratoma. J Pediatr Surg 1990;25:1287–1291.

48. Grison ER, Gauderer MWL, Wolfson RN, Jassani MN, Olsen MM. Antenatal diagnosis of sacrococcygeal teratoma: prognostic features. Pediatr Surg Int 1998;3:173–175.

49. Flake AW. Sacrococcygeal teratoma. Semin Pediatr Surg 1993;2:113–120.

50. Kapoor R, Saha MM. Antenatal sonographic diagnosis of fetal sacrococcygeal teratoma with hydrops. Austral Radiol 1989;33:285–287.

51. Kuhlmann RS, Warsof SL, Levy DL, Flake AJ, Harrison MR. Fetal sacrococcygeal teratoma. Fetal Ther 1987;1:95–100.

52. Adozick NS, Crombleholme TM, Morgan MA, Quinn TM. A rapidly growing fetal teratoma. Lancet 1997;349:538.

53. Nair R, Pai SK, Saikia TK. Malignant germ cell tumors in childhood. J Surg Oncol 1994;56:186–190.

54. Wilson RD, Johnson MP. Congenital abdominal wall defects: an update. Fetal Diagn Ther 2004;19:385–398.

55. Kitchanan S, Patole SK, Muller R, Whitehall JS. Neonatal outcome of gastroschisis and exomphalos: a 10-year review. J Paediatr Child Health 2000;36:428–430.

56. Bianchi A, Dickson AP. Elective delayed reduction and no anesthesia: "minimal intervention management" for gastrochisis. J Pediatr Surg 1998;33:1338–1340.

57. Kimble RM, Singh SJ, Bourke C, Cass DT. Gastroschisis reduction under analgesia in the neonatal unit. J Pediatr Surg 2001;36:1672–1674.

Section IV

Where Is the Evidence?

Chapter 13

Evidence-based Evaluation of the Management of Neonatal Shock

David A. Osborn, MBBS, MM, FRACP, PhD

Available Evidence that Neonatal Hypotension and/or Systemic or Cerebral Blood Flow Abnormalities Affect Mortality and Morbidity with Special Interest to Neurodevelopmental Outcome

Available Evidence that Treatment of Neonatal Hypotension and/or Systemic or Cerebral Blood Flow Abnormalities has an Impact on Mortality and Morbidity with Special Interest to Neurodevelopmental Outcome

Conclusions

References

This chapter reviews the available evidence for the effectiveness of management of neonatal shock with a special focus on the findings in preterm neonates. Brain injury and subsequent neurodevelopmental impairment remains one of the greatest burdens of premature birth. Multiple risk factors in the perinatal period are likely to impact on brain development, and contribute to brain injury. Increasing evidence now links cardiovascular maladaptation in the first day with subsequent brain injury, particularly peri/intraventricular hemorrhage (PIVH), developmental, and motor impairments. Hypotension, signs of poor tissue perfusion, and low systemic blood flow (SBF) during the immediate postnatal period have been associated with end organ dysfunction and damage, particularly in extremely premature infants and infants with severe respiratory disease, asphyxia, or infection. However, simply monitoring blood pressure and treating hypotension in preterm neonates during the first postnatal days fails to detect many infants with low SBF (1) and has not yet been associated with improvements in clinical outcome (2). Echocardiography, organ Doppler ultrasound, and other techniques for assessing or measuring organ blood flows have highlighted the potential importance of measuring systemic and organ blood flow in preterm infants. However, evidence also needs to be presented that using functional echocardiography or other techniques to assess systemic and organ blood flows improves outcome in preterm neonates.

AVAILABLE EVIDENCE THAT NEONATAL HYPOTENSION AND/ OR SYSTEMIC OR CEREBRAL BLOOD FLOW ABNORMALITIES AFFECT MORTALITY AND MORBIDITY, WITH SPECIAL INTEREST TO NEURODEVELOPMENTAL OUTCOME

Cerebral Injury in Preterm Infants

Examining the association between cardiovascular factors and cerebral injury in preterm infants is confounded by differences in modality of detection of injury and timing of measurement. Head ultrasound has proven to be a simple but rather insensitive tool for detecting cerebral injury that may be performed serially at the bedside of even the sickest infants. The two principal patterns of injury found include PIVH and periventricular white matter injury (WMI). PIVH includes a spectrum from germinal matrix or subependymal hemorrhage, intraventricular hemorrhage with or without post-hemorrhagic dilatation, to parenchymal extension of the hemorrhage (3,4). Porencephalic cysts may result subsequent to the parenchymal extension. There are two distinct patterns in timing of PIVH. Early PIVH detected on head ultrasound performed during the first hours after birth, which is predominately found in vaginally delivered infants (5), and late PIVH which occurs predominately after the first day. For late PIVH, there is strong evidence that postnatal cardiovascular maladaptation contributes the development of this form of PIVH (5–7).

White matter injuries found on ultrasound include transient and persistent periventricular echodensities ("flares") and periventricular leucomalacia (PVL). The presence of persistent fetal (8) and neonatal (9) periventricular echodensities predicts the development of cystic PVL. With the advent of MRI, term-equivalent correlates to these abnormalities detected by ultrasonography earlier in the course of affected preterm neonates have been described. Inder (9,10) described four grades of WMI in preterm infants who underwent MRI at term equivalent age: normal (grade 1); mild white matter abnormality with ventricular dilatation, focal signal change indicating focal areas of gliosis, predominately in the white matter, and thinning of the corpus callosum (grade 2); moderate white matter abnormality with more diffuse signal changes indicating extensive periventricular gliosis (grade 3); and severe white matter abnormality with extensive periventricular cystic abnormality associated with a substantial increase in subarachnoid space and reduction in cerebral gray and white matter volumes (grade 4). This latter grade with extensive periventricular cystic change is equivalent to the PVL described on ultrasound. The presence of prolonged white matter echodensities (lasting > 7 days) on neonatal head ultrasounds had a low sensitivity (26%) and positive predictive value (36%) for the presence of noncystic WMI detected on MRI at term in infants born very prematurely (9). However, all infants with cystic PVL had preceding persistent periventricular echodensities. The importance of imaging timing is that term equivalent findings on MRI may represent a combination of injuries, including insults producing PIVH as well as those associated with the production of periventricular WMI associated with cystic PVL.

Early Peri/intraventricular Hemorrhage

Up to 40% of PIVH in preterm infants is present on head ultrasound in the first few hours after birth (11). Reported risk factors for early PIVH include lower gestation (12), lower birth weight (13), lack of antenatal steroids (6,12,14), active labor (15–18), vaginal delivery (5,6,14,19), vaginal delivery in breech but not cephalic infants (17,18), breech presentation (13), low 1 min Apgar (5), and lower cord arterial pH (12).

Three studies (5,6,20) reported measures of postnatal blood flow in infants with early PIVH. Two cohorts of infants (5,6) in whom right ventricular output (RVO) and blood flow to the brain and upper body (superior vena cava [SVC] flow) were measured, reported no association between these measures of SBF and early PIVH. Ment (20) using the xenon technique, measured cerebral blood flow (CBF) at 6 h and observed that infants with early PIVH had lower CBF, needed more vigorous resuscitation at birth, had higher ventilator settings in the first 36 h and higher values of $Paco_2$ compared to infants without early PIVH. No studies have measured postnatal cardiac output or CBF prior to demonstrating early PIVH on head ultrasound. It is likely that the low CBF detected postnatally in infants with early PIVH is secondary to the cerebral injury. The timing and mechanism of the insult producing early PIVH is presently uncertain but the association of early PIVH with active labor, vaginal delivery, and depression at birth suggests the injury is occurring intrapartum.

Late Peri/Intraventricular Hemorrhage

Of infants developing PIVH, 58% develop "late" PIVH, which was not present in the first hours after birth (11). Reported risk factors for late PIVH include caesarean section (19), low CBF (7), and low blood flow from the brain and upper body (SVC flow) in the first 24 h after birth (5,6). In two sequential cohorts of infants (5,6), almost all infants developing late PIVH had preceding low SVC flow in the first day. Kluckow (6) reported a cohort of 126 infants born at < 30 weeks' gestation. Thirteen of 14 infants who developed late Papile grade 2–4 PIVH had SVC flow below the normal range before development of the PIVH. In all, PIVH occurred after SVC flow improved, with the grade of PIVH related to the severity and duration of low SVC flow. Osborn (5), in a second cohort of 128 infants born at < 30 weeks' gestation, reported that 14 of 19 infants who developed late PIVH had preceding low SVC flow identified in the first 24 h. Meek (7) measured CBF using near infrared (NIR) spectroscopy in 24 infants with a median gestation of 26 weeks in the first 24 h. Cerebral blood flow was significantly lower in infants who developed PIVH despite no difference in $Paco_2$ and a higher mean blood pressure. Infants with severe PIVH had the lowest CBF. The median CBF was 12.2 mL/100 g/min in infants without PIVH, 12.0 mL/100 g/min in infants with mild PIVH and only 5.8 mL/100 g/min in infants with severe PIVH. The PIVH developed subsequent to the measurement of lower CBF. There is now reproducible evidence in preterm infants that late PIVH is a hypoperfusion–reperfusion injury.

White Matter Injury

Clinical risk factor analyses for development of PVL in preterm infants have reported associations with first trimester bleeding (21), maternal urinary tract infection (21), histological chorioamnionitis (22–24), clinical chorioamnionitis (25–29), prolonged premature rupture of membranes (21), lack of antenatal maternal antibiotic treatment (30), multiple antenatal courses of dexamethasone but not betamethasone (31), vaginal delivery in twins (32), meconium stained liquor (21), fetal acidosis on cord blood (21), neonatal acidosis (33), high cord blood creatine kinase brain isoenzyme (34), neonatal hypocarbia in the first days (35–42), neonatal hypercarbia in the first days (43), a symptomatic ductus arteriosus (DA) (44), hypotension after the first 24 h (44), and neonatal hyperbilirubinemia (45). In infants with twin–twin transfusion syndrome, two studies (46,47) reported outcomes of donor and recipient twins separately. They found that PVL is significantly more likely to occur in the recipient, whereas the donor most commonly suffered from PIVH and PVL was uncommon. The recipient is less likely to be growth restricted but more likely to be polycythemic potentially producing cardiovascular dysfunction, disturbances in cerebral microvascular perfusion and chronic cerebral hypoxia. Interestingly, studies fail to report placental insufficiency resulting in fetal growth restriction as a risk factor for PVL (27).

Animal models have produced lesions similar to PVL from insults involving hypoxic–ischemia (48,49) and inflammation (50,51), or a combination of both (52). In preterm infants, several studies failed to demonstrate associations between hypotension in the immediate postnatal period and WMI (28,43,53). White matter injury also occurs in neonates after cardiac surgery (54,55). Risk factors for the development of post-cardiac surgery-associated PVL included prolonged cardio-pulmonary bypass with or without deep hypothermic circulatory arrest, hypotension, especially diastolic hypotension, and hypoxemia in the early postoperative period (54). In ventilated preterm infants, analysis of secondary outcomes from a trial of morphine versus placebo (44) reported adjusted risk factors for cystic PVL were a symptomatic PDA and hypotension between 25 and 72 h after start of the study infusion drug, along with maternal fever $>38.5\,°C$.

There have been relatively few studies examining the role of CBF in infants who subsequently developed PVL (56,57). Greisen (56) reported seven infants who had early low CBF (8 mL/100 g/min) and among these infants one developed parenchymal PIVH and two developed PVL. Although the relationship between low CBF and parenchymal injury was significant, the small number of infants prevents any meaningful conclusion. Okumura (57), using Doppler ultrasonography, reported the resistive index was significantly lower during the first 72 h in infants who developed PVL, but no association could be documented between the resistive index and $Paco_2$. Mean velocity did not differ significantly in infants developing PVL. This suggests an early loss of the ability to autoregulate CBF as demonstrated by no change in blood flow velocity in response to changes in $Paco_2$, and a loss of vascular resistance as measured by a reduced resistive index. However, Doppler ultrasound measurement of velocity does not measure actual CBF and, based on the timing of the assessments, these changes could well be secondary to the cerebral injury and not necessarily causative. Two studies reported on SVC blood flow in the first day and subsequent PVL. Kluckow (6) reported that three of four infants and Osborn (5) reported that two of four infants who developed PVL had low SVC flow (minimum < 41 mL/kg/min) in the first 24 h after birth. Again, the low number of patients with PVL makes these associations intriguing but inconclusive.

In contrast, as mentioned earlier several studies link markers of infection/inflammation with PVL. Infectious associations reported for the development of PVL include maternal infection (23) and urinary tract infection (21), histological chorioamnionitis (22–24) and clinical chorioamnionitis (25–29). A protective effect has been reported with use of maternal antibiotics (30). A meta-analysis of observational studies (58) examining the association between chorioamnionitis, PVL, and cerebral palsy (CP), found clinical chorioamnionitis a risk factor for both PVL (summary relative risk [RR] 3.0, 95% CI 2.2–4.0) and CP (summary RR 1.0, 95% CI 1.4–2.5), and histological chorioamnionitis a risk factor for PVL (summary RR 1.8, 95% CI 1.5–2.3) but not CP (summary RR 1.6, 95% CI 0.9–2.7). However, an important methodological weakness of this meta-analysis was the use of unadjusted relative risks from the studies, resulting in a failure of the analysis to adjust for confounding variables. Postnatal infection in premature and very premature infants has also been associated with PVL (59,60) and developmental impairments including CP (60–63). In the largest cohort study ($n = 5587$), researchers in the NICHD Neonatal Research Network found that infants with infection were significantly more likely to develop PVL (incidence: no sepsis 3%; clinical sepsis alone 5%; sepsis alone 6%; sepsis with necrotizing enterocolitis [NEC] 8%; sepsis with meningitis 8%) and subsequent developmental impairments including CP, developmental and psychomotor delays, and hearing and visual impairment (60).

Several studies in premature infants have also implicated postnatal hypocarbia in the development of PVL (35,37–42) and severe PIVH and PVL (36). Three studies (37,39,41) have reported a $Paco_2 < 25$ mm Hg in ventilated preterm infants to be strongly associated with PVL. A strong correlation between CBF measured by NIRS and $Paco_2$ has been reported in preterm infants (64). Kissack (65) reported that cerebral fractional oxygen extraction (FOE) was increased in infants with low left ventricular output (LVO) when the $Paco_2$ was low, presumably as a compensatory mechanism for low CBF. However, Kissack (66) found no association between cerebral FOE and subsequent PVL. Rather a high cerebral FOE was associated with PIVH. The timing and mechanisms linking hypocarbia with PVL are yet to be precisely elucidated, although current data suggest that infants with hypocarbia may be particularly susceptible to the effects of low CBF.

MRI studies of premature infants at term equivalent age are more accurate in detecting WMI. Inder (67) reported a cohort of 100 consecutive premature infants with MRI performed at term equivalent age. Univariate predictors for moderate to severe WMI were lower gestation, maternal fever, proven early onset sepsis, use of inotropes for hypotension, a symptomatic PDA, severe PIVH, and pneumothorax, with the presence of intrauterine growth restriction being protective. Although treatment of hypotension is associated with WMI seen on MRI at term equivalent age in this cohort, this injury is not differentiated from WMI associated with PIVH and may not differentiate risk factors for cystic PVL from those for PIVH.

In summary, clinical studies to date do not provide compelling and consistent evidence for the pathogenesis of periventricular WMI. Animal studies point to infection/inflammation as critical in the development of cystic WMI and the potential role of hypoxia–ischemia. Studies in premature infants have reported associations with infection/inflammation and hypocarbia, but not a reproducible role for postnatal hypotension or low blood flow states. However, data are now appearing (67) associating WMI seen on term equivalent MRI with maternal fever, infant sepsis and hypotension defined as use of inotropes, although this is confounded by the potential for multiple pathogenesis seen in WMI detected at term equivalent age.

Blood Pressure and Neonatal Outcomes

Population studies in preterm infants report that systolic, mean and diastolic blood pressure rapidly increases during the first postnatal week followed by a continued but slower increase during the neonatal period and early infancy (68,69). In addition, infants with asphyxia and ventilated infants have significantly lower blood pressure. However, several studies report a weak relationship between blood pressure and cardiac output in preterm infants during the immediate postnatal period (6,70–72). Kluckow (70) reported a significant but weak correlation ($r = 0.38$) between left ventricular output (LVO) and mean blood pressure. In a cohort of infants with a mean blood pressure <30 mm Hg, Pladys (72) found LVO was frequently normal or high. In a second cohort, Kluckow (6) reported an inverse relationship between systemic vascular resistance and SVC flow, a finding supported by Pladys who observed many infants with low blood pressure had a low index of resistance and normal or high LVO. It has been suggested that there may be a "critical" mean blood pressure (around 30 mm Hg), which results in loss of cerebral autoregulation and reduction in CBF in very preterm infants during the first postnatal day (73), a level associated with cerebral injury in one study (74). It has also been suggested that the forebrain may not be a "vital organ" in the extremely premature infant (65) or newborn animal (75) in the immediate postnatal period. However, loss of cerebral autoregulation is also a feature of cerebral hypoxia and may reflect preceding hypoperfusion–hypoxia. The majority of studies examining cerebral autoregulation have measured CBF or oxygenation changes in infants predominately after the first day. Further studies examining the relationship between blood pressure and CBF to determine the ability of the premature brain to autoregulate in the first day are required.

Low blood pressure has been associated with morbidity and mortality in preterm infants. Table 13-1 summarizes studies examining the association between blood pressure measurements and neurological outcomes in preterm infants. Several studies have reported significant associations between early hypotension and neurological abnormality or developmental impairment (76–79). Unfortunately, there are relatively few data from adequately designed, prospective cohort studies that adjust for appropriate perinatal confounders examining the association between early neonatal hypotension and subsequent brain injury. Neonatal practice has been influenced by observations associating a mean blood pressure <30 mm Hg with subsequent cerebral injury. Miall-Allen (74) reported a small series of 33 infants born at <31 weeks' gestation. A mean blood pressure <30 mm Hg for >1 h was associated with severe PIVH, ischemic cerebral lesions, or death. Low (77,80) reported a relationship between hypotension in the first 4 days and ultrasound detected cerebral lesions (including intraventricular hemorrhage, ventriculomegaly, or hyperechoic parenchymal lesions), as well as neurodevelopmental abnormality. The combination of hypotension and hypoxia increased the risk of abnormal outcome to over 50%. Goldstein (79) reported a cohort of 191 very low birth weight infants who had blood gas measurements to identify metabolic or respiratory acidosis including the duration of single and cumulative episodes, and to examine the interaction of acidosis with hypoxemia and hypotension. Developmental follow up was performed using the Bayley Scales of Infant Development at 6 and 24 months, corrected age. Duration of hypotension was independently correlated with developmental outcome at 6 and 24 months'. None of these studies measured systemic or cerebral blood flow.

Only one study reported simultaneous measurements of SBF and blood pressure in the first day and developmental outcomes (76). Hunt reported a cohort of 96 surviving infants born at < 30 weeks' gestation that had echocardiographic measurements of SVC flow and blood pressure measurements via an arterial line in the neonatal period, and developmental follow up at three years. No significant association was found between average mean blood pressure over the first 12 or 24 h and abnormal developmental outcome, but a significant association was reported between the percent of mean blood pressure readings (mm Hg) in first 24 h less than gestation in weeks with death and any disability, and abnormal developmental outcome. Analysis of SVC flow findings is examined in the following section on systemic and organ blood flows and neonatal outcomes.

Systemic and Organ Blood Flows and Neonatal Outcomes

Several studies have reported measures of CBF in preterm infants. Lou (81) using ^{133}Xe measured CBF in the first hours, reported that ventilated, hypotensive infants with respiratory distress syndrome (RDS) and/or asphyxia tended to have low values for CBF (< 20 mL/100 g/min), whereas relatively well normotensive infants tended to have much higher values (40 mL/100 g/min). Nine of 10 infants with low CBF developed cerebral atrophy with only one normal on developmental follow-up. Cerebral atrophy did not develop in those with flows above 20 mL/100 g/min. Meek (7) measured CBF in 24 infants in the first 24 h using NIR spectroscopy. Cerebral blood flow was significantly lower in the infants that developed PIVH

Table 13-1 Summary of Studies of the Association Between Hypotension, Mortality, and Neurological Morbidity

Study (Reference)	Infants	Methods	Hypotension	Timing of Hypotension	Outcomes	Results
Prospective cohorts						
199	n = 42 1020–3720 g 26–36 weeks Base population not reported	Intermittent BP UAC No early HUS Some infants received volume and inotrope	No definition 30 min recordings 2, 8, 16, and 24 h	First 24 h	HUS detected PIVH, PVED, and PVL before day 4	Univariate: average SBP, MBP, and DBP higher in infants with PIVH. No significant differences reported in heart rate or BP variability
76	n = 126, 103 survived to discharge <30 weeks	106 (84%) infants had arterial line Multivariate analysis 17 (17%) no Griffiths assessment 7 (7%) infants no developmental data Blinded 3-year assessment	MBP (mm Hg) < gestational age in weeks	First 24 h	3 years pediatrician examination and Griffiths Scales of Mental Development	Multivariate: no significant association between average MBP over first 24 h and abnormal developmental outcome Significant association between proportion of MBP readings (mm Hg) in first 24 h < gestation (weeks) with death and any disability, and abnormal developmental outcome
10	n = 100 <1500 g	98% of eligible infants Multivariate analysis 66 (66%) infants had invasive arterial line	Invasive arterial line MBP<30 mm Hg Inotropes used	Not reported	MRI detected WMI and GMI at term equivalent age	Univariate: MBP<30 mm Hg and inotrope use predictive of WMI. Multivariate: inotrope use (OR 2.7, 95% CI 1.5, 4.5), maternal fever and infant sepsis predictive of WMI. GMI predicted by presence of WMI only
200	n = 119 <1500 g and <32 weeks	88% eligible infants Number of infants with arterial line not reported No losses reported for MRI	Inotrope use	Not reported	MRI measured cerebral tissue volumes at term corrected age	Multivariate: no effect of inotrope use on cerebral tissue volumes after adjustment for PIVH and WMI

Table continued on following page

Table 13-1   Summary of Studies of the Association Between Hypotension, Mortality, and Neurological Morbidity (Continued)

Study (Reference)	Infants	Methods	Hypotension	Timing of Hypotension	Outcomes	Results
77	n = 98 <34 weeks	Continuous invasive BP monitoring Adjusted for multiple perinatal variables	MBP below 95% CI for population data (<1500 g and >1500 g) Hours MBP <95% CI	First 96 h	Neurologic exam and Bayley scales at 6 and 12 months' corrected age	Multivariate: hypotension, birthweight, and hypoxaemia predicted major abnormal outcome. Increasing duration of hypotension and hypoxaemia associated with increased probability of abnormal outcome
78	n = 266 <32 weeks	Base population not reported 28 died before term 211 (89%) assessed UAC (43%) or oscillometric BP	MBP <30 mm Hg on at least 2 occasions duration not reported	Not reported	Term equivalent HUS detected PIVH and PVL, Prechtl neurological exam	Univariate: hypotension predictor of PVL but not PIVH. Multivariate: hypotension predictor of neurological abnormality
74	n = 33 26–30 weeks UAC by 6 h Normal early HUS. Base population not reported	Losses not reported clinicians "blinded to data" Volume and inotropes given for "underperfusion" UAC No adjusted analysis	Lowest MBP for >1 hour grouped as <25, 25–29, 30–34, ≥35 mm Hg	Measured MBP from 2–5 h after birth, average 86 h. MBP ≤29 only occurred in first 24 h	HUS detected transient PVED, PIVH and PVL weekly to discharge	Univariate: no infant who maintained MBP ≥30 had severe cerebral lesion. Transient PVED in infants at all levels of lowest MBP
43	n = 200 <1501 g	57% had SBP measured Invasive and "indirect" BP used Unblinded study Adjusted for perinatal variables	Proportion time SBP <25, <35, <45, <55 mm Hg	Not reported	HUS detected PIVH and PVL Timing not reported	Univariate: SBP >55 mm Hg predictive of PIVH. Hypotension not related to PIVH or PVL Multivariate: hypertension not predictive of PIVH
41	n = 67 enrolled in trial of rescue high-frequency jet ventilation for severe lung	Base population not reported Arterial catheter BP at least hourly Blinded outcome measurement	Lowest MBP on day 1, 2, and 3	First 3 days	HUS by day 3, weekly to 6–8 weeks, then 2–4 weekly to discharge	Univariate: lowest MBP day 3 (not 1 or 2) predicted mortality but not cystic PVL Multivariate: only cumulative $PaCO_2$

Ref	Population	Population/losses	Definition	BP monitoring	Imaging/detection	Results
	disease <33 weeks <12 h age					<25 mm Hg predictive of cystic PVL
Retrospective cohorts						
26	*n* = 110, 25–32 weeks with clinical or histological chorio-amnionitis	101 survivors >7 days; 99 included in analysis; number of infants with BP monitoring not reported	"Hemodynamic failure" – definition not reported	Not reported	HUS detected cystic PVL and MRI confirmed non-cystic PVL.	Univariate: hemodynamic failure not associated with PVL (cystic and non-cystic)
201	*n* = 127, <36 weeks, HUS by third day	87% of eligible consecutive infants <36 weeks. Number of infants with BP measurement not reported	Hypotension/shock, definition not reported	Not reported	HUS before day 3 and every 1–2 weeks till discharge to detect postnatal white matter necrosis (PWMN)	Univariate: hypotension/shock recorded in 5 of 10 infants with PWMN – not significant
202	*n* = 232, ≤1500 g	Losses: 62/440 died before 24 h, 144 infants no BP data. 232 included	Mean BP <10th percentile for birthweight and postnatal age	>24 h BP monitoring in first 7 days	HUS detected IVH first 7 days	Univariate: low mean BP associated with PIVH, and death, not PVL. Multivariate: BP variability day 7 associated with death. PIVH associated with low BP and BP variability
203	*n* = 34, 24–33 weeks UAC, All with RDS and ventilated	Base population not reported. Losses not reported. Adjusted for birthweight gestation, and postnatal age	Umbilical artery catheter Inotrope use	Measured mean BP every 15 min for first 10 days. Used daily median mean BP in analysis	Daily HUS detected PIVH, no early HUS	Univariate: No significant differences in median mean BP found between infants with and without PIVH. Trend to higher coefficient of variation of mean BP readings on day of hemorrhage
79	*n* = 191, <1500 g	Base population not reported. 23 infants died, 44 lost to follow-up. 158 (89%) followed to 6 months, 106 (71%) to 24 months. Inotrope use not reported or adjusted for	Arterial catheter or oscillometric recording at least hourly. Infants <750g: SBP <35 mm Hg. Infants 750–1500 g: SBP <40 mm Hg	Not reported	Neurological examination and Bayley Scales of Infant Development at 6 and 24 months' corrected age	Univariate: hypotension associated with lower MDI and PDI at 6 and 24 months. Multivariate: hypotension associated with lower MDI, PDI and abnormal neurological score at 24 months

Table continued on following page

Table 13-1   Summary of Studies of the Association Between Hypotension, Mortality, and Neurological Morbidity (Continued)

Study (Reference)	Infants	Methods	Hypotension	Timing of Hypotension	Outcomes	Results
28	n = 632 <1750 g	Base population 709 infants; 77 (10.8%) excluded (66 died first 12 h); Retrospective; Indications for volume and inotrope not reported	MBP on admission; use of volume expansion or inotropes Method of measurement not reported	On admission to NICU	HUS day 2 3–5, 10–14, 28; normal HUS, grade 1 or 2 PIVH, severe PIVH, cystic PVL	Univariate: infants with grade 3 or 4 PIVH significantly lower initial MBP, received more volume and inotropes; Initial MBP not significantly different in infants with cystic PVL
204	n = 131; <1500 g; UAC or peripheral arterial catheter	Consecutively admitted Base population not reported	Hourly SBP, MBP, DBP; hypotension defined as 2 consecutive MBP readings <10th percentile for birthweight, postnatal age, and gestation	First 96 h	Daily HUS 4 days and weekly to discharge; PIVH and late detected parenchymal lesions. Physical and neurological exam and Denver Developmental Screening Test to 2 years	Univariate: PIVH, severity of PIVH, but not periventricular ischemic lesions, associated with hypotension; hypertension not associated with PIVH Multivariate: BP not related to periventricular ischemic lesions
205	n = 86 <1501 g or <34 weeks		Mean BP <30 mm Hg or volume for shock given	First week	HUS detected PIVH and PVL day 1–5, day 7, then weekly to discharge	Univariate: hypotension in 12% of infants with normal scans and 29% with PIVH. PVL not associated with hypotension
Case–control studies						
206	Base population 1606 infants 500–1500 g; Cases (n = 61: all infants with HUS detected WMD; Controls (n = 182): random	Method of BP detection not reported Retrospective flow sheet retrieval of data Unblinded Adjusted for multiple perinatal confounders	Lowest mean BP z-score quartile for gestational age	First week	HUS first 4 days, day 5–15, day 15–70 White matter echolucency	Univariate: Lowest quartile z-score BP in first week borderline significant association with echolucency Multivariate: hypotension not associated with echolucency

	sample without WMD				
207	$n = 17$ cases (cystic PVL) and 34 controls (normal HUS); <34 weeks	Case–control; infants with cystic PVL matched with 2 infants with normal HUS and 2 infants with large PIVH by selecting infant born within 2 months and ≥2 HUS; method of BP monitoring not reported; No adjusted analysis	SBP <40 mm Hg requiring colloid or dopamine; Dopamine use	Not reported	HUS daily for first week and then twice weekly till discharge; Detected cystic PVL and large PIVH detected on	Univariate: hypotension and dopamine use associated with cystic PVL. Infants with large PIVH not compared to infants with normal HUS
61	$n = 59$ cases with CP; and 234 controls; <32 weeks	Case–control; randomly selected controls from area population of infants born at <32 weeks without CP	Mean BP <30 mm Hg on at least two occasions	Not reported	CP identified from the Oxford region register of early childhood impairments	Multivariate: PDA, hypotension, transfusion, prolonged ventilation, pneumothorax, sepsis, hyponatraemia, and total parenteral nutrition associated with CP

DBP = diastolic BP; GMI = gray matter injury; HUS = head ultrasound; MBP = mean BP; MRI = magnetic resonance imaging; PIVH = peri/intraventricular hemorrhage; PVED = periventricular echodensities; PVL = periventricular leucomalacia; RDS = respiratory distress syndrome; SBP = systolic BP; WMI = white matter injury. WMD = white matter damage.

(median 7.0 mL/100 g/min) compared to those without (median 12.2 mL/100 g/min). Infants with severe PIVH had the lowest cerebral blood flows.

Two sequential cohort studies that adjusted for potential confounders have now examined the relationships between a measure of systemic blood flow (SVC flow) in the immediate postnatal period and subsequent neonatal outcomes. In a cohort of 126 preterm infants, Evans (82) reported a multivariate analysis adjusting for mean blood pressure, SVC flow, and Doppler measures of CBF for prediction of PIVH. SVC flow was the only cardiovascular risk factor to remain an independent predictor of PIVH, with mean blood pressure no longer significant in the multivariate model. Following up this cohort, Hunt (76) reported mortality and neurodevelopmental outcomes at three years. After controlling for confounding variables including gestational age, need for postnatal steroids, and level of maternal education, for every 10 mL/kg/min increase in average SVC flow in the first 24 h the odds ratio for death or survival with any disability were decreased by 28% ($P = 0.004$), abnormal development quotient decreased by 36% ($P = 0.006$), and there was a trend to reduced abnormal motor development that did not reach statistical significance ($P = 0.07$). The risk of death or survival with any disability increased significantly as the number of times (from zero to three measurements) in the first 24 h SVC flow was less than 30 mL/kg/min. All babies with two or more measurements of SVC flow <30 mL/kg/min had an abnormal developmental quotient and all babies with three low measurements had an abnormal motor score. In unpublished data (Table 13-3), when both average SVC flow and percent mean blood pressure readings less than gestational age in weeks were included in analysis, average SVC flow predicted death and significant developmental delay. There was a strong trend to reduced abnormal motor findings (cerebral palsy or motor score >2 standard deviations below population mean). The percent of mean blood pressure readings below the gestational age in weeks in the first 24 h (but not first 12 h) also maintained a significant relationship with death and significant developmental delay, but not abnormal motor findings.

In a second cohort study from the same group, Osborn (5) reported 44 of 128 (34%) infants developed low SVC flow in the first 24 h. Low SVC flow was associated with a significant increase in PIVH (20% versus 48%), severe PIVH (6% versus 27%), mortality before discharge (13% versus 57%), NEC (0% versus 9%) and severe ROP in survivors (9% versus 30%). There was no significant association with PVL (3 of 75 [4%] versus 3 of 24 [13%], $P = 0.2$). At three years, adjusted for perinatal risk factors, low SVC flow was a significant predictor for mortality (OR 3.89, 95% CI 1.23–12.13), associated with substantial reductions in the Griffiths Quotient (mean difference −16.53, 95% CI −29.45, −3.60) and personal–social, hearing and speech and performance Griffiths subscales (Table 13-2).

Table 13-2	Significant Perinatal Risk Factors in Multivariate Analysis for Early PIVH, Late PIVH, in the 1995–1996 and 1998–1999 Cohorts of Infants (5)				
Outcome	1995–1996 OR (95%CI)	P	1998–1999 OR (95%CI)	P
Early PIVH				
Gestation/week decrease	1.08 (0.69, 1.70)	0.7	0.95 (0.68, 1.34)	0.8
Vaginal delivery	13.29 (1.52, 116.35)	0.02	18.15 (3.56, 91.60)	<0.001
Apgar ≤4 at 1 min	0.58 (0.11, 3.04)	0.5	9.14 (2.23–37.49)	0.002
Late PIVH				
Gestation/week decrease	1.42 (0.99, 2.02)	0.06	1.23 (0.91, 1.67)	0.2
Low SVC flow in first 24 h	20.39 (2.54, 163.89)	0.005	5.16 (1.59, 16.71)	0.006

PIVH = peri/intraventricular hemorrhage; SVC = superior vena cava; OR = odds ratio.

Table 13-3   **Regression Analysis of the Association Between Average SVC Flow in First 24 h and Percent of MBP Readings < Gestational Age in Weeks in First 24 h for Prediction of Death and Neurological Impairments (unpublished data)**

Outcome	Average SVC first 24 h OR (95% CI) per 10 mL/kg/min	% readings MBP < gestation in weeks OR (95% CI) per 10% change
Died	0.66 (0.51, 0.85)*	1.57 (1.12, 2.12)*
Developmental quotient ≤2SD	0.69 (0.52, 0.92)*	1.58 (1.07, 2.34)*
Abnormal motor	0.75 (0.55, 1.02)	1.06 (0.70, 1.60)
Developmental quotient ≤2SD or died	0.76 (0.63, 0.92)*	1.48 (1.11, 1.98)*
Abnormal motor or died	0.74 (0.60, 0.92)*	1.28 (0.98, 1.64)

Model = Average SVC flow per 10 mL/kg/min change in first 24 h. percent mean BP readings in first 24 h < gestational age in weeks, gestational age, postnatal steroids.
*p < 0.05

Summary

There is reproducible evidence that early low systemic and organ blood flow are associated with adverse neonatal outcomes, including mortality and late PIVH (5–7,83), NEC (5) and developmental impairments (5,76). There is evidence that both blood pressure and systemic blood flow are independently associated with long-term developmental outcomes (76). The association of systemic blood flow and adverse outcomes was predominately for infants developing low systemic blood flow in the first 12 h, a high proportion of whom had blood pressure considered to be within normal limits at this time. The association between blood pressure and developmental outcomes was reported for measurements taken after the first 12 h. This would appear to describe a pattern of cardiovascular maladaptation in which infants are progressing from early compensated shock, associated with high systemic vascular resistance (6,84), poor myocardial contractility (84), and normal blood pressures, to decompensated shock which is clinically detectable as hypotension. Thus, targeting of hypotension has the potential to substantially delay cardiovascular support of infants with low systemic blood flow. In addition, many extremely premature infants who develop hypotension after the first day and infants with sepsis will have normal or high systemic blood flow and low systemic vascular resistance (71,72,85). These infants are likely to benefit from strategies of cardiovascular support that raise systemic vascular resistance, whereas increasing systemic vascular resistance in extremely premature infants who develop low SBF in the first day may further impair cardiac output in infants with poor myocardial contractility (84).

AVAILABLE EVIDENCE THAT TREATMENT OF NEONATAL HYPOTENSION AND/OR SYSTEMIC OR CEREBRAL BLOOD FLOW ABNORMALITIES HAS AN IMPACT ON MORTALITY AND MORBIDITY, WITH SPECIAL INTEREST TO NEURODEVELOPMENTAL OUTCOME

Most trials of cardiovascular interventions in preterm infants have enrolled infants with hypotension during the immediate postnatal period, with the goal of increasing blood pressure (2,86,87). These trials used varying treatment criteria, with

Table 13-4 Meta-Analysis of Trials of Early Cord Clamping Versus Delayed Cord Clamping in Preterm Infants (88)

Outcome	Studies/Participants	Effect (95% CI)
Neonatal mortality	6/278	RR 1.05 (0.41, 2.73)
Transfused for anemia	3/111	RR 2.01 (1.24, 3.27)
Transfused for low BP	2/58	RR 2.58 (1.17, 5.67)
Inotropes for low BP	3/118	RR 2.17 (0.51, 9.12)
Patent ductus arteriosus	3/118	RR 0.79 (0.36, 1.72)
PIVH	5/225	RR 1.74 (1.08, 2.81)
Severe PIVH	3/161	RR 0.86 (0.15, 4.75)
Periventricular leukomalacia	1/31	RR 0.31 (0.01, 7.15)
Respiratory distress syndrome	2/75	RR 0.83 (0.59, 1.15)
Ventilated	3/121	RR 0.91 (0.65, 1.28)
Oxygen at 36 weeks postmenstrual age	2/65	RR 0.97 (0.35, 2.69)
Necrotizing enterocolitis	2/72	RR 2.08 (0.52, 8.37)

SP = blood pressure; PIVH = peri/intraventricular hemorrhage; RR = risk ratio.

common thresholds including a mean or systolic BP $<10^{th}$ percentile for gestation or birth weight and postnatal age, or a common approximation of this being a mean blood pressure (mm Hg) below the gestational age in weeks during the first postnatal day. Additional criteria have included clinical signs of reduced tissue perfusion or disturbed organ function including increased capillary refill time, poor urine output and acidosis. Few studies have measured systemic or organ blood flow to determine which infants may benefit from cardiovascular support. Several attempts have been made to use prophylactic strategies of cardiovascular support with the goal of improving neonatal morbidity and mortality.

Delayed Cord Clamping in Preterm Infants

Systematic review of randomized controlled trials comparing early (before 30 s) with delayed (30 to 120 s) clamping of the umbilical cord for preterm infants found seven trials including 297 infants (88). The studies, although unblinded, were generally of good methodological quality but small in size. Delayed cord clamping was associated with fewer transfusions for anemia or low blood pressure and significantly reduced PIVH, but not severe PIVH, than early clamping (Table 13-4). No effect was found on infant mortality and long-term outcomes were not reported. A trial published subsequent to this review confirms the benefit of delayed cord clamping for prevention of PIVH (89). There are no data on the effect of delayed cord clamping on systemic and organ blood flows over the first day. There was a non-significant trend to reduced use of inotropes for hypotension, although numbers reported were small. Given the lack of effect on severe PIVH and data on long-term outcomes, further trials of delayed cord clamping in very preterm infants are warranted.

Cyclooxygenase Inhibitors for Closure of the Ductus Arteriosus in Preterm Infants

Cyclooxygenase inhibitors, including indomethacin and ibuprofen, are used to close the PDA in preterm infants. A large PDA has the potential to result in significant left to right shunting, increasing pulmonary blood flow and reducing flow to vital organs. A large diameter DA (> 1.6 mm at 5 h) in extremely preterm infants is a risk factor for low SVC flow and late PIVH (5,6). Although prophylactic indomethacin has been demonstrated in large randomized trials to prevent PIVH (90), no neurodevelopmental benefit has been reported from use of prophylactic indomethacin. Observational data indicate indomethacin may reduce brain blood flow Doppler velocities, increase resistive indices (91–93), and reduce NIR spectroscopy-determined CBF (94) in the short term, depending on rate of infusion. In a randomized trial (95) examining the effects of early targeted indomethacin on SVC flow in the first hours after birth, 1 h after infusion of indomethacin or placebo there was no significant difference in degree of DA constriction (indomethacin − 20% vs placebo − 15%), change in SVC flow (− 1% vs − 9%), or right ventricular output (RVO). Two hours post-indomethacin, 62 infants had uncontrolled observations at which time significant DA constriction had occurred. At this time, infants > 26 weeks had significantly greater increases in SVC flow and RVO compared to infants < 27 weeks. This supports the observation that the benefits of prophylactic indomethacin in preventing PIVH appear to be greatest in larger infants (96). Further studies are required to determine the effect of closure of the DA on systemic and organ blood flows and to identify infants likely to benefit from early DA closure.

Systematic review of randomized trials found no clinical benefit from prophylactic ibuprofen for preventing PIVH or NEC (97). Studies of the hemodynamic effects of ibuprofen have shown that ibuprofen is effective in closing the DA without reducing CBF (94,98–100) or affecting the intestinal (101) and renal circulations (99,101). Despite these positive hemodynamic observations, significant increased incidences of elevated creatinine (>140 μmol/L) and oliguria were reported in trials of prophylactic ibuprofen versus placebo (97). These observations are largely of the short-term effects of ibuprofen. There are insufficient data to determine the effect of ibuprofen on long-term neurodevelopmental outcomes. There are also insufficient data to determine if there is a benefit in terms of systemic and organ blood flows over the first day from closing a large diameter PDA in the first hours using ibuprofen.

Volume Expansion

Evidence does not support the use of volume expansion in preterm infants especially in the immediate postnatal period, either routinely or for treatment of infants with evidence of cardiovascular compromise, unless hypovolemia is strongly suspected. The observation (102,103) that clinical measures such as systemic hypotension are poorly correlated to blood volume in premature infants suggests that hypovolemia is not a substantial factor underlying the cardiovascular maladaptation of most newborn infants. Observational studies have found increases in cardiac output after albumin infusion in sick preterm infants (104) and a small increase in systemic blood pressure (102,105). However, there is also evidence of potential harm from excessive use of volume expansion in preterm infants with observational studies reporting an association with PIVH (105) and bronchopulmonary dysplasia (106) in preterm infants receiving volume expansion. A systematic review (107) of albumin infusions in critically ill patients of all ages found no benefit in mortality risk following albumin administration for hypovolemia (RR 1.01, 95% CI 0.92–1.10), a significant increase in mortality risk for patients with burns (RR 2.40, 95% CI 1.11–5.19) and no significant benefit for patients with hypoalbuminemia (RR 1.38, 95% CI 0.94–2.03). For all trials, the pooled relative risk of death with albumin administration was 1.04 (95% CI 0.95–1.13). This meta-analysis is heavily influenced by the SAFE trial, which contributed 91% of the information (108).

In preterm infants, systematic review found no evidence from randomized trials that routine volume expansion in the first day in preterm infants improves any neonatal outcome, including mortality, PIVH or neurodevelopment (86,87) (Table 13-5). However, most trials comparing volume expansion with no treatment enrolled infants on the basis of birth weight or prematurity, not cardiovascular compromise. There is insufficient evidence from randomized trials to determine

Table 13-5   Meta-Analysis of Randomized Controlled Trials of Volume Expansion Versus No Treatment in Preterm Infants (87)

Outcome	Studies/Participants	Effect (95% CI)
Death	4/940	RR 1.11 (0.88, 1.40)
PIVH, any grade	3/533	RR 0.91 (0.68, 1.23)
PIVH grade 3–4	2/493	RR 0.94 (0.50, 1.76)
Periventricular leucomalacia	1/432	RR 0.75 (0.36, 1.60)
Necrotizing enterocolitis	1/776	RR 0.64 (0.32, 1.27)
CLD (oxygen at 28 days)	1/776	RR 1.01 (0.67, 1.54)
Severe disability	1/604	RR 0.80 (0.52, 1.23)
Death or severe disability	1/773	RR 1.00 (0.80, 1.24)
Failed treatment:		
Persistent hypotension	1/644	RR 0.55 (0.24, 1.28)
Persistent low flow	0/0	
Change CBF (%)	1/25	WMD 7.8 (−19.8, 35.4)
Change in LVO (%)	1/25	WMD 26.6 (−16.7, 69.9)
Change in mean BP (%)	1/25	WMD 6.8 (−16.8, 30.4)

PIVH = peri/intraventricular hemorrhage; CLD = chronic lung disease; CBF = cerebral blood flow; LVO = left ventricular; BP = blood pressure; RR = risk ratio; WMD = white matter damage.

the effect of volume on systemic blood flow in preterm infants who had hypotension or low systemic blood flow. Where infants who had cardiovascular compromise were enrolled, different types of volume expansion (109–112) or volume versus inotrope (113) were compared (Table 13-6). One small trial enrolling hypotensive infants reported albumin was not as effective as dopamine for correcting hypotension, but there were no significant differences in short-term outcomes, including mortality, PIVH, and PVL (113). However, in trials comparing volume expansion with inotrope (usually dopamine), around 50% of hypotensive infants responded to albumin. Three trials compared the use of colloid (albumin 5%) with crystalloid (saline) in hypotensive preterm infants (109,110,112). So (109) and Oca et al. (112) reported no significant difference for outcomes, including the incidence of failed treatment (persistent hypotension). A randomized trial investigated the effect on blood pressure of 5 mL/kg 20% albumin, 15 mL/kg fresh frozen plasma (FFP), and 15 mL/kg 4.5% albumin given at a rate of 5 mL/kg/h in a total of 60 hypotensive preterm infants during the first postnatal day (111). Thus, patients in all three groups received roughly similar amounts of colloids per kg body weight.

Table 13-6   Meta-analyses of Randomized Controlled Trials of Volume versus Inotrope (Dopamine) in Preterm Infants (86)

Outcome	Studies/Participants	Effect (95% CI)
Death	2/63	RR 1.45 (0.53, 3.95)
PIVH, grade 2–4	1/39	RR 1.47 (0.96, 2.25)
Periventricular leucomalacia	1/24	Not estimable
Failed treatment:		
Persistent hypotension	1/39	RR 5.22 (1.33, 20.55)
Persistent low flow	0/0	
CLD (oxygen at 28 days)	1/39	RR 0.71 (0.39, 1.29)
Retinopathy of prematurity	1/39	RR 0.83 (0.37, 1.84)
Change CBF (%)	1/24	WMD 5.9 (−25.0, 36.8)
Change in LVO (%)	1/24	WMD 3.4 (−47.2, 54.0)
Change in mean BP (%)	1/24	WMD −13.9 (−43.6, 15.8)

PIVH = peri/intraventricular hemorrhage; CLD = chronic lung disease; CBF = cerebral blood flow; LVO = left ventricular output; BP = blood pressure; RR = risk ratio; WMD = white matter damage.

FFP and 4.5% albumin were significantly more effective for treating hypotension compared to 20% albumin after the first hour following the completion of the infusions indicating that the volume infused rather than albumin load is important in producing a more sustained increase in blood pressure. In a trial published only in abstract form, Lynch (110) reported 10 mL/kg albumin administered to hypotensive preterm infants in the first 3 days resulted in significantly greater increase in mean blood pressure than saline and a reduced requirement for vasopressor support. Effects on blood flow were not reported.

In an observational study (114), 42 infants with low SVC flow (< 41 mL/kg/min) in the first 12 h received normal saline 10 mL/kg, which produced a significant short term increase in SVC flow (mean + 43%) measured 30 min later. As all infants then received inotropes, it is not known whether this response would have been maintained. Given the potential effect of delayed cord clamping in reducing need of blood transfusion for hypotension and reducing PIVH (88), and the observations of increased systemic blood flow in response to volume (114), further studies examining the effects of early volume expansion in preterm infants with suspected hypovolemia may be warranted.

Vasopressor/Inotropes and Inotropes

Vasopressor/inotropes and inotropes used in preterm infants have included epinephrine, norepinephrine, and dopamine, and isoprenaline and dobutamine, respectively. These inotropes have varying pharmacological properties that include increased myocardial contractility and heart rate (via cardiac β- and α-adrenoreceptors), and reduced (via peripheral β-adrenoreceptors) or increased (via peripheral α-adrenoreceptors and serotoninergic receptors) vascular resistance. The cardiovascular effects of these medications are dose-dependent and depend on which receptors are stimulated. There is concern that the immature cardiovascular and autonomic nervous system of the immature newborn may alter the response of newborn infants to these agents (115,116). The immature myocardium has decreased sympathetic innervation and norepinephrine stores (117), potentially reducing the positive inotropic effects of dopamine, which stimulates noradrenaline release (118). Myocardial contractility is reduced in very preterm infants with low systemic blood flow in the first postnatal day (84), as well as shocked preterm infants (119).

Substantial practice variation exists between different neonatal intensive care units in their thresholds for treatment of hypotension, therapeutic strategies, and doses of inotrope in preterm infants (120). This is likely to be a result of a dearth of evidence demonstrating improvements in outcomes from various therapeutic strategies for circulatory support in preterm infants.

Epinephrine

Epinephrine is a naturally occurring sympathomimetic amine with cardiac and peripheral α and β adrenergic effects and therefore it is characterized as a vasopressor/inotrope. In animal research, low dose adrenaline has predominately β-adrenergic effects and produces increases in cardiac output and blood pressure (115,121,122). At doses ≥ 3.2 μg/kg/min, α-effects become significant, with increases in vascular resistance in multiple vascular beds and a trend to reduced cardiac output (121,122). Both systemic and pulmonary pressures and resistances are increased with greatest increases in the systemic circulation. In an observational study, epinephrine has been reported to be effective in treating infants with infants with hypotension refractory to other inotropes (123). In a randomized trial, epinephrine has been compared with dopamine in hypotensive preterm infants in the first day (124) (see the section "Dopamine versus epinephrine in preterm infants with hypotension" on p. 250).

Dopamine

Dopamine is a naturally occurring biochemical catecholamine precursor of epinephrine and norepinephrine (116,118) and is characterized as a vasopressor/inotrope. Dopamine hydrochloride stimulates dopaminergic, α- and β-adrenergic, and serotoninergic receptors in a dose-dependent manner. In the mature cardiovascular system, at infusion rates of 0.5 to 4 μg/kg/min, the dopaminergic receptors are stimulated with renal and mesenteric vasodilatation and little change in blood pressure. At infusion rates of 4 to 10 μg/kg/min, $β_1$- and $β_2$-adrenoreceptors are also activated and cardiac output and systolic BP increase. Total systemic vascular resistance is relatively unchanged due to peripheral vasoconstriction (α-adrenoreceptor effect) and vasodilatation ($β_2$-adrenorecpetor effect). At infusion rates above to 10 μg/kg/min, the activation of the peripheral α-receptors causes dose-dependent increases in peripheral vasoconstriction with increases in systolic and diastolic blood pressure. Dopamine has been used extensively in neonates for treatment of hypotension. In the immature cardiovascular system, the myocardial and vascular response to dopamine (and the other vasoactive amines) is affected by maturational differences in the expression of the different adrenoreceptors and dopaminergic receptors (118). In addition, down regulation of adrenergic receptors and relative adrenal insufficiency further influence the cardiovascular response to dopamine (125). Therefore, the dose–response curves established for the mature cardiovascular system do not reflect the pharmacodynamics seen in the immature neonate (116,118).

Several randomized controlled trials have examined the effect of low-dose dopamine compared to control (no treatment or placebo) in preterm infants. These studies enrolled ventilated infants with RDS (126,127), or infants receiving indomethacin (128) to determine the cardiovascular and renal effects of low dose dopamine. In ventilated infants with RDS, Cuevas (126) reported no significant difference in blood gases, acid–base status, blood pressure, glomerular filtration rates, and urine outputs in infants on low-dose dopamine. The fractional excretion of sodium was increased on infants on dopamine 1 μg/kg/min but not 2.5 μg/kg/min. There were no significant differences in mortality, chronic lung disease or duration of oxygen therapy. In normotensive preterm infants (127), dopamine 5 μg/kg/min resulted in a significant increase in blood pressure and LVO but not [131]Xe-measured CBF compared to no treatment.

In randomized trials of dopamine for prevention of renal side effects of indomethacin, three trials compared low dose dopamine at rates between 2 and 5 μg/kg/min in preterm infants being treated with indomethacin for a symptomatic DA (128). There are no results for several important clinical outcomes including mortality, PIVH, PVL or renal failure, CBF, cardiac output, or gastrointestinal complications. Dopamine was associated with a minor increase in urine output but there was no significant difference in serum creatinine, fractional sodium excretion, or incidence of oliguria.

In infants with suspected perinatal asphyxia, one trial (129) compared low-dose dopamine at 2.5 μg/kg/min with placebo in 14 term infants with a 5 min Apgar ≥ 6 and a systolic blood pressure ≥ 50 mm Hg. Although dopamine increased cardiac output, no significant differences between these two groups were found for mortality or long-term neurodevelopmental outcome. In addition, no data were found reporting outcomes in infants with clinical evidence of cardiovascular compromise. High dose dopamine (> 20 μg/kg/min) has been used in infants with refractory hypotension (130).

Dobutamine

Dobutamine is a synthetic catecholamine with predominately β-adrenergic effects but some α-effects and, because it does not produce increases in SVR, it is classified as an inotrope (116,131). Dobutamine increases myocardial contractility by direct stimulation of myocardial α- and β-adrenergic receptors and, unlike dopamine, its pharmacological action is not dependent on released norepinephrine (131). There are no published randomized controlled trials of dobutamine compared to placebo or no treatment in newborn infants, either term or preterm. Several observational studies have reported cardiovascular effects of dobutamine in newborn infants. Devictor (132) reported increased cardiac output, heart rate, and aortic blood flow velocities in six term newborn infants with severe perinatal asphyxia receiving dobutamine 10 μg/kg/min. Martinez (133) reported increases in cardiac output but no significant change in blood pressure or heart rate at infusion rates of 5 and 7.5 μg/kg/min in sick newborn infants between 27 and 42 weeks' gestation. All infants had received volume prior to dobutamine. Stopfkuchen (134) enrolled 17 ventilated preterm infants selected for dobutamine treatment on the basis of an elevated ratio of pre-ejection period to left ventricular ejection time (PEP:LVET) reflecting abnormal left ventricular function. No volume loading was given prior to infusion of dobutamine 10 μg/kg/min. Dobutamine infusion increased heart rate, decreased PEP:LVET ratio, and increased mean blood pressure. The authors conclude that dobutamine improves left ventricular performance in preterm infants with echocardiographic evidence of impaired left ventricular function.

Isoprenaline

Isoprenaline (isoproterenol) is a synthetic sympathomimetic amine that is structurally related to adrenaline and acts almost exclusively on β-adrenergic receptors. In animals, isoprenaline increased cardiac output, but caused a significantly greater increase in heart rate to achieve a similar change of cardiac output compared to dopamine and dobutamine (135). There are few published data on use of isoprenaline in premature infants, although it has been used in clinical practice. Isoprenaline infusions have been used for management of infants and children with congenital heart block, status asthmaticus, and meningococcal septicemia (136–140). There are case reports of isoprenaline infusions in infants with persistent pulmonary hypertension of the newborn (141,142).

Norepinephrine

Norepinephrine is a naturally occurring sympathomimetic amine that acts on myocardial and vascular α- and β-adrenergic receptors (118). Norepinephrine differs from epinephrine primarily in its decreased peripheral β_2-adrenoreceptor affinity and therefore it causes a more pronounced peripheral vasoconstriction (α-adrenergic action). As with epinephrine, norepinephrine has positive inotropic effects and also dilates the coronary arteries via its cardiac β-adrenergic actions. These effects result in increased systemic blood pressure and coronary artery blood flow. There are few published data on use of norepinephrine in premature infants with its use being restricted to the treatment of hypotension refractory to other vasopressor/inotropes (143).

Dopamine versus Dobutamine in Preterm Infants with Hypotension

Several randomized trials (Table 13-7) have compared dopamine with dobutamine in preterm infants (144–149). These trials enrolled infants remaining hypotensive despite a trial of volume expansion. The definitions of systemic hypotension varied but included a systolic blood pressure < 40 mm Hg (150), mean blood pressure < 30 mm Hg (149), mean blood pressure < 30 mm Hg for more than 1 h (148),

Table 13-7   Randomized Trials of Dopamine versus Dobutamine in Hypotensive Preterm Infants

Trial	Infants	Treatment Criteria/ Success	Random	Blind	Intervention 1	Intervention 2	Outcome Measures
144	1–6 days <34 weeks	Systolic BP <40 mm Hg	Y	N	Dopamine 5–15 µg/kg/min	Dobutamine 5–15 µg/kg/min	Correction of hypotension
145	2 h to 17 days Preterm	Mean BP <10th percentile	Y	N	Dopamine 10 µg/kg/min	Dobutamine 10 µg/kg/min	Change in mean BP; mortality, PIVH, PVL
146	<24 h <35 weeks	Mean BP <31 mm Hg	Y	Y	Dopamine 5–20 µg/kg/min	Dobutamine 5–20 µg/kg/min	Correction of hypotension; mortality, PIVH, PVL
148	Age unclear < 32 weeks	Mean BP <30 mm Hg	Y	Y	Dopamine 5–20 µg/kg/min	Dobutamine 5–20 µg/kg/min	Correction of hypotension; echo measured LVO; mortality, PVL
149	<24 h Preterm	Mean BP <30 mm Hg	Y	N	Dopamine 5–10 µg/kg/min	Dobutamine 5–10 µg/kg/min	Correction of hypotension

BP = blood pressure; PIVH = peri/intraventricular hemorrhage; PVL = periventricular leucomalacia; LVO = left ventricular out-put.

mean blood pressure < 31 mm Hg for 30 min (146), and mean blood pressure below 10th percentile for the normal range (145). The drugs were commenced at a median age < 24 h in most studies, except one (145), which enrolled infants up to 17 days. Both agents were administered as continuous infusions at doses between 5 and 20 µg/kg/min. All studies were randomized, with allocation concealment reported by all but one study (148). Blinding of intervention was reported by two studies (146,148). Follow up of randomized infants was complete in all studies although measurement was blinded in only two studies (145,146).

Meta-analysis (2) found no significant difference in mortality, grade 3–4 PIVH and PVL (Table 13-8). Not included in this meta-analysis were reporting of any PIVH and necrotizing enterocolitis (NEC). Meta-analysis of two studies reporting these outcomes (146,148) found no significant difference in incidence of PIVH or NEC. Dopamine resulted in significantly greater increases in blood pressure, with

Table 13-8   Meta-Analysis of Randomized Controlled Trials of Dopamine versus Dobutamine in Hypotensive Preterm Infants (2)

Outcome	Studies/Participants	Effect (95% CI)
Death	3/103	RR 1.17 (0.47, 2.92)
PIVH any grade	2/93	RR 0.75 (0.24, 2.30)
PIVH grade 3–4	2/83	RR 0.73 (0.15, 3.50)
Periventricular leukomalacia	3/103	RR 0.43 (0.12, 1.52)
Necrotizing enterocolitis	2/83	RR 0.43 (0.09, 2.06)
Failed treatment:		
Persistent hypotension	4/189	RR 0.41 (0.25, 0.65)
Persistent low flow	0	
Change CBF (%)	0	
Change in LVO (%)	1/20	WMD −35.0 (−55.8, 14.2)
Tachycardia	1/63	RR 0.74 (0.26, 2.08)

PIVH = peri/intraventricular hemorrhage; CBF = cerebral blood flow; LVO = left ventricular output; RR = risk ratio; WMD = white matter damage.

meta-analysis (four studies, 189 infants) finding a significant reduction in treatment failure defined as persistent hypotension in infants receiving dopamine. However, dobutamine was effective at treating hypotension in around 60% of infants. Three studies (146,148,149) reported no significant difference in change in heart rate between dopamine and dobutamine. As mentioned earlier, all studies pretreated infants with volume expansion. Measures of cardiac output were only reported by Roze (148), who found infants on dopamine had a statistically non-significant mean 14% reduction and infants on dobutamine a statistically significant mean 21% increase in LVO. The difference in the response in LVO was also statistically significant between the two medications. Dopamine produced a significantly greater increase in mean blood pressure than dobutamine, associated with a significantly greater increase in systemic vascular resistance. The presence and size of a DA shunt was not reported. However, nearly all the infants in this study had cardiac outputs in the normal range with baseline mean LVO 269 mL/kg/min and 245 mL/kg/min in the dobutamine and dopamine groups, respectively. Thus, this study appears to have investigated the cardiovascular effects of dopamine and dobutamine in preterm infants with normal systemic blood flow during the immediate postnatal period. However, since the presence, size and shunting across the DA was not reported in these patients, caution is warranted when characterizing the cardiovascular status of this patient population.

In summary, dopamine produces greater increases in blood pressure in hypotensive preterm infants than dobutamine. There is evidence from one study that dobutamine is better at increasing LVO, whereas dopamine produces greater increases in blood pressure and systemic vascular resistance (148). No other clinical benefit has been demonstrated from use of dopamine or dobutamine.

Dopamine versus Dobutamine in Preterm Infants with Low SVC Flow

Only one study (114) enrolled infants with low systemic (SVC) blood flow. Infants with low SVC flow (< 41 mL/kg/min) in the first 12 h received a normal saline bolus at 10 mL/kg, and were randomized to dobutamine or dopamine at a dose of 10 µg/kg/min. If low flow persisted or recurred, the dose was increased to 20 µg/kg/min, with crossover to the other agent if treatment failed to maintain SVC flow. At the highest dose reached, dobutamine produced significantly greater increases in SVC flow (Table 13-9). In contrast, dopamine produced significantly greater increases in blood pressure. Infants on dobutamine only at 24 h had higher RVO than infants on dopamine. However, 40% failed to increase or maintain SVC flow in response to either medication. No significant difference in mortality, any PIVH, PVL, and NEC was reported. However, there was a reduction in grade 3 or 4 PIVH in the dobutamine group (5% versus 35%). In 13 survivors assessed at three years, the dopamine group had significantly more disability and lower development quotients. However, since more patients died in the dobutamine group, this finding has to be viewed with caution. Combined rates of death or disability at three years were similar. The study provides evidence that dobutamine is better than dopamine at increasing SVC flow at the applied doses in preterm infants with low SVC flow in the first postnatal day. Neither inotrope was found to increase myocardial contractility as determined by the relationship between left ventricular mean velocity of circumferential fiber shortening and wall stress (84). A limitation of this study was the titration of inotrope irrespective of blood pressure (and hence systemic vascular resistance), resulting in many infants being exposed to high dose dopamine (20 µg/kg/min). The usual approach with dopamine is to treat infants with hypotension, with the dose titrated according to pharmacodynamic response (i.e. blood pressure). However, the goal of this study was to treat infants with low systemic blood

Table 13–9   Randomized Trial of Dobutamine versus Dopamine for Preterm Infants with Low SBF (114)

Outcome	Studies/ Participants	Effect (95% CI)
Mortality to discharge	1/42	RR 1.41 (0.79, 2.52)
Any PIVH	1/42	RR 1.01 (0.52, 1.97)
Late PIVH	1/42	RR 0.57 (0.22, 1.45)
PIVH grade 3–4	1/42	RR 0.39 (0.12, 1.31)
NEC	1/42	RR 2.73 (0.31, 24.14)
Cerebral palsy at 3 years	1/13	RR 0.16 (0.01, 2.64)
Deafness at 3 years	1/13	RR 0.16 (0.01, 2.64)
Griffith's general quotient >2SD below norm at 3 years	1/13	RR 0.16 (0.01, 2.64)
Disability at 3 years	1/13	RR 0.10 (0.01, 1.56)
Death or disability at 3 years	1/37	RR 0.79 (0.57, 1.11)
Griffith's general quotient at 3 years	1/13	WMD 35.00 (17.68, 52.32)
PVL	1/24	RR 6.00 (0.34, 104.89)
Renal impairment (creatinine ≥120 mmol/L)	1/42	RR 0.55 (0.15, 2.00)
Pulmonary hemorrhage	1/42	RR 0.61 (0.11, 3.26)
Chronic lung disease at 36 weeks postmenstrual age	1/19	RR 0.83 (0.27, 2.49)
Retinopathy of prematurity	1/20	RR 0.80 (0.30, 2.13)
Failed treatment (did not maintain SVC flow ≥41 mL/kg/min in first 24 h)	1/42	RR 0.58 (0.28, 1.20)
Change mean BP at 10 μg/kg/min	1/42	WMD −4.50 (−8.06−0.94)
Change mean BP at 20 μg/kg/min	1/23	WMD −4.60 (−8.74−0.46)
Change mean BP at highest dose reached	1/42	WMD −7.20 (−11.41−2.99)
Change SVC flow at 10 μg/kg/min	1/42	WMD 4.70 (−4.02, 13.42)
Change SVC flow at 20 μg/kg/min	1/23	WMD 9.70 (−3.93, 23.33)
Change SVC flow at highest reached	1/42	WMD 13.10 (2.87, 23.33)
Change RVO at 10 μg/kg/min	1/42	WMD 4.00 (−19.27, 27.27)
Change RVO at 20 μg/kg/min	1/23	WMD 1.20 (−25.35, 27.75)
Change RVO at highest dose reached	1/42	WMD 10.70 (−19.16, 40.56)

SBF = systemic blood flow; PIVH = peri/intraventricular hemorrhage; NEC = necrotizing enterocolitis; SD = standard deviation; PVL = periventricular leucomalacia; SVC = superior vena cava; BP = blood pressure; RVO = right ventricular output; RR = risk ratio; WMD = white matter damage.

flow with the dose adjusted to increase systemic blood flow, and fixed dosages selected to maintain blinding of measurement.

Dopamine Versus Epinephrine in Preterm Infants with Hypotension

Two studies (Table 13-10) have compared dopamine to epinephrine in preterm infants with hypotension (124,150). Only one has been published to date (124,151). Pellicer (124,151) reported a randomized, blinded trial of dopamine versus epinephrine in infants born < 1501 g and < 32 weeks' gestation with a mean blood pressure less than the gestational age in the first postnatal day. Dopamine (2.5, 5, 7.5, or 10 μg/kg/min) or adrenaline (0.125, 0.250, 0.375, or 0.5 μg/kg/min) was titrated every 20 min to achieve a mean blood pressure ≥ gestational age in weeks. Initial successful treatment of hypotension was reported for 97% of patients on dopamine and 94% on epinephrine. Subsequent hypotension resulted in 33% of infants on dopamine and 38% on epinephrine receiving rescue treatment. Both dopamine and epinephrine increased measures of cerebral perfusion using NIR spectroscopy, as indicated by the increase in both cerebral blood volume and oxygenation. Neonatal mortality was not significantly different (dopamine 11%

Table 13-10   Randomized Trials of Dopamine versus Adrenaline in Hypotensive Preterm Infants

Trial (references)	Infants	Treatment Criteria/ Success	Random	Blind	Intervention 1	Intervention 2	Outcome Measures
150	<24 h Mean 34– 36 weeks	Mean BP <1 SD below mean for weight	Y	Y	Dopamine 5– 20 μg/kg/min	Adrenaline 0.125–0.5 μg/ kg/min	Correction hypotension; echo measured LVO, RVO
124, 151	<24 h <32 weeks <1501 g	Mean BP, mmHg < gestation weeks	Y	Y	Dopamine 2.5– 10 μg/kg/min	Adrenaline 0.125–0.5 μg/ kg/min	NIR spectroscopy measured CBF; correction hypotension

BP = blood pressure; SD = standard deviation; LVO = left ventricular output; RVO = right ventricular output; CBF=cerebral blood flow.

versus adrenaline 19%). Unfortunately, incidences of cerebral ischemic lesions (56% overall) were not reported according to group assignment. Although changes in CBF were followed, no measure of cardiac output or systemic blood flow was reported. In summary, similar treatment success rates from use of dopamine and epinephrine in hypotensive preterm infants in the first postnatal day were reported. Short-term measures of cerebral perfusion improved with increases in mean blood pressure. However, subsequent treatment failure rates were high as were morbidity and mortality.

Milrinone for Prevention of Low SVC Blood Flow in Preterm Infants

Milrinone is a selective class III phosphodiesterase inhibitor that, in children and adults, increases myocardial contractility and reduces systemic and pulmonary vascular resistance. However, it is not known, if class III phosphodiesterase inhibitors have positive inotropic effects in the immature animal or preterm neonate (152–154). In a pilot study (155,156), an optimized dose regimen for Milrinone in preterm infants was determined that fulfilled a therapeutic goal of maintaining SVC flow in the first 24 h when started within 6 h of birth. In a subsequent double-blind randomized placebo controlled trial (157), 90 infants at high risk of low SVC flow were enrolled within 6 h of birth including all infants born at ≤ 27 weeks' gestation and infants at 28 to 29 weeks' gestation with mean airway pressure ≥ 8 cm H_2O and $Fio_2 \geq 0.3$. Normal saline 15 mL/kg was given and infants randomized to milrinone (0.75 μg/kg/min for 3 h then 0.2 μg/kg/min until 18 h after birth) or placebo. No significant difference was observed in mean SVC flow in the first 24 h, incidences of low SVC flow (milrinone: 17% vs placebo: 19%), low RVO (14% vs 23%), or need for vasopressor/inotrope (45% vs 35%). There was no significant difference in PIVH (19% vs 15%) or mortality (19% vs 19%). The incidence of low systemic blood flow was lower than predicted in this study. However, there is no evidence of benefit from use of Milrinone for prevention of low systemic blood flow in sick very preterm neonates during the first postnatal day.

Postnatal Corticosteroids in Hypotensive Preterm Infants

There is increasing interest in the use of postnatal corticosteroids for stabilizing the cardiovascular status of preterm infants (115,116). The evidence for postnatal corticosteroids improving the cardiovascular status of preterm infants comes from observations of the effects of both antenatal and postnatal corticosteroids. A systematic review (158) of randomized trials of antenatal corticosteroids given prior to preterm birth found a significant reduction in neonatal death, respiratory distress syndrome, PIVH (RR 0.54, 95% CI 0.43–0.69) and NEC (RR 0.46, 95% CI 0.29–0.74). However, the incidence of hypotension, low blood flows, and use of inotrope support was not reported. In observational studies, antenatal corticosteroids have been reported to reduce the need for postnatal dopamine for hypotension (159), and reduce the incidence of failure of response to dobutamine or dopamine for infants with low SVC flow (114).

Several randomized trials (160–164) have reported increases in systemic blood pressure and reduced need for vasopressor/inotrope support in hypotensive preterm infants treated with postnatal corticosteroids. Gaissmaier (161) randomized 20 preterm infants with hypotension, refractory to colloid and vasopressor/inotrope, to dexamethasone 0.25 mg/kg or placebo (Table 13-11). Epinephrine was discontinued in five of eight infants treated with dexamethasone and one of nine on placebo. Osiovich (163) compared hydrocortisone 5 mg/kg/dose for four doses to placebo in hypotensive infants born <1250 g in the first 48 h. Dopamine use was reduced in the hydrocortisone group. No difference was reported for clinical outcomes (data not given – published in abstract form only). Efird (160) randomized extremely low birth weight infants to five days' prophylactic hydrocortisone or placebo starting in the first three postnatal hours. Vasopressor/inotrope use for hypotension was reduced in the hydrocortisone group on day 1 (25% versus 44%) and day 2 (7% versus 39%, $P < 0.05$). However, effects on systemic and organ blood flow have not been reported. Ng (164) reported a randomized controlled blinded trial of a five-day course of stress dose hydrocortisone (3 mg/kg/day) in VLBW neonates started on the first postnatal day. Hydrocortisone resulted in a decrease in cumulative doses of vasopressor, inotropes and volume expanders, and a reduction in the number of infants on support after 72 h. The mean blood pressure was significantly and consistently higher in the hydrocortisone group, although clinical outcomes were not affected.

In a systematic review (165) of randomized trials of early (<96 h age) postnatal corticosteroids for preventing chronic lung disease, 21 trials enrolling 3072 infants were included with most trials enrolling ventilated low birth weight infants. Meta-analysis found early postnatal corticosteroids resulted in earlier extubation, decreased incidence of chronic lung disease, death or chronic lung disease, DA and severe ROP. No significant difference was found in mortality, infection, severe PIVH, PVL, NEC, or pulmonary hemorrhage. Early postnatal corticosteroids were associated with significant adverse effects including increased rates of gastrointestinal hemorrhage and intestinal perforation. Cardiovascular effects included increased hypertension and hypertrophic cardiomyopathy. In trials reporting late outcomes, some adverse neurological effects were found, including increased rates of developmental delay, cerebral palsy, and abnormal neurological examination in a patients who had received corticosteroids in the form of dexamethasone. Other late outcomes were not significantly different, including major neurosensory disability and combined death or major neurosensory disability. Incidences of hypotension, low cardiac output, or organ blood flow and use of inotropes were not reported.

Echocardiographic studies of postnatal corticosteroids in newborn infants have focussed on the long-term effects of corticosteroids in producing myocardial septal hypertrophy and reduced left ventricular end-diastolic dimensions (165,166). Evans (166) reported a reduction in pulmonary artery time to peak velocity to right ventricular ejection time ratio in a small observational study of infants being treated with dexamethasone, suggesting a reduction in pulmonary artery pressures. There are no published data of the effects of postnatal corticosteroids on cardiac outputs or organ blood flows in the first days after birth.

Table 13-11   **Randomized Trials of Corticosteroids in Hypotensive Preterm Infants**

Trial (References)	Infants	Treatment Criteria/ Success	Random	Blind	Intervention 1	Intervention 2	Outcome Measures
167	<7 days <1500 g	Mean BP <25, 30 mm Hg at <750g and 750–1500g, respectively	Y	N	Hydrocortisone 2.5 mg/kg q4h × 2 then q6h	Dopamine 5–20 μg/kg/min	Correction of hypotension; PIVH, NEC, CLD, DA, mortality
161	1–20 days Preterm	Mean BP mm Hg unresponsive to volume and dopamine: 23 (<750 g), 25 (750–999), 28–30 (1–2000), 35 (2–3000), 40 (>3000)	Y	Y	Dexamethasone 0.25 mg/kg	Placebo	Cessation of adrenaline infusion; NEC, PIVH, PVL, mortality
164	VLBW 8–15 h hypotension refractory to dopamine >10 μg/kg/min	Mean BP < gestation in weeks	Y	Y	Hydrocortisone 1 mg/kg q8h	Placebo	Correction of hypotension, duration and quality of cardiovascular support

BP = blood pressure; VLBW = very low birth weight; PIVH = peri/intraventricular hemorrhage; NEC = necrotizing enterolcolitis; CLD = chronic lung disease; DA = ductus arteriosus; PVL = periventricular leukomalacia.

Postnatal Corticosteroids versus Dopamine in Hypotensive Preterm Infants

One randomized controlled trial (167) compared dopamine starting at 5 μg/kg/min and titrated up to 20 μg/kg/min to hydrocortisone 2.5 mg/kg in hypotensive preterm infants < 1500 g in the first postnatal week (Table 13-11). No significant difference was reported in treatment failure rate (absence of hypotension) in infants receiving dopamine compared to hydrocortisone (0% versus 19%, $P = 0.1$). There were no significant differences in mortality (5% versus 10%), CLD (11% versus 26%), NEC (5% versus 19%), PIVH grades 2–4 (16% versus 24%), or sepsis (32% versus 19%). Measures of cardiac output and organ blood flow were not reported.

Inhaled Nitric Oxide in Preterm Infants

Inhaled nitric oxide (iNO) in infants with respiratory disease results in improvement in oxygenation due to reductions in pulmonary vascular resistance (168) and improvements in pulmonary blood flow velocities in infants with low pulmonary blood flow velocity (169). However, there are inadequate data to determine the effect of iNO on systemic blood flow in preterm infants. Systematic review (170) of randomized trials of iNO enrolling preterm infants found seven trials. An additional two trials have been published subsequently (171,172). Trial eligibility criteria varied and included infants at high risk of chronic lung disease (171,173), routine use of early iNO in ventilated preterm infants (174) and infants with high predicted mortality due to poor oxygenation indices (172,175–179). Meta-analyses (Table 13-12) of the nine trials found no significant benefit from use of iNO on mortality, but a significant reduction in CLD measured at 36 weeks postmenstrual age and combined death or CLD. There was no significant difference in incidence of PIVH or severe PIVH, although individual studies have reported significant reductions in cerebral abnormalities in infants randomized to iNO. In particular, Schreiber (174), enrolling preterm infants at a mean age around 12.9 to 14 h, reported a significant reduction in severe PIVH or PVL (RR 0.53, 95% CI 0.28–0.98), and Kinsella (172), enrolling infants at a mean age of 30 h, reported a significant reduction in severe PIVH, PVL or ventriculomegaly (RR 0.73, 95% CI 0.55–0.98). Two studies to date have reported developmental outcomes with Field (175) reporting no significant difference (iNO 7 of 55 versus control 3 of 53) in incidence of major disability (defined as no/minimal head control or inability to sit unsupported or no/minimal responses to visual stimuli) at one year of age. This trial

Table 13-12	**Meta-Analysis of Randomized Trials of Nitric Oxide Versus No Treatment in Preterm Infants**	
Outcome	**Studies/ Participants**	**Effect (95% CI)**
Death before discharge	9/2455	RR 0.96 (0.85, 1.08)
Death before 36 weeks postmenstrual age	5/460	RR 0.96 (0.77, 1.18)
BPD at 36 weeks postmenstrual age	9/1931	RR 0.91 (0.85, 0.98)
Death or BPD	9/2441	RR 0.93 (0.89, 0.98)
PIVH all grades	2/214	RR 0.98 (0.71, 1.35)
Grade 3 or 4 IVH	4/1426	RR 1.05 (0.86, 1.29)
PIVH (Grade 3 or 4) or PVL	7/1714	RR 0.93 (0.78, 1.10)
Neurodevelopmental disability	1/138	RR 0.53 (0.33, 0.87)
Cerebral palsy	1/138	RR 1.13 (0.40, 3.20)
Bayley MDI or PDI ≥2SD below norms	1/138	RR 0.56 (0.33, 0.93)

BPD = bronchopulmonary dysplasia; PIVH = peri/intraventricular hemorrhage; IVH = intraventricular hemorrhage; PVL = periventricular leukomalacia; MDI = mental developmental index; PDI = psychomotor developmental index.

enrolled infants with severe respiratory failure in the first 28 days. However, Schreiber (174), in a single center study, reported a significant reduction in neuro-developmental disability (RR 0.53, 95% CI 0.33–0.87). Of note is that this is the only trial to enrol infants predominately in the first day, a time when postnatal systemic blood flow might be expected to be falling or at its lowest (5,6,83). Infants with more severe RDS ($FiO_2 > 0.5$) and fatal RDS have been shown to have echocardiographic evidence of increased pulmonary artery pressures, suggesting a relationship between severity of RDS, pulmonary hypertension, and outcome. In addition, in term infants with severe respiratory disease, including those with pulmonary hypertension, low ventricular outputs are a common echocardiographic finding (180). The study raises the possibility that reducing pulmonary vascular resistance in preterm infants with nitric oxide has the potential to prevent cerebral injury.

In summary, trials of iNO in preterm infants have predominately used iNO for treatment of severe respiratory disease after the first day. One single-center trial (174) enrolling infants in the first day reported a reduction in severe cerebral lesions (grade 3–4 PIVH or PVL) and developmental disability while the findings of another large multicenter study (172) suggest that early iNO may be neuroprotec-tive. Trials of early, targeted iNO in preterm infants are needed.

Infants with Perinatal Asphyxia

Low-cardiac output states occur in newborns that have perinatal asphyxia (180). Such infants have reduced myocardial contractility (181) and variable degrees of pulmonary hypertension (180). Evidence for treatment is sparse. There are no data to support use of volume expansion in infants with suspected asphyxia (182), although the occasional infant will have coexistent hypovolemia (183). One randomized trial (184) compared use of sodium bicarbonate infusion versus 5% dextrose in asphyxiated newborn infants. No evidence of an effect on mortality, (RR 1.04, 95% CI 0.49–2.21), abnormal neurological examination at discharge, or a composite outcome of death or abnormal neurological examination at discharge was reported. There was no significant difference in the incidence of encephalo-pathy, PIVH, and neonatal seizures. Long-term neurodevelopmental outcomes were not assessed. One observational study (132) reported increases in cardiac output, heart rate, and aortic blood flow velocities in six term infants with severe perinatal asphyxia receiving dobutamine 10 µg/kg/min. A similar response was observed in another study using dopamine (185). No benefit was reported from use of low-dose dopamine versus placebo in infants with severe asphyxia but without evidence of cardiovascular compromise (129). There is inadequate evidence to make strong recommendations regarding the cardiovascular support of infants with perinatal asphyxia.

Pulmonary Hypertension

Newborns with high oxygen and ventilator-support requirements with or without pulmonary hypertension frequently have low cardiac outputs (180). Among pre-term infants, the incidence of low ventricular outputs (particularly RVO) in the first days after birth increases with worsening respiratory distress (186). The incidence of right to left ductal shunting indicating severe pulmonary hypertension was signifi-cantly increased in infants who had fatal respiratory distress syndrome. The treat-ment of choice for improving oxygenation in term infants with hypoxemic respiratory failure is iNO. Systematic review of randomized trials in term and late preterm infants found a significant reduction in combined death or need for extracorporeal membrane oxygenation (ECMO) (187). Mortality was not reduced, although this may be attributed to the use of ECMO. Oxygenation improved in around 50% of infants receiving iNO. There are inadequate data in newborn infants to determine the effect of iNO on measures of systemic blood flow, although iNO increases pulmonary blood flow velocities in infants with low pulmonary blood flow velocity (169). Since the introduction of iNO, there are no trials of vasopressor/inotrope or inotrope use in infants with persistent pulmonary hypertension of the newborn (PPHN) to guide therapy. Oral sildenafil resulted in a significant reduction in mortality in a small trial in infants with PPHN where iNO was not available (188). No significant effects on blood pressure were noted. In centers with ECMO available, trials of ECMO have demonstrated significant reductions in mortality (RR 0.44, 95% CI 0.31–0.61) restricted largely to infants without diaphragmatic hernia. The UK trial reported a significant reduction in death and disability at one year (RR 0.56, 95% CI 0.40–0.78) and four years (RR 0.62, 95% CI 0.45–0.86). The UK trial reported that an ECMO policy was as cost-effective as other intensive care technologies in common use. However, these trials preceded the use of iNO and the UK trial was a trial of transport to an ECMO center and ECMO versus no transport, limiting the generalizability of this study.

There are inadequate data to determine the effect of vasopressor/inotropes or inotropes in infants with PPHN. Small case series document responses to dopamine (189) and milrinone (190), with no adverse effect on blood pressure from milrinone use reported. The focus of management for infants with PPHN has been to maintain an adequate systemic blood pressure, the use of ventilator and pharmacologic measures to increase pulmonary vasodilatation and decrease pulmonary vascular resistance, with the goal of increasing blood and tissue oxygenation and normalization of blood pH (191). However, apart from use of iNO, sildenafil, and ECMO, trials are currently lacking to guide specific treatments.

Infants with Sepsis

Low cardiac outputs and hypotension are common in septic infants. In children, low-output states associated with high systemic vascular resistance ("nonhyperdynamic" sepsis) and high-output states characterized by low systemic vascular resistance ("vasodilatory shock") have been described (192,193). A substantial capillary leak can occur with subsequent hypovolemia. Unfortunately, most of this information is derived from infants beyond the newborn period. In adult patients, a randomized trial of "goal-directed therapy" for severe sepsis and septic shock has provided guidance for the aggressive management of these patients (194). The approach involves adjustments of cardiac preload, afterload, and contractility to balance oxygen delivery with oxygen demand using information derived from vital signs monitoring, laboratory data, cardiac monitoring, pulse oximetry, urinary catheterization, arterial and central venous catheterization. Of note is that a target of mixed venous saturation ≥70% was used for targeting therapy. Mortality to 60 days was significantly reduced in patients with goal-directed therapy (RR 0.67, 95% CI 0.46–0.96). Many of these monitoring strategies are not feasible in newborn infants.

There is some evidence from a non-randomized study enrolling a large number of children and neonates with septic shock, that early and aggressive volume-therapy improves survival and outcomes even in the neonatal patient population (195). There are no randomized trial data in newborn infants with sepsis to guide inotrope treatment for infants with sepsis. However, in preterm infants, pentoxifylline, a phosphodiesterase inhibitor might hold some promise. Meta-analysis (196) of two small randomized trials (197,198) of pentoxifylline in preterm infants with suspected sepsis after the first postnatal week, found a significant reduction in mortality (RR 0.14, 95% CI 0.03–0.76). However, pentoxifylline has anti-inflammatory properties and there are inadequate data to attribute these potential benefits to its cardiovascular effects. Further trials of pentoxifylline and other vasopressor/inotropes are needed in infants with suspected or proven sepsis tailored to the hemodynamic profile of the cardiovascular disturbance (vasoconstriction with low cardiac output or vasodilation with hyperdynamic myocardial function).

CONCLUSIONS

1. The mechanisms of cerebral injury in preterm infants remain incompletely understood. In particular, research is required to determine the antenatal, intrapartum, and immediate postpartum factors that affect cerebral perfusion in the premature fetus/newborn.

2. Early low systemic blood flow (5,6) or low CBF (7) have been associated with cerebral injury in premature infants, particularly late PIVH and subsequent developmental disability.

3. Low systemic blood flow in preterm infants in the first 24 h is predominately found in ventilated infants and is associated with lower gestation, early large diameter DA, higher mean airway pressures, higher systemic vascular resistance, and poor myocardial contractility (5,6,84). Many preterm infants with low systemic blood flow in the first 12 h will have blood pressure in the normal range at this time (compensated shock) (1).

4. Findings of retrospective studies indicate that hypotension is associated with increased mortality and morbidity in the VLBW population. However, causation has not been documented. Prospectively collected data indicate that low mean blood pressure in the second 12h after birth is associated with abnormal neurodevelopmental outcome (76). However, targeting *blood pressure alone* has the potential to delay treatment for infants with low systemic blood flow.

5. Evidence suggests that delayed cord clamping (>30 s) in infants born prematurely may reduce need for subsequent blood transfusion for anemia and hypotension, and PIVH (88,89). Further trials are required to determine the effect of delayed cord clamping on SBF and long-term outcomes.

6. Trials of volume expansion have predominately enrolled infants selected on the basis of birth weight or prematurity (86,87). There is no evidence that routine volume expansion improves clinical outcomes in preterm infants. In hypotensive infants, over 50% will respond to volume expansion, although volume expansion is not as effective as dopamine for increasing blood pressure (86).

7. In preterm infants with low systemic blood flow in the first day, dobutamine at 10 or 20 μg/kg/min is better than dopamine at the same doses at increasing systemic blood flow based on measurements of SVC flow (114). However, no significant difference in clinical outcomes and neurodevelopment was reported.

8. In hypotensive preterm infants, dopamine is better than dobutamine at increasing blood pressure (2). However, changes in systemic blood flow were not assessed in the majority of these studies. One trial found medium doses of dobutamine increased LVO whereas medium-to-high doses of dopamine resulted in a trend to decrease LVO (148). However, no significant difference in other clinical outcomes was reported.

9. In hypotensive preterm infants, dopamine and epinephrine produce similar increases in blood pressure and CBF (124,151). Effects on systemic blood flow were not reported. There were inadequate data to determine the effects on other neonatal outcomes.

10. In infants with asphyxia that are at risk of low systemic blood flow (180) and poor myocardial contractility, dobutamine increases cardiac output (132).

11. In infants with hypotension refractory to volume and/or vasopressor/inotropes, responses have been reported with high dose dopamine (130), norepinephrine (143), and corticosteroids (161,164). Other clinical benefits have not been reported from the use of early postnatal corticosteroids.

12. Further research is needed to determine how to prevent low systemic blood flow in preterm infants, and the optimal cardiovascular treatment strategies for infants with hypotension and/or low systemic blood flow. In addition, cardiovascular treatment strategies for infants with suspected perinatal asphyxia, PPHN, and sepsis need evaluation. Finally, the relationship between systemic blood flow and CBF needs to be rigorously studied especially in preterm neonates during the immediate postnatal period.

REFERENCES

1. Osborn DA, Evans N, Kluckow M. Clinical detection of low upper body blood flow in very premature infants using blood pressure, capillary refill time, and central–peripheral temperature difference. Arch Dis Child, Fetal Neonatal Ed 2004;89:F168–F173.
2. Subhedar NV, Shaw NJ. Dopamine versus dobutamine for hypotensive preterm infants. Cochrane Database Syst Rev 2003;CD001242.
3. Tortorolo G, Luciano R, Papacci P, Tonelli T. Intraventricular hemorrhage: past, present and future, focusing on classification, pathogenesis and prevention. Childs Nerv Syst 1999;15:652–661.
4. Papile LA, Burstein J, Burstein R, Koffler H. Incidence and evolution of subependymal and intraventricular hemorrhage: a study of infants with birth weights less than 1,500 gm. J Pediatr 1978;92:529–534.
5. Osborn DA, Evans N, Kluckow M. Hemodynamic and antecedent risk factors of early and late periventricular/intraventricular hemorrhage in premature infants. Pediatrics 2003;112:33–39.
6. Kluckow M, Evans N. Low superior vena cava flow and intraventricular haemorrhage in preterm infants. Arch Dis Child, Fetal Neonatal Ed 2000;82:F188–F194.
7. Meek JH, Tyszczuk L, Elwell CE, Wyatt JS. Low cerebral blood flow is a risk factor for severe intraventricular haemorrhage. Arch Dis Child, Fetal Neonatal Ed 1999;81:F15–F18.
8. Yamamoto N, Utsu M, Serizawa M, et al. Neonatal periventricular leukomalacia preceded by fetal periventricular echodensity. Fetal Diagn Ther 2000;15:198–208.
9. Inder TE, Anderson NJ, Spencer C, Wells S, Volpe JJ. White matter injury in the premature infant: a comparison between serial cranial sonographic and mr findings at term. AJNR, Am J Neuroradiol 2003;24:805–809.
10. Inder TE, Wells SJ, Mogridge NB, Spencer C, Volpe JJ. Defining the nature of the cerebral abnormalities in the premature infant: a qualitative magnetic resonance imaging study. J Pediatr 2003;143:171–179.
11. Paneth N, Pinto-Martin J, Gardiner J, et al. Incidence and timing of germinal matrix/intraventricular hemorrhage in low birth weight infants. Am J Epidemiol 1993;137:1167–1176.
12. Leviton A, Pagano M, Kuban KC, Krishnamoorthy KS, Sullivan KF, Allred EN. The epidemiology of germinal matrix hemorrhage during the first half-day of life. Dev Med Child Neurol 1991;33:138–145.
13. Ment LR, Oh W, Philip AG, et al. Risk factors for early intraventricular hemorrhage in low birth weight infants. J Pediatr 1992;121:776–783.
14. Ment LR, Oh W, Ehrenkranz RA, Philip AG, Duncan CC, Makuch RW. Antenatal steroids, delivery mode, and intraventricular hemorrhage in preterm infants. Am J Obstet Gynecol 1995;172:795–800.
15. Anderson GD, Bada HS, Sibai BM, et al. The relationship between labor and route of delivery in the preterm infant. Am J Obstet Gynecol 1988;158:1382–1390.
16. Meidell R, Marinelli P, Pettett G. Perinatal factors associated with early-onset intracranial hemorrhage in premature infants. A prospective study. Am J Dis Child 1985;139:160–163.
17. Tejani N, Verma U, Hameed C, Chayen B. Method and route of delivery in the low birth weight vertex presentation correlated with early periventricular/intraventricular hemorrhage. Obstet Gynecol 1987;69:1–4.
18. Tejani N, Verma U, Shiffman R, Chayen B. Effect of route of delivery on periventricular/intraventricular hemorrhage in the low-birth-weight fetus with a breech presentation. J Reprod Med 1987;32:911–914.
19. Shaver DC, Bada HS, Korones SB, Anderson GD, Wong SP, Arheart KL. Early and late intraventricular hemorrhage: the role of obstetric factors. Obstet Gynecol 1992;80:831–837.

20. Ment LR, Duncan CC, Ehrenkranz RA, et al. Intraventricular hemorrhage in the preterm neonate: timing and cerebral blood flow changes. J Pediatr 1984;104:419–425.

21. Spinillo A, Capuzzo E, Stronati M, Ometto A, De Santolo A, Acciano S. Obstetric risk factors for periventricular leukomalacia among preterm infants. BJOG 1998;105:865–871.

22. Yoon BH, Romero R, Park JS, Kim CJ, Kim SH, Choi JH, Han TR. Fetal exposure to an intra-amniotic inflammation and the development of cerebral palsy at the age of three years. Am J Obstet Gynecol 2000;182:675–681.

23. Leviton A, Paneth N, Reuss ML, et al. Maternal infection, fetal inflammatory response, and brain damage in very low birth weight infants. Developmental epidemiology network investigators. Pediatr Res 1999;46:566–575.

24. De Felice C, Toti P, Laurini RN, et al. Early neonatal brain injury in histologic chorioamnionitis. J Pediatr 2001;138:101–104.

25. Bass WT, Schultz SJ, Burke BL, White LE, Khan JH, Karlowicz MG. Indices of hemodynamic and respiratory functions in premature infants at risk for the development of cerebral white matter injury. J Perinatol 2002;22:64–71.

26. Baud O, Ville Y, Zupan V, et al. Are neonatal brain lesions due to intrauterine infection related to mode of delivery? BJOG 1998;105:121–124.

27. Zupan V, Gonzalez P, Lacaze-Masmonteil T, Boithias C, d'Allest AM, Dehan M, Gabilan JC. Periventricular leukomalacia: risk factors revisited. Dev Med Child Neurol 1996;38:1061–1067.

28. Perlman JM, Risser R, Broyles RS. Bilateral cystic periventricular leukomalacia in the premature infant: associated risk factors. Pediatrics 1996;97:822–827.

29. Resch B, Vollaard E, Maurer U, Haas J, Rosegger H, Muller W. Risk factors and determinants of neurodevelopmental outcome in cystic periventricular leucomalacia. Eur J Pediatr 2000;159:663–670.

30. Paul DA, Coleman MM, Leef KH, Tuttle D, Stefano JL. Maternal antibiotics and decreased periventricular leukomalacia in very-low-birth-weight infants. Arch Pediatr Adolesc Med 2003;157:145–149.

31. Spinillo A, Viazzo F, Colleoni R, Chiara A, Maria Cerbo R, Fazzi E. Two-year infant neurodevelopmental outcome after single or multiple antenatal courses of corticosteroids to prevent complications of prematurity. Am J Obstet Gynecol 2004;191:217–224.

32. Salomon LJ, Duyme M, Rousseau A, Audibert F, Paupe A, Zupan V, Ville Y. Periventricular leukomalacia and mode of delivery in twins under 1500 g. J Matern Fetal Neonatal Med 2003;13:224–229.

33. Low JA, Froese AF, Galbraith RS, Sauerbrei EE, McKinven JP, Karchmar EJ. The association of fetal and newborn metabolic acidosis with severe periventricular leukomalacia in the preterm newborn. Am J Obstet Gynecol 1990;162:977–981.

34. Amato M, Gambon R, Von Muralt G, Huber P. Neurosonographic and biochemical correlates of periventricular leukomalacia in low-birth-weight infants. Pediatr Neurosci 1987;13:84–89.

35. Calvert SA, Hoskins EM, Fong KW, Forsyth SC. Etiological factors associated with the development of periventricular leukomalacia. Acta Paediatr Scand 1987;76:254–259.

36. Erickson SJ, Grauaug A, Gurrin L, Swaminathan M. Hypocarbia in the ventilated preterm infant and its effect on intraventricular haemorrhage and bronchopulmonary dysplasia. J Paediatr Child Health 2002;38:560–562.

37. Giannakopoulou C, Korakaki E, Manoura A, Bikouvarakis S, Papageorgiou M, Gourgiotis D, Hatzidaki E. Significance of hypocarbia in the development of periventricular leukomalacia in preterm infants. Pediatr Int 2004;46:268–273.

38. Kubota H, Ohsone Y, Oka F, Sueyoshi T, Takanashi J, Kohno Y. Significance of clinical risk factors of cystic periventricular leukomalacia in infants with different birthweights. Acta Paediatr 2001;90:302–308.

39. Liao SL, Lai SH, Chou YH, Kuo CY. Effect of hypocapnia in the first three days of life on the subsequent development of periventricular leukomalacia in premature infants. Acta Paediatr Taiwan 2001;42:90–93.

40. Okumura A, Hayakawa F, Kato T, et al. Hypocarbia in preterm infants with periventricular leukomalacia: the relation between hypocarbia and mechanical ventilation. Pediatrics 2001;107:469–475.

41. Wiswell TE, Graziani LJ, Kornhauser MS, Stanley C, Merton DA, McKee L, Spitzer AR. Effects of hypocarbia on the development of cystic periventricular leukomalacia in premature infants treated with high-frequency jet ventilation. Pediatrics 1996;98:918–924.

42. Resch B, Jammernegg A, Vollaard E, Maurer U, Mueller WD, Pertl B. Preterm twin gestation and cystic periventricular leucomalacia. Arch Dis Child, Fetal Neonatal Ed 2004;89:F315–F320.

43. Trounce JQ, Shaw DE, Levene MI, Rutter N. Clinical risk factors and periventricular leucomalacia. Arch Dis Child 1988;63:17–22.

44. Hall RW, Kronsberg SS, Barton BA, Sieibert JJ, Anand KJ. Pathways to periventricular leukomalcia: Secondary results from the neopain trial. Pediatr Res 2005;57:A2585.

45. Ikonen RS, Janas MO, Koivikko MJ, Laippala P, Kuusinen EJ. Hyperbilirubinemia, hypocarbia and periventricular leukomalacia in preterm infants: relationship to cerebral palsy. Acta Paediatr 1992;81:802–807.

46. Haverkamp F, Lex C, Hanisch C, Fahnenstich H, Zerres K. Neurodevelopmental risks in twin-to-twin transfusion syndrome: preliminary findings. Eur J Paediatr Neurol 2001;5:21–27.

47. Senat MV, Deprest J, Boulvain M, Paupe A, Winer N, Ville Y. Endoscopic laser surgery versus serial amnioreduction for severe twin-to-twin transfusion syndrome. N Engl J Med 2004;351:136–144.

48. Marumo G, Kozuma S, Ohyu J, et al. Generation of periventricular leukomalacia by repeated umbilical cord occlusion in near-term fetal sheep and its possible pathogenetical mechanisms. Biol Neonate 2001;79:39–45.

49. Ohyu J, Marumo G, Ozawa H, et al. Early axonal and glial pathology in fetal sheep brains with leukomalacia induced by repeated umbilical cord occlusion. Brain & Development 1999;21:248–252.

50. Duncan JR, Cock ML, Scheerlinck JP, Westcott KT, McLean C, Harding R, Rees SM. White matter injury after repeated endotoxin exposure in the preterm ovine fetus. Pediatr Res 2002;52:941–949.

51. Mallard C, Welin AK, Peebles D, Hagberg H, Kjellmer I. White matter injury following systemic endotoxemia or asphyxia in the fetal sheep. Neurochem Res 2003;28:215–223.

52. Hagberg H, Peebles D, Mallard C. Models of white matter injury: Comparison of infectious, hypoxic–ischemic, and excitotoxic insults. Mental Retardation & Developmental Disabilities Research Reviews. 2002;8:30–38.

53. Argyropoulou MI, Xydis V, Drougia A, et al. MRI measurements of the pons and cerebellum in children born preterm; associations with the severity of periventricular leukomalacia and perinatal risk factors. Neuroradiology 2003;45:730–734.

54. Galli KK, Zimmerman RA, Jarvik GP, et al. Periventricular leukomalacia is common after neonatal cardiac surgery. J Thor Cardiovasc Surg 2004;127:692–704.

55. Gaynor JW. Periventricular leukomalacia following neonatal and infant cardiac surgery. Seminars in Thoracic & Cardiovascular Surgery Pediatric Cardiac Surgery Annual 2004;7:133–140.

56. Greisen G, Pryds O. Low CBF, discontinuous EEG activity, and periventricular brain injury in ill, preterm neonates. Brain & Development 1989;11:164–168.

57. Okumura A, Toyota N, Hayakawa F, et al. Cerebral hemodynamics during early neonatal period in preterm infants with periventricular leukomalacia. Brain & Development 2002;24:693–697.

58. Wu YW, Colford Jr JM. Chorioamnionitis as a risk factor for cerebral palsy: a meta-analysis. JAMA 2000;284:1417–1424.

59. Faix RG, Donn SM. Association of septic shock caused by early-onset group b streptococcal sepsis and periventricular leukomalacia in the preterm infant. Pediatrics 1985;76:415–419.

60. Stoll BJ, Hansen NI, Adams-Chapman I, Fanaroff AA, Hintz SR, Vohr B, Higgins RD, and the National Institute of Child Health and Human Development Neonatal Research. Neurodevelopmental and growth impairment among extremely low-birth-weight infants with neonatal infection. JAMA 2004;292:2357–2365.

61. Murphy DJ, Hope PL, Johnson A. Neonatal risk factors for cerebral palsy in very preterm babies: case–control study. BMJ 1997;314:404–408.

62. Msall ME, Buck GM, Rogers BT, Merke DP, Wan CC, Catanzaro NL, Zorn WA. Multivariate risks among extremely premature infants. J Perinatol 1994;14:41–47.

63. Wheater M, Rennie JM. Perinatal infection is an important risk factor for cerebral palsy in very-low-birthweight infants. Dev Med Child Neurol 2000;42:364–367.

64. Tyszczuk L, Meek J, Elwell C, Wyatt JS. Cerebral blood flow is independent of mean arterial blood pressure in preterm infants undergoing intensive care. Pediatrics 1998;102:337–341.

65. Kissack CM, Garr R, Wardle SP, Weindling AM. Cerebral fractional oxygen extraction in very low birth weight infants is high when there is low left ventricular output and hypocarbia but is unaffected by hypotension. Pediatr Res 2004;55:400–405.

66. Kissack CM, Garr R, Wardle SP, Weindling AM. Postnatal changes in cerebral oxygen extraction in the preterm infant are associated with intraventricular hemorrhage and hemorrhagic parenchymal infarction but not periventricular leukomalacia. Pediatr Res 2004;56:111–116.

67. Inder TE, Wells SJ, Mogridge NB, Spencer C, Volpe JJ. Defining the nature of the cerebral abnormalities in the premature infant: a qualitative magnetic resonance imaging study. J Pediatr 2003;143:171–179.

68. Hegyi T, Carbone MT, Anwar M, et al. Blood pressure ranges in premature infants. I. The first hours of life. J Pediatr 1994;124:627–633.

69. Nuntnarumit P, Yang W, Bada-Ellzey HS. Blood pressure measurements in the newborn. Clin Perinatol 1999;26:981–996.

70. Kluckow M, Evans N. Relationship between blood pressure and cardiac output in preterm infants requiring mechanical ventilation. J Pediatr 1996;129:506–512.

71. Lopez SL, Leighton JO, Walther FJ. Supranormal cardiac output in the dopamine- and dobutamine-dependent preterm infant. Pediatr Cardiol 1997;18:292–296.

72. Pladys P, Wodey E, Beuchee A, Branger B, Betremieux P. Left ventricle output and mean arterial blood pressure in preterm infants during the 1st day of life. Eur J Pediatr 1999;158:817–824.

73. Munro MJ, Walker AM, Barfield CP. Hypotensive extremely low birth weight infants have reduced cerebral blood flow. Pediatrics 2004;114:1591–1596.

74. Miall-Allen VM, de Vries LS, Whitelaw AG. Mean arterial blood pressure and neonatal cerebral lesions. Arch Dis Child 1987;62:1068–1069.

75. Hernandes MJ, Brennan RW, Bowman GS. Autoregulation of cerebral blood flow in the newborn dog. Brain Res 1980;184:199–201.

76. Hunt RW, Evans N, Rieger I, Kluckow M. Low superior vena cava flow and neurodevelopment at 3 years in very preterm infants. J Pediatr 2004;145:588–592.

77. Low JA, Froese AB, Galbraith RS, Smith JT, Sauerbrei EE, Derrick EJ. The association between preterm newborn hypotension and hypoxemia and outcome during the first year. Acta Paediatr 1993;82:433–437.

78. Martens SE, Rijken M, Stoelhorst GM, et al. Follow-up project on prematurity TN. Is hypotension a major risk factor for neurological morbidity at term age in very preterm infants? Early Hum Dev 2003;75:79–89.

79. Goldstein RF, Thompson Jr RJ, Oehler JM, Brazy JE. Influence of acidosis, hypoxemia, and hypotension on neurodevelopmental outcome in very low birth weight infants. Pediatrics 1995;95:238–243.

80. Low JA, Froese AB, Smith JT, Galbraith RS, Sauerbrei EE, Karchmar EJ. Hypotension and hypoxemia in the preterm newborn during the four days following delivery identify infants at risk of echosonographically demonstrable cerebral lesions. Clin Invest Med – Medecine Clinique et Experimentale 1992;15:60–65.

81. Lou HC, Lassen NA, Friis-Hansen B. Impaired autoregulation of cerebral blood flow in the distressed newborn infant. J Pediatr 1979;94:118–121.

82. Evans N, Kluckow M, Simmons M, Osborn D. Which to measure, systemic or organ blood flow? Middle cerebral artery and superior vena cava flow in very preterm infants. Arch Dis Child, Fetal Neonatal Ed 2002;87:F181–F184.

83. Evans N, Kluckow M. Early ductal shunting and intraventricular haemorrhage in ventilated preterm infants. Arch Dis Child, Fetal Neonatal Ed 1996;75:F183–F186.

84. Osborn D, Evans N, Kluckow M. Left ventricular contractility in extremely premature infants in the first day and response to inotropes. Pediatr Res 2007;61:335–40.

85. Gaytan Becerril A, Olvera Hidalgo C, Vieto Rodriguez EE, Chavez Angeles DS, Elena Salas M. [Cardiac index, oxygen and serum lactate consumption in infants with hypovolemic and septic shock]. Bol Med Hosp Infant Mex 1980;37:11–22.

86. Osborn DA, Evans N. Early volume expansion versus inotrope for prevention of morbidity and mortality in very preterm infants. Cochrane Database Syst Rev 2001;CD002056.

87. Osborn DA, Evans N. Early volume expansion for prevention of morbidity and mortality in very preterm infants. Cochrane Database Syst Rev 2004;CD002055.

88. Rabe H, Reynolds G, Diaz-Rossello J. Early versus delayed umbilical cord clamping in preterm infants. Cochrane Database Syst Rev 2004;CD003248.

89. Mercer JS, Vohr BR, McGrath MM, Padbury JF, Wallach M, Oh W. Delayed cord clamping in very preterm infants reduces the incidence of intraventricular hemorrhage and late-onset sepsis: a randomized, controlled trial. Pediatrics 2006;117:1235–1242.

90. Fowlie PW, Davis PG. Prophylactic intravenous indomethacin for preventing mortality and morbidity in preterm infants. Cochrane Database Syst Rev 2002;CD000174.

91. Christmann V, Liem KD, Semmekrot BA, van de Bor M. Changes in cerebral, renal and mesenteric blood flow velocity during continuous and bolus infusion of indomethacin. Acta Paediatr 2002;91:440–446.

92. Benders MJ, van de Bor M, van Bel F. Doppler sonographic study of the effect of indomethacin on cardiac and pulmonary hemodynamics of the preterm infant. Eur J Ultrasound 1999;9:107–116.

93. Yanowitz TD, Yao AC, Werner JC, Pettigrew KD, Oh W, Stonestreet BS. Effects of prophylactic low-dose indomethacin on hemodynamics in very low birth weight infants. J Pediatr 1998;132:28–34.

94. Patel J, Roberts I, Azzopardi D, Hamilton P, Edwards AD. Randomized double-blind controlled trial comparing the effects of ibuprofen with indomethacin on cerebral hemodynamics in preterm infants with patent ductus arteriosus. Pediatr Res 2000;47:36–42.

95. Osborn DA, Evans N, Kluckow M. Effect of early targeted indomethacin on the ductus arteriosus and blood flow to the upper body and brain in the preterm infant. Arch Dis Child, Fetal Neonatal Ed 2003;88:F477–F482.

96. Clyman RI. Recommendations for the postnatal use of indomethacin: an analysis of four separate treatment strategies. J Pediatr 1996;128:601–607.

97. Shah SS, Ohlsson A. Ibuprofen for the prevention of patent ductus arteriosus in preterm and/or low birth weight infants. Cochrane Database Syst Rev 2006;CD004213.

98. Mosca F, Bray M, Lattanzio M, Fumagalli M, Tosetto C. Comparative evaluation of the effects of indomethacin and ibuprofen on cerebral perfusion and oxygenation in preterm infants with patent ductus arteriosus. J Pediatr 1997;131:549–554.

99. Romagnoli C, De Carolis MP, Papacci P, et al. Effects of prophylactic ibuprofen on cerebral and renal hemodynamics in very preterm neonates. Clin Pharmacol Ther 2000;67:676–683.

100. Naulaers G, Delanghe G, Allegaert K, et al. Ibuprofen and cerebral oxygenation and circulation. Arch Dis Child, Fetal Neonatal Ed 2005;90:F75–F76.

101. Pezzati M, Vangi V, Biagiotti R, Bertini G, Cianciulli D, Rubaltelli FF. Effects of indomethacin and ibuprofen on mesenteric and renal blood flow in preterm infants with patent ductus arteriosus. J Pediatr 1999;135:733–738.

102. Barr PA, Bailey PE, Sumners J, Cassady G. Relation between arterial blood pressure and blood volume and effect of infused albumin in sick preterm infants. Pediatrics 1977;60:282–289.

103. Bauer K, Linderkamp O, Versmold HT. Systolic blood pressure and blood volume in preterm infants. Arch Dis Child 1993;69:521–522.

104. Pladys P, Wodey E, Betremieux P, Beuchee A, Ecoffey C. Effects of volume expansion on cardiac output in the preterm infant. Acta Paediatr 1997;86:1241–1245.

105. Bignall S, Bailey PC, Bass CA, Cramb R, Rivers RP, Wadsworth J. The cardiovascular and oncotic effects of albumin infusion in premature infants. Early Hum Dev 1989;20:191–201.

106. Van Marter LJ, Leviton A, Allred EN, Pagano M, Kuban KC. Hydration during the first days of life and the risk of bronchopulmonary dysplasia in low birth weight infants. J Pediatr 1990;116:942–949.

107. Alderson P, Bunn F, Lefebvre C, Li WP, Li L, Roberts I, Schierhout G, Albumin R. Human albumin solution for resuscitation and volume expansion in critically ill patients. Cochrane Database Syst Rev 2004;CD001208.

108. Finfer S, Bellomo R, Boyce N, French J, Myburgh J, Norton R, Investigators SS. A comparison of albumin and saline for fluid resuscitation in the intensive care unit. N Engl J Med 2004;350:2247–2256.

109. So KW, Fok TF, Ng PC, Wong WW, Cheung KL. Randomised controlled trial of colloid or crystalloid in hypotensive preterm infants. Arch Dis Child, Fetal Neonatal Ed 1997;76:F43–F46.

110. Lynch SK, Stone CS, Graeber J, Polak MJ. Colloid vs. cystalloid therapy for hypotension in neonates. Pediatr Res 2002;51:384A.

111. Emery EF, Greenough A, Gamsu HR. Randomised controlled trial of colloid infusions in hypotensive preterm infants. Arch Dis Child 1992;67:1185–1188.

112. Oca MJ, Nelson M, Donn SM. Randomized trial of normal saline versus 5% albumin for the treatment of neonatal hypotension. J Perinatol 2003;23:473–476.

113. Gill AB, Weindling AM. Randomised controlled trial of plasma protein fraction versus dopamine in hypotensive very low birthweight infants. Arch Dis Child 1993;69:284–287.

114. Osborn D, Evans N, Kluckow M. Randomized trial of dobutamine versus dopamine in preterm infants with low systemic blood flow. J Pediatr 2002;140:183–191.

115. Seri I, Evans J. Controversies in the diagnosis and management of hypotension in the newborn infant. Curr Opin Pediatr 2001;13:116–123.

116. Seri I. Circulatory support of the sick preterm infant. Semin Neonatol 2001;6:85–95.

117. Friedman WF, Pool PE, Jacobowitz D, Seagren SC, Braunwald E. Sympathetic innervation of the developing rabbit heart. Biochemical and histochemical comparisons of fetal, neonatal, and adult myocardium. Circ Res 1968;23:25–32.

118. Seri I. Cardiovascular, renal and endocrine actions of dopamine in neonates and children. J Pediatr 1995;126:333–344.

119. Gill AB, Weindling AM. Echocardiographic assessment of cardiac function in shocked very low birthweight infants. Arch Dis Child 1993;68:17–21.

120. Dempsey EM, Barrington KJ. Diagnostic criteria and therapeutic interventions for the hypotensive very low birth weight infant. J Perinatol 2006;26:677–681.

121. Barrington K, Chan W. The circulatory effects of epinephrine infusion in the anesthesized piglet. Pediatr Res 1993;33:190–194.

122. Barrington KJ, Finer NN, Chan WK. A blind, randomized comparison of the circulatory effects of dopamine and epinephrine infusions in the newborn piglet during normoxia and hypoxia. Crit Care Med 1995;23:740–748.

123. Heckmann M, Trotter A, Pohlandt F, Lindner W. Epinephrine treatment of hypotension in very low birthweight infants. Acta Paediatr 2002;91:566–570.

124. Pellicer A, Valverde E, Elorza MD, Madero R, Gaya F, Quero J, Cabanas F. Cardiovascular support for low birth weight infants and cerebral hemodynamics: a randomized, blinded, clinical trial. Pediatrics 2005;115:1501–1512.

125. Noori, S, Friedlich P, Wong P, Ebrahimi M, Siassi B, Seri I. Hemodynamic changes following low-dose hydrocortisone administration in vasopressor-treated neonates. Pediatrics 2006;118:1456–1466.

126. Cuevas L, Yeh TF, John EG, Cuevas D, Plides RS. The effect of low-dose dopamine infusion on cardiopulmonary and renal status in premature newborns with respiratory distress syndrome. Am J Dis Child 1991;145:799–803.

127. Lundstrom K, Pryds O, Greisen G. The haemodynamic effects of dopamine and volume expansion in sick preterm infants. Early Hum Dev 2000;57:157–163.

128. Barrington K, Brion LP. Dopamine versus no treatment to prevent renal dysfunction in indomethacin-treated preterm newborn infants. Cochrane Database Syst Rev 2002;CD003213.

129. DiSessa TG, Leitner M, Ti CC, Gluck L, Coen R, Friedman WF. The cardiovascular effects of dopamine in the severely asphyxiated neonate. J Pediatr 1981;99:772–776.

130. Perez CA, Reimer JM, Schreiber MD, Warburton D, Gregory GA. Effect of high-dose dopamine on urine output in newborn infants. Crit Care Med 1986;14:1045–1049.

131. Ruffolo Jr RR, Spradlin TA, Pollock GD, Waddell JE, Murphy PJ. Alpha and beta adrenergic effects of the stereoisomers of dobutamine. J Pharmacol Exp Ther 1981;219:447–452.

132. Devictor D, Verlhac S, Pariente D, Huault G. [Hemodynamic effects of dobutamine in asphyxiated newborn infants]. Arch Fr Pediatr 1988:45:467–470.

133. Martinez AM, Padbury JF, Thio S. Dobutamine pharmacokinetics and cardiovascular responses in critically ill neonates. Pediatrics 1992;89:47–51.

134. Stopfkuchen H, Schranz D, Huth R, Jungst BK. Effects of dobutamine on left ventricular performance in newborns as determined by systolic time intervals. Eur J Pediatr 1987;146:135–139.

135. Driscoll DJ, Gillette PC, Lewis RM, Hartley CJ, Schwartz A. Comparative hemodynamic effects of isoproterenol, dopamine, and dobutamine in the newborn dog. Pediatr Res 1979;13:1006–1009.

136. Deloof E, Devlieger H, Van Hoestenberghe R, Van den berghe K, Daenen W, Gewillig M. Management with a staged approach of the premature hydropic fetus due to complete congenital heart block. Eur J Pediatr 1997;156:521–523.

137. Kantoch MJ, Qurashi MM, Bulbul ZR, Gorgels AP. A newborn with a complex congenital heart disease, atrioventricular block, and torsade de pointes ventricular tachycardia. Pacing Clin Electrophysiol 1998;21:2664–2667.

138. Liu YL. [Isoproterenol in the treatment of fulminating meningococcemia in children complicated by shock. An analysis of 181 cases]. Zhonghua Yi Xue Za Zhi 1974;214:766–770.

139. Quek SC, Low KT, Sim EK, Joseph R. A case report on the perinatal management of a 30-week preterm baby with congenital complete heart block. Ann Acad Med Singapore 2000;29:510–513.

140. Wood DW, Downes JJ, Scheinkopf H, Lecks HI. Intravenous isoproterenol in the management of respiratory failure in childhood status asthmaticus. J Allergy Clin Immunol 1972;50:75–81.

141. Drummond WH. Use of cardiotonic therapy in the management of infants with pphn. Clin Perinatol 1984;11:715–728.

142. Kulik TJ, Lock JE. Pulmonary vasodilator therapy in persistent pulmonary hypertension of the newborn. Clin Perinatol 1984;11:693–701.

143. Derleth DP. Clinical experience with norepinephrine infusions in critically ill newborns. Pediatr Res 1997;41:145A.

144. Greenough A, Emery EF. Randomized trial comparing dopamine and dobutamine in preterm infants. Eur J Pediatr 1993;152:925–927.

145. Hentschel R, Hensel D, Brune T, Rabe H, Jorch G. Impact on blood pressure and intestinal perfusion of dobutamine or dopamine in hypotensive preterm infants. Biol Neonate 1995;68:318–324.

146. Klarr JM, Faix RG, Pryce CJ, Bhatt-Mehta V. Randomized, blind trial of dopamine versus dobutamine for treatment of hypotension in preterm infants with respiratory distress syndrome. J Pediatr 1994;125:117–122.

147. Miall-Allen VM, Whitelaw AG. Response to dopamine and dobutamine in the preterm infant less than 30 weeks gestation. Crit Care Med 1989;17:1166–1169.

148. Roze JC, Tohier C, Maingueneau C, Lefevre M, Mouzard A. Response to dobutamine and dopamine in the hypotensive very preterm infant. Arch Dis Child 1993;69:59–63.

149. Ruelas-Orozco G, Vargas-Origel A. Assessment of therapy for arterial hypotension in critically ill preterm infants. Am J Perinatol 2000;17:95–99.

150. Phillipos EZ, Robertson MA. A randomized double blinded controlled trial of dopamine vs epinephrine for inotropic support in premature infants < 1750 grams. Pediatr Res 2000;47:425A.

151. Valverde E, Pellicer A, Madero R, Elorza D, Quero J, Cabanas F. Dopamine versus epinephrine for cardiovascular support in low birth weight infants: analysis of systemic effects and neonatal clinical outcomes. Pediatrics 2006;117:e1213–e1222.

152. Klitzner TS, Shapir Y, Ravin R, Friedman WF. The biphasic effect of amrinone on tension development in newborn mammalian myocardium. Pediatr Res 1990;27:144.

153. Binah O, Legato MJ, et al. Developmental changes in the cardiac effects of amrinone in the dog. Circ Res 1983;52:747–752.

154. Akita T, Joyner RW, Lu C, Kumar R, Hartzell HC. Developmental changes in modulation of calcium currents of rabbit ventricular cells by phosphodiesterase inhibitors. Circulation 1994;90:469–78.

155. Paradisis M, Evans N, Kluckow M, Osborn D, McLachlan AJ. Pilot study of milrinone for low systemic blood flow in very preterm infants. J Pediatr 2006;148:306–313.

156. Paradisis M, Jiang X, McLachlan AJ, Evans N, Kluckow M, Osborn D. Population pharmacokinetics and dosing regimen design of milrinone in preterm infants. Arch Dis Child, Fetal Neonatal Ed 2007;92:204–209.

157. Paradisis M, Evans NJ, Kluckow MR, Osborn DA. Randomized trial of milrinone versus placebo for prevention of low systemic blood flow in very preterm infants. Pediatr Res 2007. Abstract 752932.

158. Roberts D, Dalziel S. Antenatal corticosteroids for accelerating fetal lung maturation for women at risk of preterm birth. Cochrane Database Syst Rev 2006;3:CD004454.

159. Moise AA, Wearden ME, Kozinetz CA, Gest AL, Welty SE, Hansen TN. Antenatal steroids are associated with less need for blood pressure support in extremely premature infants. Pediatrics 1995;95:845–850.

160. Efird MM, Heerens AT, Gordon PV, Bose CL, Young DA. A randomized-controlled trial of prophylactic hydrocortisone supplementation for the prevention of hypotension in extremely low birth weight infants. J Perinatol 2005;25:119–124.

161. Gaissmaier RE, Pohlandt F. Single-dose dexamethasone treatment of hypotension in preterm infants. J Pediatr 1999;134:701–705.

162. Gerstmann D,S.M, Stoddard R, et al. Cardiovascular instability (cvi) in ventilated neonates: a double-blind controlled trial of hydrocortisone supplementation. Pediatr Res 1998;43:198A.

163. Osiovich H, Phillipos EZ, Lemke RP. A short course of hydrocortisone in hypotensive neonates < 1250 g in the first 24 hours of life:A randomized, double blind controlled trial. Pediatr Res 2000;47:422A.

164. Ng PC, Lee CH, Bnur FL, Chan IH, Lee AW, Wong E, Chan HB, Lam CW, Lee BS, Fok TF. A double-blind, randomized, controlled study of a "stress dose" of hydrocortisone for rescue treatment of refractory hypotension in preterm infants. Pediatrics 2006;117:367–375.

165. Halliday HL, Ehrenkranz RA, Doyle LW. Early postnatal (< 96 hours) corticosteroids for preventing chronic lung disease in preterm infants. Cochrane Database Syst Rev 2003;CD001146.

166. Evans N. Cardiovascular effects of dexamethasone in the preterm infant. Arch Dis Child, Fetal Neonatal Ed 1994;70:F25–F30.

167. Bourchier D, Weston PJ. Randomised trial of dopamine compared with hydrocortisone for the treatment of hypotensive very low birthweight infants. Arch Dis Child, Fetal Neonatal Ed 1997;76:F174–F178.

168. Subhedar NV, Shaw NJ. Changes in oxygenation and pulmonary haemodynamics in preterm infants treated with inhaled nitric oxide. Arch Dis Child, Fetal Neonatal Ed 1997;77:F191–F197.

169. Desandes R, Desandes E, Droulle P, Didier F, Longrois D, Hascoet JM. Inhaled nitric oxide improves oxygenation in very premature infants with low pulmonary blood flow. Acta Paediatr 2004;93:66–69.

170. Barrington KJ, Finer N. Inhaled nitric oxide for respiratory failure in preterm infants. Cochrane Database Syst Rev 2006CD000509.

171. Ballard RA, Truog WE, Cnaan A, et al. Inhaled nitric oxide in preterm infants undergoing mechanical ventilation. N Engl J Med 2006;355:343–353.

172. Kinsella JP, Cutter GR, Walsh WF, et al. Early inhaled nitric oxide therapy in premature newborns with respiratory failure. N Engl J Med 2006;355:354–364.

173. Subhedar NV, Ryan SW, Shaw NJ. Open randomised controlled trial of inhaled nitric oxide and early dexamethasone in high risk preterm infants. Arch Dis Child, Fetal Neonatal Ed 1997;77:F185–F190.

174. Schreiber MD, Gin-Mestan K, Marks JD, Huo D, Lee G, Srisuparp P. Inhaled nitric oxide in premature infants with the respiratory distress syndrome. N Engl J Med 2003;349:2099–2107.

175. Field D, Elbourne D, Truesdale A, et al. Neonatal ventilation with inhaled nitric oxide versus ventilatory support without inhaled nitric oxide for preterm infants with severe respiratory failure: the innovo multicentre randomised controlled trial. Pediatrics 2005;115:926–936.

176. Hascoet JM, Fresson J, Claris O, et al. The safety and efficacy of nitric oxide therapy in premature infants. J Pediatr 2005;146:318–323.

177. Kinsella JP, Walsh WF, Bose CL, et al. Inhaled nitric oxide in premature neonates with severe hypoxaemic respiratory failure: A randomised controlled trial. Lancet 1999;354:1061–1065.

178. NINOS. Early compared with delayed inhaled nitric oxide in moderately hypoxaemic neonates with respiratory failure: a randomised controlled trial. The Franco-Belgium collaborative no trial group. Lancet 1999;354:1066–1071.

179. Van Meurs KP, Wright LL, Ehrenkranz RA, et al. Inhaled nitric oxide for premature infants with severe respiratory failure. N Engl J Med 2005;353:13–22.

180. Evans N, Kluckow M, Currie A. Range of echocardiographic findings in term neonates with high oxygen requirements. Arch Dis Child, Fetal Neonatal Ed 1998;78:F105–F111.

181. Van Bel F, Walther FJ. Myocardial dysfunction and cerebral blood flow velocity following birth asphyxia. Acta Paediatr Scand 1990;79:756–762.

182. Kecskes Z, Kent A, Reynolds G. Treatment of pulmonary hypertension with Sildenafil in a neonate with spondyloepiphyseal dysplasia congenita. J Matern Fetal Neonatal Med 2006;19:579–582.

183. Evans N. Volume expansion during neonatal intensive care: Do we know what we are doing? Semin Neonatol 2003;8:315–323.

184. Lokesh L, Kumar P, Murki S, Narang A. A randomized controlled trial of sodium bicarbonate in neonatal resuscitation-effect on immediate outcome. Resuscitation 2004;60:219–223.

185. Walther FJ, Siassi B, Ramadan NA, Wu PY. Cardiac output in newborn infants with transient myocardial dysfunction. J Pediatr 1985;107:781–785.

186. Evans N, Kluckow M. Early determinants of right and left ventricular output in ventilated preterm infants. Arch Dis Child, Fetal Neonatal Ed 1996;74:F88–F94.

187. Finer NN, Barrington KJ. Nitric oxide for respiratory failure in infants born at or near term. Cochrane Database Syst Rev 2006;CD000399.

188. Baquero H, Soliz A, Neira F, Venegas ME, Sola A. Oral sildenafil in infants with persistent pulmonary hypertension of the newborn: a pilot randomized blinded study. Pediatrics 2006;117:1077–1083.

189. Fiddler GI, Chatrath R, Williams GJ, Walker DR, Scott O. Dopamine infusion for the treatment of myocardial dysfunction associated with a persistent transitional circulation. Arch Dis Child 1980;55:194–198.

190. McNamara PJ, Laique F, Muang-In S, Whyte HE. Milrinone improves oxygenation in neonates with severe persistent pulmonary hypertension of the newborn. J Crit Care 2006;21:217–222.

191. Ostrea EM, Villanueva-Uy ET, Natarajan G, Uy HG. Persistent pulmonary hypertension of the newborn: Pathogenesis, etiology, and management. Paediatr Drugs 2006;8:179–188.

192. Sparrow A, Willis F. Management of septic shock in childhood. Emerg Med Australas 2004;16:125–134.

193. Carcillo JA, Fields AI. Clinical practice parameters for hemodynamic support of pediatric and neonatal patients in septic shock. Crit Care Med 2002;30:1365–1378.

194. Rivers E, Nguyen B, Havstad S, et al. Early goal-directed therapy in the treatment of severe sepsis and septic shock. N Engl J Med 2001;345:1368–1377.

195. Han YY, Carcillo JA, Dragotta MA, Bills DM, Watson RS, Westerman ME, Orr RA. Early reversal of pediatric–neonatal septic shock by community physicians is associated with improved outcome. Pediatrics 2003;112:793–799.

196. Haque K, Mohan P. Pentoxifylline for neonatal sepsis. Cochrane Database Syst Rev 2003;CD004205.

197. Lauterbach R, Zembala M. Pentoxifylline reduces plasma tumour necrosis factor-alpha concentration in premature infants with sepsis. Eur J Pediatr 1996;155:404–409.

198. Lauterbach R, Pawlik D, Kowalczyk D, Ksycinski W, Helwich E, Zembala M. Effect of the immunomodulating agent, pentoxifylline, in the treatment of sepsis in prematurely delivered infants: a placebo-controlled, double-blind trial. Crit Care Med 1999;27:807–814.

199. Gronlund JU, Korvenranta H, Kero P, Jalonen J, Valimaki IA. Elevated arterial blood pressure is associated with peri-intraventricular haemorrhage. Eur J Pediatr 1994;153:836–841.

200. Inder TE, Warfield SK, Wang H, Huppi PS, Volpe JJ. Abnormal cerebral structure is present at term in premature infants. Pediatrics 2005;115:286–294.

201. Bejar RF, Vaucher YE, Benirschke K, Berry CC. Postnatal white matter necrosis in preterm infants. J Perinatol 1992;12:3–8.

202. Cunningham S, Symon AG, Elton RA, Zhu C, McIntosh N. Intra-arterial blood pressure reference ranges, death and morbidity in very low birthweight infants during the first seven days of life. Early Hum Dev 1999;56:151–165.

203. D'Souza SW, Janakova H, Minors D, et al. Blood pressure, heart rate, and skin temperature in preterm infants: associations with periventricular haemorrhage. Arch Dis Child, Fetal Neonatal Ed 1995;72:F162–F167.

204. Watkins AM, West CR, Cooke RW. Blood pressure and cerebral haemorrhage and ischaemia in very low birthweight infants. Early Hum Dev 1989;19:103–110.

205. Weindling AM, Wilkinson AR, Cook J, Calvert SA, Fok TF, Rochefort MJ. Perinatal events which precede periventricular haemorrhage and leukomalacia in the newborn. BJOG 1985;92:1218–1223.

206. Dammann O, Allred EN, Kuban KC, Van Marter LJ, Pagano M, Sanocka U, Leviton A, Developmental epidemiology N. Systemic hypotension and white-matter damage in preterm infants. Dev Med Child Neurol 2002;44:82–90.

207. de Vries LS, Regev R, Dubowitz LM, Whitelaw A, Aber VR. Perinatal risk factors for the development of extensive cystic leukomalacia. Am J Dis Child 1988;142:732–735.

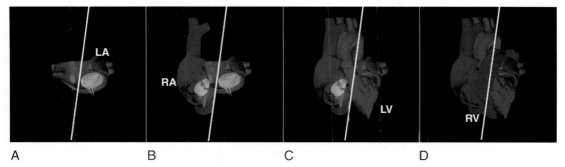

A   B   C   D

FIGURE 5-1 These four frames show the chambers of the heart being progressively added from back to front. The white line shows where the ultrasound beam will transect the heart. (A) The left atrium (LA) at the back of heart with two pulmonary veins coming in each side posteriorly. (B) The right atrium (RA), which is to the right and slightly in front of the LA. (C) The endocardial surface of the left ventricle (LV), which receives blood towards the apex through the mitral valve and ejects it into the ascending aorta, which runs towards the right shoulder in front of the LA. (D) The anterior nature of the right ventricle, which wraps in front of the LV outflow tract before ejecting blood posteriorly into the pulmonary artery.

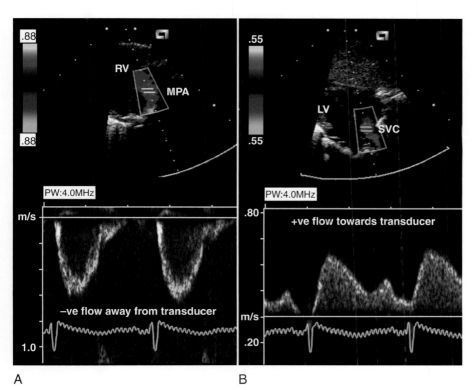

A   B

FIGURE 5-4 Pulsed Doppler assesses flow velocity at a defined location (= sign on 2-D image). Flow away from the transducer is negative (A) and towards the transducer positive (B). Color Doppler maps those signals onto the 2-D image with flow away coded blue (A) and towards coded red (B).

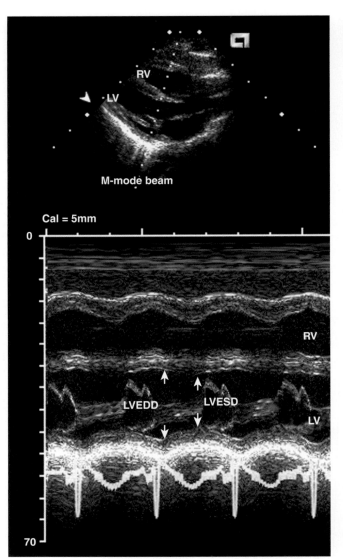

Cal = 5mm

FIGURE 5-3 M-mode plots the ultrasound signals from the single beam (shown on a 2-D image) against time. This allows movement and dimensions to be more accurately measured. The LV end diastolic diameter (LVEDD) and LV end systolic diameter (LVESD) are shown.

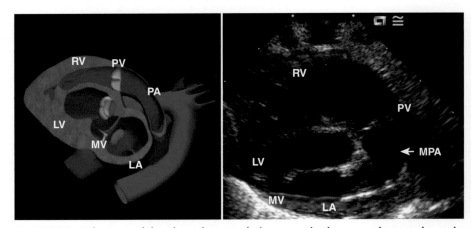

FIGURE 5-2 A heart model and an ultrasound picture cut in the same plane as shown in Fig. 5-1. The RV is seen at the front connecting with the posteriorly directed pulmonary artery. Behind the RV is the LV outflow tract and the LA and mitral valve.

FIGURE 5-5 A model of the heart viewed from the left-hand side. It can be seen that the ductus arteriosus is a continuation of the pulmonary artery and describes an arch into the descending aorta. It is slightly offset to the left reflecting the need to connect with the left-sided descending aorta.

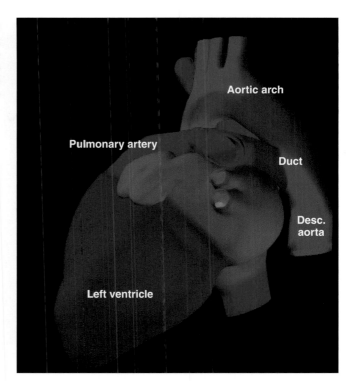

FIGURE 5-6 A 2-D image of a patent duct adjacent to the root of the left pulmonary artery, which is seen this section as a diverticulum inferior to the duct. The duct describes an arch that is in continuity with the anterior wall of the main pulmonary artery.

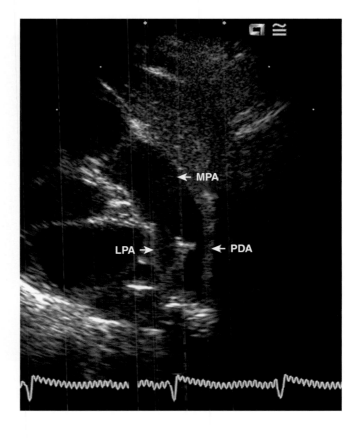

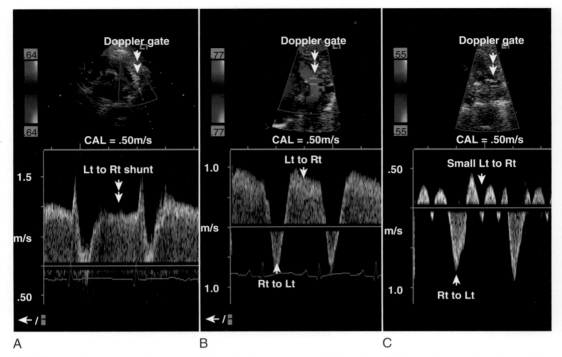

FIGURE 5-8 The range of pattern of ductal shunt on pulsed Doppler. (A) Shows the positive (towards the transducer) trace of a pure left to right shunt. (B) Shows a bidirectional shunt with both left to right (positive) and right to left (negative) components. (C) Shows a predominantly right to left (negative) shunt but with some left to right shunt in diastole. Pure right to left ductal shunts are uncommon.

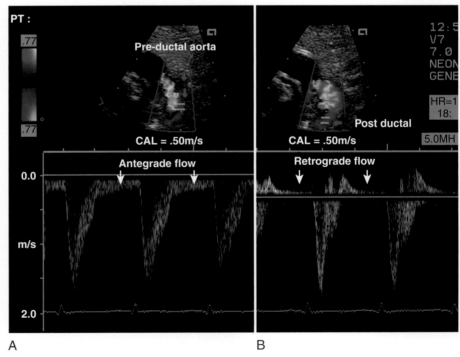

FIGURE 5-9 Compares the normal forward diastolic flow (A), which is also seen with a Patent ductus arferiosus (PDA) in the pre-ductal aorta with the retrograde diastolic flow seen in the post ductal aorta in the presence of a significant PDA.

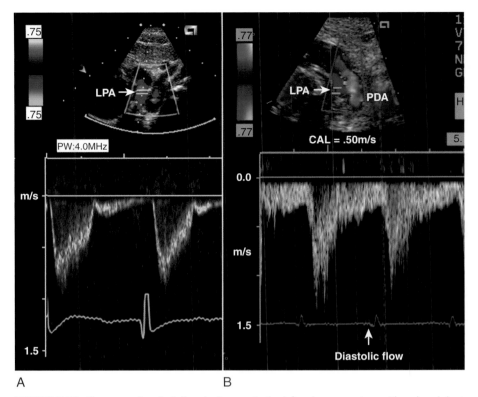

A   B

FIGURE 5-10 Compares the diastolic velocity seen in the left pulmonary artery with a closed duct with the increased diastolic velocity (in this case 0.5 m/s) seen with a significant PDA.

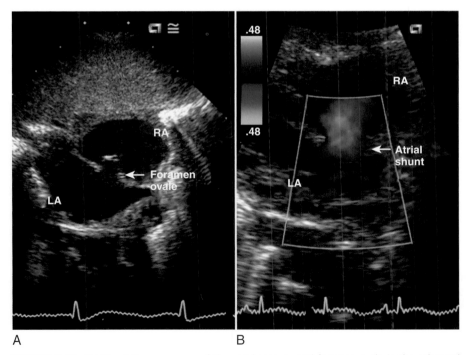

A   B

FIGURE 5-11 (A) The 2-D appearance of the atrial septum and foramen ovale in the subcostal four chamber view. (B) The color Doppler of a left to right shunt through an incompetent foramen ovale.

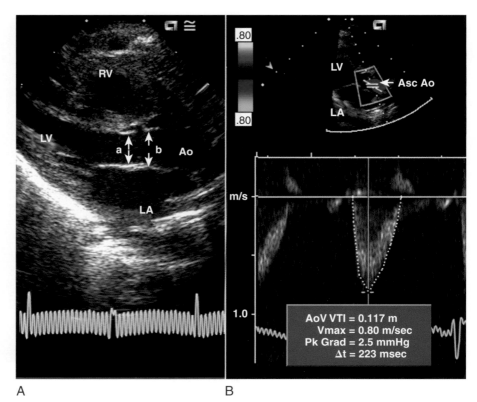

FIGURE 5-15 (A) Shows the site of measurement of aortic diameter. Some authors recommend measurement of valve ring or leaflet separation (a); we usually use the internal diameter beyond the coronary sinus (b). (B) Shows pulsed Doppler assessment of ascending aortic velocity from the apical long axis view. Velocity time integral (VTI) is derived by tracing around the systolic spectral envelope (VTI = 0.117 m in this case).

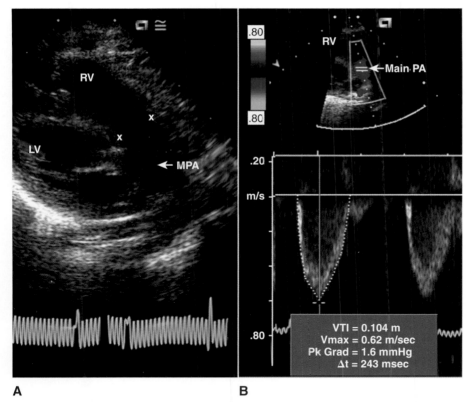

FIGURE 5-17 (A) Shows the site of measurement of pulmonary artery diameter, in end-systole at the valve hinge points. (B) Shows pulsed Doppler assessment of main pulmonary artery velocity with the range gate just beyond the valve. Velocity time integral (VTI) is derived by tracing around the systolic spectral envelope (VTI = 0.104 m in this case).

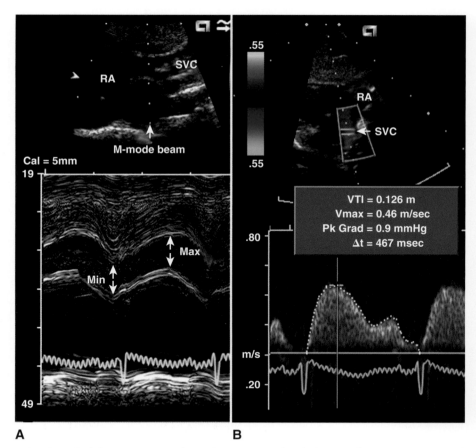

A

B

FIGURE 5-18 (A) Measurement of superior vena cava (SVC) diameter from a mid-parasternal sagittal view. The M-mode beam is dropped through the SVC at the point that is starts to funnel out into the RA. Diameter is averaged from a maximum (max) and minimum (min) diameter. (B) Pulsed Doppler assessment of SVC velocity from a low subcostal view. Velocity time integral (VTI) is derived by tracing around the systolic spectral envelope including any negative trace if present (VTI = 0.126 m in this case).

FIGURE 5-20 Shows the normal neonatal pulsed Doppler velocity trace of mitral valve flow that is used to measure diastolic function. The E-wave represents early filling due to active ventricular relaxation while the A-wave represents filling due to atrial systole. Act E-wave shows the acceleration time of early diastolic filling.

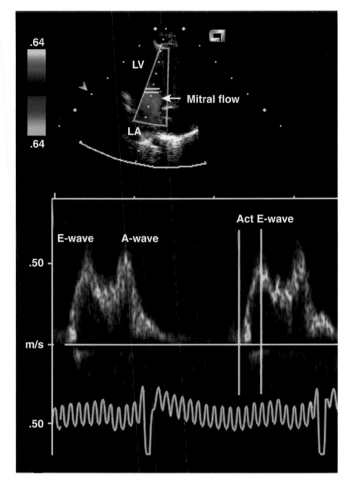

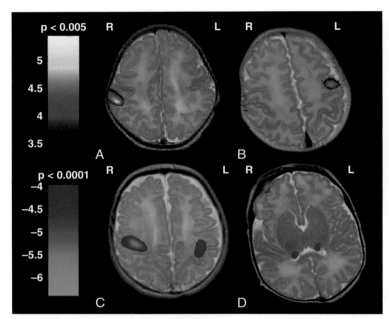

FIGURE 7-7 **Changes in sensorimotor areas and thalamus from passive extension and flexion stimulation.** (A) Contralateral activation from left-hand stimulation of a 40-week gestation female (at 42-week postmenstrual age) newborn. (B) Right-hand stimulation of a 26-week gestation female (at 39-week postmenstrual age) newborn. Findings are comparable to adult results for sensorimotor activation. (C) Bi-hemispheric BOLD changes (36.4% during left-hand task and 31.3% during right hand of the population), which are unique for the newborn. Bilateral deactivation in a 40-week gestational age male (at 43 weeks postmenstrual age) newborn from left-hand stimulation. Additional significant BOLD changes have been found in frontal lobe and thalamus (41.7% of the population). (D) Thalamic deactivation in both hemispheres in a 39-week gestational age male (at 42 weeks postmenstrual age) newborn from left-hand stimulation.

Section V

Cardiology

Chapter 14

Prevalence of Congenital Heart Disease

Joel I. Brenner, MD

Introduction
Prevalence of CCVM
Prevalence of HLH
Impact of Prenatal Diagnosis
Conclusion
References

INTRODUCTION

Technological advancement has played a vital role in the maturation of the field of pediatric cardiology. Description of congenital cardiac malformations (CCVM) has moved from the anatomic pathology laboratory of the first half of the twentieth century to the cardiac catheterization laboratory, the echocardiographic laboratory, and now to the molecular biology laboratory. Indeed, concepts about the nature of cardiac malformations and understanding of the etiologic mechanisms of CCVM have progressed during this evolution. Along with tools permitting more precise, invasive, and now non-invasive diagnosis of anatomic detail has come an evolution in the cultural attitudes about the provision of medical care to *all* infants and children, even those with complex, noncardiac birth defects and many of those with non-lethal chromosomal abnormalities.

The next element which made recognition of potentially life-threatening CCVM vital was the ability to alter the natural history of serious malformations, which had hitherto led to progressive disability and premature death. The advent of the palliative Blalock–Taussig shunt, in 1945, opened an era of therapeutic intervention leading to open-heart surgical repair of even the most complex lesions in children and now in infants as well. The last element in this evolution is the process of understanding the genetic and environmental factors which contribute to the phenotypic expression of cardiac malformations and other birth defects. This last frontier enlivens the hope of clinicians and scientists alike, for with this understanding comes the ability to prevent CCVM, the most common of birth defects and the largest contributor to infant mortality caused by birth defects.

PREVALENCE OF CCVM

It is in this context that the concept of prevalence of CCVM can best be understood. To be optimal both the *numerator* (those with the disease of interest) and the *denominator* (the entire cohort) have to be carefully defined and meticulously in particular genetic factors that may play an important role in the evaluation and management of the patient *and* the family. The finding of cardiac disease, even the most straightforward lesion, may have implications for the nuclear and extended family unit. Collaboration between obstetricians, pediatric cardiologists, and geneticists will continue to enlighten our appreciation of the complexity of the phenotypic expression of CCVM and offer the possibility of genotypic identification and, ultimately, prevention of this most common birth defect.

REFERENCES

1. Mitchell SC, Sellman AH, Westphal MC, Park J. Etiologic correlates in a study of congenital heart disease in 56, 109 births. Am J Cardiol 1971;28:637–653.
2. Fyler DC. Report of the New England Regional Infant Cardiac Program. Pediatrics 1980;65(suppl):375–461.
3. Fixler DE, Pastor P, Chamberlin M, Sigman E, Eifler CW. Trends in congenital heart disease in Dallas county births, 1971–1984. Circulation 1990;81:137–142.
4. Rubin JD, Ferencz C, Brenner JI, Neill CA, Perry LW. Early detection of congenital cardiovascular malformations in infancy. AJDC 1987;141:1218–1220.
5. Ferencz C, Loffredo CA, Magee CA. Epidemiology of Congenital Heart Disease: The Baltimore–Washington Infant Study, 1981–1989. Mt Kisko, NY: Futura, 1993.
6. Ferencz C, Loffredo CA, Correa-Villasenor A, Wilson PD. Genetic and environmental risk factors of Major Cardiovascular Malformations: the Baltimore-Washington Infant Study, 1981–1989. Armonk, NY: Futura, 1997.
7. Martin GR, Perry LW, Ferencz C. Increased prevalence of ventricular septal defect: epidemic or improved diagnosis? Pediatrics 1989;83:200–203.
8. Lurie IW, Ferencz C, Brenner JI. Heart disease in infancy: a window to the world of fetal cardiology. Progress in Pediatric Cardiology 1996;5:73–78.
9. Forrester MB, Merz RD. Descriptive epidemiology of selected congenital heart defects, Hawaii, 1986–1999. Paediatr Perinat Epidemiol, 2004;18:415–424.
10. Goldmuntz E. The genetic contribution to congenital heart disease. In Wernovsky G, ed. From fetus to Young Adult: Contemporary Topics in Pediatric Cardiovascular Disease. Pediatric Clinics of North America. Elsevier Saunders 2004;51:1721–1737.
11. Belmont JW, Mohapatra B, Towbin JA, Ware SM. Molecular genetics of heterotaxy syndrome. Curr Opin Cardiol 2004;19:216–220.
12. Megarbane A, Salem N, Stephan E, Ashoush R, Lenoir D, et al. X-linked transposition of the great arteries and incomplete penetrance among males with a nonsense mutation in ZIC3. Eur J Hum Genet 2000;8:704–708.
13. Wilson DI, Burn J, Scambler P, Goodship J. DiGeorge Syndrome: part of CATCH 22. J. Med Genet 1993;30:852–856.
14. Brenner JI, Berg KA, Schneider DS, Clark EB, Boughman JA. Cardiac malformations in relatives of infants with hypoplastic left-heart syndrome. AJDC 1989;143:1492–1494.
15. Loffredo CA, Chokkalingam A, Sill AM, Boughman JA, Clark EB, Scheel J, Brenner JI. Prevalence of congenital cardiovascular malformations among relatives of infants with hypoplastic left heart, coarctation of the aorta, and d-transposition of the great arteries. Am J Med Genet 2004;123:225–230.
16. Cripe L, Andelfinger G, Martin LJ, Shooner K, Benson DW. Bicuspid aortic valve is heritable. J Am Coll Cardiol 2004;44:138–143.

Chapter 15

Impact of Congenital Heart Disease and Surgical Intervention on Neurodevelopment

Mary T. Donofrio, MD, FAAP, FACC, FASE

INTRODUCTION

Congenital heart disease occurs in five to eight per 1000 live births (1), making it a significant cause of childhood morbidity and mortality. With improvements in cardiac surgical techniques and postoperative intensive care over the last two decades, most babies with congenital heart disease today will survive; however, a significant percentage of these infants may have multiple handicaps, either related to associated birth defects or to neurodevelopmental compromise. Attention has now turned to the potential for neurologic injury during the surgical repair or palliation, in which cerebral perfusion may be compromised during cardiopulmonary bypass and deep hypothermic circulatory arrest. The issue at hand is to determine how much of observed impairment in neurodevelopmental outcome is related to congenital neurologic defects or to prolonged cyanosis after birth and how much is related to potential insult during the operative procedure. Recent studies suggest that blood flow and altered oxygen delivery in fetuses and newborns with congenital heart disease may have an important impact on the development of the brain and central nervous system.

This chapter will review the following topics.

- Intrauterine growth, neurodevelopment, and cerebral blood flow autoregulation in fetuses with congenital heart disease.

- Congenital brain abnormalities and abnormal neurologic findings in babies with heart disease.
- Intraoperative cerebral monitoring during surgery for congenital heart disease.
- Effects of surgical intervention on cerebral perfusion.
- Neurodevelopmental outcome after surgical repair of congenital heart disease.

INTRAUTERINE FACTORS WHICH AFFECT DEVELOPMENT

Somatic Intrauterine Growth in Fetuses with Congenital Heart Disease

The association of complex congenital heart disease with intrauterine growth retardation is well established (2–13). The etiology of this finding is speculative, although two theories have been proposed. First, fetuses with altered growth may have an increased risk of developing cardiac abnormalities (6). Second, and perhaps more likely, the altered circulation that occurs as a result of the specific structural cardiac abnormality can lead to flow disturbances which may affect normal growth (2–5). In 1972, the concept that intrauterine blood flow is altered in the presence of congenital heart disease was introduced (2). In 1995, supporting biometric data from a regional, population-based, case-controlled study that tracked infants with congenital heart disease was published (5). Birth weights, lengths, and head circumferences were compared between infants with specific congenital heart defects and matched control subjects. The study demonstrated that infants with transposition of the great arteries (TGA) had normal birth weights, but small head circumferences relative to birth weight. Newborns with hypoplastic left heart (HLH) syndrome had birth weights, lengths, and head circumferences that were less than normal, and had head volumes that were disproportionately small relative to birth weight. Finally, infants with tetralogy of Fallot had normal proportions, but birth weights, lengths, and head circumferences that were less than normal. The authors (5) theorized that the circulatory abnormalities created by the anatomic cardiac defects likely caused the alterations in intrauterine growth and neurodevelopment.

Blood Flow Characteristics in Normal and Compromised Fetuses

Fetal lamb studies (4) have shown that right ventricular output is twice left ventricular output, and oxygen saturation of blood delivered to the cerebral circulation is higher than that delivered to the body through the ductus arteriosus. Deoxygenated blood from the superior vena cava is directed into the right ventricle, across the ductus arteriosus, and to the placenta. The Eustachian valve and atrial septum move together to direct deoxygenated blood from the hepatic inferior vena cava into the right ventricle, and oxygenated blood from the ductus venosus across the foramen ovale, through the left ventricle, to the aorta and cerebral circulation. In the human fetus, the path the blood takes through the heart is identical. Right ventricular output is greater than left, though the difference is not as substantial as in the fetal lamb (Figure 15-1(A)).

In 1979, Peeters (14) demonstrated in an animal model that there is a redistribution of blood flow to the brain in fetuses with diminished arterial oxygen content. Arbeille (15) also documented this occurrence in lambs and showed that there is a relationship between fetal oxygenation and cerebral blood flow as represented by Doppler waveform tracings. In the human fetus, cerebral Doppler

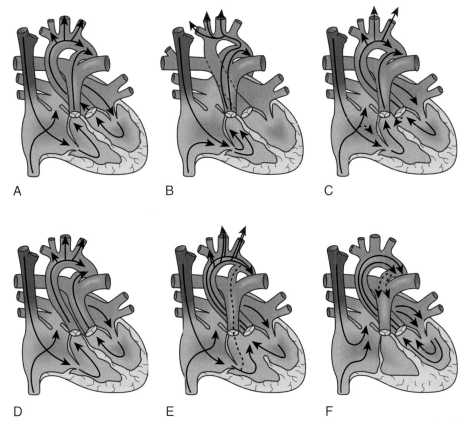

FIGURE 15–1 **(A)** Normal fetal blood flow; **(B)** Hypoplastic left heart (HLH) syndrome; **(C)** Left ventricular outflow obstruction; **(D)** Transposition of the great arteries (TGA); **(E)** Tetralogy of Fallot; **(F)** Hypoplastic right heart. Red arrows, oxygenated blood; blue arrows, deoxygenated blood.

ultrasound has demonstrated that many fetuses with intrauterine growth retardation have a change in the diastolic velocity profile suggesting increased flow to the brain (17–23). This hemodynamic phenomenon, termed "brain sparing," is represented by increased diastolic flow in the cerebral arteries and decreased diastolic flow in the descending aorta and umbilical arteries.

Resistance and pulsatility indices can both be calculated from Doppler waveform tracings of the cerebral vessels obtained during imaging of the fetus. The *resistance index* is defined as the systolic flow velocity minus the diastolic velocity divided by the systolic velocity, and the *pulsatility index* is defined as the systolic flow velocity minus the diastolic velocity divided by the mean velocity. These indices are considered to be representative of the resistance to flow distal to the point of measurement. Cerebral resistance and pulsatility indices have been studied in human fetuses without heart disease (17–23). In a study by Rizzo (19), of high-risk women with hypertension and placental insufficiency, a fetal cerebral pulsatility index more than standard deviations (SD) below the mean compared with normal predicted poor neonatal neurologic outcome and post-asphyxia encephalopathy with a sensitivity of 78%, a specificity of 87%, and an accuracy of 90%. Mari (18) showed that the cerebral pulsatility index is parabolic through gestation, suggesting a maximum cerebral vascular resistance at about 24 weeks' gestation that decreased after about 26 weeks' gestation. In his study of small-for-gestational-age fetuses, an abnormally low cerebral pulsatility index was found in 27%. Thirty-three percent of fetuses with an abnormal index died, compared with only 12% of those with a normal index.

a significantly longer recovery time to the first reappearance of normal EEG activity, and a statistically greater release of brain isoenzymes immediately after surgery. The duration of circulatory arrest also was associated with worse outcome. Definite seizures were strongly statistically associated with a longer period of circulatory arrest in a logistic-regression model in which the time in minutes of arrest and the diagnosis (intact ventricular septum versus ventricular septal defect) were used as predictors. All infants with an arrest time >35 min had clinical seizures. Abnormalities found during the neurologic examination at discharge were not related to the support method used. In the combined group, 20% had an abnormal neurologic examination with the most common finding being hypotonia. Specific findings of focal or lateralized abnormalities were present in 10% and discrepancies in ability to control extensor posture were found in 16%. The perioperative results of this study suggested that low-flow bypass should be used instead of circulatory arrest with alpha stat and low hematocrit hemodilution when possible. Limiting circulatory arrest periods to <30 min is ideal for brain protection.

The cohort of infants enrolled in the BCAT has been followed longitudinally and assessed at one, four, and eight years postsurgery. Developmental outcome, as measured by the Bayley scales of infant development at one year, and IQ testing, as assessed by the Wechsler test at four and eight years, have been reported by Bellinger et al. (70), Wang et al. (71), and Bellinger et al. (72). Neurodevelopmental outcome at one year of age differed when comparing deep hypothermic circulatory arrest and low-flow bypass. The PDI was significantly lower in the circulatory arrest group than in the low-flow group (27% versus 12% scoring <80) and was inversely correlated with the duration of circulatory arrest. The risk of neurologic abnormalities significantly increased with the duration of circulatory arrest as calculated by logistic regression. The MDI trended toward being lower in the circulatory arrest group; however, it did not reach statistical significance. The method of support was not associated with brain abnormalities on MRI scan. Seizures postoperatively were associated with abnormalities on MRI and lower psychomotor testing scores. By four years of age IQ scores and neurologic status were not associated with the method of support; however, the circulatory arrest group did score significantly lower on some subtests of motor function and had more severe speech abnormalities. Perioperative seizures were associated with lower mean IQ and an increased risk of neurologic abnormalities. At eight years of age the group as a whole was closer to normal compared with the population mean. Deficits were found in visual-spatial and visual-memory skills as well in executive functioning skills such as attention, language, memory, hypothesis generation, and coordination skills to perform complex operations. Interestingly, the low-flow bypass group had more behavioral difficulties and the circulatory arrest group more motor and speech deficits. This unique longitudinal study demonstrates that multiple factors influence neurodevelopmental outcome, and that abnormalities may change over time. These data support minimizing the use of circulatory arrest in favor of low-flow bypass where possible.

Two other studies have suggested a direct relationship between the duration of circulatory arrest and developmental testing scores. Wells and colleagues (75) compared 31 patients who underwent heart surgery, with hypothermic circulatory arrest, with their siblings. Patients were evaluated with the McCarthy scale. The study suggests that each additional minute of circulatory arrest was associated with a decrease of 0.53 points on developmental testing. In a similar evaluation of 114 patients, Oates et al. (76) found a decrease of three to four IQ points for each additional 10 minutes of circulatory arrest.

These studies demonstrate that neurodevelopmental outcome in infants and children with complex congenital heart disease is influenced by intraoperative factors which include the method of bypass, pH management strategy, and hematocrit (66–68). These data are encouraging because these factors can all be controlled so that neurologic outcome may be optimized for these high-risk patients.

NEURODEVELOPMENTAL OUTCOME AFTER SURGICAL REPAIR OF CONGENITAL HEART DISEASE

Between 10% and 30% of infants with congenital heart disease are found to have significant neurological abnormalities following cardiac surgery (77). Neurological sequelae that have been reported include cognitive deficits, seizures, choreoathetosis, spastic quadriparesis, bilateral motor deficits, and hemiparesis (77–81). Miller et al. (79) performed postoperative neurologic examinations in 91 infants who had undergone heart surgery and found 15% had clinical seizures, 34% had hypotonia, 7% had hypertonia, 5% had asymmetry of tone, and 19% had decreased alertness at hospital discharge. Limperopoulos and colleagues (49) prospectively studied 131 infants with congenital heart disease, excluding HLH syndrome. Preoperative abnormalities were found in >50% of infants. Postsurgical evaluation in 98 children at one to three years of age revealed gross and fine motor abnormalities in 42%. Mild to moderate deficits were noted in >50% of infants evaluated.

Neurodevelopmental Outcomes in Children with Transposition of the Great Arteries

The most extensively studied group of children with heart disease is the cohort enrolled in the BCAT (72–74). The details of this study, relating to the method of bypass, have been discussed; however, in analyzing the children with TGA as a whole, the group was found to have significant neurologic and neurodevelopmental abnormalities. Abnormalities in academic achievement, fine motor, visual-spatial, and higher language skills, memory, hypothesis generating, and sustaining attention were present in a significant number of children. Full-scale IQ scores were similar to the population mean (97 versus 100); mean performance IQ scores were significantly lower than mean verbal IQ scores (95 versus 100).

Neurodevelopmental Outcomes in Children with Single Ventricles

Children with a single functioning ventricle who undergo a series of palliative surgical procedures culminating in the Fontan operation are at the highest risk of developmental compromise. In addition to being at risk for cerebral hypoxia and hypoperfusion in fetal life, postnatally they may also have hemodynamic compromise with hypotension, chronic hypoxia, failure to thrive, and thromboembolic events. In addition, multiple operations involving bypass and circulatory arrest are often necessary. Children with HLH syndrome are at particular risk for neurodevelopmental abnormalities, in part because the repair involves a period of hypothermic circulatory arrest that in the past has been longer than 30 to 40 min. There have been several studies reporting neurodevelopmental outcomes in these patients. Wernovsky et al. (82) evaluated 133 patients who had a Fontan operation between the years 1972 and 1991, and the mean full-scale IQ of 96 was lower than the population mean. Mental retardation was found in eight percent. Children with HLH syndrome scored lower on all parameters when compared with children with other single-ventricle lesions. Mahle and colleagues (83) reported results for the period between 1984 and 1991. In 28 children the median full-scale IQ was 86, lower than the general population mean. Performance IQ was lower than verbal (83 versus 90). Full-scale IQ scores in the mental retardation range were found in 18%. Neurologic evaluation in 23 children revealed that only

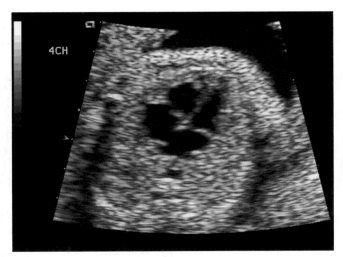

FIGURE 16–1 A normal four-chamber view of the fetal heart from the apex. The two atria are of equal size and the two ventricles are of equal size. The foramen ovale is visible in the atrial septum.

PRENATAL SCREENING FOR CARDIAC DEFECTS

The majority of pregnant women in the USA undergo at least one ultrasound examination (3). The standard of care for an ultrasound examination of the fetus as described by the American College of Radiology, the American Institute of Ultrasound in Medicine, and the American College of Obstetricians and Gynecologists is to include an evaluation of the four-chamber view and its axis at the time of a routine prenatal ultrasound (4–6) (Figure 16–1). This allows for a general examination of the basic anatomy of the heart, the atrioventricular connections, and its orientation in the fetal chest. The fetal heart is best imaged at 18 to 22 weeks of gestation, which corresponds to the optimal time to examine fetal anatomy during pregnancy (7). The detection of major heart defects in the second trimester offers obstetricians time for counseling and time for patients to consider termination if they decide that continuing the pregnancy is not their best option. Although not endorsed by the American College of Obstetricians and Gynecologists, universal screening for congenital heart disease in the second trimester of pregnancy offers a reasonable approach to detect major cardiac anomalies before birth.

Unfortunately, the ability of the basic four-chamber view to detect anomalies varies widely. In the large Routine Antenatal Diagnostic Imaging with Ultrasound (RADIUS) trial of low-risk women in the USA, only 23% of fetuses with heart defects were detected using the four-chamber view in tertiary care centers and no cardiac malformations were detected in non-tertiary sites before 24 weeks of gestation (8). Overall, the four-chamber view has been shown to identify 40% to 50% of cardiac anomalies in low-risk populations (1). Multiple factors affect the ability to detect heart defects prenatally, including the skill of examiner, the experience of the physician interpreting the study, the gestational age of the fetus, the fetal position during the examination, maternal weight, maternal abdominal scarring from prior surgery, and amniotic fluid volume. In addition, the four-chamber view does not allow for visualization of the great vessels. Studies have shown that including views of the outflow tracts increases the sensitivity of cardiac screening to over 60% in low-risk populations (9,10) (Figure 16–2 (A) and Figure 16–2 (B)). In high-risk populations, the detection of major heart anomalies is reported to be even higher when screening is done in experienced tertiary-level

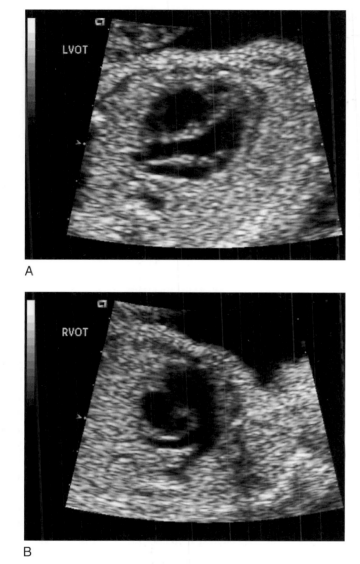

FIGURE 16–2 **(A)** Long-axis view of the left ventricular outflow tract (LVOT). The ventricular septum is contiguous with the wall of the ascending aorta. **(B)** Short-axis view of the right ventricular outflow tract (RVOT). The branching of the RVOT into the ductus arteriosus and the pulmonary artery may be appreciated.

referral centers (11). However, this level of screening is not available for most obstetric patients and the majority of congenital heart disease occurs in pregnancies without identifiable risk factors. These are additional arguments for universal cardiac screening of both low- and high-risk pregnancies, and recognition that improvements in screening are needed.

INDICATIONS FOR FETAL ECHOCARDIOGRAPHY

The American College of Cardiology, American Heart Association, and the American Society of Echocardiography have defined reasons to obtain an echocardiogram during pregnancy (7,12) (Table 16–1). A positive family history of congenital heart disease is a common indication for fetal echocardiography. While a previously affected pregnancy has a low rate of recurrence at one percent to three percent, the risk may be as high as 5% to 15% when multiple siblings have been

Table 16–1	Indications for Fetal Echocardiography (7,12)

Abnormal-appearing fetal heart on routine obstetric ultrasound examination
Fetal tachycardia, bradycardia, or persistent irregular rhythm on clinical or ultrasound examination
Parent, sibling, or first-degree relative with congenital heart disease
Maternal diabetes
Maternal systemic lupus erythematosus
Teratogen exposure during first trimester
Other fetal system abnormalities, including chromosomal, structural, enlarged nuchal translucency
Performance of transplacental therapy or presence of a history of significant but intermittent arrhythmia

affected or when the parent has a congenital heart defect (13). Despite the identification of high-risk factors for congenital heart disease, over 90% of heart defects occur in low-risk pregnancies (14). Interestingly, an abnormal cardiac screen at the time of routine obstetric ultrasound has become the most common reason for referral for fetal echocardiography and the most predictive of congenital heart disease (13). A fetal echocardiogram is a more extensive examination of the heart which evaluates multiple views and connections utilizing M-mode, color, and pulsed wave Doppler technologies. The goal of a screening fetal echocardiogram is to demonstrate normal fetal cardiac anatomy, and normal fetal heart rate and rhythm. In cases of an abnormal cardiac screening exam, fetal echocardiography is expected to confirm the presence of a defect and to more completely define the features of the lesion and its impact on heart function.

An enlarged nuchal translucency is a recently recognized indication for fetal echocardiography. The fetal nuchal translucency refers to the subcutaneous space between the skin and the cervical spine observed in the first trimester of pregnancy (15). Although nuchal translucency assessment is used primarily with maternal serum markers for aneuploidy screening, an increased nuchal translucency alone has been found to be associated with fetal malformations including congenital heart disease (Figure 16–3).

The reported sensitivities of increased nuchal translucency for major cardiac defects have steadily decreased since the initial studies in the late 1990s (Table 16–2). In the recently completed First And Second Trimester Evaluation of Risk (FASTER) trial, nuchal translucency assessment in the first trimester lacked the characteristics of a good screening tool for major congenital heart disease in a

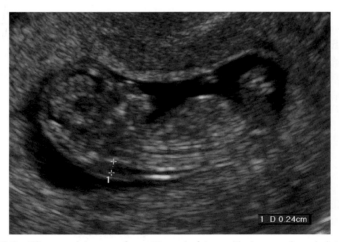

FIGURE 16–3 Ultrasound image of an 11-week fetus with increased nuchal translucency thickness measuring 2.4 mm.

Table 16–2 Nuchal Translucency (NT) Screening and Detection of Congenital Heart Disease

Study (year)	Type	n	Incidence of major CHD (per 1000)	NT threshold	Sensitivity (%)	Positive predictive value (%)
Hyett et al. (1999) (38)	Single-center	29,154	1.7	95th percentile	56	1.5
	99th percentile	40	6.3			
Makrydimas et al. (2003) (39)	Meta-analysis	58,492	2.8	95th percentile	37	3
	99th percentile	31	6			
Hafner et al. (2003) (40)	Single-center	12,978	2.1	95th percentile	25.9	1.1
Bahado-Singh et al. (BUN) (2004) (41)	Multicenter	8167	2.6	95th percentile	23.8	0.8
Simpson et al. (FASTER) (2004) (16)	Multicenter	33,968	1.3	2.0 MoM	18.6	1.5
	2.5 MoM	16.3		3.7		
	3.0 MoM	11.6		5.4		

large, unselected population (16). However, nuchal translucency measurement more than two multiples of the median was a marker for major cardiac defects with almost a fifth of major heart anomalies found in this group. While most congenital heart disease will occur in cases of normal nuchal translucency, an enlarged nuchal translucency does warrant referral for fetal echocardiography.

Regardless of the indication for referral, the results of the fetal echocardiogram are very important in managing pregnancies complicated by congenital heart disease. The distinction between a simple and a complex cardiac malformation can assist with making decisions about the appropriate delivery hospital. For example, the detection of a small ventricular septal defect may permit a patient to deliver in her community hospital rather than transfer for delivery in a tertiary care center. The type of cardiac anomaly can also be useful in counseling patients about the likelihood of chromosomal abnormalities or associated genetic syndromes. Complex heart lesions are more likely to be affected by hemodynamic compromise and the development of hydrops fetalis. As a result, serial echocardiograms for repeat assessments of cardiac function and monitoring of potentially progressive lesions are recommended when managing these pregnancies.

MANAGEMENT FOLLOWING THE DIAGNOSIS OF AN ABNORMAL FETAL HEART

The optimal management of fetuses with congenital heart disease involves a multidisciplinary team of obstetricians, pediatric cardiologists, geneticists, pediatric cardiothoracic surgeons, and neonatologists. Ideally, this multidisciplinary approach should occur in a single center during a single visit so that comprehensive information can be provided to the patient and her family in a timely fashion. Several large referral hospitals have dedicated centers that function to coordinate the care of these complicated pregnancies.

A number of important issues must be addressed when an abnormal fetal heart is found: Is it simple or complex? Is not isolated or associated with multiple anomalies? Does the fetus have a normal or abnormal karotype? Is the lesion associated with hemodynamic compromise or are there no functional implications?

Table 16–2 Nuchal Translucency (NT) Screening and Detection of Congenital Heart Disease

Study (year)	Type	n	Incidence of major CHD (per 1000)	NT threshold	Sensitivity (%)	Positive predictive value (%)
Hyett et al. (1999) (38)	Single-center	29,154	1.7	95th percentile	56	1.5
	99th percentile	40	6.3			
Makrydimas et al. (2003) (39)	Meta-analysis	58,492	2.8	95th percentile	37	3
	99th percentile	31	6			
Hafner et al. (2003) (40)	Single-center	12,978	2.1	95th percentile	25.9	1.1
Bahado-Singh et al. (BUN) (2004) (41)	Multicenter	8167	2.6	95th percentile	23.8	0.8
Simpson et al. (FASTER) (2004) (16)	Multicenter	33,968	1.3	2.0 MoM	18.6	1.5
	2.5 MoM	16.3		3.7		
	3.0 MoM	11.6		5.4		

large, unselected population (16). However, nuchal translucency measurement more than two multiples of the median was a marker for major cardiac defects with almost a fifth of major heart anomalies found in this group. While most congenital heart disease will occur in cases of normal nuchal translucency, an enlarged nuchal translucency does warrant referral for fetal echocardiography.

Regardless of the indication for referral, the results of the fetal echocardiogram are very important in managing pregnancies complicated by congenital heart disease. The distinction between a simple and a complex cardiac malformation can assist with making decisions about the appropriate delivery hospital. For example, the detection of a small ventricular septal defect may permit a patient to deliver in her community hospital rather than transfer for delivery in a tertiary care center. The type of cardiac anomaly can also be useful in counseling patients about the likelihood of chromosomal abnormalities or associated genetic syndromes. Complex heart lesions are more likely to be affected by hemodynamic compromise and the development of hydrops fetalis. As a result, serial echocardiograms for repeat assessments of cardiac function and monitoring of potentially progressive lesions are recommended when managing these pregnancies.

MANAGEMENT FOLLOWING THE DIAGNOSIS OF AN ABNORMAL FETAL HEART

The optimal management of fetuses with congenital heart disease involves a multidisciplinary team of obstetricians, pediatric cardiologists, geneticists, pediatric cardiothoracic surgeons, and neonatologists. Ideally, this multidisciplinary approach should occur in a single center during a single visit so that comprehensive information can be provided to the patient and her family in a timely fashion. Several large referral hospitals have dedicated centers that function to coordinate the care of these complicated pregnancies.

A number of important issues must be addressed when an abnormal fetal heart is found: Is it simple or complex? Is not isolated or associated with multiple anomalies? Does the fetus have a normal or abnormal karotype? Is the lesion associated with hemodynamic compromise or are there no functional implications?

Table 16–3 Classification of Congenital Heart Disease by Risk

Low risk	Moderate risk	High risk
Long-term survival likely with low morbidity	Potential impact on long-term survival with moderate morbidity	Significant impact on long-term survival with potential high morbidity
Ventricular septal defect	Complete and corrected TGA	Truncus arteriosus
Atrial septal defect	Tetralogy of Fallot	HLH syndrome
Mild pulmonic stenosis	Atrioventricular septal defect	Hypoplastic right ventricle
Mild aortic stenosis	Double outlet right ventricle	Tetralogy of Fallot with pulmonary atresia
	Coarctation	Critical aortic stenosis
	Ebstein anomaly	Atrioventricular canal with double outlet right ventricle and right isomerism
	Isolated total anomalous pulmonary venous return	Atrioventricular canal with congenital heart block and left isomerism
		Ebstein anomaly with severe cardiomegaly
		Total anomalous pulmonary venous return with obstruction or with isomerism syndrome

Modified from Allan LD and Huggon. Counseling following a diagnosis of congenital heart disease. Prental Diagn 2004;24:1136–1142.

Will the infant be a candidate for surgical intervention or is comfort care an option? Counseling about corrective and palliative surgical options, genetics, obstetric management and delivery plans, neonatal management, long-term survival, and expected quality of life should all be part of the discussion with the parents (17). Maternal mental health should also be the focus of obstetric management. The involvement of social services and consultation with an experienced psychologist or psychiatrist can provide the level of support many patients and their families need during this time.

The details of the counseling will depend on the specific diagnosis (Table 16-3). It is important to recognize that the diagnosis can change or be modified during the antepartum period or after birth. Reported long-term outcomes also vary for different cardiac anomalies and can differ depending on whether prenatal or postnatal clinical studies are considered (18). Certain heart defects are expected to have a more favorable antenatal course and perinatal outcome. For example, fetuses with two ventricles, normal chromosomes, and no other significant anomalies typically have a better prognosis than a fetus with a single ventricle (17,19,20). Overall, poor prognostic indicators include complex cardiac lesions, abnormal karyotype, extracardiac malformations, intrauterine growth restriction, and hydrops fetalis (21–23). In general, major congenital heart disease has a 5% to 12% rate of intrauterine fetal demise (11,24,25).

Although a multidisciplinary approach is ideal, the managing obstetrician often serves as the coordinating physician for the patient's care. Obstetric management of fetuses with congenital heart disease should include an evaluation for extracardiac anomalies, chromosomal abnormalities, pregnancy option considerations, serial growth scans, antenatal fetal testing, and scheduled delivery of major heart defects at experienced centers.

NON-CARDIAC STRUCTURAL ANOMALIES

Once the diagnosis of a cardiac anomaly is confirmed, an assessment of the remainder of the fetal anatomy should be performed. This may involve a review of a previously performed comprehensive ultrasound or referral for a repeat fetal survey in a more experienced ultrasound practice. Major extracardiac malformations are found in over 30% of prenatally diagnosed cases (22,23,26). Multiple structural defects often imply the presence of fetal syndromes which frequently are associated with abnormal development of the heart and less-favorable outcomes. Certain combinations of congenital defects may also suggest the diagnosis of a specific genetic syndrome that may have a poorer prognosis than would be expected for the same isolated cardiac defect. The accurate detection of associated structural anomalies is important for pregnancy counseling as well as for ongoing antepartum and intrapartum care. In addition to a potential to influence a patient's decision to continue the pregnancy, the severity of extracardiac malformations may affect the amount of antenatal testing, monitoring during labor, and route of delivery.

CHROMOSOMAL ABNORMALITIES

It is estimated that the etiology of 90% of congenital heart disease is multifactorial, the result of some yet undefined interaction of genetic and environmental factors (27). Previous studies have suggested that three percent of all congenital heart defects are caused by single gene mutations, seven percent by chromosomal aberrations, and the remainder by a host of other factors (28). However, in some prenatal series, 17% to 38% of fetuses diagnosed with cardiac anomalies have an underlying abnormality in their chromosomes (29). While the risk of a karyotypic abnormality is significant when congenital heart disease is associated with multiple non-cardiac malformations, this risk is reduced to 15% or less if the cardiac defect is isolated (23). Cases of known fetal aneuploidy should also be screened carefully for congenital heart disease. It is well-recognized that 40% to 50% of fetuses with trisomy 21 and more than 90% of fetuses with trisomy 18 will have structural cardiac anomalies (1).

Fetal karyotyping by amniocentesis, placental bed biopsy, or fetal blood sampling should be considered for most cases of prenatally diagnosed heart defects. Although some heart lesions, such as complete transposition of the great vessels (TGA), are rarely reported to be associated with chromosomal abnormalities, routine discussions about fetal karyotyping at the time of diagnosis will decrease the risk of missing a chromosomally abnormal fetus or the need for invasive procedures later in pregnancy when additional findings or disease progression make an abnormal fetal karyotype more likely. For patients who decline fetal chromosomal analysis, this may be accomplished at the time of pregnancy termination or following delivery of a live or stillborn infant. The results of the chromosomal testing can be valuable for genetic counseling about the current and future pregnancies.

Although specific gene abnormalities have not yet been identified for all heart defects, a microdeletion of the short arm of chromosome 22 (22q11) has been associated with conotruncal anomalies. These include truncus arteriosus, malaligned ventricular septal defects, tetralogy of Fallot, and interrupted aortic arch. This microdeletion has been linked to DiGeorge syndrome and velocardiofacial syndrome (30). Unfortunately, the phenotype can be variable and its effect on neurodevelopment uncertain. Fluorescence in-situ hybridization (FISH) at the time of fetal karyotyping may be used to make the diagnosis prenatally. Referral to an experienced geneticist is important in order to provide accurate information about the implications of a 22q11 microdeletion.

PREGNANCY OPTIONS

Whilst pregnancy options can be difficult to discuss with the patient and her family, the managing obstetrician often has the most established relationship with the patient and the best understanding of available options for pregnancy termination. A comprehensive assessment of the case, with input from all the subspecialists, is important as parents decide whether to end or continue a pregnancy. Ideally, the diagnosis is made early enough to give the patient ample time to consider her options. Although the patient and her family may ask for specific recommendations, non-directive counseling is optimal. Termination of pregnancy is never an easy decision for a patient but she must be the one to make that decision.

The incidence of a pregnancy termination varies with the severity of the cardiac defect, gestational age at diagnosis, and geographic location. There is a high rate of termination when severe congenital heart disease is detected in the second trimester of pregnancy. In some European countries, 50% to 80% of fetuses affected by serious cardiac malformations are terminated following early diagnosis (9,25,31). It is speculated that the termination rate might be even higher if prenatal screening for congenital heart disease was improved. The acceptance of pregnancy termination in the USA also varies by region. In a small study in Boston, 31% of congenital heart disease was diagnosed prior to 24 weeks' gestation and 22% of eligible patients chose the option of pregnancy termination (13). In contrast, only 13% of patients were diagnosed before 24 weeks' gestation in a New York series but 55% of eligible women chose to end their pregnancies (32). It is clear that universal screening and improved early prenatal detection of congenital heart disease could have a significant impact on pregnancy management.

ANTEPARTUM CARE

In addition to routine prenatal care, serial growth scans are often done for the early detection of poor fetal growth when a fetus has a known cardiac defect. While there is some controversy over the strength of the association between congenital heart disease and intrauterine fetal growth restriction, in many cases is it higher than the expected 10% background risk. The recognition of poor intrauterine fetal growth impacts obstetric management with respect to antenatal surveillance and timing of delivery. This may also decrease the risk of fetal demise because early delivery is undertaken if non-reassuring testing occurs or lack of growth is identified.

Unfortunately, intrauterine fetal demise and stillbirth are still more common in pregnancies affected by *in utero* congenital heart disease (31). Although some fetal deaths may be the result of poor growth, lesion progression with the development of hydrops fetalis is another cause of stillbirth. For example, an obstructed vessel or chamber may lag behind the growth of the rest of the fetus, resulting in hypoplasia of the affected part. Aortic stenosis or coarctation may progress to hypoplastic left ventricle, pulmonary stenosis can result in right ventricular hypoplasia, and pulmonary or aortic stenosis can progress to atresia. Hemodynamic compromise with chamber dilation, atrioventricular valve regurgitation, and cardiomegaly can eventually lead to fetal hydrops (17). Once hydrops develops, the prognosis for the fetus with congenital heart disease decreases significantly with only rare survivors (31). For these reasons, serial ultrasounds and echocardiograms are often planned every two to four weeks to monitor the fetus with a major heart anomaly.

Although there is no direct evidence that antenatal fetal testing improves outcomes in congenital heart disease, many managing obstetricians advocate for weekly fetal surveillance in the third trimester. Twice-weekly testing is recommended when intrauterine fetal growth restriction is diagnosed, which may be increased to daily testing depending on the umbilical artery Doppler assessments.

Although daily fetal surveillance with a nonstress test or biophysical profile, or both, is recommended when the diastolic flow is absent, delivery should be considered if the umbilical artery end-diastolic flow is reversed. The role of routine fetal testing in the absence of intrauterine growth restriction is uncertain. Whilst antenatal fetal testing may not benefit the fetus with a lesion judged to be incompatible with long-term survival, this should be thoroughly discussed with the members of the multidisciplinary team and with the parents. Parental decisions concerning care and the management plan should be clearly documented in the antenatal record.

INTRAPARTUM MANAGEMENT

The most critical aspect of intrapartum management is a planned delivery in a hospital capable of caring for an infant with congenital heart disease. Whereas smaller community hospitals may be appropriate for the birth of an infant with a small isolated ventricular septal defect, most cases of major congenital heart disease should be delivered at a tertiary-level center. Although definitive evidence that delivery in a tertiary care hospital improves outcome is lacking, a scheduled delivery in a center experienced in handling the medical, surgical, and supportive interventions that may be necessary for the newborn with a cardiac anomaly makes the process easier for the patient, her family, and the multidisciplinary team (33). In certain circumstances, survival may be improved by prenatal detection and delivery in a referral hospital. For example, the prenatal diagnosis of hypoplastic left heart (HLH) syndrome has been associated with decreased preoperative acidosis and improved survival compared with those diagnosed after birth (34). This has also been observed in neonates diagnosed with lesions amenable to biventricular repair (17).

In addition to delivery in the appropriate setting, a major goal of intrapartum management is to minimize the possibility of fetal hypoxemia and metabolic acidosis, which can lead to multi-organ failure and neurological handicap in the newborn. When the correct diagnosis has been made prenatally, potential problems can be identified and appropriate measures taken to support the neonate until corrective surgery can be performed (11,24,35). The prenatal detection of ductal-dependent lesions such as complete TGA with an intact ventricular septum or total anomalous pulmonary venous return, can result in life-saving measures in the immediate postnatal period (36). Anticipation of potential interventions, such as prostaglandin administration, emergency balloon valvuoplasty, or atrial septostomy, or utilization of extracorporeal membrane oxygenation (ECMO), may reduce confusion and chaos during the intrapartum period.

In contrast, a request for nonintervention may be made when the likelihood of long-term survival is small. It is optimal that these decisions be made in consultation with the multidisciplinary team prior to labor and delivery. In these circumstances, parents may opt for no intrapartum fetal monitoring, no Cesarean delivery for nonreassuring fetal testing, and no neonatal interventions apart from comfort care. Experienced care-providers in a comforting setting can make the birthing process less distressing even when lethal fetal anomalies are present (37).

Fortunately, most fetuses with major congenital heart disease tolerate labor and delivery without incident. Continuous intrapartum fetal monitoring with Cesarean delivery for standard obstetric indications is appropriate management in the majority of cases. Scheduling delivery at 39 weeks' gestation is ideal if the patient has a favorable cervix or when a Cesarean delivery is required. An established delivery plan provides an opportunity to have the various specialists involved in the patient's care available for the birth. This is comforting to the patient and her family, and, it is hoped, improves the immediate and long-term outcome of the infant with major congenital heart disease.

CONCLUSIONS

In summary, the obstetric management of a fetus with congenital heart disease involves a multidisciplinary approach which takes into account the needs of both the parents and the infant. Information about the severity of the defect, associated extracardiac anomalies, and chromosomal abnormalities is valuable for planning appropriate care of the patient during the antepartum, intrapartum, and neonatal periods.

REFERENCES

1. Simpson LL. Screening for congenital heart disease. Obstet Gynecol Clin North Am 2004;31:51–59.
2. Randall P, Brealey S, Hahn S, et al. Accuracy of fetal echocardiography in the routine detection of congenital heart disease among unselected and low-risk populations: a systematic review. Br J Obs Gynae 2005;112:24–30.
3. American Institute of Ultrasound in Medicine. Practice guideline for the performance of an antepartum obstetric ultrasound. J Ultrasound Med 2003;22:1116–1125.
4. American Society of Echocardiography. Guidelines and standards for performance of the fetal echocardiogram. J Am Soc Echocardiogr 2004;17:803–819.
5. American College of Obstetricians and Gynecologists. Ultrasonography in Pregnancy, Practice Bulletin, Number 58. Washington, DC American College of Obstetricians and Gynecologists, 2004.
6. American Institute of Ultrasound in Medicine. Guidelines for the performance of the antepartum obstetrical ultrasound examination. J Ultrasound Med 1991;10:576–578.
7. Rychik J, Ayres N, Cuneo B, et al. American Society of Echocardiography guidelines and standards for performance of the fetal echocardiogram. J Am Soc Echocardiogr 2004;17:803–810.
8. Crane JP, LeFevre ML, Winborn RC, et al. A randomized trial of prenatal ultrasonographic screening: impact on the detection, management, and outcome of anomalous fetuses. The RADIUS Study Group. Am J Obstet Gynecol 1994;171:392–399.
9. Bull C. Current and potential impact of fetal diagnosis on prevalence and spectrum of serious congenital heart disease at term in the UK. British Paediatric Cardiac Association. Lancet 1999;354:1242–1247.
10. Rustico MA, Benettoni A, D'Ottavio G, et al. Fetal heart screening in low-risk pregnancies. Ultrasound Obstet Gynecol 1995;6:313–319.
11. Copel JA, Tan AS, Kleinman CS. Does a prenatal diagnosis of congenital heart disease alter short-term outcome? Ultrasound Obstet Gynecol 1997;10:237–241.
12. American College of Cardiology/American Heart Association. Guidelines for the Clinical Application of Echocardiography. Number 71-0103. J Am Coll Cardiol, 1997.
13. Simpson LL, Marx GR, D'Alton, ME. The detection of congenital heart disease in a tertiary care ultrasound practice. Am J Obstet Gynecol 1995;172:253–456.
14. Maher JE, Colvin EV, Samdarshi TE, et al. Fetal echocardiography in gravidas with historic risk factors for congenital heart disease. Am J Perinatol 1994;11:334–336.
15. Devine PC, Simpson LL. Nuchal translucency and its relationship to congenital heart disease. Semin Perinatol 2000;24:343–351.
16. Simpson LL, Malone F, Bianchi D, et al. Nuchal translucency and the risk of congenital heart disease – a population-based screening study (the FASTER trial). Am J Obstet Gynecol 2004;191:376–383.
17. Allan LD, Huggon IC. Counselling following a diagnosis of congenital heart disease. Prenat Diagn 2004;24:1136–1142.
18. Simpson LL. Structural cardiac anomalies. Clin Perinatol 2000;27:839–863.
19. Allan LD, Apfel HD, Printz BF. Outcome after prenatal diagnosis of the hypoplastic left heart syndrome. Heart 1998;79:371–373.
20. Rodriguez JG, Holmes R, Martin R, et al. Prognosis following prenatal diagnosis of heart malformations. Early Hum Dev 1998;52:13–20.
21. Allan LD, Crawford DC, Anderson RH, et al. Spectrum of congenital heart disease detected echocardiographically in prenatal life. Br Heart J 1985;54:523–526.
22. Respondek ML, Binotto CN, Smith S, et al. Extracardiac anomalies, aneuploidy, and growth retardation in 100 consecutive fetal congenital heart defects. Ultrasound Obstet Gynecol 1994;4:272–278.
23. Smythe JF, Copel JA, Kleinman CS. Outcome of prenatally detected cardiac malformations. Am J Cardiol 1992;69:1471–1474.
24. Brick DH, Allan LD. Outcome of prenatally diagnosed congenital heart disease: an update. Pediatr Cardiol 2002;23:449–453.
25. Fesslova V, Villa L, Kustermann A. Long-term experience with the prenatal diagnosis of cardiac anomalies in high-risk pregnancies in a tertiary center. Ital Heart J 2003;4:855–864.
26. Copel JA, Pilu G, Kleinman CS. Congenital heart disease and extracardiac anomalies: associations and indications for fetal echocardiography. Am J Obstet Gynecol 1986;154:1121–1132.

27. Awane-Yeboa K. Genetics of congenital heart disease. In Gersony W, Rosenbaum M eds. Congenital Heart Disease: Adult. New York, NY McGraw-Hill, 2000:281–294.

28. Welch KK, Brown SA. The role of genetic counseling in the management of prenatally detected congenital heart defects. Semin Perinatol 2000;24:373–379.

29. Moore JW, Binder GA, Berry R. Prenatal diagnosis of aneuploidy and deletion 22q11.2 in fetuses with ultrasound detection of cardiac defects. Am J Obstet Gynecol 2004;191:2068–2073.

30. Goldmuntz E, Clark BJ, Mitchell LE, et al. Frequency of 22q11 deletions in patients with conotruncal defects. J Am Coll Cardiol 1998;32:492–498.

31. Sharland GK, Lockhart SM, Chita SK, et al. Factors influencing the outcome of congenital heart disease detected prenatally. Arch Dis Child 1991;66:284–287.

32. Shevell T, Perez-Delboy A, Simpson L. Prenatal diagnosis of congenital heart disease and voluntary termination: experience of a single tertiary care center. Am J Obstet Gynecol 2001;185:S70–S288.

33. Simpson LL, Harvey-Wilkes K, D'Alton ME. Congenital heart disease: the impact of delivery in a tertiary care center on SNAP scores (scores for neonatal acute physiology). Am J Obstet Gynecol 2000;182:184–191.

34. Tworetzky W, Wilkins-Haug L, Jennings RW, et al. Balloon dilation of severe aortic stenosis in the fetus: potential for prevention of hypoplastic left heart syndrome: candidate selection, technique, and results of successful intervention. Circulation 2004;110:2125–2131.

35. Allan L, Benacerraf B, Copel JA, et al. Isolated major congenital heart disease. Ultrasound Obstet Gynecol 2001;17:370–379.

36. Kohl T, Sharland G, Allan LD, et al. World experience of percutaneous ultrasound-guided balloon valvuloplasty in human fetuses with severe aortic valve obstruction. Am J Cardiol 2000;85:1230–1233.

37. Spinnato JA, Cook VD, Cook CR, et al. Aggressive intrapartum management of lethal fetal anomalies: beyond fetal beneficence. Obstet Gynecol 1995;85:89–92.

38. Hyett J, Perdu M, Sharland G, et al. Using fetal nuchal translucency to screen for major congenital cardiac defects at 10-14 weeks of gestation: population based cohort study. Br Med J 1999;318:81–85.

39. Makrydimas G, Sotiriadis A and Ioannidis JP. Screening performance of first-trimester nuchal translucency for major cardiac defects: a meta-analysis. Am J Obstet Gynecol 2003;189:1330–1335.

40. Hafner E, Schuller T, Metzenbauer M, et al. Increased nuchal translucency and congenital heart defects in a low-risk population. Prenat Diagn 2003;23:985–989.

41. Bahado-Singh RO, Wapner R, Thom E, et al. Elevated first-trimester nuchal translucency increases the risk of congenital heart defects. Am J Obstet Gynecol 2005;192:1357–1361.

Chapter 17

Fetal Cardiac Intervention

Mark K. Friedberg, MD • Norman H. Silverman, MD DSc (Med) FACC FASE • Frank L. Hanley, MD • Vadiyala Mohan Reddy, MD • Craig T. Albanese, MD, MBA

INTRODUCTION

Advances in ultrasound and fetal imaging have enhanced our understanding of how cardiac form follows function, with development *in utero* to exert secondary developmental effects which create lesions of greater severity and complexity after birth. The hypoplastic left heart (HLH) syndrome exemplifies this model. Obstruction to left ventricular inflow or outflow in fetal life may cause progressive hypoplasia of the left ventricle (1), but the characteristics of the fetal circulation permit continuing extracardiac development. After birth, however, the lesion is almost uniformly fatal unless treated. The aim of fetal intervention is therefore to curtail the pathological process *in utero* and to allow for normal fetal development, thereby:

- improving fetal outcomes
- decreasing the severity of congenital heart disease and its effects on other organ systems
- improving postnatal outcome.

Advances in our understanding of these processes, alongside technical advances and capabilities, have allowed the realistic pursuit of these goals. At present, however, the risk:benefit ratio remains very high. Fetal cardiac intervention is currently practiced only in select centers, on select lesions, and much progress remains to be made with regard to patient selection, pathology amenable to intervention, and technical hurdles to be overcome before cardiac fetal intervention becomes a routine and widespread therapeutic modality. This chapter will address some of the major advances, as well as the inherent risks, of fetal surgery. Table 17–1 summarizes some of the current applications of fetal surgery. We do not address all lesions summarized in the table, but, rather, focus on a number of lesions that have had a major impact on this field; we also address the specific issues that these surgeries present for the fetal cardiovascular system and that the cardiovascular

Table 17–1   Summary of Applications of Fetal Surgery

Defect	Effect on development	Open	Minimal access
Lethal			
Placental vascular anomalies			
Twin–twin transfusion syndrome (TTTS)	Vascular steal through placenta → Fetal hydrops/demise		Photocoagulation of chorangiopagus
Surviving twin with severe morbidity	→	Fetectomy	Fetectomy
Twin reversed arterial perfusion syndrome (TRAP)	Normal co-twin heart pumps for both twins → High output cardiac failure, hydrops		Selective reduction via umbilical cord ligation or radiofrequency needle
Obstructive uropathy	Hydronephrosis → Renal failure →	Vesicostomy	Vesicoamniotic shunt; Valve ablation
Congenital diaphragmatic hernia	Lung hypoplasia → Pulmonary failure	Complete repair; Temporary tracheal occlusion (PLUG)	Temporary tracheal occlusion
Cystic adenomatoid malformation/sequestration	Lung hypoplasia or hydrops → Respirator insufficiency	Pulmonary lobectomy	Radiofrequency ablation
Sacrococcygeal teratoma	High-output heart failure → Fetal hydrops/demise	Debulk; Complete resection	Laser vascular occlusion
Complete heart block	Low-output failure → Fetal hydrops/demise	Pacemaker	Pacemaker
Pulmonary/aortic stenosis	Ventricular hypertrophy → Heart failure; Single ventricle physiology	Valvuloplasty	Catheter valvuloplasty
Pericardial teratoma	Heart failure → Fetal hydrops/demise	Resection	—
Ebstein's anomaly	Heart failure → Fetal hydrops/demise	Valve repair and atrial reduction	—
Congenital high airway obstruction syndrome	Pulmonary hypoplasia; Overdistention by lung fluid → Pulmonary failure; Fetal hydrops/demise; EXIT strategy	Tracheostomy	Tracheostomy
Obstructive hydrocephalus	Hydrocephalus → Brain damage	Ventriculoamniotic shunt; Ventriculoperitoneal shunt	Ventriculoamniotic shunt
Nonlethal			
Myelomeningocele	Chiari formation → Paralysis	Repair	Repair

Table continued on following page

Table 17–1   Summary of Applications of Fetal Surgery (Continued)

Defect	Effect on development	Open	Minimal access
	Explosed spinal cord		Neurogenic bladder/bowel Orthopedic anomalies
Tension hydrothorax	Hydrocephalus Lung hypoplasia	↑	Respiratory failure – Serial thoracenteses Thoracoamniotic shunt
Previable premature rupture of membranes	Preterm labor	↑	Fetal demise – Amniopatch
Gastoschisis	Bowel exteriorization	↑	Fetal/maternal infection – Bowel perivisceritis – Prolonged ileus Amniograft Amnioexchange
Amniotic bands	Limb/digit/umbilical cord constriction	↑	Limb/digit deformity or amputation – Fetal demise (cord occlusion) Laser separation of bands
Other Stem cell/enzyme defects	Hemoglobinopathy Immunodeficiency Storage diseases	↑	Anemia – Infection Neurological impairment Stem cell transplants Gene therapy

From Malladi P, Sylvester KG and Albanese CT. Outcomes in fetal surgery. In: Stringer M, Oldham K, Mouriquand P (eds). Longterm Outcomes in Paediatric Surgery and Urology. Cambridge: Cambridge University Press, in press.

system presents to these surgeries. We present problems related to cardiopulmonary bypass and cardiac imaging in anticipation of the advent of routine fetal cardiac surgery in the not too distant future.

CATHETER-BASED TECHNIQUES

As catheter techniques have pioneered fetal intervention in congenital heart disease, a brief overview is of their development is warranted here.

The pioneering work of Rudolph and colleagues in delineating fetal physiology and the pathophysiologic effects of cardiovascular disease in experimental models of cardiac disease in the sheep fetus laid the foundation for these interventions. Chronic instrumentation of sheep fetuses determined the changes in cardiovascular hemodynamics through the course of gestation (2) and demonstrated that flow is a key factor in normal growth and development of the cardiovascular system (3).

The observation that HLH syndrome may develop over the second trimester and that pulmonary atresia with intact ventricular septum is a relatively late event in fetal development led to the premise that relief of outflow obstruction would increase blood flow through the affected chambers, resulting in normal chamber size and function (4–6). Early animal studies supported this hypothesis. Alteration in blood flow in the chick embryonic heart led to HLH syndrome (7–9) and obstructing left ventricular inflow in the baboon fetal heart, by inflating a balloon in the left atrium, diminished left ventricular size and mass. The longer the balloon was left inflated in the left atrium, the more severe the left ventricular hypoplasia (10). Creation of left ventricular outflow obstruction by placement of an ascending aorta band caused initial left ventricular hyperplasia, followed, after one to two months of aortic stenosis, by severe left ventricular hypoplasia. The degree of hypoplasia was proportional to the degree of aortic stenosis. These early experiments provided the rationale for the assumption that relief of valvular obstruction would increase flow through the distal chamber, thereby stimulating normal fetal growth of that chamber and achievement of a two-ventricle heart after birth.

The first balloon valvuloplasty in a human fetus was reported by Maxwell and colleagues (11) in 1991, who ballooned the aortic valve in two fetuses. Experience continued in the subsequent decade (12), although the numbers of interventions were small and morbidity and mortality remained high. Further advances in maternal anesthesia, fetal imaging, and interventional techniques prompted an expanded fetal intervention program at a few centers, notably at the Children's Hospital in Boston (13–16). In a review of 20 aortic balloon valvuloplasties in fetuses of 21 to 29 weeks' gestation 14 were technically successful, but, of these, only three babies achieved a two-ventricle circulation after birth. Six children were born with HLH syndrome and five fetuses succumbed *in utero*.

Candidate selection, maternal anesthesia, fetal imaging, and technical abilities continue to be important factors in catheter-based fetal interventions, while current developments include a combined surgical–catheter approach to allow for optimal positioning of the fetus.

Pulmonary valvuloplasty in pulmonary atresia and intact ventricular septum is now being performed to treat the fetus with a hypoplastic right ventricle; however, experience remains limited as compared to the wider experience that has been accumulated in ballooning the aortic valve (17,18).

FETAL SURGERY

Several trends culminated in the advent of fetal surgery in past decades. The development of ultrasound and, more recently, magnetic resonance imaging (MRI) has allowed documentation of prenatal pathology and its evolution over gestation. In addition, the creation of animal models of congenital pathologies has permitted study of the pathogenesis, evolution, and treatment of these lesions. Fetal positioning has facilitated both superior imaging and improved surgical access, while advances in anesthesia of the mother and the fetus have permitted fetal surgery and have reduced its risks. Surgical advances in technique and instrumentation have advanced from open uterine surgery in the initial period, to laparoscopic and other minimally invasive techniques today. Resultant reduction in the major risks of fetal intervention, including preterm labor, chorioamniotic membrane separation, preterm premature rupture of the membranes, and altered fetal homeostasis have shifted the risk:benefit ratio to a more beneficial one. Lastly, the advent of randomized clinical trials to evaluate fetal interventions now provide answers to many key questions and allow for a more objective assessment of the efficacy and safety of these procedures.

SURGICAL INTERVENTIONS FOR SPECIFIC LESIONS

We will now consider some of the key pathologies for which significant progress in fetal interventions have been made.

Congenital Diaphragmatic Hernia

High postnatal mortality rates, despite prenatal diagnosis and optimal postnatal care, provided the impetus for fetal surgery for congenital diaphragmatic hernia (CDH) (19,20). Fetal surgery, initially performed in sheep and primates, demonstrated that lung growth, pulmonary function, and neonatal survival were improved (21–23). Surgical repair through a hysterotomy with partial fetal delivery and repair of the diaphragmatic defect was demonstrated to be feasible in humans in 1990 (20). Many problems, however, including preterm premature rupture of the membranes, preterm labor, and fetal morbidity, precluded surgery for CDH from becoming a routine procedure.

In 1997, a prospective study revealed similar survival rates of fetuses undergoing prenatal open repair compared with standard postnatal care (75% versus 86%, respectively) (24), leading to the conclusion that less severely affected fetuses prenatally diagnosed with CDH (i.e. those without liver herniation through the diaphragmatic hernia and a normal lung:head ratio) should be treated with standard postnatal care. However, the optimum treatment for more severely affected fetuses, that is, those with liver herniation through the CDH and a small lung:head ratio remained unanswered.

The observation that fetal lungs do not grow when drained of fluid, whereas prevention of fluid efflux from the lungs via tracheal obstruction promotes lung growth (25) created the rationale for reversible tracheal occlusion, several methods of which were subsequently developed. These included placement of an intratracheal plug or external tracheal clips at open surgery (26). Complications of these procedures included tracheomalacia and impaired lung function after birth, even in fetuses with dramatic lung growth following the procedure (27). These complications were attributed to various factors, including infant prematurity, impaired number and function of type II pneumocytes (28–30), and abnormal lymphatic drainage. Further progress came in the form of video-assisted fetal endoscopy (FETENDO), designed to reduce uterine trauma and its resultant complications (31,32,33). This technique is performed through a small (5 mm) hysterotomy, and has evolved from clips placed externally on the fetal trachea, through various devices, to placement of a detachable balloon that occludes the tracheal lumen. FETENDO improved fetal and postnatal survival over previous experience, and was encouragingly high at 77% at 90 days after procedure, although problems arising from infant prematurity as well as other complications remained. Issues that continue to be actively studied include optimal timing for tracheal occlusion, occlusion duration, and developments in instrumentation. However, outcomes for many fetuses with CDH continue to be poor (34), especially for fetuses with a small lung:head ratio and those with herniated liver through the defect. In some populations pregnancy termination after fetal diagnosis of CDH is high (34).

Twin–twin Transfusion Syndrome

Twin–twin transfusion syndrome (TTTS), defined by polyhydramnios in the recipient twin's sac and oligohydramnios in the donor twin's sac (35) results from an imbalance in net blood flow between the twins owing to abnormal placental vascular communications that occur in 10% of monochorionic pregnancies (36). This flow imbalance leads to increased cardiac afterload in the donor and increased cardiac preload in the recipient. It has been hypothesized that a placental vasculopathy is responsible for the pathophysiology of TTTS and several humoral mediators have been implicated in its pathogenesis (37–39). As a result of high vascular resistance mediated by endothelin, the renin–angiotensin axis and the shunting of blood, the donor twin develops hypovolemia and oligohydramnios. On the other hand, the recipient has low vascular resistance and develops polyhydramnios and cardiac remodeling.

The recipient twin is the most severely afflicted by the cardiac sequelae of this condition. Initially, the right ventricle dilates and hypertrophies in response to the increased volume load, but the fetal heart tolerates volume loading poorly, and right ventricular dysfunction and tricuspid regurgitation develop, leading to progressive hydrops. Flow through the ductus venosus decreases and flow reversal in the ductus venosus may follow. With worsening fetal condition, increased right atrial pressure may cause pulsations in the umbilical vein through an abnormally relaxed ductus venosus sphincter. Diastolic umbilical arterial flow, normal or even increased initially, will also eventually decrease. The increased vascular resistance, decreased cardiac output, and decreased flow across the right ventricular outflow may lead to pulmonary stenosis and even pulmonary atresia with intact ventricular septum. These severe hemodynamic abnormalities will cause fetal demise in a high proportion of affected fetuses. Although the donor is usually less severely affected, and usually has normal left and right ventricular size and function, without intervention, both twins will die in 80% to 100% of cases (36,40). Risk factors for poor outcome (41) include no urine in the donor twin bladder after 60 min of observation and abnormal Doppler flow studies in either twin (absent or reversed end-diastolic velocity in the umbilical artery, pulsatile umbilical venous flow, and flow reversal in the ductus venosus). Cardiac failure, manifested by hydrops in either twin, is an extremely poor prognostic indicator, and death of one twin usually portends death of the other or neurological impairment in survivors.

Treatment options for TTTS have included expectant management in low-risk cases or cases discovered late in pregnancy, selective fetocide, amniotic fluid reduction, amniotic septostomy, laser photocoagulation of abnormal communicating vessels in the placenta, and umbilical cord occlusion.

Serial amniocentesis to reduce amniotic fluid volume in the recipient sac prolongs pregnancy and improves survival of at least one twin to 79% and survival of both twins to 50% (42). The mechanism by which serial amniocentesis works is unknown (43,44). Fetoscopy guided Nd-YAG laser photocoagulation of placental vessels crossing the intertwin membrane was first performed for TTTS in 1990 (45–47). One technique targets all vessels crossing the intertwin membrane while a second selectively targets unpaired arterial vessels (in these vessels the vein returns to the recipient fetus). Similar survival rates to those reported for serial amniocentesis have been reported for photocoagulation (47), although laser therapy might increase survival of both twins (46), lessen intrauterine deaths, decrease brain abnormalities, prolong pregnancy, and lead to higher birth weights in comparison with serial amniocentesis. Despite improvements in neonatal outcome after laser treatment of TTTS, outcomes still remain poor as compared with monochorionic twins without TTTS (48).

Umbilical cord occlusion is usually undertaken only in cases where intrauterine death of one twin is likely. A falling blood pressure in the dying twin causes acute hemorrhage from the healthy twin into the dying one, which may cause neurologic damage or death in the previously relatively healthy twin (49). Umbilical cord occlusion by ligating (50,51) or cauterizing (52,53) the umbilical cord of the dying twin limits the amount of blood transfused between the fetuses. Survival after umbilical cord ligation is somewhat lower than that after photocoagulation (41,53). Furthermore, the incidence of cerebral palsy may also be lower with umbilical cord ligation (35).

Septostomy, first described in 1995, equalizes volumes in each fetal sac and minimizes the number of invasive procedures (54). A needle is used to puncture the intertwin membrane, allowing fluid to accumulate around the oligohydramniotic fetus. Survival rates in the range of 83% are comparable with those for more invasive methods. However, it should be noted that some authors believe that as there is no pressure differential between the two sacs, septostomy lacks physiologic rationale and is a poor treatment option (55,56). On the other hand, complications of septostomy can be significant and may include cord entanglement and fetal demise (35).

Sacrococcygeal Teratoma

Sacrococcygeal teratoma (SCT), a usually but not always benign tumor (57), arises from extragonadal germ cells around the sacrum, occurring in one out of 35,000 to 40,000 live births, four times more frequently in females than males (58). Fetuses with SCT, especially those with large, rapidly growing, solid, vascular SCT, are at high risk for hydrops and high-output cardiac failure because of the high blood flow through the tumor (19,59). Fetal cardiac output may be calculated using echocardiography, by multiplying the Doppler velocity time-integral of the right ventricular outflow tract by the right-ventricular outflow cross-sectional area and heart rate. The normal average fetal cardiac output, indexed for weight, was found to be 553 ± 153 mL/min·kg in one study (60) and 429 ± 100 mL/min·kg in another (61). Schmidt and colleagues (62) found a cardiac index as high as 1200 mL/min·kg in three fetuses with SCT. Fetal demise is not uncommon in this scenario, although if the SCT is resected the prognosis is usually excellent. Other potential complications from the SCT itself may include tumor rupture, preterm labor, and dystocia (63–65).

The goal of fetal intervention is to interrupt the high-flow circulation through the tumor (66). Initially accomplished by open hysterotomy with tumor debulking or complete resection, fetal intervention has evolved to intrauterine therapy, often with resolution of hydrops. Cyst aspiration to reduce uterine irritability, maternal discomfort, or tumor rupture at time of delivery is a less invasive approach (67,68), but generally works only in relatively avascular, cystic tumors. Cyst–amniotic shunts have been used when the SCT has caused obstructive uropathy (69,70). Minimally invasive approaches for highly vascular tumors in fetuses with heart failure have included tumor embolization, balloon occlusion, sclerosis, endoscopic snaring of the tumor neck, laser ablation, thermocoagulation, and radio-frequency ablation. Fetoscopically guided Nd-YAG laser treatment to reduce bloodflow to the tumor in a 20-weeks' gestation fetus with polyhydramnios has been reported (71), as has attempted thermocoagulation of the tumor neck in one fetus, although this fetus did not survive (72). Percutaneous radio-frequency ablation of large SCT is yet another approach. In a report of this procedure in four fetuses, two fetuses survived and two others succumbed (73). Survivors suffered large soft-tissue defects that necessitated further postnatal surgery. A more focused field of ablation to limit collateral heat production should reduce this complication. Combined radio-frequency ablation and angiography with embolization before surgery has also been performed (74).

SCT leads to profound hemodynamic changes in the fetus at time of surgery (75). Before surgery the fetal heart faces increased preload and afterload, determined by the combined vascular resistances of the fetus, placenta, and low-resistance SCT. After resection of the SCT there is an abrupt reduction in the preload, a large increase in afterload, but no immediate change in the cardiac ventricular mass, leading to a diminished ventricular cavity and relative increase in myocardial wall thickness, a substrate for diastolic dysfunction (75).

Congenital Cystic Adenomatoid Malformation

Congenital cystic adenomatoid malformation (CCAM) is a focal pulmonary dysplasia, involving proliferation of the terminal respiratory bronchioles at the expense of alveoli development, leading to cysts of various sizes. CCAM represents 25% of all congenital lung malformations and its course is highly variable ranging from complete *in utero* regression to severe fetal hydrops and fetal demise.

In the normal fetus, the collapsed lungs and relatively noncompliant chest wall restrict preload, limiting cardiac stroke volume. A large CCAM further reduces the already limited preload by impeding ventricular filling, thus limiting stroke volume and cardiac output, producing tamponade-like physiology and diastolic dysfunction (76,77). This diastolic dysfunction may lead to fetal hydrops and eventual fetal demise. Surgical removal of the CCAM leads to resolution of fetal hydrops and subsequent survival of the fetus (78,79), providing the rationale for fetal intervention in severe cases of CCAM. However, fetal surgery for CCAM is fraught with risk, as fetuses with CCAM were found to be the sickest of all patient groups at the time of surgery (75). Rychick and colleagues (75) have recently summarized their institution's experience with fetal surgery for CCAM. Before surgery, fetuses with CCAM were commonly hydropic and had low cardiac output. At surgery, fetuses with CCAM demonstrated profound hemodynamic changes, including a 50% drop in cardiac output: to as low as 200 mL/kg·min, severe ventricular and valvar dysfunction, and bradycardia. These changes occurred immediately after removal of the mass through the thoracotomy incision, necessitating resuscitation with cardiac compressions along with infusion of fluids and medications. Operative mortality was high: only seven of 15 fetuses surviving beyond 24 h after surgery. These authors also noticed prominent proximal coronary arteries in two fetuses which died whilst undergoing CCAM removal, and theorized that this finding may be related to the sudden decrease in intrathoracic pressure when the CCAM is removed from the chest, leading to an increased gradient necessary for coronary perfusion. This group therefore recommends extracting the CCAM very slowly, while monitoring the ventricular cavity volume as a measure of preload. Volume infusion is given as the mass is removed, guided by the echocardiographic appearance of the ventricular cavities.

CARDIOPULMONARY BYPASS FOR FETAL SURGERY

Fetal cardiac bypass was first reported by Bradley and colleagues in 1992 (80). This early experimental work in the fetal lamb showed that it was technically possible to place the fetus on separate cardiopulmonary bypass (CPB) (80,81), although most animals died within hours of the procedure as a result of placental dysfunction and fetal stress – the two major challenges to successful fetal CPB (80–83).

Placental dysfunction after CPB is characterized by elevated fetal partial carbon dioxide pressure (pCO_2), progressive acidosis, and elevated placental vascular resistance. Suggested mechanisms for placental dysfunction have included diminished or nonpulsatile placental blood flow, hypothermia, cytokines, neutrophils, nitric oxide (NO), and endothelin-1 (84–92). Stimuli for placental dysfunction may include fetal stress in response to the procedure, use of priming substances in the CPB circuit, exposure of fetal blood to extracorporeal surfaces, and the flow characteristics of the circuit itself. These induce endothelial dysfunction, as demonstrated by a reduced response of umbilical arterial flow to direct vasodilator injection after fetal cardiac bypass (89), by cardiac bypass-induced endothelial dysfunction of the umbilical artery and hemodynamic deterioration as a result of metabolic acidosis (93), and by exaggerated sensitivity to vasoconstrictors such as endothelin-1. Fetal serum concentrations of endothelin-1 are elevated after CPB, causing an elevation in placental vascular resisistance and a decrease in placental blood flow. This response is blocked by administration of endothelin-1-blocking agents. A second axis in this pathophysiologic response is mediated through secretion of prostaglandin E2 and thromboxane A2. This effect is ameliorated by indomethacin or corticosteroids and these pharmacologic agents have been shown to improve placental function after fetal CPB (83,94). Further support for vascular endothelial dysfunction as the basis for placental dysfunction has come from the demonstration that pulsatile bypass flow preserved endothelial NO synthesis more efficiently than nonpulsatile flow (91).

To overcome this placental dysfunction, significant modifications have been made to CPB technique and equipment. The "hemopump," a system that ignores priming volume and utilizes an inline axial pump to decrease extracorporeal surface area, is advantageous to the conventional roller-pump method. The hemopump yielded better hemodynamic results associated with lower placental vascular resistance, increased placental blood flow, and improved survival (from 42% to 88.9% in one study as compared with the conventional roller-pump) (95).

Fetal responses to CPB and surgery include catecholamine secretion and myocardial depression, which lead to low cardiac output and metabolic acidosis. Immature fetal cardiac cellular components differ both in morphology and function from the mature form in adult myocytes. The sarcoplasmic reticulum (SR) content in fetal myocytes is markedly reduced (96) and contains low concentrations of calcium ATPase and the calcium storage protein calsequestran (97). In addition, functional differences exist between fetal and adult forms of phospholamban, a SR membrane calcium transport protein (97). These differences lead to impaired fetal myocyte calcium uptake and release (98), yielding the fetal heart extremely sensitive to calcium concentrations in cardioplegia solutions. Hence, hypocalcemic cardioplegia may optimize fetal myocardial protection, and several studies have demonstrated improved post-ischemic recovery with normocalcemic cardioplegia and profound post-ischemic myocardial dysfunction with hypercalcemic cardioplegia (99,100). Bolling and colleagues (101) reported equivalent protection of the neonatal myocardium with different calcium cardioplegic concentrations under normal conditions, but improved protection of the hypoxic myocardium with hypocalcemic cardioplegia. Hypocalcemic cardioplegia improved post-ischemic systolic function of both fetal ventricles, although right ventricular diastolic function was not improved. The right ventricle may be more compliant than the left, and thus may be less prone to ischemic diastolic dysfunction. As the fetal right ventricle contributes two-thirds of the combined ventricular output this finding holds potentially significant implications for myocardial protection in the fetus. Calcium influx has been implicated in cellular damage during reperfusion injury, and immature fetal myocardial calcium regulation magnifies the deleterious effects of increased intracellular calcium during periods of ischemia. It is evident that the fetal myocardial response to ischemia and the response to calcium metabolism are intricately connected. The fetal heart is especially sensitive to ischemic stress (102), and as ischemic stress is intricately related to myocyte calcium metabolism, hypocalcemic cardioplegia may provide better fetal cardioprotection.

Myocyte contractile proteins also influence fetal myocardium vulnerability to CPB and fetal surgery. Immature isoforms of contractile proteins, such as heavy chain myosin, predominate in the fetal ventricle (103). The adult form of heavy chain myosin, found only in atrial tissue during fetal life, begins to be expressed in the ventricle only after birth (103). This histology may underlie the impaired Frank–Starling mechanism and diastolic compliance of the fetal ventricle (81).

Volatile anesthesia administered to the mother is another potential cause of fetal myocardial depression. Relatively high levels of isoflurane are necessary to provide an appropriate degree of uterine relaxation. At these high levels isoflurane can decrease maternal cardiac output and uterine blood flow by up to 30% (104). Diminished uterine blood flow reduces oxygen delivery to the utero–placental unit, causing fetal hypoxia (105). Halothane has been shown to increase placental and total vascular resistance, potentially limiting gas exchange and increasing afterload on the fetal heart (106). This increased afterload is deleterious to the fetal myocardium owing to its altered myocardial compliance as compared with the mature myocardium (107). Therefore, fetal hypoxia, altered afterload, or direct myocardial depression by the anesthetic agent may decrease systolic function and decrease cardiac output. Decreased cardiac output induces metabolic acidosis, which, in turn, further compromises cardiac function. These explanations, largely derived from animal models, need further confirmation in the human fetus.

Fetal bradycardia has been observed in various types of fetal surgery (75), and may result from fetal hypoxia as the fetal response to hypoxia is bradycardia (108). Mechanical compression of the umbilical cord or uterine vessels may also induce bradycardia (109).

INTRA-AMNIOTIC ULTRASOUND FOR FETOSCOPY

Fetal cardiac interventions have traditionally been guided by transabdominal fetal echocardiography. Adequate fetal position, high imaging quality, and sufficient acoustic windows are critical to the success of these procedures. Dorso-anterior fetal position, inadequate ultrasound windows, or ultrasound scatter from interventional devices might hinder adequate visualization of the procedure (110). Fetal transesophageal echocardiography using intravascular ultrasound probes has also been used to monitor fetal cardiac anatomy and hemodynamics during experimental procedures (110–114). However, intraesophageal placement of the intravascular ultrasound probes may be precluded in very small fetuses, may not be successful owing to unfavorable fetal position, and has the potential to cause esophageal trauma. These problems mean that minimally invasive fetoscopic procedures for fetal cardiac intervention are being developed in sheep as an alternative to existing imaging methods (111,112,115,116). Intra-amniotic fetal echocardiography with a phased-array intravascular ultrasound catheter has been used in the assessment of fetal cardiac anatomy and hemodynamics in sheep, and in the future may also be used to precisely define the incision site on the fetal chest (115). Insertion of the catheter is achieved by use of a modified Seldinger approach and has been found safe in animal studies (115). Owing to its intra-amniotic position the phased-array catheter permits detailed two-dimensional fetal echocardiography as well as color, pulsed, and continuous-wave Doppler interrogation of the fetal cardiovascular and feto–placental system, and may supplant transcutaneous imaging for monitoring of fetal cardiac anatomy and hemodynamics during fetoscopic interventions. In the future, intra-amniotic imaging may also be indicated in the assessment of high-risk fetuses when sufficient images cannot be obtained by conventional maternal trans-abdominal or transvaginal imaging techniques. This detailed two-dimensional and Doppler imaging also allows hemodynamic monitoring inside a gas-insufflated uterus during fetoscopic interventions. However, low insonance angles may be difficult to achieve for all cardiac, great vessel, and feto–placental flows during an individual study, limiting the physician's ability to estimate pressure gradients, flow volumes, and valvar regurgitation. Despite these limitations, important fetal circu-lation-flow profiles can be obtained, including pathologic signals such as retrograde flow in the ductus venosus, umbilical vein pulsatile flow, absent or reversed umbil-ical artery end-diastolic flow, and flow disturbance across stenotic valves. Potential hazards of intra-amniotic imaging include injury to the fetus, umbilical cord or placenta, infection, premature rupture of the membranes, amniotic fluid leakage, and premature induction of labor. The operator therefore needs to be especially cautious when manipulating the intra-amniotic catheter. Because of this invasive nature intra-amniotic imaging should be reserved for fetoscopic interventions and high-risk fetuses in whom conventional imaging methods have failed. Similar-sized devices introduced into the amniotic cavity, such as fetoscopes and vesico–amniotic shunts, hold a risk as high as 10% for premature rupture of membranes and induction of labor (117) and it would be reasonable to assume that intra-amniotic imaging holds similar risks. These potential risks may be offset by virtue of the intra-amniotic ultrasound as a monitoring tool that minimizes the risks of the intervention itself, as well as by the fact that the catheter can be placed with minimal uterine injury. Therefore, intra-amniotic ultrasound may hold less risk than would have been expected otherwise (111) and as smaller-caliber catheters become available it is likely that the risks of intra-amniotic imaging will be even less in the near future.

CONCLUSION

Ongoing and future directions in this area pertain to development of biplane and multiplane intravascular ultrasound catheters and assessment of high-risk pregnancies for recognition of abnormal fetal phenotypes.

REFERENCES

1. Rudolph AM. Congenital Diseases of the Heart: Clinical–Physiological Considerations. Armonk, NY Futura, 2001.
2. Rudolph AM, Heymann MA. Circulatory changes during growth in the fetal lamb. Circ Res 1970;26:289–299.
3. Rudolph AM, Spitznas U. Hemodynamic considerations in the development of narrowing of the aorta. Am J Cardiol 1972;30:514–525.
4. Danford CA, Cronican P. Hypoplastic left heart syndrome: progression of left ventricular dilation and dysfunction to left ventricular hypoplasia in utero. Am Heart J 1992;123:1712–1713.
5. Simpson JM, Sharland GK. Natural history and outcome of aortic stenosis diagnosed prenatally. Heart 1997;77:205–210.
6. Hornberger LK, Sanders SP, Rein AJ, Spevak PJ, Parness IA, Colan SD. Left heart obstructive lesions and left ventricular growth in the midtrimester fetus. A longitudinal study. Circulation 1995;92:1531–1538.
7. Harh JY, Paul MH, Gallen WJ, Friedberg DZ, Kaplan S. Experimental production of hypoplastic left heart syndrome in the chick embryo. Am J Cardiol 1973;31:51–56.
8. Hogers B, De Ruiter MC, Gittenberger-de Groot AC, Poelmann RE. Unilateral vitelline vein ligation alters intracardiac blood flow patterns and morphogenesis in the chick embryo. Cric Res 1997;80:473–481.

9. Hove JR, Koster RW, Forouhar AS, Acevedo-Bolton G, Fraser SE, Gharib M. Intracardiac fluid forces are an essential epigenetic factor for embryonic cardiogenesis. Nature 2003;421:172–177.

10. Fishman NH, Hof RB, Rudolph AM, Heyman MA. Models of congenital heart disease in fetal lambs. Circulation 1978;58:254–364.

11. Maxwell D, Allan L, Tynan MJ. Balloon dilatation of the aortic valve in the fetus: a report of two cases. Br Heart J 1991;65:256–258.

12. Kohl T, Sharland G, Allan LD, et al. World experience of percutaneous ultrasound-guided balloon valvuloplasty in human fetuses with severe aortic valve obstruction. Am J Cardiol 2000;85:1230–1233.

13. Marshall AC, van der Velde ME, Tworetzky W, et al. Creation of an atrial septal defect in utero for fetuses with hypoplastic left heart syndrome and intact or highly restrictive atrial septum. Circulation 2004;110:253–258.

14. Tworetzky W, Marshall AC. Balloon valvuloplasty for congenital heart disease in the fetus. Clin Perinatol 2003;30:541–550.

15. Tworetzky W, Wilkins-Haug L, Jennings RW, et al. Balloon dilation of severe aortic stenosis in the fetus: potential for prevention of hypoplastic left heart syndrome: candidate selection, technique, and results of successful intervention. Circulation 2004;110:2125–2131.

16. Marshall AC, Tworetzky W, Bergersen L, et al. Aortic valvuloplasty in the fetus: technical characteristics of successful balloon dilatation. J Pediatr 2005;147:535–539.

17. Arzt WTG, Aigner M, Mair R, Hafner E. Invasive intrauterine treatment of pulmonary atresia/intact ventricular septum with heart failure. Ultrasound Obstet Gynecol 2003;21:186–188.

18. Tulzer G, Arzt W, Franklin RC, Loughna PV, Mair R, Gardiner HM. Fetal pulmonary valvuloplasty for critical pulmonary stenosis or atresia with intact septum. Lancet 2002;360:1567–1568.

19. Bond SJ, Harrison MR, Schmid KG, et al. Death due to high-output cardiac failure in fetal sacrococcygeal teratoma. J Pediatr Surg 1990;25:1287–1291.

20. Harrison MR, Adzick NS, Longaker MT, et al. Successful repair in utero of a fetal diaphragmatic hernia after removal of herniated viscera from the left thorax. N Engl J Med 1990;322:1582–1584.

21. Harrison MR, Bressack MA, Churg AM, de Lorimer AA. Correction of congenital diaphragmatic hernia in utero. II. Simulated correction permits fetal lung growth with survival at birth. Surgery 1980;88:260–268.

22. Harrison MR, Jester JA, Ross NA. Correction of congenital diaphragmatic hernia in utero. I. The model: intrathoracic balloon produces fatal pulmonary hypoplasia. Surgery 1980;88:174–182.

23. Harrison MR, Ross NA, de Lorimer AA. Correction of congenital diaphragmatic hernia in utero. III. Development of a successful surgical technique using abdominoplasty to avoid compromise of umbilical blood flow. J Pediatr Surg 1981;16:934–942.

24. Harrison MR, Adzick NS, Bullard KM, et al. Correction of congenital diaphragmatic hernia in utero. VII. A prospective trial. J Pediatr Surg 1997;32:1637–1642.

25. Carmel JA, Friedman F, Adams RH. Fetal tracheal ligation and lung development. Am J Dis Child 1965;109:452–456.

26. Harrison MR, Adzick NS, Flake AW, et al. Correction of congenital diaphragmatic hernia in utero. VIII. Response of the hypoplastic lung to tracheal occlusion. J Pediatr Surg 1996;31:1339–1348.

27. Flake AW, Crombleholme TM, Johnson MP, Howell LJ, Adzick NS. Treatment of severe congenital diaphragmatic hernia by fetal tracheal occlusion: clinical experience with fifteen cases. Am J Obstet Gynecol 2000;183:1059–1066.

28. Benachi A, Chailly-Heu B, Delezoide AL, et al. Lung growth and maturation after tracheal occlusion in diaphgragmatic hernia. Am J Respir Crit Care Med 1998;157:921–927.

29. Bin Saddiq W, Piedboeuf B, Laberge JM, et al. The effects of tracheal occlusion and release on type II pneumocytes in fetal lambs. J Pediatr Surg 1997;32:834–838.

30. O'Toole SJ, Karamanoukian HL, Irish MS, Sharma A, Holm BA, Glick PA. Tracheal ligation: the dark side of in utero congenital diaphragmatic hernia treatment. J Pediatr Surg 1997;32:407–410.

31. Skarsgard ED, Meuli M, Vander Wall KJ, Bealer JF, Adzick NS, Harrison MR. Fetal endoscopic tracheal occlusion ('Fetendo-PLUG') for congenital diaphragmatic hernia. J Pediatr Surg 1996;31:1335–1338.

32. Vander Wall KJ, Skarsgard ED, Filly RA, Eckert J, Harrison MR. Fetendo-clip: a fetal endoscopic tracheal clip procedure in a human fetus. J Pediatr Surg 1997;32:970–972.

33. Harrison MR, Mychaliska GB, Albanese CT, et al. Correction of congenital diaphragmatic hernia in utero. IX. Fetuses with poor prognosis (liver herniation and low lung-to-head ratio) can be saved by fetoscopic temporary tracheal occlusion. J Pediatr Surg 1998;33:1017–1022, discussion 1022–1023.

34. Colvin J, Bower C, Dickinson JE, Sokol J. Outcomes of congenital diaphragmatic hernia: a population-based study in Western Australia. Pediatrics 2005;116:e356–e363.

35. Quintero RA. Twin–twin transfusion syndrome. Clin Perinatal 2003;30:591–600.

36. Machin GA, Keith LG. Can twin-to-twin transfusion syndrome be explained, and how is it treated? Clin Obstet Gynecol 1998;41:104–113.

37. Bajoria R, Gibson MJ, Ward S, Sooranna SR, Neilson JP, Westwood M. Placental regulation of insulin-like growth factor axis in monochorionic twins with chronic twin–twin infusion syndrome. J Clin Endocrinol Metab 2001;86:3150–3156.

38. Mahieu-Caputo D, Dommergues M, Delezoide AL, et al. Twin-to-twin transfusion syndrome. Role of the fetal renin-angiotensin system. Am J Pathol 2000;156:629–636.

39. Mahieu-Caputo D, Meulemans A, Martinovic J, et al. Paradoxic activation of the rennin-angiotensin system in twin–twin transfusion syndrome: an explanation for cardiovascular disturbances in the recipient. Pediatr Res 2005;58:685–688.

319

40. Weir PE, Ratten GJ, Beischer NA. Acute polyhydraminos – a complication of monozygous twin pregnancy. Br J Obstet Gynaecol 1979;86:849–853.

41. Quintero RA, Comas C, Bornick PW, Allen MH, Kruger M. Selective versus non-selective laser photocoagulation of placental vessels in twin-to-twin transfusion syndrome. Ultrasound Obstet Gynaecol 2000;16:230–236.

42. Johnsen SL, Albrechtsen S, Pirhonen J. Twin–twin transfusion syndrome treated with serial amniocenteses. Acta Obstet Gynecol Scand 2004;83:326–329.

43. Saunders NJ, Snijders RJ, Nicolaides KH. Therapeutic amniocentesis in twin–twin transfusion syndrome appearing in the second trimester of pregnancy. Am J Obstet Gynecol 1992;166:820–824.

44. Trespidi L, Boschetto C, Caravelli E, Villa L, Kustermann A, Nicholini U. Serial amniocentesis in the management of twin–twin transfusion syndrome: when is it valuable:? Fetal Diagn Ther 1997;12:15–20.

45. De Lia JE, Cruickshank DP, Keye WR, Jr. Fetoscopic neodymium: YAG laser occlusion of placental vessels in severe twin–twin transfusion syndrome. Obstet Gynecol 1990;75:1046–1053.

46. Hecher K, Plath H, Bregenzer T, Hansmann M, Hackloer BJ. Endoscopic laser surgery versus serial amnioamcenteses in the treatment of severe twin-to-twin transfusion syndrome. Am J Obstet Gynecol 1999;180:717–724.

47. Ville Y, Hecher K, Gagnon A, Sebire N, Hyett J, Nicolaides K. Endoscopic laser coagulation in the management of severe twin-to-twin transfusion syndrome. Br J Obstet Gynaecol 1998;105:446–453.

48. Lopriore E, Sueters M, Middeldorp JM, Oepkes D, Vandenbussche FP, Walther FJ. Neonatal outcome in twin-to-twin transfusion syndrome treated with fetoscopic laser occlusion of vascular anastomoses. J Pediatr 2005;147:597–602.

49. De Lia J, Fisk N, Hecher K, et al. Twin-to-twin transfusion syndrome – debates on the etiology, natural history and management. Ultrasound Obstet Gynecol 2000;16:210–213.

50. Lemery DJ, Vanlieferinghen P, Gasq M, Finkeltin F, Beaufrere AM, Beytout M. Fetal umbilical cord ligation under ultrasound guidance. Ultrasound Obstet Gynecol 1994;4:399–401.

51. Quintero RA, Romero R, Reich H, et al. In utero per cutaneous umbilical cord ligation in the management of complicated monochorionic multiple gestations. Ultrasound Obstet Gynecol 1996;8:16–22.

52. Deprest JA, Audibert F, Van Schoubroeck D, Hecher K, Mahieu-Caputo D. Bipolar coagulation of the umbilical cord in complicated monochorionic twin pregnancy. Am J Obstet Gynecol 2000;182:340–345.

53. Taylor MJ, Shalev E, Tanawattanacharoen S, et al. Ultrasound-guided umbilical cord occlusion using bipolar diathermy for Stage III/IV twin–twin transfusion syndrome. Prenatal Diag, 2002;22:70–76.

54. Saade GR, Belfort MA, Berry DL, et al. Amniotic septostomy for the treatment of twin oligohydramnios–polyhydramnois sequence. Fetal Diagn Ther 1998;13:86–93.

55. Hartung J, Chqaoui R, Bollmann R. Amniotic fluid pressures in both cavities of twin–twin transfusion syndrome: a vote against septostomy. Fetal Diagn Ther 2000;15:79–82.

56. Quintero RQL, Morales W. Amniotic fluid pressures in severe twin–twin transfusion syndrome. Prenat Neonat Med 1998;3:607–610.

57. Altman RP, Randolph JG, Lilly JR. Sacrococcygeal teratoma: American Academy of Pediatrics Surgical Section Survey – 1973. J Pediatr Surg 1974;9:389–398.

58. Rescorla FJ, Sawin RS, Coran AG, Dillon PW, Azizkhan RG. Long-term outcome for infants and children with sacrococcygeal teratoma: a report from the Children's Cancer Group. J Pediatr Surg 1998;33:171–176.

59. Silverman NH, Schmid KG. Ventricular volume overload in the human fetus: observations from fetal echocardiography. J Am Soc Echocardiogr 1990;3:20–29.

60. De Smedt MC, Visser GH, Meijboom EJ. Fetal cardiac output estimated by Doppler echocardiography during mid- and late gestation. Am J Cardiol 1987;60:338–342.

61. Mielke G, Benda N. Cardiac output and central distribution of blood flow in the human fetus. Circulation 2001;103:1662–1668.

62. Schmidt KG, Silverman NH, Harrison MR, Callan PW. High-output cardiac failure in fetuses with large sacrococcygeal teratoma: diagnosis by echocardiography and Doppler ultrasound. J Pediatr 1989;114:1023–1028.

63. Flake AW, Harrison MR, Adzick NS, Laberge JM, Warsof SL. Fetal sacrococcygeal teratoma. J Pediatr Surg 1876;21:563–566.

64. Gross SJ, Benzie RJ, Sermer M, Skidmore MB, Wilson SR. Sacrococcygeal teratoma: prenatal diagnosis and management. Am J Obstet Gynecol 1987;156:393–396.

65. Musci MN, Jr, Clark MJ, Ayres RE, Finkel MA. Management of dystocia caused by a large sacrococcygeal teratoma. Obstet Gynecol 1983;63(3 Suppl.):10s–12s.

66. Langer JC, Harrison MR, Schmidt KG, et al. Fetal hydrops and death from sacrococcygeal teratoma: rationale for fetal surgery. Am J Obstet Gynecol 1989;160:1145–1150.

67. Hedrick HL, Flake AW, Crombleholme TM, et al. Sacrococcygeal teratoma: prenatal assessment, fetal intervention, and outcome. J Pediatr Surg 2004;39:430–438.

68. Kay S, Khalife S, Laberge JM, Shaw K, Morin L, Flageole H. Prenatal percutaneous needle drainage of cystic sacrococcygeal teratomas. J Pediatr Surg 1999;34:1148–1151.

69. Garcia AM, Morgan WM, III, Bruner JP. In utero decompression of a cystic grade IV sacrococcygeal teratoma. Fetal Diagn Ther 1998;13:305–308.

70. Jouannic JM, Doimmergues M, Auber F, Bessis R, Nihoul-Fekete C, Dumez Y. Successful intrauterine shunting of a sacrococcygeal teratoma (SCT) causing fetal bladder obstruction. Prenat Diagn 2001;21:824–826.

71. Hecher K, Hackeloer BJ. Intrauterine endoscopic laser surgery for fetal sacrococcygeal teratoma. Lancet 1996;347:470.

72. Lam YH, Tang MH, Shek TW. Thermocoagulation of fetal sacrococcygeal teratoma. Prenat Diagn 2002;22:99–101.

73. Paek BW, Jennings RW, Harrison MR, et al. Radiofrequency ablation of human fetal sacrococcygeal teratoma. Am J Obstet Gynecol 2001;184:503–507.

74. Cowles RA, Stolar CJ, Kandel JJ, Weintraub JL, Susman J, Spigland NA. Preoperative angiography with embolization and radiofrequency ablation as novel adjuncts to safe surgical resection of a large, vascular sacrococcygeal teratoma. Pediatr Surg Int 2006;6:554–556.

75. Rychik J, Tian Z, Cohen MS, et al. Acute cardiovascular effects of fetal surgery in the human. Circulation 2004;110:1549–1556.

76. Mahle WT, Rychik J, Tian ZY, et al. Echocardiographic evaluation of the fetus with congenital cystic adenomatoid malformation. Ultrasound Obstet Gynecol 2000;16:620–624.

77. Rice HE, Estes JM, Hedrick MH, Bealer JF, Harrison MR, Adzick NS. Congenital cystic adenomatoid malformation: a sheep model of fetal hydrops. J Pediatr Surg 1994;29:692–696.

78. Adzick NS, Harrison MR, Crombleholme TM, Flake AW, Howell LJ. Fetal lung lesions: management and outcome. Am J Obstet Gynecol 1998;179:884–889.

79. Adzick NS, Harrison MR, Flake AW, Howell LJ, Golbus MS, Filly RA. Fetal surgery for cystic adenomatoid malformation of the lung. J Pediatr Surg 1993;28:806–812.

80. Bradley SM, Hanley FL, Duncan BW, et al. Fetal cardiac bypass alters regional blood flows, arterial blood gases, and hemodynamics in sheep. Am J Physiol 1992;263:H919–928.

81. Hanley FL. Fetal cardiac surgery. Adv Card Surg 1994;5:47–74.

82. Malhotra SP, Thelitz S, Riemer RK, Reddy VM, Suleman S, Hanley FL. Induced fibrillation is equally effective as crystalloid cardioplegia in the protection of fetal myocardial function. J Thorac Cardiovasc Surg 2003;125:1276–1282.

83. Sabik JF, Assad RS, Hanley FL. Prostaglandin synthesis inhibition prevents placental dysfunction after fetal cardiac bypass. J Thorac Cardiovasc Surg 1992;103:733–741, discussion 741–742.

84. Champsaur G, Parisot P, Martinot S, et al. Pulsatility improves hemodynamics during fetal bypass. Experimental comparative study of pulsatile versus steady flow. Circulation 1994;90(5 Pt 2):II47–II50.

85. Champsaur G, Vedrinne C, Martinot S, et al. Flow-induced release of endothelium-derived relaxing factor during pulsatile bypass: experimental study in the fetal lamb. J Thorac Cardiovasc Surg 1997;114:738–744, discussion 744–745.

86. Hawkins JA, Clark SM, Shaddy RE, Gay WA, Jr. Fetal cardiac bypass: improved placental function with moderately high flow rates. Ann Thorac Surg 1994;57:293–296, discussion 296–297.

87. Hawkins JA, Paape KL, Adkins TP, Shaddy RE, Gay WA, Jr. Extracorporeal circulation in the fetal lamb. Effects of hypothermia and perfusion rate. J Cardiovasc Surg 1991;32:295–300.

88. Parry AJ, Petrossian E, McElhinney DB, Reddy VM, Hanley FL. Neutophil degranulation and complement activation during fetal cardiac bypass. Ann Thorac Surg 2000;70:582–589.

89. Parry AJ, Petrossian E, McElhinney DB, et al. Role of the endothelium in placental dysfunction after fetal cardiac bypass. J Thorac Cardiovasc Surg 1999;117:343–351.

90. Reddy VM, McElhinney DB, Rajasinghe HA, Rodriguez JL, Hanley FL. Cytokine response to fetal cardiac bypass. J Mat–Fetal Invest 1998;8:46–49.

91. Vedrinne C, Tronc F, Martinot S, et al. Better preservation of endothelial function and decreased activation of the fetal renin-angiotensin pathway with the use of pulsatile flow during experimental fetal bypass. J Thorac Cardiovasc Surg 2000;120:770–777.

92. Vedrinne C, Tronc F, Martinot S, et al. Effects of various flow types on maternal hemodynamics during fetal byass: is there nitric oxide release during pulsatile perfusion? J Thorac Cardiovasc Surg 1998;116:432–439.

93. Oishi Y, Masuda M, Yasutsune T, et al. Impaired endothelial function of the umbilical artery after fetal cardiac bypass. Ann Thorac Surg 1999–2003;discussion 2004.

94. Sabik JF, Heinemann MK, Assad RS, Hanley FL. High-dose steroids prevent placental dysfunction after fetal cardiac bypass. J Thorac Cardiovascular Surg 1994;107:116–124, discussion 124–125.

95. Reddy VM, Liddicoat JR, Klein JR, McElhinney DB, Wampler RK, Hanley FL. Fetal cardiac bypass using an in-line axial flow pump to minimize extracorporeal surface and avoid priming volume. Ann Thorac Surg 1996;62:393–400.

96. Friedman WF, Pool PE, Jacobwitz D, Seagren SC, Brunwald E. Sympathetic innervations of the developing rabbit heart. Biochemical and histochemical comparisons of fetal, neonatal, and adult myocardium. Circ Res 1968;23:25–32.

97. Pegg W, Michalak M. Differentiation of sarcoplasmic reticulum during cardiac myogenesis. Am J Physiol 1987;525:H22–H31.

98. Mahony L. Maturation of calcium transport in cardiac sarcoplasmic reticulum. Pediatr Res 19881;24:639–643.

99. Corno AF, Bethancourt DM, Laks H, et al. Myocardial protection in the neonatal heart. A comparison of topical hypothermia and crystalloid and blood cardioplegic solutions. J Thorac Cardiovasc Surg 1987;93:163–172.

100. Pearl JM, Laks H, Drinkwater DC, et al. Normocalcemic blood or crystalloid cardioplegia provides better neonatal myocardial protection than does low-calcium cardioplegia. J Thorac Cardiovasc Surg 1993;105:201–206.

101. Bolling K, Kronon M, Allen BS, et al. Myocardial protection in normal and hypoxically stressed neonatal hearts: the superiority of hypocalcemic versus normocalcemic blood cardioplegia. J Thorac Cardiovasc Surg 1996;112:1193–1200, discussion 1200–1201.

102. Lee JC, Halloran KH, Taylor JF, Downing SE. Coronary flow and myocardial metabolism in newborn lambs: effects of hypoxia and acidemia. Am J Physiol 1973;224:1381–1387.

103. Mahdavi V, Izumo S, Nadal-Ginard B. Developmental and hormonal regulation of sarcomeric myosin heavy chain gene family. Circ Res 1987;60:804–814.

104. Palahnuik RJ, Shnider SM. Maternal and fetal cardiovascular and acid-base changes during halothane and isofluane anesthesia in the pregnant ewe. Anesthesiol 1974;41:462–472.

105. Toubas PL, Silverman NH, Heymann MA, Rudolph AM. Cardiovascular effects of acute hemorrhage in fetal lambs. Am J Physiol 1981;240:H45–48.

106. Sabik JF, Assad RS, Hanley FL. Halothane as an anesthetic for fetal surgery. J Pediatr Surg 1993;28:542–546, discussion 546–547.

107. Grant DA, Fauchere JC, Eede KJ, Tyberg JV, Walker AM. Left ventricular stroke volume in the fetal sheep is limited by extracardiac constraint and arterial pressure. J Physiol 2001;535:231–239.

108. Rudolph AM. The fetal circulation and its response to stress. J Dev Physiol 1984;6:11–19.

109. Tchirikov M, Hecher K, Deprest J, Zikulnig L, Devlieger R, Schroder HJ. Doppler ultrasound measurements in the central circulation of anesthetized fetal sheep during obstruction of umbilical–placental blood flow. Ultrasound Obstet Gynaecol 2001;18:656–661.

110. Kohl T, Hartlage MG, Westphal M, et al. Intra-amniotic multimodal fetal echocardiography in sheep: a novel imaging approach during fetoscopic interventions and for assessment of high-risk pregnancies in which conventional imaging methods fail. Ultrasound Med Biol 2002;28:731–736.

111. Kohl T, Stelnicki EJ, Vander Wall KJ, et al. Transesophageal echocardiography in fetal sheep. A monitoring tool for open and fetoscopic cardiac procedures. Surg Endosc 1996;10:820–824.

112. Kohl T, Suda K, Reckers J, Scheld HH, Vogt J, Silverman NH. Fetal transesophageal echocardiography utilizing a 10-F, 10-MHz intravascular ultrasound catheter – comparison with conventional maternal transabdominal fetal echocardiography in sheep. Ultrasound Med Biol 1999;25:939–946.

113. Kohl T, Szabo Z, Vander Wall KJ, et al. Experimental fetal transesophageal and intracardiac echocardiography utilizing intravascular ultrasound technology. Am J Cardiol 1996;77:899–946.

114. Kohl T, Westphal M, Strumper D, et al. Multimodal fetal transesophageal echocardiography for fetal cardiac intervention in sheep. Circulation 2001;104:1757–1760.

115. Kohl T, Strumper D, Witteler R, et al. Fetoscopic direct fetal cardiac access in sheep: an important experimental milestone along the route to human fetal cardiac intervention. Circulation 2000;192:1602–1604.

116. Kohl T, Szabo Z, Suda K, et al. Fetoscopic and open transumbilical fetal cardiac catheterization in sheep. Potential approaches for human fetal cardiac intervention. Circulation 1997;95:1048–1053.

117. Morales RAQ, WJ. Percutaneous fetoscopically guided interventions. In Harrison MR, Adzick NS, Holzgreve W (eds). The Unborn Patient. Philadelphia, PA WB Saunders 2001;199–211.

Chapter 18

Impact of Prenatal Diagnosis on the Management of Congenital Heart Disease

Charles S. Kleinman, MD

Introduction
Continuation versus Termination of Pregnancy
Impact of Prenatal Cardiac Diagnosis on the Prevalence of Congenital
Heart Disease
Does a Prenatal Cardiac Diagnosis Enhance Neonatal Survival?
Prenatal Cardiac Diagnosis and *In Utero* Medical Therapy
Prenatal Cardiac Diagnosis and Fetal Intervention
The Impact of Prenatal Cardiac Diagnosis on Informed Consent
Conclusion
References

INTRODUCTION

Thirty years ago, when our laboratory first became involved in echocardiographic examination of the human fetal heart, it was hoped that these studies might provide added insight into the anatomic and physiologic development of the human cardiovascular system. It was our intention to take a systematic approach to the development of the human fetus in order to determine whether we could use fetal echocardiography to compare human cardiac development with the studies of chronically instrumented fetal lambs that served as the foundation for our understanding of fetal cardiovascular development. Our first publication documented the utility of the technique to measure the growth of cardiac structures through the second and third trimesters, recognized relative right ventricular volume overload as a normal feature of the fetal human heart, and established the potential for studies to identify congenital cardiac malformations among fetuses identified to be at higher than normal risk for congenital heart disease (1). At that time we were intrigued with the research potential of the technique, but Dr Helen B. Taussig, who was present at our initial presentation at the 1977 annual meeting of the Society for Pediatric Research, enthusiastically welcomed the potential for the prenatal diagnosis of congenital heart disease. Dr Taussig, who had devoted her life to the care of children with congenital heart disease, and who shared in the development of the first surgical procedure for the palliation of tetralogy of Fallot, emphasized the potential for the use of prenatal cardiac diagnostic studies to identify candidates for termination of pregnancy, in order to avoid devastating disability and pain. At the time of our presentation we had decided to avoid mention of termination of pregnancy, owing to the emotional controversy and the risk that such discussion could eclipse the remainder of the content of the presentation. Dr Taussig, however, in characteristic fashion was prescient and unflinching in offering her observations.

Today, fetal echocardiography has become a fundamental aspect of perinatal care throughout the developed world. Routine visualization of the fetal heart has become a standard of care for obstetrical ultrasound, and the prenatal diagnosis of major forms of congenital heart disease is now commonplace. It has taken these 30 years, however, to define the clinical role that prenatal diagnosis has in the management of pregnancies which are complicated by congenital heart disease.

Prenatal diagnosis for genetic, skeletal, neurologic, gastrointestinal, pulmonary and urological malformations, and certain metabolic diseases has been commonplace for many decades. Furthermore, there are widely accepted standardized, diagnostic, counseling, and treatment protocols in place. However, there is little consensus concerning the most appropriate response to specific prenatal cardiac diagnoses. Indisputably, the answer to the question of whether prenatal cardiac diagnosis "makes a difference" is an emphatic "yes." In this chapter the various options offered by the prenatal recognition of congenital heart disease will be discussed (2,3,4).

CONTINUATION VERSUS TERMINATION OF PREGNANCY

Given its prevalence (approximately eight per 1000 live births) consumption of healthcare resources (approximately four per 1000 will require medical or surgical therapy during the first year of life), and its mortality rates, congenital heart disease is one of the most dominant birth defects (5). Survivors may fare quite well, but often with significant chronic disabilities, requiring ongoing medical care, special education resources, and vocational and other social supports.

Although most frequently found in isolation, congenital heart disease does occur in association with extracardiac anomalies, frequently in recognizable malformation syndromes or in association with an abnormal karyotype (6). Studies in our laboratory in the 1980s suggested that the diagnosis of congenital heart disease by echocardiography during the second trimester was associated with an abnormal karyotype in almost 30% of affected fetuses (7). This is consistent with expectations based on the incidence of abnormal karyotype in patients who are diagnosed with congenital heart disease at term and the expected incidence of spontaneous fetal wastage of affected neonates during late gestation. Therefore, we recommend careful genetic screening in all fetuses diagnosed prenatally with congenital heart disease.

Whilst discussions of termination of pregnancy are complicated by religious, emotional, moral, legal, and political considerations it is important to recognize that families face the question of whether termination of pregnancy is a reasonable option for their situation. Many families, faced with the reality of a diagnosis of congenital heart disease, may decide to terminate the pregnancy. An additional complicating factor is that antenatal diagnosis of congenital heart disease is confined to fetuses beyond 10 weeks' gestational age, with the vast majority of these diagnoses established during the second trimester. The decision to terminate a pregnancy at this stage can be wrenching. Careful counseling, including discussion of the degree of certainty of the diagnosis, detailed discussion of the nature of the cardiac lesion, including management options, expected survival, and functional outcomes (prediction of activity level, academic performance, long-term survival, and reproductive capacity), and the potential for recurrence in future offspring should be made clear. While no two families use the same decision-making formula, the most common considerations are as follows.

Gestational Age

Some individuals faced with congenital cardiac malformations, in isolation or associated with defined syndromes incompatible with life, have sought late-term abortion. The counseling of the majority of patients is based on local abortion laws, most of which limit this option to 20–24 weeks of gestation. Although it might seem intuitive that the abortion option would be chosen more frequently in earlier gestation, the literature is somewhat contrary on this point (8). A recent publication, offering a mathematical model to calculate the impact of prenatal cardiac diagnosis on the prevalence of congenital heart disease uses a factor of 1.4 to account for an increased likelihood of the abortion option being chosen during early gestation (9).

- *Nature of the lesion*: isolated congenital heart disease may most often be addressed with surgical strategies that result in long-term palliation, if not a definitive "cure." For a long time, we have used a linear scale of severity, from one to 10, when counseling families about the complexity of heart disease in their fetuses. We consider lesions that may be repaired or palliated into a two-ventricular physiology as inherently "simpler" than abnormalities that will require univentricular palliation, passing through cavopulmonary connection, or orthotopic cardiac transplantation. To be sure, we may encounter hearts with biventricular circulations (e.g. complex atrioventricular discordant hearts, persistent truncus arteriosus with important truncal valve regurgitation) which represent daunting surgical or medical problems. The specter of a minimum of two – and often more – complex open heart procedures in the first years of life, with the known potential complications of the Fontan circulation (10) has weighted the parental decision to seek termination of pregnancy.

Neurodevelopmental Potential

Although the literature is not completely consistent on this point, it appears that children who are subjected to open heart surgery during early infancy are at higher risk for neurodevelopmental delay (11). This has been a particular concern in the follow-up of children with complete transposition of the great arteries (TGA). This subgroup of patients is of particular interest. A large-scale long-term follow-up study at the Boston Children's Hospital (12) has focused particular attention on the impact of deep hypothermic cardiac arrest on neurodevelopmental outcomes by following a large cohort of patients with simple transposition and transposition with ventricular septal defect. The study randomized patients into two groups: one with a deep hypothermic cardiac arrest strategy and one with a bypass strategy involving the use of low-flow bypass. Neurodevelopmental testing demonstrated an advantage among children managed with low-flow bypass, with further data suggesting that the differences in neurodevelopmental outcome between the two groups could be ameliorated with the use of early intervention educational strategies. Whilst considerable attention has been focused on the effect of circulatory support strategy during cardiac bypass as the cause of neurodevelopmental disability it is important to note that both experimental groups in the Boston Deep Hypothermic Arrest Trial (BDHAT) fell below the neurodevelopmental scores of normal infants. This suggests that there could be a global disadvantage of cardiac bypass *per se* on neurodevelopmental outcome, or that these infants may have poor neurodevelopmental potential, based on the presence of congenital heart disease. We have been interested in the study of Rosenthal (13), which suggest that neonates with congenital heart disease associated with impaired systemic perfusion or cyanotic congenital heart disease tend to have smaller head versus abdominal circumferences. We postulated that this disturbed growth pattern might reflect altered blood flow distribution during fetal development, which results in a relative shortfall of cerebral substrate or oxygen delivery, or both. A multicenter preliminary study demonstrated that patients with cyanotic lesions (i.e. tetralogy of Fallot, tricuspid atresia, and TFA (or lesions associated with retrograde perfusion of the aortic arch and cerebral circulation, such as hypoplastic left heart (HLH) syndrome)) tended to have reversal of the cerebro:placental resistance ratio, in a manner that parallels the altered resistance ratio of fetuses with placental insufficiency and "brain-sparing" growth restriction (14). In these patients there is lower than normal systemic resistance in the cerebral circulation, reflecting an autoregulatory "centralization" of systemic blood flow. Neurodevelopmental studies of growth-restricted neonates suggest that these children are at a disadvantage despite their centralization of blood flow, since there may be a shortfall in cerebral oxygen or substrate delivery, or both (15). Fouron and colleagues (16) have demonstrated that retrograde perfusion of the aortic isthmus is associated with impaired neurocognitive outcomes in fetuses with congenital heart disease. We have postulated that the detection of reversed cerebro:placental resistance ratio, in the presence of congenital heart disease, may be an indicator of poor neurodevelopmental potential, regardless of the circulatory support strategy that is used during open-heart surgery. We have not yet included this in our patient counseling, since our experience is only preliminary. We are in the process of testing this hypothesis in a multicenter study of HLH syndrome, and anticipate that such studies will be expanded to include a wider spectrum of congenital cardiac malformations.

Associated Malformations

Although usually found as isolated birth defects, congenital cardiac malformations are often part of a multi-organ constellation of abnormalities that may include the skeletal, gastrointestinal, urogenital, and neurologic systems. In some cases there may be a predictable pattern of multisystem involvement. Such syndromic associations are found in infants with:

- **VACTERL** association (Vertebral, Anal, Cardiac, Tracheal, Esophageal, Renal, and Limb anomalies).
- **CHARGE** association (Coloboma, Heart abnormalities, Atresia choanae, Retarded growth and development and/or central nervous system anomalies, Genital hypoplasia, and Ear anomalies).
- Karyotypic abnormalities such as trisomy 21, trisomy 18, and trisomy 134) in fetuses with partial deletions from the short arm of chromosome 22 (e.g. velocardiofacial or DiGeorge syndrome) which occurs in approximately 25% of fetuses diagnosed with conotruncal malformations, including interrupted aortic arch type B (between the carotid arteries), persistent truncus arteriosus, tetralogy of Fallot, and/or fetuses with isolated aortic arch anomalies such as double aortic arch and right aortic arch. Whilst the manifestations of the velocardiofacial syndrome may be pleomorphic, making accurate counseling difficult, the recent suggestion that this syndrome may be associated with schizophrenia in adolescence or early adulthood in as many as 25% of affected patients has resulted in an increase in the frequency with which termination of pregnancy is chosen for the management of fetuses who have this microdeletion (17–28).

Cardiopulmonary Interaction

A substantial subgroup of fetuses with congenital heart disease are prone to associated pulmonary hypoplasia, airway obstruction, pulmonary lymphangiectasis, and/or pulmonary hypertension that may threaten survival, even in situations in which the anatomy of the heart may be amenable to surgical repair. For example, fetuses with intrathoracic space-occupying masses may have lung hypoplasia on the side of the mass. In addition, shift of the mediastinal mass into the contralateral thoracic cavity may result in concomitant hypoplasia of that lung. This has been well-established in clinical cases of congenital diaphragmatic hernia as well as in fetal animal models. The association of congenital diaphragmatic hernia with congenital heart disease may be particularly malignant, and while we have had some experience with performing ex utero intrapartum treatment (EXIT) procedures to establish extracorporeal membrane oxygenation (ECMO) support (29), the overall result for children with this combination of lesions has been disappointing. The subgroup of patients with tetralogy of Fallot with Absent Pulmonary Valve syndrome may be at a severe disadvantage, owing to aneurismal dilation of the main and proximal branch pulmonary arteries, resulting in compression of the carina and proximal tracheal tree (30). In addition, some of these fetuses have morphologically abnormal distal plexiform arborization patterns of the pulmonary arteries, resulting in pulmonary hypertension. Approximately 25% of these fetuses also have the DiGeorge or velocardiofacial syndromes. Our experience suggests that parental response to counseling regarding the potential outcome for tetralogy of Fallot with Absent Pulmonary Valve syndrome will often be to choose termination of pregnancy. Pulmonary lymphangiectasis may result from severe *in utero* obstruction to pulmonary venous return (31). There are some cardiac lesions associated with critical obstruction to pulmonary venous return. These include total anomalous pulmonary venous return with obstruction and HLH syndrome with premature obstruction of the foramen ovale. Diagnosis of isolated anomalies of pulmonary venous return may be difficult in the mid-trimester fetus, and our experience with the prenatal diagnosis of total anomalous pulmonary venous return has largely been in patients with complex congenital heart disease in the setting of right atrial isomerism and asplenia (32,33). Parents faced with this constellation of anomalies will often choose to terminate the pregnancy. Fetuses with HLH syndrome, complicated by premature closure of the foramen ovale, represent a subgroup of patients with an extremely poor prognosis. These fetuses are usually born with severe respiratory distress and severe hypoxemia (33,34,35). Despite aggressive neonatal management, including immediate surgical palliation or neonatal radio-frequency wire perforation of the atrial septum with subsequent stenting of the septum, mortality rates approach 50%. The latter appears to relate to irreversible prenatal development of pulmonary vascular changes. These poor neonatal outcomes have served as the impetus for the effort to develop a protocol for intrauterine stenting of the atrial septum. It is not surprising that parents faced with the reality of a fetus with HLH syndrome that will require heroic prenatal or neonatal intervention, only to be placed on the pathway through Norwood and Fontan palliation will often choose to terminate these pregnancies.

IMPACT OF PRENATAL CARDIAC DIAGNOSIS ON THE PREVALENCE OF CONGENITAL HEART DISEASE

The impact of prenatal cardiac diagnosis on the prevalence of congenital heart disease was reviewed in a recent publication by Germanakis and Sifakis (36). These authors enumerated the factors that are considered by parents in their decision-making and reviewed the literature in an effort to determine the frequency with which pregnancy termination is chosen for specific malformations. They offer a mathematical model to determine the impact of prenatal diagnosis on prevalence and suggest that the product of the probability that prenatal cardiac ultrasound screening will be performed ($P_{evaluation}$), the probability that congenital heart disease, if present, will be detected ($P_{detection}$), and the probability that a decision will be made to terminate the affected pregnancy ($P_{decision}$), subtracted from unity, represents the impact of prenatal cardiac diagnosis on the prevalence of congenital heart disease (1.0). This model is certainly accurate; however, the specific impact of prenatal cardiac diagnosis will differ from locale to locale, and will vary for specific cardiac malformations according to local surgical experience. For example, the authors suggest that $P_{evaluation}$ approximates 1.0, based on the widely held European standard of at least one, if not multiple, mandated ultrasound examinations during uncomplicated pregnancies and the recommendation that all such studies include fetal cardiac imaging. In the USA the standard of care still does not call for routine ultrasound examination of every pregnant woman, although the American Institute of Ultrasound in Medicine, the American College of Obstetrics and Gynecology, and the American College of Radiology all have established four-chamber and outflow tract views of the fetal heart as the standard of care during any general ultrasound study of the fetus. Depending upon the community being considered, $P_{evaluation}$ in the USA is probably in the range of 0.5 to 0.8. The authors estimate that $P_{detection}$ is approximately 0.47, based on a review of the literature. Our experience suggests that a detection rate of 47% is a best-case scenario, with the standard of care in many communities considerably lower. In addition, the authors estimate a $P_{decision}$ of ~0.35. Based on these estimates the overall impact of prenatal cardiac diagnosis on the prevalence of congenital heart disease was estimated to be a 14% reduction, with the estimate increasing to 21%, assuming an overall factor of 1.4 may be applied owing to earlier gestational diagnosis. Our own experience has suggested that $P_{decision}$ may vary greatly. At Morgan Stanley Children's Hospital of New York – Presbyterian $P_{decision}$ has hovered in the 0.10 range for the past three years. This almost certainly reflects the referral patterns to our laboratory. Our Section of Maternal–Fetal Medicine is actively involved in Level III fetal echocardiographic studies for prescreening. Many patients do not seek further counseling once they have been informed of the presence of congenital heart disease as part of multiorgan malformation complexes or in association with karyotypic abnormalities. To be sure, the local surgical philosophy and the social mores of a particular community will have a profound impact on the way in which even the most complex abnormalities are managed. This may be witnessed by examining the extremely high frequency of termination of pregnancy in the series reported by Dr Lindsey Allen when she described her experience in London compared with her experience with the same cardiac lesions when diagnosed in New York City. The suggested mathematical model may be useful for assessing the impact of prenatal diagnosis on the prevalence of individual cardiac malformations, but the results will clearly differ depending on the community of patients and physicians.

DOES A PRENATAL CARDIAC DIAGNOSIS ENHANCE NEONATAL SURVIVAL?

Our assumption, from the time of our first prenatal cardiac diagnosis (tricuspid atresia, ventricular septal defect, and pulmonary stenosis) was that advance knowledge of the presence of congenital heart disease, especially lesions that render the neonate dependent upon persistent patency of the ductus arteriosus for ongoing pulmonary or systemic blood flow, would quickly be shown to enhance survival. In fact, it has taken over 20 years, and multiple studies, to demonstrate a statistically significant enhancement in survival for such children.

Our initial assessment of the impact of fetal echocardiographic diagnosis of congenital heart disease on survival, demonstrated a survival advantage for neonates who had been diagnosed prenatally with lesions that could be managed using a two-ventricular management strategy. Infants who would ultimately require Fontan palliation of single ventricle variants did not appear to enjoy a survival advantage. This was initially a surprise, since most of these neonates required some form of neonatal surgery, most frequently associated with ductal-dependent lesions. In retrospect, our numbers were relatively small, and our local experience with HLH syndrome was such that the statistics could not detect an enhancement of survival likelihood related to antenatal diagnosis. Other centers investigating the same question drew similar conclusions, related either to uniformly dismal surgical outcomes for HLH syndrome, or, alternatively, such uniformly excellent results that the studies lacked the statistical power to adequately investigate the hypothesis at hand.

More recent studies, from large pediatric cardiac surgical centers took into account variables such as the impact of prenatal diagnosis on *intention to treat*, and demonstrated a relatively profound impact of prenatal diagnosis on the survival likelihood of lesions such as HLH syndrome, complete transposition of the great arteries, and coarctation of the aorta (2,3,4). Of interest is the fact that a recent report from the Children's Hospital of Philadelphia failed to demonstrate a significant survival advantage imparted by the prenatal diagnosis of visceral heterotaxy. This, in part, is related to the uniformly poor prognosis for this syndrome, which appears virtually unmanageable in a significant percentage of fetuses and neonates, regardless of the application of aggressive management strategies (37).

A recent publication established the importance surgical volume plays in the outcome for neonates undergoing surgical palliation of HLH syndrome. Survival is directly proportional to surgical volume at such centers, independent of the operating surgeon at each institution (38). Although not examined for other neonatal surgical procedures, it seems logical that the same phenomenon will hold for a wide variety of complex surgical procedures. This raises an obvious question when considering the potential impact of prenatal diagnosis on neonatal surgical survival: What is the impact of such diagnoses in allowing patients to be referred for delivery at particular high-volume pediatric cardiac centers with demonstrated excellence in the performance of specific procedures? With the proliferation of fetal cardiac diagnostic centers throughout our geographic area we have noted a selective process of referral to our center for specific high-risk procedures. We anticipate that such a collaborative approach to neonatal cardiac surgical management will be adopted in an increasing number of centers as regionalization of care for "super-specialties" such as neonatal cardiac surgery is mandated, either by clinical necessity, by medical governing boards, or by economic reality.

Our first study of the impact of prenatal diagnosis of congenital heart disease on survival did note a significant decrease in the frequency of metabolic acidosis in neonates with a variety of critical congenital heart diseases who had been diagnosed antenatally (39). This finding was confirmed in a study from Columbus Children's Hospital which focused on fetuses with left heart obstructive lesions, although they did not detect a survival advantage among these children (40). In a subsequent multicenter study involving our group at Yale, the University of Maryland and the University of Utrecht, in the Netherlands, prenatal cardiac diagnosis was found to virtually eliminate the risk of preoperative metabolic acidosis in the presence of critical congenital heart disease (41), presumably by allowing anticipatory treatment to avoid hypoxemia and ischemia secondary to neonatal closure of the ductus arteriosus or the initiation of inotropic support, or both, for fetuses with impaired ventricular pump function. The neurocognitive advantage imparted by avoidance of metabolic acidosis has previously been demonstrated in premature infants. It remains to be seen whether a similar phenomenon can be demonstrated for mature infants with congenital heart disease (42).

In our study we attempted to demonstrate an economic advantage that could be attributed to prenatal cardiac diagnosis. Naïvely, we assumed that prenatal diagnosis would facilitate neonatal surgery, improve surgical outcomes, and shorten hospitalizations. Retrospectively, it seems obvious that we should have anticipated no such impact in the subgroup of patients for whom prenatal diagnosis had no significant impact on survival (e.g. patients with single ventricle variants). In patients in whom there was a survival advantage, costs were significantly *increased* owing to the increased cost of hospitalization of the surviving children. We could, however, demonstrate significantly lower costs if we factored in the savings to the medical care delivery system associated with termination of pregnancy, and if it can be proven that prenatal cardiac diagnosis contributes to an improvement in neurodevelopmental outcome. The substantial costs per surgical survivor may be dwarfed by the costs incurred for the care of survivors with chronic disabilities. Of course it is difficult, if not impossible, to perform an accurate cost:benefit analysis, since we cannot adequately assign a value to a given child's survival.

PRENATAL CARDIAC DIAGNOSIS AND *IN UTERO* MEDICAL THERAPY

At the time of our initial publication concerning prenatal cardiac diagnosis we commented on the use of M-mode echocardiography to detect and analyze disturbances in fetal cardiac rhythm. Among the arrhythmias that were described were isolated extrasystoles, one case of complete heart block in the fetus of a mother with a history of collagen vascular disease and a high titer of anti-nuclear antibodies, and a hydropic fetus with left atrial isomerism, complex atrioventricular canal defect, atrial flutter, and complete heart block. We quickly realized that fetal extrasystoles were a frequent and relatively benign rhythm disturbance. However, they may serve to initiate reciprocating atrioventricular tachycardia in fetuses who have an underlying anatomic substrate (an accessory atrioventricular connection and decremental conduction in the atrioventricular node). The risk of juxtaposition of appropriately timed extrasystoles and appropriate anatomic substrate appears to occur in 0.5% to 2% of neonates with supraventricular ectopic beats, and in a similar percentage of fetuses with extrasystoles.

In the early 1980s we focused our attention on the frequency with which idiopathic non-immune hydrops fetalis could be attributed to primary fetal cardiovascular disease, including congenital heart disease associated with atrioventricular or semilunar valve regurgitation. In hydropic fetuses, the edema is thought to be secondary to the limited reserve of fetal myocardium, in which increased preload results in a dramatic increase in systemic venous pressure, with a limited augmentation of systolic output. Increased systemic venous pressure, translates into increased hydrostatic pressure at the capillary level of the fetus. This results in a rapid accumulation of interstitial and third-spaced fluid (hydrops) in fetuses with lower oncotic pressure, interstitial tissue pressure, and greater vascular permeability than the mature organism. The normal fetus produces considerably more lymphatic fluid per unit of body weight than the mature child. An increase in outflow pressure from the thoracic duct beyond a critical level will result in a relatively abrupt cessation of lymphatic drainage. This results in the development of anasarca. In the adult sheep the "closing pressure" to lymphatic drainage is in the range of 25 mm Hg, whereas in the fetal lamb this critical pressure is in the range of 12 mmHg to 15 mmHg. Significantly increased systemic venous pressure, therefore, leads to a marked increase in extravasated water and an abrupt decrease in lymphatic drainage. It should be no surprise that hydrops fetalis is the final common pathway for a variety of structural and functional abnormalities that lead to increased venous pressure or diminished lymphatic drainage in the fetus (46).

Romero (47) and Friedman (48), studying fetal and mature sheep hearts and isolated muscle strips, demonstrated that fetal myocardium is less compliant and generates less contractile force when stimulated at any given preload than mature myocardium. This is reflected in the Doppler diastolic filling waveforms from both ventricular inflow tracts and longitudinal myocardial tissue velocities from both lateral atrioventricular valve rings that demonstrate E/A (and E'/A') ratios <1.0. This indicates the reliance of ventricular diastolic filling on coordinated active atrial contraction. The loss of a coordinated atrial contraction results in "cannon" a-waves, which are reflected in retrograde pulsations in the inferior vena cava, ductus venosus, and, in most severe cases, the umbilical vein. These cannon a-waves may result in a sufficient increase in capillary hydrostatic pressure to cause hydrops fetalis.

Fetuses with atrial tachyarrhythmias have foreshortened diastolic filling periods, often resulting in inadequate atrial emptying. In addition, fetuses with atrioventricular reciprocating tachycardia may have ineffective atrial contractions, depending upon the ventriculoatrial conduction time. In the presence of short ventriculoatrial conduction time, the active atrial contraction may occur so soon after the ventricular depolarization that it may interfere with atrial, rather than facilitate ventricular, filling. This results in a-wave reversal in the inferior vena cava, ductus venosus, and, possibly, the umbilical vein. In the presence of atrial flutter there will typically be multiple retrograde a-wave pulsations in the fetal systemic venous system that will be associated with elevated mean venous and capillary hydrostatic pressure. These findings account for the rapid development of hydrops fetalis in fetuses with sustained atrial tachyarrhythmias. Krapp and colleagues (49) have suggested that prolonged atrial retrograde flow in the ductus venosus after conversion of atrial tachycardia to sinus rhythm may be used to define the presence of tachycardia-induced cardiomyopathy. The latter may result in atrial compromise rather than a disturbance in ventricular pump function and may delay the resolution of hydrops fetalis, despite the re-establishment of normal sinus rhythm (50).

Whilst it has been demonstrated that the administration of ß-mimetic agents may increase fetal heart-rate, there has been little evidence that this resolves hydrops fetalis. The latter may well require establishment of atrioventricular synchrony, and may have an impact on efforts to develop protocols for fetal pacemaker therapy. Our experience with the use of absorbable corticosteroid in a small group of patients with complete heart block suggested that the anti-inflammatory effect of such therapy improves fetal hemodynamics, and may partially ameliorate immune complex-mediated damage to the atrioventricular node (51). This finding has led to a multicenter study of the effect of corticosteroid for the treatment of complete heart block associated with high maternal titers of anti-Ro or anti-La antibodies. Jaeggi and colleagues (52) have presented data to suggest a remarkable improvement in the prognosis of fetuses with complete heart block since they introduced routine administration of corticosteroid for these fetuses.

In a review of 4838 consecutive fetal echocardiograms Copel et al. (53) found that 595 (12.3%) had been referred for arrhythmia evaluation. Three hundred thirty

(55.4%) of these fetuses were in normal sinus rhythm at the time of initial evaluation, whereas 255 (42.9%) had isolated extrasystoles at initial examination. Ten fetuses (1.7%) had sustained atrial tachyarrhythmias. Of the 330 fetuses in normal sinus rhythm at the time of initial evaluation five (1.5%) subsequently developed supraventricular tachycardia (during later gestation or the neonatal period). Of the 10 fetuses in which sustained atrial tachyarrhythmias were diagnosed on initial evaluation there was one death, in a fetus with congenital heart disease and atrial flutter.

Although algorithms for the evaluation and treatment of fetal tachyarrhythmias remain in flux, it is clear that a detailed risk:benefit analysis must take place prior to initiating transplacental treatment of fetal arrhythmias. The complexities of treating a patient within a patient make it advisable to bring a range of subspecialists to the table when considering antiarrhythmic treatment. The team should include experts in fetal cardiac ultrasound, developmental electrophysiology, neonatology, perinatology, and adult cardiology. The decision-making algorithm should include accurate diagnosis of the nature of the arrhythmia, its hemodynamic consequences, fetal gestational age and pulmonary maturity, and the potential risks and benefits of antiarrhythmic therapy on the fetus and mother. Both members of the complex patient "unit" require careful monitoring. There is a lack of unanimity concerning the role of antiarrhythmic therapy in the management of fetuses with intermittent tachycardia. On the other hand, we believe that supraventricular tachyarrhythmia, associated with hydrops fetalis, in a previable or extremely premature fetus, warrants transplacental antiarrhythmic therapy.

PRENATAL CARDIAC DIAGNOSIS AND FETAL INTERVENTION

The role of fetal intervention for the management of selected fetuses with aortic stenosis has intrigued the pediatric cardiology community since the early 1990s. The initial descriptions of transplacental introduction of balloon catheters for balloon aortic valvuloplasty were stimulated by poor outcomes among neonates with valvar aortic stenosis at that time. The low success rate of such interventions and the parallel improvement in neonatal surgical and catheter intervention for this condition resulted in a moratorium for such procedures (54,55). Recently, however, there has been a renaissance in the degree of interest in this technique as a means of preventing progressive left ventricular hypoplasia in fetuses with aortic stenosis, left ventricular fibro-elastosis and retrograde perfusion of the aortic arch and ascending aorta. The subgroup of patients with HLH syndrome and premature closure of the foramen ovale have a particularly malignant course, due to pulmonary insufficiency and lymphangiectasia (54–56). The same investigative group has used catheter therapy, and more recently stent implantation, to relieve pulmonary venous hypertension in such patients. Additionally, catheter-based therapy has been applied for the palliation of membranous fetal pulmonary atresia with intact ventricular septum. While the initial report of successful pulmonary balloon valvuloplasty suggested that each of the two fetuses faced an immediate future of hydrops fetalis, based on the detection of atrial flow reversal in the ductus venosus (57), subsequent experience has suggested that such flow reversal is the rule, rather than the exception, in fetuses with pulmonary outflow obstruction (58). The status of the foramen ovale may well be a determinant of the presence or absence of hydrops fetalis in this subgroup of patients.

While the impact of such interventions on the management of fetuses with congenital heart disease remains to be defined, the lessons that are being learned and applied to the treatment of the fetus are likely to produce a quantum leap in our understanding of the fetal and transitional circulation.

THE IMPACT OF PRENATAL CARDIAC DIAGNOSIS ON INFORMED CONSENT

While we have reached a level of sophistication in prenatal diagnosis that allows most major forms of congenital heart disease to be diagnosed reliably between approximately 12 weeks' and term gestation, even the busiest fetal cardiac centers appear to have reached a plateau in the frequency with which diagnoses are made prenatally. Our own experience has suggested that 45% to 55% of the neonates who pass through our neonatal intensive care unit with a primary diagnosis of congenital heart disease will have been diagnosed prenatally. We estimate this figure to approximate >85% among patients who are followed by our full-time obstetrical faculty, whereas the figure among referral centers outside the New York – Presbyterian Health Care System is significantly lower.

In a study that was recently conducted in our laboratory, Williams et al. (59) used a written instrument to measure the level of maternal understanding. The mothers of fetuses who were diagnosed prenatally to have congenital heart disease demonstrated a significantly enhanced degree of understanding compared with the level of understanding demonstrated by the mothers of children with similar conditions, who were not diagnosed until after birth.

CONCLUSION

The field of pediatric cardiology has seen significant change over the past 30 years. One of the most fundamental differences is the change of focus: from neonatal through school-age patients constituting >90% of clinical activities in 1977 to more than 50% of patient activity involving the care of young adults and fetuses with congenital heart disease.

As discussed above, the prenatal diagnosis of congenital heart disease has had profound implications for the clinical care of neonates with congenital heart disease. The challenge that we now face is to extend fetal cardiology beyond the academic medical center and to demonstrate that prenatal cardiac diagnosis has a positive impact on the functional outcome of our patients.

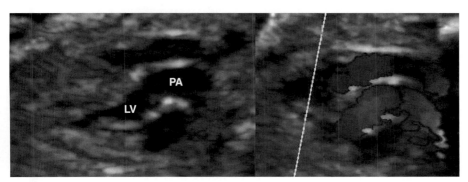

FIGURE 18-1 Mid-trimester fetal heart with complete (d-) transposition of the great arteries (TGA). Bifurcating pulmonary artery (PA) arises from left ventricle (LV). Parallel course of proximal great arteries may be demonstrated using color flow or Doppler power imaging.

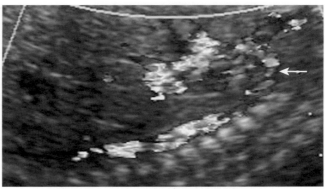

FIGURE 18–2 Retrograde flow (in orange) in aortic arch of fetus with complex double outlet right ventricle, with aortic outflow tract obstruction with aortic arch hypoplasia. Fouron and colleagues (16) have demonstrated that retrograde perfusion of the aortic arch through the aortic isthmus is associated with a high risk of unfavorable neurocognitive outcome.

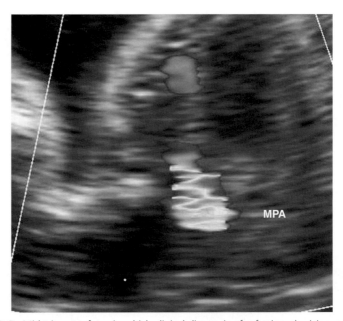

FIGURE 18–3 Mid-trimester fetus in which clinical diagnosis of referring physician, of valvar pulmonary stenosis, was confirmed. Previous counseling had focused on neonatal pulmonary balloon valvuloplasty, with possible later aortopulmonary shunting. Somewhat to our surprise, in light of absence of ventricular septal defect, fetus was noted to have polyhydramnios with persistently absent stomach bubble. In addition, ectopic pelvic kidneys, with probable horseshoe deformity, and kyphoscoliosis, with several hemivertebrae were diagnosed. Apparent diagnosis is previously unsuspected VACTERL with esophageal atresia component. Counseling has included management of esophageal atresia with probable TE fistula, and probable insertion of stent into ductus arteriosus at the time of pulmonary valvuloplasty, in order to avoid need for two thoracotomies during the neonatal period.

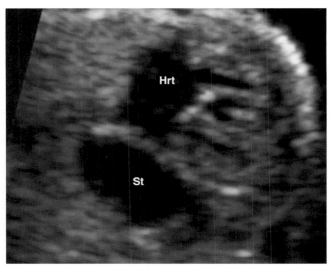

FIGURE 18–4 Fetus with large left-sided diaphragmatic hernia. Stomach bubble is seen alongside heart. Latter is displaced far to the right chest wall. The left lung, on the side of the hernia, is hypoplastic, as is the lung on the right side, where the heart and mediastinum are functioning as space-occupying masses. There is some controversy about the prognostic accuracy of lung:head ratios for prediction of adequacy of neonatal pulmonary function.

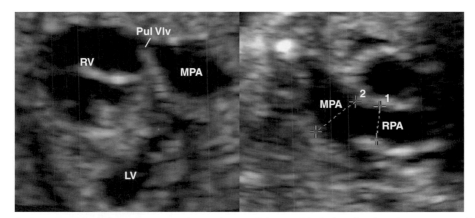

FIGURE 18–5 Fetus with absent pulmonary valve syndrome. Right ventricle (RV) and main pulmonary artery (MPA) are dilated. Pulmonary annulus is guarded by dysplastic tissue that results in moderate pulmonary outflow obstruction and severe pulmonary regurgitation (Pul Vlv). Right-hand panel demonstrates aneurismal dilation of MPA and right pulmonary artery (RPA). Aneurisma pulmonary arteries result in significant large airway compression. This fetus had acquired premature closure of the ductus arteriosus.

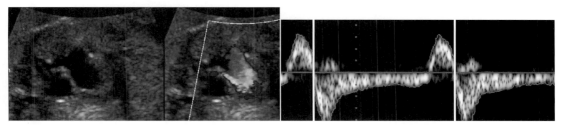

FIGURE 18–6 Discordant atrial volumes in fetus developing hypoplastic left heart (HLH) syndrome. Upper panels demonstrate smaller left atrium with narrow jet of left-to-right shunting across atrial septum into relatively dilated right atrial chamber. In panel below pulsed Doppler waveform in pulmonary vein demonstrates "to-and-fro" flow pattern that presages severe respiratory insufficiency in the delivery room, secondary to pulmonary venous obstruction and secondary pulmonary edema. Such fetuses require emergency decompression of the pulmonary veins.

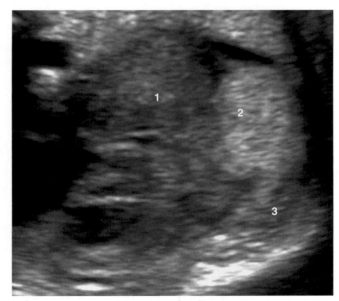

FIGURE 18–7 Fetal heart demonstrating multiple, large, homogeneous, sessile masses at the apex of the left ventricle (1–3), the interventricular septum, and the right ventricular free wall. This is the typical appearance of ventricular rhabdomyomata. These are associated with a high (~80%) likelihood of tuberous sclerosis. A careful family history, including genetic screening for one of the tuberous sclerosis-associated genes is indicated.

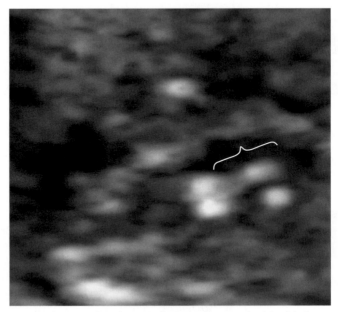

FIGURE 18–8 Multiple intensely echogenic foci are demonstrated in this fetus at 20 weeks' gestation. The echocardiographic signal is virtually as intense as that from adjacent boney structures. There are multiple foci, most involving the papillary muscles of the mitral valve (bracket), with a single focus associated with a tricuspid papillary muscle. These foci do not represent cardiac neoplasms. There presence increases the odds ratio of the Down syndrome by a factor of five to six. These findings must be taken into consideration during general counseling of families regarding fetal wellbeing, and the need for amniocentesis.

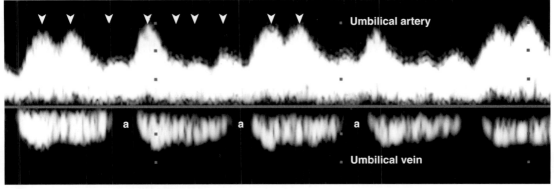

FIGURE 18–9 Fetus with hydrops fetalis had chaotic rhythm reflected in umbilical vessels with extremely rapid and irregular ventricular pulse and marked, regular, slower, a-wave pulsatility. This fetus had protracted episodes of ventricular tachycardia. Image reproduced with permission from Moss and Adam's Heart Disease in Infants, Children and Adolescents. Including the Fetus and Young Adult, 2 volume set, Lippincott Williams & Wilkins, Fedilion (October 1, 2007).

REFERENCES

1. Kleinman CS, et al. Echocardiographic studies of the diagnosis of congenital heart disease and cardiac dysrhythmias. Pediatrics 1980;65:1059–1067.
2. Tworetzky W, et al. Improved surgical outcome after fetal diagnosis of hypoplastic left heart syndrome. Circulation 2001;103:1269–1273.
3. Franklin O, et al. Prenatal diagnosis of coarctation of the aorta improves survival and reduces morbidity. Heart 2002;87:67–69.
4. Bonnet D, et al. Detection of transposition of the great arteries reduces neonatal morbidity and mortality. Circulation 1999;99:916–918.
5. Hoffman JI, Kaplan S, Libathson RR. Prevalence of congenital heart disease. Am Heart J 2007;147:425–439.
6. Wladimiroff JW, et al. Prenatal diagnosis and management of congenital heart defect: significance of associated fetal anomalies and prenatal chromosome studies. Am J Med Genet 1985;21:285–290.
7. Copel JA, et al. The frequency of aneuploidy in prenatally diagnosed congenital heart disease: an indication for fetal karyotyping. Am J Obstet Gynecol 1988;158:409–413.
8. Evans MI, Sobiecki MA, Krivchenia EL, et al. Parental decisions to terminate/continue following abnormnal cytogenetic prenatal diagnosis: "what" is still more important than "when". Am J Med Genet 1996;61:353–355.
9. Germanakis I, Sifakis S. The impact of fetal echocardiography on the prevalence of liveborn congenital heart disease. Pediatr Cardiol 2006;27:465–472.
10. Driscoll DJ. Long-term results of the Fontan operation. Pediatr Cardiol 2007;28:438–442.
11. Miatton M, De Wolf D, Francois K, Thiery E, Vingerhoets G. Neuropsychological performance in school-age children with surgically corrected congenital heart disease. J Pediatr 2007;151:73–78.
12. McGrath E, Wypji D, Rappaport LA, Newburger JW, Bellinger DC. Prediction of IQ and achievement at age 8 years from neurodevelopmental status at age 1 year in children with D-transposition of the great arteries. Pediatrics 2004;114:572–576.
13. Rosenthal GL. Patterns of prenatal growth among infants with cardiovascular malformations: possible hemodynamic effects. Am J Epidemiol 1996;143:505–513.
14. Donofrio MT, Bremer YA, Schieken RM, et al. Autoregulation of cerebral blood flow in fetuses with congenital heart disease: the brain sparing effect. Pediatr Cardiol 2003;24:436–443.
15. Leitner Y, Fattal-Valevski A, Geva R, et al. Neurodevelopmental outcome of children with intrauterine growth retardation: a longitudinal, 10-year prospective study. J Child Neurol 2007;22:580–587.
16. Fouron JC, Gosselin J, Raboisson MJ, et al. The relationship between an aortic isthmus blood flow velocity index and the postnatal neurodevelopmental status of fetuses with placental circulatory insufficiency. Am J Obstet Gynecol 2005;192:497–503.
17. Fogel M, et al. Congenital heart disease and fetal thoracoabdominal anomalies: associations in utero and the importance of cytogenetic analysis. Am J Perinatol 1991;8:411–416.
18. Copel JA, Pilu G, Kleinman CS. Congenital heart disease and extracardiac anomalies: associations and indications for fetal echocardiography. Am J Obstet Gynecol 1986;154:1121–1132.
19. Paladini D, et al. The association between congenital heart disease and Down syndrome in prenatal life. Ultrasound Obstet Gynecol 2000;15:104–108.
20. Fasnacht MS, Jaeggi ET. Fetal and genetic aspects of congenital heart disease. Ther Umsch 2001;58:70–75.
21. Moyano D, Huggon IC, Allan LD. Fetal echocardiography in trisomy 18. Arch Dis Child Fetal Neonatal Ed 2005;90:F520–F522.
22. Nicolaides KH, Sebire NJ, Snijders RJ. Down's syndrome screening with nuchal translucency. Lancet 1997;349:438.

23. Hyett JA, et al. Intrauterine lethality of trisomy 21 fetuses with increased nuchal translucency thickness. Ultrasound Obstet Gynecol 1996;7:101–103.

24. Cheng PJ, et al. First-trimester nuchal translucency measurement and echocardiography at 16 to 18 weeks of gestation in prenatal detection for trisomy 18. Prenat Diagn 2003;23:248–251.

25. Kelly D, et al. Confirmation that the velo-cardio-facial syndrome is associated with haplo-insufficiency of genes at chromosome 22q11. Am J Med Genet 1993;45:308–312.

26. Goldmuntz E, et al. Microdeletions of chromosomal region 22q11 in patients with congenital conotruncal cardiac defects. J Med Genet 1993;30:807–812.

27. Driscoll DA, et al. Prevalence of 22q11 microdeletions in DiGeorge and velocardiofacial syndromes: implications for genetic counselling and prenatal diagnosis. J Med Genet 1993;30:813–817.

28. Shprintzen RJ. Velocardiofacial syndrome and DiGeorge sequence. J Med Genet 1994;31:423–424.

29. Hedrick HL. Ex utero intrapartum therapy. Semin Pediatr Surg 2003;12:190–195.

30. Brown JW, Ruzmetov M, Vijay P, et al. Surgical treatment of absent pulmonary valve syndrome associated with bronchial obstruction. Ann Thorac Surg 2006;82:2221–2226.

31. Holcomb RG, Tyson RW, Ivy DD, et al. Congenital pulmonary venous stenosis presenting as persistent pulmonary hypertension of the newborn. Pediatr Pulmonol 1999;28:301–306.

32. Taketazu M, Lougheed J, Yoo SJ, et al. Spectrum of cardiovascular disease, accuracy of diagnosis, and outcome in fetal heterotaxy syndrome. Am J Cardiol 2006;97:720–724.

33. Cohen MS, Schultz AM, Tian ZY, et al. Heterotaxy syndrome with functional single ventricle: does prenatal diagnosis improve survival? Ann Thorac Surg 2006;82:1629–1636.

34. Taketazu M, Barrea C, Smallhorn JF, et al. Intrauterine pulmonary venous flow and restrictive foramen ovale in fetal hypoplastic left heart syndrome. J Am Coll Cardiol 2004;43:1902–1907.

35. Weidenbach M, Caffier P, Hamisch T, Daehnert I. Hypoplastic left heart syndrome with intact atrial septum – attempt of an interventional palliation by ductal and interatrial stent implantation. Clin Res Cardiol 2006;95:110–114.

36. Germanakis I, Sifakis S. The impact of fetal echocardiography on the prevalence of liveborn congenital heart disease? Pediatr Cardiol 2006;27:465–472.

37. Cohen MS, Schultz AH, Tian ZY, et al. Heterotaxy syndrome with functional single ventricle: does prenatal diagnosis improve survival? Ann Thorac Surg 2006;85:1629–1636.

38. Bazzani LG, Mancin SP. Case volume and mortality in pediatric surgery patients in California1978–2003. Circulation 2007;115:2652–2659.

39. Smythe JF, Copel JA, CS Kleinman. Outcome of prenatally detected cardiac malformations. Am J Cardiol 1992;69:1471–1474.

40. Eapen RS, Rowland DG, Franklin WH. Effect of prenatal diagnosis of critical left heart obstruction on perinatal morbidity and mortality. Am J Perinatol 1998;15:237–242.

41. Verheijen PM, et al. Prenatal diagnosis of congenital heart disease affects preoperative acidosis in the newborn patient. J Thorac Cardiovasc Surg 2001;121:798–803.

42. Lavrijsen SW, et al. Severe umbilical cord acidemia and neurological outcome in preterm and full-term neonates. Biol Neonate 2005;88:27–34.

43. Isaacs H Jr. Fetal and neonatal cardiac tumors. Pediatr Cardiol 2004;25:287–298.

44. Sotiriadis A, Makrydimas G, Joannidis JP. Diagnostic performance of intracardiac echogenic foci for Down syndrome: a meta-analysis. Obstet Gynecol 2003;101:1009–1016.

45. Bromley B, et al. Significance of an echogenic intracardiac focus in fetuses at high and low-risk for aneuploidy. J Ultrasound Med 1998;17:127–131.

46. Rudolph AM. Congenital Diseases of the Heart, second edn. Armonk, NY Futura 2001.

47. Friedman WF. The intrinsic physiologic properties of the developing heart. Prog Cardiovasc Dis 1972;15:87–111.

48. Friedman WF, Kirkpatrick SE. In situ physiological study of the developing heart. Recent Adv Stud Card Struct Metab 1975;5:497–504.

49. Krapp M, Gembruch U, Baumann P. Venous blood flow pattern suggesting tachycardia-induced "cardiomyopathy" in the fetus. Ultrasound Obstet Gynecol 1997;10:32–40.

50. Kleinman CS, Nehgme RA. Cardiac arrhythmias in the human fetus. Pediatr Cardiol 2004;25:234–251.

51. Copel JA, Buyon JP, Kleinman CS. Successful in utero therapy of fetal heart block. Am J Obstet Gynecol 1995;173:1384–1390.

52. Jaeggi ET, et al. Transplacental fetal treatment improves the outcome of prenatally diagnosed complete atrioventricular block without structural heart disease. Circulation 2004;110:1542–1548.

53. Copel JA, Liang RI, Demasio K, et al. The clinical significance of the irregular fetal heart rhythm. Am J Obstet Gynecol 2000;182:813–817, discussion 817–819.

54. Allan LD, et al. Survival after fetal aortic balloon valvuloplasty. Ultrasound in Obstet Gynecol 1995;5:90–91.

55. Kohl T, et al. World experience of percutaneous ultrasound-guided balloon valvuloplasty in human fetuses with severe aortic valve obstruction. Am J Cardiol 2000;85:1230–1233.

56. Wilkins-Haug LE, et al. In utero intervention for hypoplastic left herart syndrome – a perinatologist's perspective. Ultrasound Obstet Gynecol 2005;26:481–486.

57. Tulzer G, et al. Fetal pulmonary valvuloplasty for critical pulmonary stenosis or atresia with intact septum. Lancet 2002;360:1567–1568.

58. Berg C, Kremer C, Geipel A, et al. Ductus venosus blood flow alterations in fetuses with obstructive lesions of the right heart. Ultrasound Obstet Gynecol 2006;28:137–142.

59. Williams IA, et al. The impact of prenatal diagnosis on parental understanding of congenital heart disease. Ultrasound Obstet Gynecol 2007;30:408.

Chapter 19

Neonatal Interventional Catheterizations

Carl P. Garabedian, MD • William E. Hellenbrand, MD

INTRODUCTION

Historically, cardiac catheterizations have been an essential technique for diagnosing cardiac lesions in newborn infants. Cardiac catheterizations were performed on virtually all infants, and children who were suspected of having a cardiac anomaly, to provide vital hemodynamic and anatomic information to direct further therapy. Recent advances in echocardiography have significantly decreased the need for diagnostic catheterizations (1). Two-dimensional echocardiography has been refined so that accurate delineation of intracardiac and extracardiac anatomy may be accomplished noninvasively. With the addition of Doppler analysis and advancements in computer processing, a routine echocardiogram can also provide accurate hemodynamic information, which, in the past, necessitated diagnostic catheterization. Today most neonatal cardiac surgery is performed without the neonate ever undergoing cardiac catheterization.

Magnetic resonance angiography (MRA) is a new noninvasive technique that can accurately delineate the intracardiac and extracardiac anatomy in neonates (2). MRA is especially useful in neonates with complex ventricular malformations and aortic arch abnormalities (including vascular rings) to delineate central and distal pulmonary artery abnormalities and supravalvular stenosis. These new noninvasive techniques have decreased the need for catheterization and avoid the risks associated with radiation, contrast agents, sedation, cold stress, blood loss, arrhythmias, and vascular complications, which are inherent during neonatal catheterization (3,4).

Although this noninvasive revolution has decreased the need for routine diagnostic catheterization the catheterization laboratory has also undergone a revolution of its own. With the development by Rashkind and Miller (5) of balloon atrial septostomy, in 1966, the catheterization laboratory became an area where interventional procedures could easily be performed. Such interventions can palliate and even "cure" various congenital heart diseases with equal and even better success than the previously performed surgical procedures, often with less morbidity and mortality (6). The remainder of this chapter will discuss the various interventional techniques currently employed in neonates and, when surgical options are available, we will discuss the advantages and disadvantages of the various options.

CREATION OF AN ATRIAL SEPTAL DEFECT

Transcatheter creation of an atrial septal defect (ASD) was initially developed to palliate neonates with transposition of the great arteries (TGA) who were deeply cyanotic with unremitting metabolic acidosis secondary to poor mixing of the parallel circulations (5). Previous surgical techniques performed in these critically ill neonates carried an extremely high mortality rate. This stimulated Rashkind and Miller (6), in 1966, to develop a technique for creating an ASD using a balloon-tipped catheter. Immediately after creation of the ASD by balloon atrial septostomy (BAS) these deeply cyanotic neonates have a rapid improvement in their oxygen saturation valves and resolution of the hypoxia-induced metabolic acidosis.

The success of BAS for TGA has led to the application of this procedure for other types of cardiac anomalies with obligatory interatrial shunts, such as hypoplastic left heart (HLH) syndrome, tricuspid atresia, and total anomalous venous return (7). In infants with HLH syndrome and a restrictive ASD, emergent enlargement of the atrial defect may be needed before surgical palliation. BAS has not met the same degree of success in these types of anomalies as that achieved in TGA. This is, in part, because the atrial septum in these anomalies is typically thickened and abnormal in position. Other techniques have been developed to create these defects in these neonates, such as blade atrial septostomy and atrial septoplasty (8,9).

BALLOON ATRIAL SEPTOSTOMY

BAS creates or enlarges an ASD by first passing a special balloon-tipped catheter from the right to left atrium across the patent foramen ovale. The catheter's balloon is inflated in the left atrium and withdrawn rapidly into the right atrium tearing the septum primum and enlarging the ASD. BAS can be performed under fluoroscopic guidance in the catheterization laboratory or under echocardiographic guidance in the neonatal intensive care unit (NICU). Performing a BAS under echocardiographic guidance was first described in 1982 by Allan and colleagues (10).

Echocardiography allows the technique to be performed at the neonate's bedside, with direct visualization of the catheter as it crosses the atrial septum.

This bedside procedure may be performed via the umbilical or femoral vein. Umbilical access is preferred in neonates older than 48 hours of life since femoral access frequently causes permanent occlusion of the vein after BAS (11). An umbilical venous catheter is placed into the right atrium and then replaced with a sheath over a wire. The septostomy catheter is then advanced through the sheath into the right atrium. Asfaq and Houston (11) reported successful umbilical cannulation in 27 of 37 neonates who were more than 48 hours old by use of echocardiographic guidance. If umbilical venous access is not feasible, right femoral venous assess is obtained. Under echocardiographic guidance the catheter tip is advanced from the right atrium through the patent foramen ovale into the left atrium and filled with saline (Figure 19-1 (A)). Echo guidance ensures that the balloon is inflated in the left atrium and not within the pulmonary veins or mitral valve apparatus. When performed in the catheterization laboratory the balloon is filled with dilute contrast under biplane fluoroscopy to assure proper positioning within the left atrium (Figure 19-1 (B)). The size of the tear and the degree of atrial shunting may be assessed by echocardiography and by the neonate's improved oxygen saturation valve (Figure 19-1 (c) and Figure 19-1 (D)).

Once the position of the inflated balloon in the left atrium is confirmed the catheter is pulled with a sharp and forceful tug into the right atrium with immediate release to prevent inferior vena cava obstruction and tears (Figure 19-2 (A), Figure 19-2 (B)). The balloon is deflated and the procedure may be repeated several times with a larger balloon.

Complications of BAS include damage to the mitral or tricuspid valve apparatus, pulmonary venous perforation, inferior vena cava tears, heart block, stroke, and femoral venous obstruction. Damage to the atrioventricular valves and pulmonary veins can almost always be avoided by the use of echocardiographic guidance prior to and during balloon inflation.

After creation of an ASD by BAS in infants with TGA, intracardiac mixing improves and support medications, such as prostaglandin 1 (PGE₁), may be stopped. These defects rarely re-obstruct acutely. Before the advent of the arterial switch operation for TGA these defects would remain patent for six months to two years, until a Mustard or Senning procedure could be performed.

BLADE ATRIAL SEPTOSTOMY

Blade atrial septostomy has been used to create an ASD in neonates and older children in whom BAS has not been successful. This occurs in infants older than one month in whom the septum is less pliable or thickened. The blade septostomy catheter has a specially designed angled tip with a retractable blade. The procedure is performed by advancing the catheter tip up the inferior vena cava from the femoral vein and into the left atrium across the atrial septum. Whilst in the left atrium the blade is extended (Figure 19-3 (A)). The use of biplane angiography is imperative to prevent a laceration of the left atrium during blade extension. The catheter is slowly withdrawn on biplane into the right atrium (Figure 19-3 (B)). This is usually sufficient to create an adequate ASD, but this may be further enlarged by BAS.

A multicenter center study by Park et al. (8) had a 10% incidence of major complications with blade septostomy, including lacerations to the heart. Improvements in the design of blade catheters have led to prevention of some of these inadvertent lacerations. A subsequent study by Atz et al. (9) attempted to use this technique in the preoperative management of neonates with HLH syndrome with restrictive atrial septums. The results of this study were disappointing with two of three neonates suffering cardiac perforation, cardiac tamponade, and death. This occurred in part because these neonates have small left atria; thus, this technique is not applicable to this lesion. We believe that blade atrial septostomy carries a high complication and failure rate in these neonates, regardless of the diagnosis, and this technique is currently not recommended in this age group.

ATRIAL SEPTOPLASTY

Atrial septoplasty enlarges a small ASD by positioning an angioplasty balloon catheter across the defect and tearing the septum with one or multiple inflations. If no ASD is present a trans-septal puncture is first performed, with subsequent angioplasty. To perform an atrial septoplasty access is achieved via the right femoral

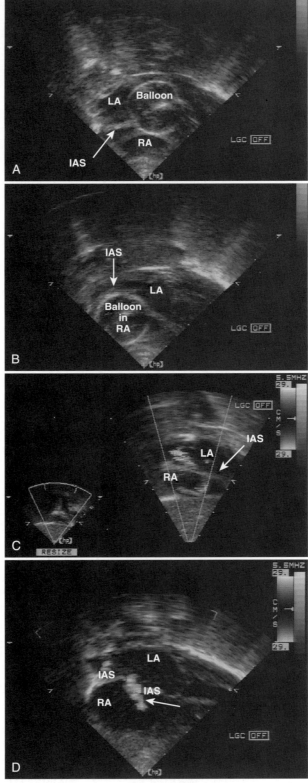

FIGURE 19–1 (A) Subcostal long-axis view of BAS catheter through the patent foramen ovale and inflated in the left atrium. **(B)** The catheter is pulled into the right atrium. Color doppler imaging of the atrial septum **(C)** prior to septostomy and **(D)** following septostomy, arrow pointing to the increased bidirectional shunting through the defect. LA, left atrium; RA, right atrium, IAS, interatrial septum.

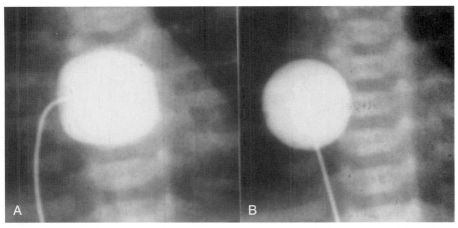

FIGURE 19–2 (A) Fluoroscopic image of an inflated BAS balloon in the left atrium. **(B)** Fluoroscopic image of the BAS catheter after being pulled into the right atrium.

vein and the neonate is fully anticoagulated. If the atrial septum is intact pulmonary artery angiography is performed and the position of the atrial septum is delineated upon levophase. A trans-septal puncture is effected by advancing a 6 French trans-septal sheath and needle to the presumed position of the atrial septum. The position of the atrial septum may be confirmed by staining the septum with contrast and or echocardiography. A trans-septal puncture is performed in the mid-portion of the septum and the sheath advanced into the left atrium. The needle is withdrawn and an 18-gauge torque wire is advanced into the left atrium (if an ASD is present the wire is placed across the defect with an end-hole catheter). The sheath is pulled down to the level of the inferior vena cava and a balloon catheter is passed over the guide wire and one or several dilations are performed with appropriately sized balloons. Echocardiography is helpful during inflations to define the anatomy (Figure 19-4) and to confirm the result (Figure 19-5).

Atrial septoplasty has been used to create an ASD in neonates, with significantly less morbidity and mortality than blade septostomy. Atz et al. (9) performed the technique in 16 neonates with HLH syndrome and a restrictive atrial septum. All 16 infants had successful relief of pulmonary venous obstruction without procedure-related mortality (one infant required stenting of the atrial septum). Atrial septoplasty produces a temporary unobstructed ASD in these neonates and is the procedure of choice in neonates with a restrictive atrial septum which is not amenable to BAS.

Surgical open septectomy may also provide adequate relief of atrial obstruction, but is significantly more invasive and carries a higher morbidity and mortality in these critically ill neonates. We feel atrial septoplasty can safely and adequately provide relief of interatrial obstruction and should be used in cases where temporary relief is required before surgical palliation. Implantation of a stent in the septum may be accomplished if angioplasty is not successful, but is not recommended for long-term creation of an ASD. Surgical septectomy should be performed expeditiously for creation of a long-term ASD.

Regardless of the technique chosen for creation of an ASD the status of the septum must be monitored closely for critical re-obstruction.

CRITICAL AORTIC STENOSIS

The management of neonates with critical aortic stenosis is challenging for cardiologists and cardiac surgeons (12,13). The lack of heterogeneity of this population

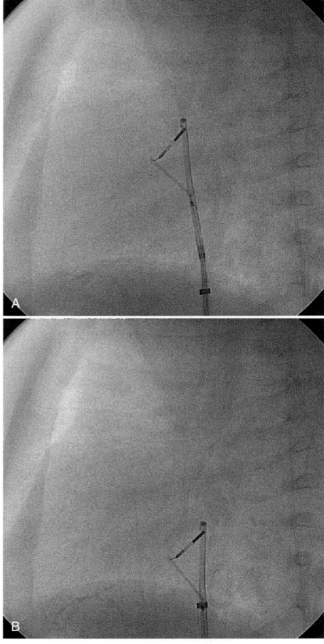

FIGURE 19–3 **(A)** Lateral fluoroscopic image of blade-tipped catheter across an atrial septal defect with the blade extended in the left atrium. **(B)** The catheter is pulled into the right atrium.

of neonates has made algorithms of treatment options elusive. Over the years it has become apparent that, regardless of the initial treatment chosen, it is only palliative, making repeat catheterizations and operations inevitable. The status of the left ventricle has proved to be the most critical issue in the long-term management of these children. Neonates with severely hypoplastic left ventricles or significant endocardial fibro-elastosis (EFE), or both, must have a single-ventricle palliation or cardiac transplantation should considered for the initial palliation if real long-term survival can be expected. A "bail-out" Norwood palliation after unsuccessful balloon dilation carries an extremely high mortality.

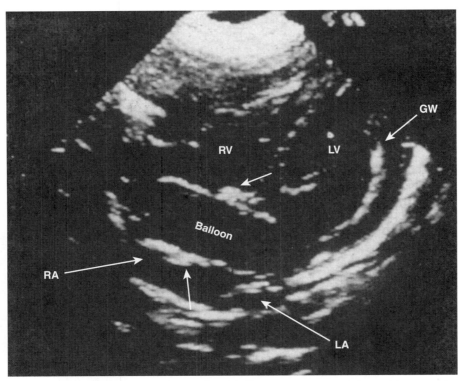

FIGURE 19–4 Echocardiographic image of an inflated balloon across an restrictive atrial septum in an infant with hypoplastic left heart. RA, right atrium; LA, left atrium; RV, right ventricle; LV, left ventricle; GW, guide-wire.

The initial attempts at transcatheter dilation of critical aortic stenosis was attempted in the setting of poor surgical outcome (12). Zeevi et al. (14) reported two matched cohorts of neonates undergoing surgical valvulotomy versus balloon dilation for critical aortic stenosis. This group included patients with hypoplastic left ventricles. Both groups had a poor outcome with no significant difference in mortality (50% surgery and 43% valvuloplasty). Both groups were also left with significant residual disease (aortic stenosis and insufficiency) which required multiple re-interventions. Patients with isolated aortic stenosis appear to have significantly better outcome than neonates with more complex lesions (small left ventricle, small aortic annulus, small mitral valve, subvalvular stenosis) (12)[1]. Over the years improved patient selection as well as improved surgical and catheter techniques have provided long-term survival results of 90% and 88%, respectively (15,16). Thus, the *initial palliative* procedure of choice for critical aortic stenosis is balloon valvuloplasty. Despite the improved results, nearly all of these neonates will go on to need multiple re-interventions, with eventual aortic valve replacement or Ross procedure.

Neonates who present in shock and severe congestive heart failure should be stabilized by use of ventilation, inotropic support, and PGE_1 before undergoing cardiac catheterization. PGE_1 will open the patent ductus arteriosus, ensuring adequate systemic blood flow. Access for percutaneous retrograde dilation of the aortic valve may be obtained via the umbilical artery, femoral artery, or the right carotid artery. The most challenging aspect of the procedure is passage of a catheter across the stenotic valve. Early reports demonstrated a high incidence of vascular complications when using the femoral artery approach (13,17). Thus, currently, we recommend trying the umbilical artery (in neonates more than 72 hours of age) before gaining femoral arterial access. The carotid artery approach has the theoretical risk of causing strokes and long-term circulation problems, and is reserved for

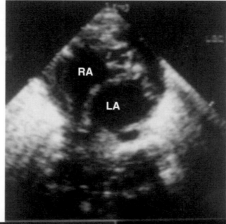

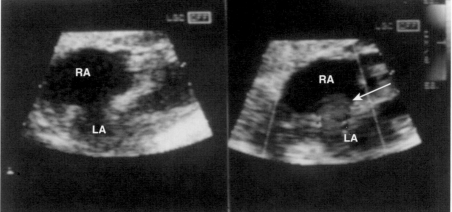

FIGURE 19–5 Echocardiographic image of a infant with hypoplastic left heart (HLH) syndrome and a restrictive atrial septum before septoplasty (top). Echocardiographic images (below) demonstrating a larger defect with arrow pointing to the increased color Doppler flow after septoplasty. RA, right atrium; LA, left atrium.

special circumstances where passage of a wire across the stenotic aortic valve is impossible via other routes (18). After complete heparinization of the neonate, a complete right and left heart catheterization is performed; this includes simultaneous measurements of left ventricular (via the foramen ovale) and ascending aortic pressures to assess the valve gradient before dilation. Biplane angiography of the left ventricle is performed to allow measurements of the aortic valve annulus, and assessment of left ventricular size and function. In addition, it allows other cardiac anomalies to be documented (Figure 19-6 (A)).

Aortic valve dilation is usually performed retrograde. A soft-tipped 0.018 in guide-wire is passed across the valve and a catheter advanced into the ventricle. The soft-tipped wire is then exchanged for an 0.021 in to 0.025 in guide-wire with a preformed tip curled in the left ventricular apex. Next, a low pressure balloon-tipped catheter is positioned across the stenotic valve. The balloon is filled with one-third-strength contrast to allow rapid inflation and deflation (which is kept under five seconds) to minimize the time the left ventricular outflow tract is obstructed. The inflation is performed by hand with pressures of three to eight atmospheres, or until the waist disappears, and the balloon is then withdrawn into the aorta (Figure 19-6 (B)). High-pressure inflations are not needed to relieve the obstruction and balloon rupture has been associated with transverse aortic valve tears even when using undersized balloons (19). Dilation is repeated several times to ensure adequate relief of the obstruction. After dilation is complete left

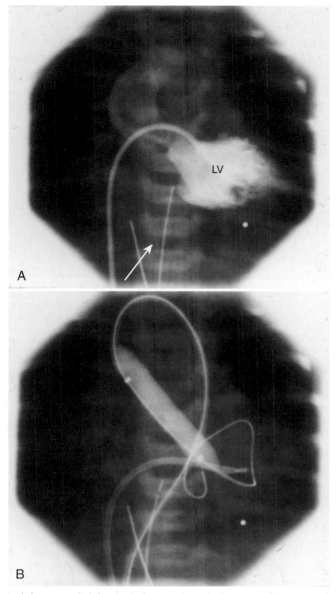

FIGURE 19–6 **(A)** Antegrade left ventriculogram through the patent foramen ovale demonstrating severe aortic valve stenosis with a discrete jet (arrow) through the narrowed valve orifice. **(B)** Balloon inflation across the stenotic aortic valve with no waist seen at the valve. LV, left ventricle.

ventricular and ascending aortic pressures are measured and an ascending aortic injection is performed to evaluate the amount of aortic regurgitation.

Aortic valve dilation may also be performed antegrade. To do this, a 5F Cook biopsy sheath is placed across the patent foramen ovale through the mitral valve and into the left ventricular apex. If no hemodynamically compromising mitral regurgitation is present an end-hole catheter is directed out of the sheath to the ascending aorta with the aid of a tip-deflecting guide-wire. The tip-deflecting guide-wire is exchanged with a J-wire preformed to curve in the ventricular apex. A balloon catheter is advanced over the wire across the aortic valve and inflated as previously described. After the dilation is complete left ventricular and ascending aortic pressures are measured, and an ascending aortic injection is performed to evaluate the amount of residual aortic regurgitation.

Valve morphology has been shown to be an important factor in predicting the outcome of balloon dilation with respect to residual obstruction and regurgitation (20). Thick and dysmorphic valves tend to have a higher incidence of residual obstruction when compared with thinner valves. Uni-commissural valves are typically left with more regurgitation in comparison with bi-commissural and tri-commissural valves. The mechanism of relief of valvular obstruction is the creation of tears along the lines of commissural fusion. The recommended balloon size is 80% to 90% of the aortic annulus diameter, which provides adequate relief of obstruction while minimizing residual regurgitation. Regardless of the initial result nearly all neonates will require further interventions, with a recent study reporting an 88% survival rate and a 64% freedom from re-intervention rate at 8.3 years of age (16).

Complications that have been reported following this procedure include loss of femoral pulse, perforation or avulsion of an aortic valve cusp, transient left bundle branch block, excessive blood loss, life-threatening arrhythmias, residual aortic valve disease, and death. These complications are becoming less frequent and balloon dilation of critical aortic stenosis remains the initial procedure of choice for neonates with adequate left ventricular size and minimal associated cardiac anomalies.

PULMONARY VALVULOPLASTY

Critical Pulmonary Stenosis

Most neonates born with critical pulmonary stenosis present in the neonatal period with cyanosis upon closure of the patent ductus arteriosus. The systolic ejection murmur of pulmonary stenosis may not be present with severe stenosis and minimal antegrade pulmonary blood flow. Initial management consists of administration of PGE_1 to maintain the patency of the ductus arteriosus and augment pulmonary blood flow. The right ventricle and tricuspid valve may be hypoplastic with a severely hypertrophied non-compliant myocardium. After successful dilation most patients have enough antegrade pulmonary blood flow to allow cessation of PGE_1 with arterial saturations of >85%. With time these saturations increase to normal levels and the hypoplastic ventricles grow to near-normal size (21). Typically, pulmonary insufficiency develops after dilation but is well tolerated and may promote ventricular growth (22). In cases with significantly hypertrophied and non-compliant ventricles cyanosis will persist even after relief of the valvar obstruction secondary to right-to-left atrial shunting. Thus, these neonates may require prolonged prostaglandin therapy (up to four weeks) until arterial saturations improve. During this time the hypertrophy regresses, improving compliance of the right ventricle, decreasing the right-to-left atrial shunt and improving arterial saturations. In cases where significant cyanosis persists three to four weeks after valvar relief, a Blalock–Taussig shunt (BTS) is surgically placed to augment pulmonary blood flow. This shunt may be closed percutaneously when right ventricular size and compliance becomes sufficient to maintain the full cardiac output, typically at six months to one year of age.

Pulmonary valve dilation is performed via the femoral venous route with continuous arterial pressure monitoring. The neonate is given a continuous infusion of prostaglandin prior to and during the procedure, which provides hemodynamic stability. A right ventriculogram is performed to assess the size of the cavity and to measure the valve annulus on straight lateral projection (Figure 19-7A). The pulmonary valve is initially crossed with an end-hole catheter. The catheter is placed below the pulmonary valve and a 0.018 in floppy wire is used to cross the valve. The end-hole catheter is then advanced over the wire into the main

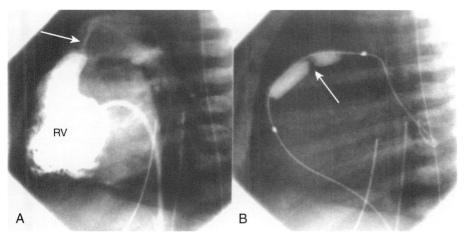

FIGURE 19–7 (A) Straight lateral projection of a right ventricular angiogram demonstrating a normal-sized right ventricle and a jet of dye (arrow) through the stenotic pulmonary valve. **(B)** A balloon inflated across the stenotic vale with a discrete "waist" (arrow) at the level of the valve. RV, right atrium.

pulmonary artery where the wire can be advanced down the descending aorta or left pulmonary artery. A balloon-tipped catheter with a diameter of 100% to 130% of the measured valve annulus is advanced over the wire and positioned across the pulmonary valve. The balloon is filled with one-third-strength contrast to allow rapid inflation and deflation of the balloon. The balloon is inflated by hand until the "waist" disappears (Figure 19-7 (B)).

The inflation–deflation time is kept under 10 sec. The balloon catheter is removed and the transvalvular gradient measured. With the patent ductus arteriosus open this gradient cannot be used to quantify the residual valvar stenosis, but may indicate the need for repeat valvar dilation if the ventricular pressure is suprasystemic. Finally, a right ventricular angiogram is performed to assess for residual obstruction or damage to the pulmonary artery or right ventricular outflow tract, or all of these.

Percutaneous balloon dilation is the procedure of choice for children with pulmonary valve stenosis. This procedure has been shown to safely and effectively relieve valvar stenosis, leaving minimal significant residual disease, obviating the need for surgical valvulotomy, and rarely necessitating re-intervention (23,24). Results of pulmonary valvuloplasty in neonates and infants have not been as spectacular as those seen in older children, partially because this group of patients may have both a hypoplastic right ventricle and tricuspid valve (25,26). We recently reviewed 45 consecutive neonates undergoing pulmonary valvuloplasty in the first month of life at our institution between July 1989 and April 2000. In six patients, early on in the series, the pulmonary valve could not be crossed, whilst the last 28 neonates all had successful dilation. There was one death early on in the series secondary to perforation of the right ventricular outflow tract (RVOT). Of the remaining 38 patients who underwent successful dilation five required placement of a BTS (two with associated surgical valvulotomy) and two required valvulotomy alone in the neonatal period. At follow-up five patients required repeat balloon valvuloplasty (two of whom had had a previous valvulotomy). Thus, 74% of infants who underwent successful valvuloplasty required no further intervention. Infants requiring surgical intervention had a small tricuspid valve and significantly smaller right ventricle than those undergoing successful dilation. The mean saturation at discharge for neonates who had not received a BTS was 89%. Multiple follow-up studies in these children demonstrate excellent right ventricle growth with time and only occasional cases may need a one-and-a-half-ventricle repair. Radtke and colleagues (27) recently reviewed a similar group of neonates and reported similar results. These workers also used transcatheter techniques to close BTS and residual ASDs, which may be left when right-to-left atrial shunts are performed (27).

Complications associated with pulmonary valve dilation include perforation of the right ventricular outflow tract, transient arrhythmias, right bundle branch block, infection, and femoral arterial and venous occlusion.

PULMONARY ATRESIA WITH INTACT SEPTUM

Management of neonates with pulmonary atresia with intact septum in the absence of coronary artery sinusoids has classically entailed placement of a RVOT patch and placement of a BTS. This procedure allows growth of the hypoplastic ventricle to allow for eventual biventricular repair. Recently, transcatheter perforation of the pulmonary valve has been performed in neonates with clear membranous pulmonary atresia and hypoplastic right ventricles and tricuspid valves. After perforation and valvuloplasty these ventricles increase in size and are able to support a two-ventricle circulation (28). In cases where the pulmonary annulus is severely hypoplastic a surgical outflow patch is preferred and felt to carry less morbidity and mortality.

The technique of pulmonary valvulotomy is nearly identical to that for critical pulmonary stenosis with the addition of transcatheter perforation of the pulmonary valve. The perforation is carried out either by puncture with the stiff end of a wire carefully directed toward the pulmonary valve via an end-hole catheter. Alternatively, perforation of the valve may be accomplished using a radio-frequency or laser-tipped wire (29,30,31). Following this procedure a standard valvuloplasty is performed. Complications of this procedure may include perforation of the pulmonary artery and RVOT.

OTHER LESIONS WITH DECREASED PULMONARY BLOOD FLOW

Lesions with significant cyanosis secondary to valvar pulmonary stenosis which require eventual surgical repair may be temporally improved by use of percutaneous balloon dilation. Lesions which have successful palliation with balloon dilation include tetralogy of Fallot, TGA with a ventricular septal defect and pulmonary stenosis, and complex single ventricles and PS. For these lesions to be palliated the pulmonary valve must be the limiting factor to pulmonary blood flow with no significant distal obstruction. The balloon chosen is usually smaller than the annulus to limit excessive pulmonary blood flow after the procedure. In neonates with tetralogy of Fallot this may delay the need for surgical intervention for up to one year. In neonates with single ventricle or complex transposition physiology, valvar dilation may obviate the need for a shunt.

COARCTATION OF THE AORTA

Coarctation of the aorta in neonates is associated with cardiac anomalies such as ventricular septal defects, diffuse arch hypoplasia, hypoplastic left ventricles, aortic stenosis, and bicuspid aortic valves. Initial short-term results of balloon angioplasty for native coarctation in neonates with simple coarctation yielded a significant reduction in the arch gradients (32). Longer-term follow-up studies have demonstrated an unacceptably high incidence of recoarctation (31% to 80%), aneurysm formation, and pulse loss (33,34). Thus, this procedure is only recommended in neonates under special circumstances where surgical repair of the coarctation cannot be accomplished.

Balloon dilation for recoarctation after neonatal arch repair is safe and effective, with less morbidity and mortality than surgical repair (35). This has been particularly true in infants who develop obstruction following Norwood I palliation and other complex arch reconstructions (Figure 19-8). Maheshwari et al. (36) recently reviewed 22 infants who underwent balloon dilation for recoarctation with an overall initial success rate of 95%. Seventy-six percent of the infants required no further intervention, with a median follow-up time of 56 months (0.6 to 12 years).

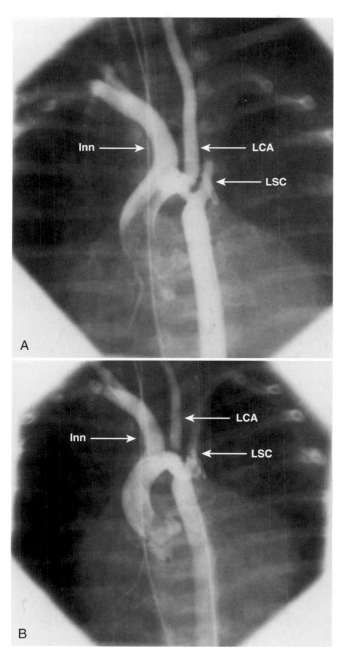

FIGURE 19–8 **(A)** An angiogram of a recurrent coarctation between the left subclavian and left carotid arteries of a surgically repaired critical coarctation in the neonatal period prior to angioplasty. **(B)** An angiogram following angioplasty at eight weeks of age demonstrated an increased diameter of the coarctation site. Inn, innominate artery; LCA, left common carotid artery; LSC, left subclavian artery.

COIL EMBOLIZATION OF VESSELS

Aberrant vessels off the aorta may be multiple and diffuse. These vessels are difficult to surgically ligate because they are typically not within the surgical field. Vessels arising from the aorta which are not critical to pulmonary blood flow or are part of a hemodynamically significant arteriovenous fistula may be embolized in the catheterization laboratory (37,38,39). Neonates with Scimitar syndrome provide an excellent example of a vascular structure needing coil embolization. These neonates have a pulmonary sequestration supplied by arteries from the descending aorta. The sequestration has little to no functioning lung tissue, acts only as arterial–venous fistula, and may be associated with pulmonary hypertension. Elimination of a sequestration may improve the pulmonary hypertension is these neonates (Figure 19-9). This sequestration is difficult to address during surgical repair for the associated cardiac lesions and embolization in the catheterization laboratory is preferred.

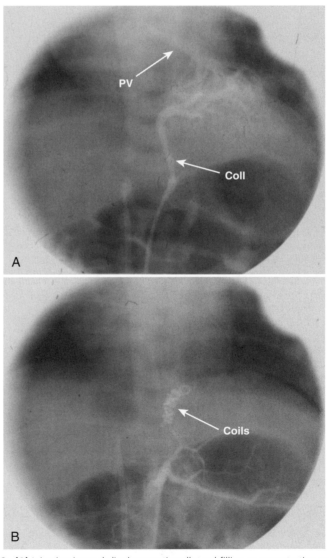

FIGURE 19–9 **(A)** Injection in a subdiaphragmatic collateral filling a sequestration and draining to the left atrium. **(B)** Following coil occlusion no flow to the sequestration can be seen. PV, pulmonary vein; Coll, collateral.

Stainless steel helical coils covered with Dacron strands are used to thrombose the vessels. The abnormal vessel is entered with an end-hole catheter. Floppy guidewires may be needed to enter the vessel distally and advance the catheter. Once an embolization position is achieved the coil is pushed out the end of the catheter using a soft-tipped wire. Multiple coils may be needed to cause complete thrombosis of the vessel.

NEONATAL ENDOVASCULAR STENTS

Endovascular stents have very limited use in neonates. Stents currently available for placement in neonatal situations have maximal diameters considerably smaller than the eventual diameter of the vessels needing stenting. Thus, stents are not routinely used in neonates except in novel and special circumstances. Several authors have reported stenting of the patent ductus arteriosus in experimental models and neonates (40,41). Neonates who may benefit from this procedure include those with HLH syndrome who are awaiting heart transplant and neonates with small pulmonary arteries who need significant pulmonary artery growth before surgical repair. This can prevent the long-term complications of prostaglandin therapy and may even permit these neonates to be discharged from the hospital while awaiting transplant or definitive surgical repair.

REFERENCES

1. Rice MJ, Seward JB, Hagler DJ, et al. Impact of 2-dimensional echocardiography on the management of distressed newborns in whom cardiac disease is suspected. Am J Cardiol 1983;51:288–292.
2. Bisset GS. Magnetic resonance imaging of congenital heart disease in the pediatric patient. Radiol Clin North Am 1991;29:279–291.
3. Cohn HE, Freed MD, Hellenbrand WE, et al. Complications and mortality associated with cardiac catheterization in infants under one year: a prospective study. Pediatr Cardiol 1985;1:123–131.
4. Stanger P, Heymann MA, Tarnoff H, et al. Complications of cardiac catheterization of neonates, infants, and children. A three-year study. Circulation 1974;50:595–608.
5. Rashkind WJ, Miller WM. Creation of an atrial septal defect without thoracotomy: a palliative approach to transposition of the great arteries. JAMA 1966;196:991–992.
6. Beekman RH, Rocchini AP. Transcatheter treatment of congenital heart disease. Prog Cardiovasc Dis 1989;32:1–30.
7. Neches WH, Mullins CE, McNamara DG. Balloon atrial septostomy in congenital heart disease in infancy. Am J Dis Child 1973;125:371–375.
8. Park SC, Neches WH, Mullins CE, et al. Blade atrial septostomy: collaborative study. Circulation 1982;66:258–266.
9. Adz AM, Einstein JA, Jonas RA, et al. Preoperative management of pulmonary venous hypertension in hypoplastic left heart syndrome with restrictive atrial septal defect. Am J Cardiol 1999;83:1224–1228.
10. Allan LD, Leanage R, Wainwright R, et al. Balloon atrial septostomy under two dimensional echocardiographic control. Br Heart J 1982;47:41–43.
11. Ashfaq M, Houston AB, Gnanapragasam SP, et al. Balloon atrial septostomy under echocardiographic control: six years' experience and evaluation of the practicability of cannulation via the umbilical vein. Br Heart J 1991;65:148–151.
12. Karl TR, Sano S, Brawn WJ, et al. Critical aortic stenosis in the first month of life: surgical results in 26 infants. Ann Thorac Surg 1990;50:105–150.
13. Rocchini AP, Beekman RH, Ben Shachar G, et al. Balloon aortic valvuloplasty: results of the valvuloplasty of congenital anomalies registry. Am J Cardiol 1990;65:784–789.
14. Zeevi B, Keane JF, Castaneda AR, et al. Neonatal critical valvar aortic stenosis: a comparison of surgical and balloon dilation therapy. Circulation 1989;80:831–839.
15. Turley K, Bove EL, Amato JJ, et al. Neonatal aortic stenosis. J Thorac Cardiovasc Surg 1990;99:679–684.
16. Egito EST, Moore P, O'Sullivan J, et al. Transvascular balloon dilation for neonatal critical aortic stenosis: early and midterm results. J Am Coll Cardiol 1997;29:442–447.
17. Vogel M, Benson LN, Burrows P, et al. Balloon dilation of congenital aortic valve stenosis in infants and children: short term and intermediate results. Br Heart J 1989;62:148–153.
18. Fischer DR, Ettedgui JA, Park SC, et al. Carotid artery approach for balloon dilation of aortic valve stenosis in the neonate: a preliminary report. J Am Coll Cardiol 1990;15:1633–1636.
19. Waller BF, Giroed DA, Dillon JC. Transverse aortic wall tears in infants after balloon angioplasty for aortic valve stenosis: relation of aortic wall damage to diameter of inflated angioplasty balloon and aortic lumen in seven necropsy cases. J Am Coll Cardiol 1984;4:1235–1241.

20. Scholler GF, Keane JF, Stanton SB, et al. Balloon dilation of congenital aortic valve stenosis: results and influence of technical and morphological features on outcome. Circulation 1988;78:351–360.

21. Velvis H, Raines KH, Bensky AS, et al. Growth of the right heart after balloon valvuloplasty for critical pulmonary stenosis in the newborn. Am J Cardiol 1997;79:982–984.

22. Berman W, Fripp RR, Raisher BD, et al. Significant pulmonary valve incompetence following oversize balloon pulmonary valveplasty in small infants: a long-term follow-up study. Cathet Cardiovasc Intervent 1999;48:61–65.

23. McCrindle BW, Kan JS. Long-term results after balloon pulmonary valvuloplasty. Circulation 1991;83:1915–1922.

24. Stanger P, Cassidy SC, Girod DA, et al. Balloon pulmonary valvuloplasty: results of the valvuloplasty and angioplasty of congenital anomalies. Am J Cardiol 1990;65:775–783.

25. Ladusans EJ, Quresji SA, Parsons JM, et al. Balloon dilation of critical stenosis of the pulmonary valve in neonates. Br Heart J 1990;63:362–367.

26. Rey C, Marache P, Francart C, et al. Percutaneous transluminal balloon valvuloplasty of congenital pulmonary valve stenosis, with a special report on infants and neonates. J Am Coll Cardiol 1988;11:815–820.

27. Radtke WAK, Balaguru D, Wiles HB, et al. Improved efficacy and long-term outcome of balloon valvuloplasty for critical pulmonary stenosis in newborns. J Am Coll Cardiol 2000;35(2 Suppl.A):519A–520A.

28. Ovaert C, Qureshi SA, Rosenthal E, et al. Growth of the right ventricle after successful transcatheter pulmonary valvotomy in neonates and infants with pulmonary atresia and intact ventricular septum. J Thorac Cardiovasc Surg 1998;115:1055–1062.

29. Qureshi SA, Rosenthal E, Tynan M, et al. Transcatheter laser-assisted balloon pulmonary valve dilation in pulmonic valve atresia. Am J Cardiol 1990;67:428–431.

30. Hijazi ZM, Patel H, Cao Q, et al. Transcatheter retrograde radio-frequency perforation of the pulmonic valve in pulmonary atresia with intact ventricular septum, using a 2 French catheter. Cathet Cardiovasc Diagn 1998;45:151–154.

31. Wang JK, Wu MH, Chang CI, et al. Outcomes of transcatheter valvotomy in patients with pulmonary atresia and intact ventricular septum. Am J Cardiol 1999;84:1055–1060.

32. Tynan M, Finley JP, Fontes V, et al. Balloon angioplasty for the treatment of native coarctation: results of valvuloplasty and angioplasty of congenital anomalies registry. Am J Cardiol 1990;65:790–792.

33. Fletcher SE, Nihill MR, Grifka RG, et al. Balloon angioplasty of native coarctation of the aorta: midterm follow-up and prognostic factors. J Am Coll Cardiol 1995;25:730–734.

34. Shaddy RE, Boucek MM, Sturtevant JE, et al. Comparison of angioplasty and surgery for unoperated coarctation of the aorta. Circulation 1993;87:793–799.

35. Hellenbrand WE, Allen HD, Golinko RJ, et al. Balloon angioplasty for aortic recoarctation: results of valvuloplasty and angioplasty of congenital anomalies registry. Am J Cardiol 1990;65:793–797.

36. Maheshwari S, Bruckheimer E, Fahey JT, et al. Balloon angioplasty of postsurgical recoarctation in infants; the risk of restenosis and long-term follow-up. J Am Coll Cardiol 2000;35:209–213.

37. Fletcher SE, Cheatham JP, Bolam DL. Primary transcatheter treatment of congenital pulmonary arteriovenous malformation causing cyanosis of the newborn. Cathet Cardiovasc Intervent 2000;50:48–51.

38. Hosono S, Ohno T, Kimoto H, et al. Sucessful transcatheter arterial embolization of a giant hemangioma associated with high-output cardiac failure and Kasabach–Merritt syndrome in a neonate: a case report. Cath Cardiovasc Intervent 1999;27:399–403.

39. Furman BP, Bass JL, Castaneda-Zuniga W, et al. Coil embolization of congenital thoracic vascular anomalies in infants and children. Circulation 1984;70:285–289.

40. Coe JY, OlleyPM. A novel method to maintain ductus arteriosus patency. J Am Coll Cardiol 1991;18:837–841.

41. Schneider M, Zartner P, Sidiropouls A, et al. Stent implantation of the arterial duct in newborns with duct-dependent circulation. Eur Heart J 1998;19:1401–1409.

Chapter 20

Cardiac Surgery in the Neonate with Congenital Heart Disease

Ryan R. Davies, MD • Jonathan M. Chen, MD •
Jan M. Quaegebeur, MD, PhD • Ralph S. Mosca, MD

Introduction
Palliative Operations
Specific Lesions
Mechanical Circulatory Support in the Neonate
Summary
References

INTRODUCTION

In 1952, scarcely more than 50 years ago, the first operation on the open human heart under direct vision – repair of an atrial septal defect (ASD) in a five-year old girl – was performed at the University of Minnesota (1). This operation was accomplished using in-flow occlusion and moderate total body hypothermia. With the development of cardiopulmonary bypass over the course of the next decade this success could be extended to a wider variety of more complex lesions. Refinements in surgical technique, medical technology, and perioperative care have since resulted in excellent survival after the repair of even the most complex types of congenital heart disease (CHD) in increasingly smaller children. Further, with the growing availability and accuracy of prenatal diagnosis by fetal echocardiography, the postnatal management of these complicated newborns can often be anticipated and planned. Future work will continue to analyze and improve the short- and long-term morbidity associated with repair of CHD, in particular with regard to long-term functional status, neurodevelopmental outcomes, and need for ongoing follow-up and re-intervention, with the attendant psychologic and financial burden this imposes on both the patient and their family.

Initially, most operations for CHD performed in the neonatal period were extracardiac palliative procedures. Despite initial success with repair of intracardiac lesions by use of cross-circulation, most early attempts to use mechanical cardiopulmonary bypass (CPB) could not duplicate these results: surgical equipment and technology were unrefined (2,3). Thus, palliative procedures not requiring CPB were used either permanently, or to defer repair until children were older. These procedures are still employed, but since the 1980s there has been a growing trend toward primary repair of CHD early in life. This trend has been spurred on by the recognition of the potentially deleterious effects of palliation upon cardiac and pulmonary physiology, neurological development, and pulmonary artery anatomy, as well as by advancements in the technology and perioperative management of CPB. In this brief overview we will discuss those common congenital heart conditions for which surgical intervention in the neonatal period is most common. Emerging techniques, both catheter-based and surgical (or a hybrid thereof), continue to modify this list and improve the outcomes of these newborns.

PALLIATIVE OPERATIONS

Pulmonary Artery Banding

Historically, pulmonary artery banding was widely used in patients with large left-to-right shunts or single ventricle physiology, to limit pulmonary blood flow and pressure, and permit somatic growth and potential clinical improvement before subsequent staged repair. More recently, primary repair in the neonatal period has replaced staged surgery as the treatment of choice for many of these diagnoses. As a result, pulmonary artery banding is now performed infrequently.

Isolated pulmonary artery banding is best performed through a median sternotomy. In the procedure, a non-absorbable material is used to surround the main pulmonary artery (Figure 20-1). This "band" is secured gradually, thereby limiting pulmonary blood flow so that the pulmonary artery pressures distal to the band range are between one-third and one-half of the systemic blood pressure; care is taken to avoid substantial arterial desaturation or impairment of cardiac output. The Trusler formula provides a guideline for the proper band circumference depending upon the patient's weight and physiology (4). Contraindications to pulmonary artery banding include significant atrioventricular valve regurgitation and a potential for significant sub-aortic obstruction with single-ventricle defects.

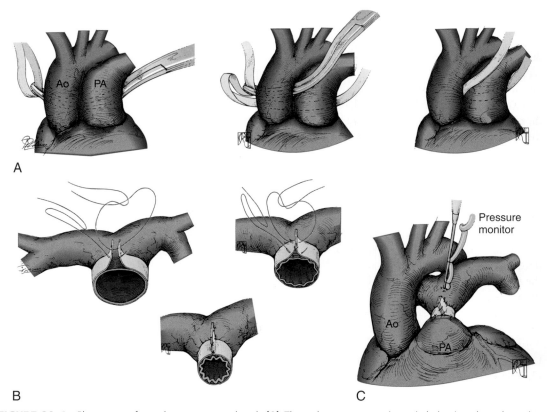

FIGURE 20–1 Placement of a pulmonary artery band. **(A)** The pulmonary artery is encircled using the subtraction technique. **(B)** Sutures are placed to tighten the band. **(C)** Pressure measurement in the pulmonary artery distal to the site of band placement to assess band tightness. Ao, aorta; PA, pulmonary artery. *From Backer and Mavroudis (5).*

Once optimal band tightness is achieved, the band is secured to the adventitia of the pulmonary artery to prevent movement, taking care so as not to impinge upon either branch of the pulmonary artery or the pulmonary valve (if pulmonary valve function is to be preserved).

Complications with pulmonary artery banding mostly relate to technical problems, including bands that are either too tight or too loose, or band migration. Permanent damage to the pulmonary valve may result from too proximal a band, leading to impingement upon pulmonary valve leaflet motion. Conversely, a band placed too far distally may produce branch pulmonary artery stenosis. At the subsequent staged procedure, band removal can be performed with facility for either reconstruction of the stenotic banding site or oversewing of the pulmonary outflow tract as indicated.

Aortopulmonary Shunts (Blalock–Taussig Shunt)

As with pulmonary artery banding, the increasing preference for primary repair of congenital cardiac defects in the neonatal period has led to a decrease in the use of isolated aortopulmonary shunts. First used in 1945 to augment pulmonary blood flow (6), the classic Blalock–Taussig (BT) shunt (creation of a subclavian artery-to-pulmonary artery anastomosis) was used as a palliative procedure for staged repair of several defects, including tetralogy of Fallot.

Later modifications to the original technique of aortopulmonary shunting include the descending aorta-to-left pulmonary artery (Potts) shunt, the ascending aorta-to-right pulmonary anastomosis (Waterston shunt), the ascending aorta-to-main pulmonary artery ("central") shunt, and the use of prosthetic graft material such as Gore-tex® (modified BT shunt). All these techniques aim to produce a controlled increase in pulmonary blood flow, which enables appropriate oxygenation in patients with cyanotic defects. Division of the main pulmonary artery in combination with a BT shunt may be utilized as an alternative to pulmonary artery banding in single-ventricle lesions to both maintain oxygenation and limit pulmonary artery pressure.

The modified Blalock–Taussig shunt (Figure 20-2) may be performed via thoracotomy or sternotomy. The benefits of thoracotomy include preservation of the median sternotomy approach for future repair and avoidance of cardiopulmonary bypass in the neonatal period, with its attendant risks, whereas the benefits of the sternotomy include access to the great vessels should emergent cardiopulmonary bypass prove necessary, the ability to ligate the ductus arteriosus at the time of shunt creation, and more proximal access to the branch pulmonary artery. In general, the shunt is performed on the side opposite to the insertion of the ductus arteriosus into the pulmonary artery. In doing so, the surgeon may clamp the branch pulmonary artery for the anastomosis, without affecting "antegrade" pulmonary blood flow via the ductus arteriosus. In the case of a right aortic arch, the shunt may still be performed from a right thoracotomy; however, if the origin is from the ascending aorta it may function more similarly to a central shunt than a modified Blalock–Taussig shunt taken off the subclavian artery (i.e. this location may mandate the use of a smaller shunt).

Complications of shunt insertion relate to: (1) the shunt material and operative technique (kinking, thrombosis); (2) anatomy (chylothorax, injury to the vagus or phrenic nerves); and (3) sequelae from the operation itself (e.g. branch pulmonary stenosis at the shunt insertion site). When shunts are "taken down" during the later staged procedure they are rarely completely removed, but, rather, are ligated and sometimes divided. Shunts may also be closed percutaneously in the catheterization laboratory with coils. Many surgeons prefer aspirin for anticoagulation in an effort to reduce platelet activation and shunt thrombosis.

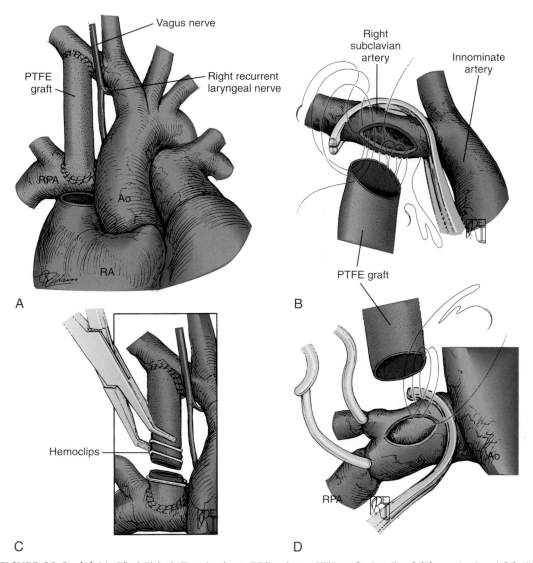

Vagus nerve

PTFE graft

Right recurrent laryngeal nerve

RPA

Ao

RA

A

Right subclavian artery

Innominate artery

PTFE graft

B

Hemoclips

C

RPA

Ao

D

FIGURE 20–2 **(A)** Modified Blalock–Taussig shunt (BTS) using a PTFE graft. Details of **(B)** *proximal* and **(C)** *distal* anastomosis for modified BTS. **(D)** Take-down of modified BTS with hemoclips and shunt division. Ao, aorta; PTFE, polytetraflouroethylene; RA, right atrium; RPA, right pulmonary artery. *From Backer and Mavroudis (5).*

SPECIFIC LESIONS

Left-to-Right Shunt Lesions

Ventricular Septal Defect

Infants with a large ventricular septal defect (VSD) and severe, intractable conges-tive heart failure may require surgical closure of the VSD during infancy; however, it is rare to require attention in the neonatal period. Occasionally, neonates born with so-called "Swiss-cheese"-like defects (multiple muscular VSDs that are poorly amenable to surgical repair but whose cumulative shunt fraction may be large) require pulmonary artery banding (see above) to limit pulmonary blood flow if they do not respond to aggressive medical management.

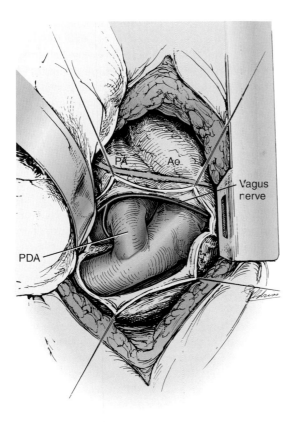

FIGURE 20–3   Operative exposure of a PDA through a left thoracotomy. The mediastinal pleura is opened and reflected anteriorly and posteriorly. The vagus and recurrent laryngeal nerves are identified and preserved by retracting them medially. Ao, aorta; PA, pulmonary artery; PDA, patent ductus arteriosus. *From Hillman et al. (9).*

Patent Ductus Arteriosus of Botalli

The presence of a large patent ductus arteriosus (PDA) in an infant may be suspected whenever the clinical symptoms of a large left-to-right shunt are identified, including the presence of a heart murmur, bounding pulses, tachycardia, hyperdynamic precordial impulse, widened pulse pressure, and worsening respiratory status (7). More common in premature infants, PDAs are unlikely to close spontaneously after the first few weeks of life. Where symptoms are present closure should be performed immediately, but, in infants without symptoms, elective closure should be planned within three months.

In preterm infants, persistence of the PDA has been associated with increased mortality (8). In general, initial medical therapy with a course (three doses) of indomethacin (ibuprofen) for PDA closure is preferred if the child exhibits no signs of renal insufficiency, necrotizing enterocolitis (NEC), or a bleeding diathesis. Contraindications to indocin use or failure of this therapy is an indication for surgical ligation. Left-to-right shunting of a magnitude to cause abdominal end-organ hypoperfusion (renal failure, NEC) and insufficiency is not infrequent.

Ligation of the patent ductus is performed through a thoracotomy, most often left-sided (Figure 20-3). In most neonates this may be achieved with the application of a permanent stainless steel hemoclip, which permits a minimially invasive incision and reduces both the need for manipulation of the fragile ductal tissue and the extent of surgical dissection required. In larger infants and children, a large PDA may require a double ligature, division, and oversewing. An echocardiogram performed as part of the preoperative analysis must demonstrate arch sidedness (which may dictate the side of the surgical incision), absence of other intracardiac lesions requiring surgical attention, and the directionality (left to right) of shunting across the ductus arteriosus. If the PDA is shunting from right to left this suggests either significant pulmonary hypertension or ductal dependency of the systemic circulation, each of which is a contraindication to closure. After the PDA is ligated the systemic diastolic pressure will often rise substantially. Complications of the procedure include damage to the recurrent laryngeal nerve, damage to the thoracic duct, ductal recanalization, and the possibility of significant hemorrhage.

Truncus Arteriosus

The primary abnormality of truncus arteriosus is the presence of a single arterial outflow from both ventricles (supplying the systemic, coronary, and pulmonary circulations) in association with a VSD. Physiologically, this results in a large left-to-right shunt that progressively worsens as pulmonary vascular resistance falls in the neonatal period. In addition, truncal valve insufficiency may exacerbate this volume load on the ventricles.

Although the occasional child may develop mild increases in pulmonary vascular resistance, which balance the pulmonary and systemic circulation enabling medium-term survival, most infants have a poor prognosis if left unrepaired. Untreated patients have 65% one-month and 75% one-year mortality, with early onset of severe congestive heart failure (10). Consequently, repair is advocated in the neonatal period to prevent heart failure and myocardial ischemia, and to protect the lungs from accelerated pulmonary vascular obstructive disease. Repair at approximately five to seven days of age as the pulmonary vascular resistance falls (heralded by tachypnea) is optimal.

Repair consists of separating ("septating") the great vessels, closing the VSD, and establishing right ventricle (RV) to pulmonary artery (PA) continuity with either a valved homograft or non-valved conduit, or direct anastomosis of the RV to the PA confluence by use of a variety of materials (so-called "direct connection") (11).

Several authors have reported excellent long-term survival in neonates, with survival frequently exceeding 90% (11,12). Assiduous follow-up to assess for truncal valve insufficiency, ventricular failure, or the effects of somatic growth on conduit function and branch pulmonary growth is required, with early intervention (either operative or catheter-based), as indicated, to maintain function or to replace the conduit.

Aortopulmonary Window

A rare congenital defect, aortopulmonary window results from failure of complete septation of the truncus arteriosus into pulmonary artery and aorta. Repair is advocated upon diagnosis, except in very rare cases with a small, physiologically well-tolerated defect in which elective repair may be completed during infancy. In general, patch closure of the defect is performed, as the use of simple ligation was associated both with an increased risk of fatal postoperative bleeding and eventual recanalization of the defect.

Obstructive Lesions

Pulmonary Stenosis and Pulmonary Atresia

A variety of congenital defects may coexist with some degree of right ventricular outflow tract obstruction. Patients with pulmonary atresia with intact ventricular septum have little or no connection between the right ventricle and the pulmonary artery, and are largely dependent on the left ventricle for both systemic and pulmonary blood flow (via the ductus or other aorto–pulmonary collateral vessels). Consequently, closure of the ductus arteriosus in these patients may result in rapid hemodynamic collapse. Without medical therapy and surgical intervention, mortality is high: 50% within two weeks of life and up to 85% at six months (13).

Initial medical therapy should be directed at maintaining ductal patency during the diagnostic work-up. Appropriate surgical treatment may include decompression of the right ventricle via valvotomy or transannular patch, use of an aortopulmonary shunt to achieve pulmonary blood flow, or a combination of these two techniques. Strategies range from univentricular staged repair, or a hybrid ("one and a half ventricular") repair, to a biventricular repair depending on the right ventricular size and function (often best estimated by the relative size of the tricuspid valve annulus) and the presence of right ventricle dependent coronary vessels, depending on the morphology of the lesion.

Isolated pulmonary stenosis may present at any age depending on the severity of the stenotic lesion. When it is manifest as cyanosis in the neonatal period, it is commonly referred to as "critical pulmonary stenosis" (13). Cardiac output is generally maintained through an atrial right-to-left shunt. If ductal closure occurs, progressive cyanosis and hemodynamic failure ensue. As with patients with pulmonary atresia, initial medical management should be directed at maintaining ductal patency. After the diagnosis of pulmonary stenosis, neonates may often be managed initially with transcatheter balloon valvuloplasty for right ventricular decompression. Four-year survival in the largest series is approximately 80% (14). Often, if the obstruction represents a composite of valvar and subvalvar (i.e. muscular or infundibular) obstruction, a further surgical procedure is warranted. Surgery for this condition consists of placement of a patch across the annulus of the pulmonary valve and onto the right ventricular outflow tract (so-called "transannular patch"). Although this procedure creates obligate pulmonary insufficiency, it produces an unobstructed right ventricular outflow tract and represents the best chance for growth in right ventricular size (Figure 20-4).

Aortic Stenosis

Valvar aortic stenosis is a common congenital cardiac defect with a wide range of morphologic and clinical variants, from bicuspid aortic valves which may be asymptomatic through adulthood to neonates with critical aortic stenosis requiring early operative intervention. When critical aortic stenosis presents in the neonate it may be associated with severely dysmorphic aortic valve leaflets. As with right ventricular outflow tract obstruction, neonates with severe aortic stenosis may have ductal dependent cardiac output (PDA flow right-to-left to provide lower body perfusion).

In neonates, the onset of hemodynamic collapse with the advent of ductal closure signals the need for urgent intervention. During evaluation and planning, ductal patency should be maintained with prostaglandin E_1 (PGE_1) infusion. Additional preoperative interventions to optimize oxygenation and systemic perfusion include endotracheal intubation and mechanical ventilation, inotropic support, and management of fluid and electrolyte imbalances.

Appropriate intervention depends largely on the morphology of the left ventricle and aortic valve: patients with a hypoplastic left heart may require a Norwood-type single ventricle repair or cardiac transplantation, whereas those with a ventricle likely to be able to support the systemic circulation may be treated with surgical or interventional aortic valvotomy (16,17).

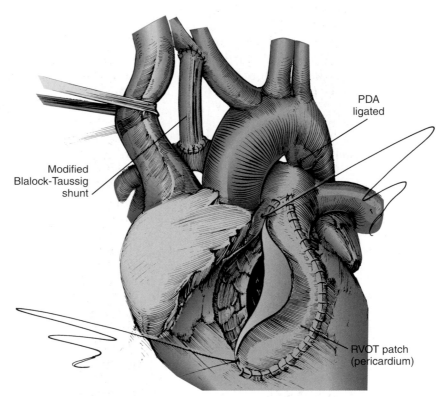

PDA
ligated

Modified
Blalock-Taussig
shunt

RVOT patch
(pericardium)

FIGURE 20–4 Placement of a transannular patch to enlarge the right ventricular outflow tract. The modified Blalock–Taussig shunt is also shown. RVOT, right ventricular outflow tract; PDA, patent ductus arteriosus. *From Casteneda et al. (15).*

A variety of techniques is available for both surgical and balloon valvotomy (including recent attempts to mitigate the left ventricular changes associated with aortic stenosis through in utero interventional aortic valvotomy (18). Recent series have reported operative survival of 90% or higher following valvotomy in patients with critical aortic stenosis in the absence of hypoplastic left heart (HLH) syndrome (17). However, valvotomy should be considered a palliative procedure, as most patients will need reoperation for aortic valve insufficiency, stenosis, or both (19,20). At present, for neonates in whom the aortic valve is irreparably dysmorphic, the Ross procedure is most commonly performed, in which the patient's pulmonary valve is used as an "autograft" to replace the aortic valve, and a cadaveric homograft is placed into the right ventricular outflow tract to establish right ventricle to pulmonary artery continuity. Naturally, because the pulmonary homograft is of a limited size, with no growth potential, it may necessitate several reoperations for homograft exchange throughout the lifetime of the patient.

Coarctation of the Aorta

"Coarctation" refers to a narrowing of the descending aorta adjacent to the insertion of the ductus arteriosus (so-called "juxtaductal") and may represent the effect of fetal development and abnormal flow dynamics, or the presence of "extra-anatomic" ductal tissue which narrows abnormally with ductal closure (Figure 20-5). Coarctation often coexists with generalized hypoplasia of the entire transverse aortic arch, the presence of which mandates a more complicated arch reconstruction at the time of repair.

As with other obstructive lesions, the natural history of aortic coarctation depends upon the degree to which systemic perfusion is dependent on a patent

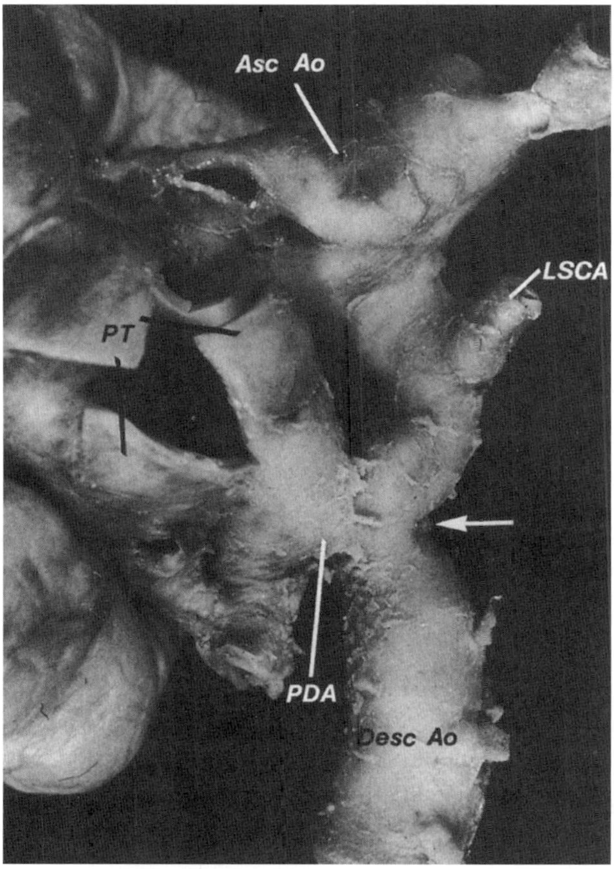

FIGURE 20–5 Autopsy specimen from a six-week-old girl, showing juxtaductal coarctation by localized shelf with typical external deformity of the aorta at the site of narrowing. Asc Ao, ascending aorta; Desc Ao, descending aorta; LSCA, left subclavian artery; PDA, patent ductus arteriosus; PT, pulmonary trunk. *From Kouchoukos et al. (21).*

ductus arteriosus. In patients who tolerate closure of the ductus, symptoms generally develop later as a consequence of the proximal systemic hypertension. These patients are at risk for a significant number of complications, but unoperated survival can extend into adulthood.

In contrast, patients with severe aortic coarctation may present in the first week of life with the onset of cardiovascular collapse at the time of ductal closure. In this population, collateral blood flow is insufficient to provide adequate perfusion to the abdominal organs and lower extremities, resulting in progressive organ ischemia and acidosis. Intravenous infusion of PGE_1 in these patients often maintains ductal patency, restoring perfusion of the lower body. In some cases, additional inotropic agents may be required to optimize perfusion and provide adequate resuscitation prior to operative repair.

TILIsolated coarctation of the descending aorta may be repaired through a left posterior-lateral thoracotomy, and involves mobilization of the descending aorta, resection of the coarctation segment, and end-to-end anastomosis. Because of problems with recurrence noted early in the history of this repair, currently a so-called "extended end-to-end anastomosis" (Figure 20-6) is more commonly performed. Here, the proximal descending aortic segment is spatulated and anastomosed proximally to the underside of the mid-transverse aortic arch in an effort to remove all the abnormal ductal tissue thought to be a major contributor to recurrence.

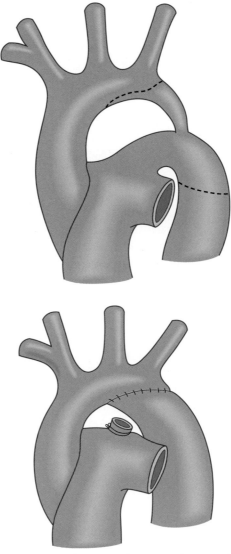

FIGURE 20–6 Extended resection and end-to-end anastomosis. Key technical points: (1) beveled anastomosis, brought up under the transverse arch; (2) extended as far proximally as deemed necessary to achieve relief of stenosis; (3) no prosthetic material used; (4) if the arch hypoplasia extends proximal to the left cartoid artery and would require clamping of the innominate artery then the repair is approached through a mediansternotomy and deep hypothermic circulatory arrest is used; otherwise, the repair is performed through a lateral thoracotomy. *From Wright et al. (49).*

For those neonates in whom the transverse aortic arch is also severely hypoplastic, the repair must be performed via median sternotomy using cardiopulmonary bypass. In particular, this aortic arch reconstruction and coarctation repair requires deep hypothermic circulatory arrest (DHCA), in which the infants are cooled to 18 °C and the circulation is discontinued for the duration of repair, or, alternatively, low-flow bypass with regional perfusion. Depending upon the degree and location of the hypoplastic transverse aortic arch, this reconstruction may or may not require exogenous tissue (generally autologous pericardium or homograft tissue) for arch augmentation.

Risks of the coarctation repair either via thoracotomy or median sternotomy include infection, bleeding, death (one to three percent nationally), damage to the recurrent laryngeal nerve (which surrounds the ductus arteriosus and aorta) or the thoracic duct (less commonly), and paralysis (from spinal ischemia) during the time of aortic occlusion for the anastomosis. Repair with DHCA additionally includes those risks of cardiopulmonary bypass and DHCA, such as neurologic damage and stroke. In all neonates undergoing coarctation repair there is a five to 10 percent likelihood of late recurrence requiring balloon dilatation.

Interrupted Aortic Arch

A condition similar to severe aortic coarctation is interrupted aortic arch, in which there is no continuity between the transverse and descending aorta; this may occur at different locations along the transverse aortic arch. The preferred surgical procedure is direct arch reconstruction and anastomosis, involving ligation and resection of the ductus arteriosus. Operative mortality from this procedure is low, and long-term mortality appears to be similarly low (22,23,24). Because of the important association with DiGeorge syndrome, vigilance in the perioperative period and beyond for hypocalcemia or susceptibility to infection, or both, is important. Over the long term, approximately 20 to 30% of patients will require re-intervention for left heart obstructive lesions, which may range from subaortic resection to more extensive procedures designed to expand the left ventricular outflow tract (22,25).

Hypoplastic Left Heart (HLH) Syndrome

HLH syndrome consists of a range of congenital defects of the left ventricle, aorta, and associated valves, all resulting in a right ventricular-dependent systemic circulation (Figure 20-7). In its most severe forms HLH syndrome exists in the context of critical aortic stenosis: left ventricular cardiac output is minimal or absent, and the entire arch and coronary vessels are perfused retrograde via the ductus arteriosus.

HLH syndrome is invariably fatal without surgical repair, and before the 1980s, most infants would expire within the first month. In the modern era, after diagnosis of HLH syndrome two primary options are available: the staged Norwood reconstruction and cardiac transplantation. Transplantation has the advantage of restoring normal circulatory physiology, but the limited number of donor organs available precludes its use in all patients and represents a therapeutic strategy that is epidemiologically non-viable. In contrast, staged reconstruction requires multiple operations (usually three) and results in Fontan circulation, with the pulmonary and systemic circulations in series. Although perioperative survival following the Norwood procedure has improved, one-year survival after stage I repair remains only 85 to 90% in the best series (26,27). Early postoperative survival after cardiac transplantation often approaches 90%; however, the complexities and outcomes of transplantation in the neonatal period are variable (and are discussed in a subsequent chapter) (28,29).

The Norwood reconstruction involves: (1) augmentation of the hypoplastic aortic arch; (2) the creation of a common arterial outflow from the heart; (3) an atrial septectomy; and (4) the establishment of controlled pulmonary blood flow with either a modified BT shunt, or a so-called "Sano" right ventricle–pulmonary artery connection with a Gore-tex® tube (Figure 20-8). Specific technical difficulties of the procedure involve accurate arch reconstruction without twisting or kinking (with a native aorta that can be as small as 1–2 mm), residual distal arch obstruction, shunt-related problems, and, in the case of Sano patients, progressive stenosis at the distal pulmonary artery anastomosis requiring early advancement to the cavopulmonary shunt procedure.

Because HLH syndrome includes a range of anatomic defects, attempts at improving outcomes with staged reconstruction have focused on improved patient selection and perioperative management based on preoperative anatomic and physiologic factors predictive of poor outcomes after repair. Such research has identified several factors which increase the risk to children undergoing the Norwood procedure. Patients aged more than one month have poor outcomes

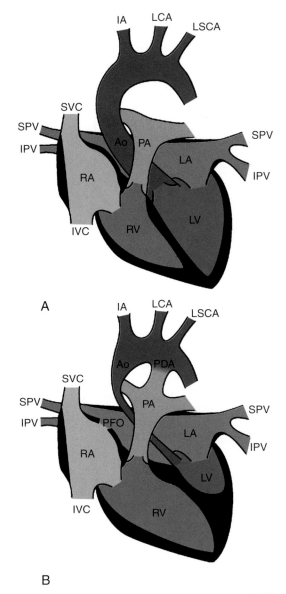

FIGURE 20–7 Schematic diagram of **(A)** normal cardiac anatomy and **(B)** hypoplastic left heart (HLH) syndrome. Note the atretic aortic and hypoplastic left ventricle. Systemic blood flow is from the right ventricle through the patent ductus arteriosus into the aortic arch. Pulmonary venous return crosses from the left atrium to the right atrium through a patent foramen ovale. SPV, superior pulmonary vein; IPV, inferior pulmonary vein; LA, left atrium; LV, left ventricle; Ao, aorta; IA, innominate artery; LCA, left carotid artery; LSCA, left subclavian artery; SVC, superior vena cava; IVC, inferior vena cava; RA, right atrium; RV, right ventricle; PA, pulmonary artery; PDA, patent ductus arteriosus; PFO, patent foramen ovale.

compared with those undergoing operation in the neonatal period (27,31) and patients with increased pulmonary venous return (PVR) are prone to lethal pulmonary vascular crises (32). A variety of other risk factors have been identified for poor outcomes after Stage I reconstruction (16,27,28,31,33,34,35,36,37,38). However, potentially correctable surgical technical problems resulted in a significant proportion of Stage I mortality in early studies (34), thus explaining the improved survival in the most recent series. This improved survival in contemporary Stage I repair should be translated into dramatically better long-term survival as these patients go on to subsequent stages (27,39).

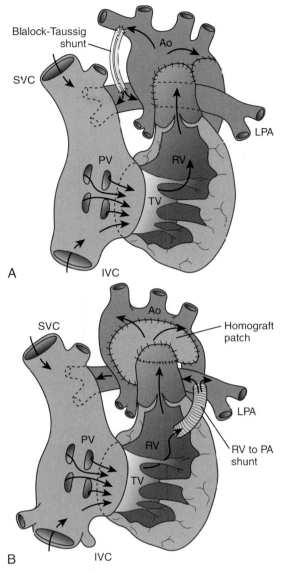

FIGURE 20–8 The Norwood reconstruction is shown using **(A)** a modified Blalock–Taussig (BT) shunt and **(B)** the so-called "Sano" right ventricule-to-pulmonary artery connection. *Reprinted from Griselli, et al. (30).*

Cyanotic Heart Lesions

Transposition of the Great Arteries

Transposition of the great arteries (TGA) consists of a reversal of the normal anatomic position of the great vessels so that the aorta represents the outflow of the right ventricle and the pulmonary artery serves as the left ventricular outflow. This results in distinct and parallel systemic and pulmonary circulations connected through some form of obligate mixing between the circulations either via a VSD, aortopulmonary flow through a PDA, or, most often (and most effective), shunting through a patent foramen ovale (PFO). Patients with marginal systemic oxygenation and restrictive atrial communication may benefit from a bedside balloon atrial septostomy.

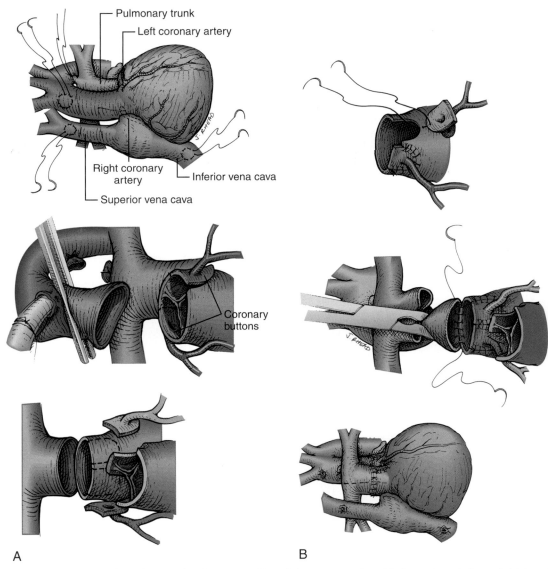

FIGURE 20–9 Arterial switch operation for transposition of the great arteries with the aorta anterior and rightward and usual coronary anatomy. *From Kouchoukos et al. (21).*

Depending on the degree of mixing and the associated cardiac anomalies, the degree of cyanosis in the neonate with TGA may vary widely. As with other congenital heart defects, initial medical management should be directed at optimizing acid-base, electrolyte, and oxygenation status. Early repair is advocated to enable development and growth of the cardiac chambers under the appropriate pressure loads: systemic pressure load on the left ventricle; pulmonary pressure load on the right ventricle. Prolonged "deconditioning" of the left ventricle may lead to muscular regression so that the left ventricle cannot support the systemic circulation and requires "training" before repair.

The procedure of choice in the current era is an arterial switch operation with concurrent coronary transfer (Figure 20-9). In this operation, the great vessels are "switched" after the coronary arteries are implanted on the neo-aorta, thus providing both an anatomic and physiologic solution to the condition.

Improvements in both operative technique and perioperative management have resulted in excellent short- and long-term outcomes with the arterial switch procedure (40,41). Overall, one-month, one-year, and five-year survival in patients undergoing arterial switch for TGA have been excellent, approaching 95% in most recent series (42). Specific challenges to repair are generally related to anatomic variations of the coronary arteries, the geometric relationship of the great vessels and ventricles, and the integrity of the pulmonic (neoaortic) valve.

Total Anomalous Pulmonary Venous Connection

Disruption of any of the complex sequence of events in the development of the pulmonary venous system may result in significant abnormalities of pulmonary venous anatomy. Total anomalous pulmonary venous connection (TAPVC), also known as anomalous venous drainage or return, occurs when these abnormalities result in return of oxygenated blood from the pulmonary circulation to the right side of the heart rather than the left atrium. An ASD or PFO is required in order for these infants to survive. The most common types of TAPVC include supracardiac connection with drainage into the left innominate vein, cardiac level connection to the coronary sinus, or infracardiac connection through the portal vein.

The clinical presentation of these patients is variable; many present with cyanosis, but the severity of the hemodynamic compromise depends not on the route of blood flow, but on the presence of other anomalies, the presence and severity of obstruction to pulmonary venous drainage, and the degree of obstruction across the atrial septum (43). Patients without obstruction to pulmonary venous return and unrestricted atrial septal communication may develop symptoms during or after the neonatal period with progressive tachypnea, cyanosis, and right-sided heart failure caused by increased pulmonary blood flow and volume load on the right ventricle.

At the opposite end of the clinical spectrum are those patients with severe obstruction of PVR. These patients develop high pulmonary pressures early in the neonatal period in combination with elevated and labile pulmonary vascular resistance. Pulmonary edema combined with progressive decrease in pulmonary blood flow leads to severe hypoxemia and hemodynamic collapse. In these instances, extracorporeal membrane oxygenation (ECMO) or emergent intervention with surgery is often required.

Preoperative preparation of the neonate with TAPVC and pulmonary venous obstruction should be directed at resuscitation and expedited operative repair, and includes intubation with 100% fraction of inspired oxygen, and inotropic support to assist the failing right ventricle. Inhaled nitric oxide should not be used in an attempt to augment systemic oxygen saturation, as this only provides for more pulmonary blood flow, thereby exacerbating pulmonary edema owing to the restriction to pulmonary venous drainage. Where these therapies are not successful, ECMO may be required in order to correct severe metabolic derangement prior to operative repair, often for as long as 48 to 72 hours.

Mortality without operative repair in TAPVC exceeds 80% at one year (44), therefore repair should be performed soon after diagnosis. Patients without obstruction to PVR may be managed with urgent rather than emergency surgery, but those with obstruction require either emergency surgery or rapid initiation of ECMO to support oxygenation and correct end-organ dysfunction prior to definitive repair.

Operative repair techniques vary depending on the anatomy of the venous connections, but all involve some connection of the pulmonary venous drainage into the left atrium and ligation of the anomalous connection ("vertical vein") to the systemic venous circulation. Usually, a single confluent vein drains all four anomalous pulmonary veins and this may be connected through as large an anastomosis as possible to the left atrium. More complex repairs may be required where anomalous pulmonary veins drain in pairs ("mixed"). Those infants with diffuse pulmonary venous atresia are generally considered inoperable.

Outcomes after repair are excellent, with operative mortality in the most recent series ranging from five to nine percent (45). Pulmonary hypertension in the immediate postoperative phase may require inhaled nitric oxide, and ECMO may be continued following surgical repair to maintain systemic oxygenation and allow for cardiac recovery. A subset of patients will require reoperation, often for pulmonary venous stenosis, which may occur in six to 11% of patients, most commonly those with infracardiac or mixed-type TAPVC. Long term, patients may be expected to grow normally with return of normal right ventricular function, resolution of right ventricular dilatation, and reversal of pulmonary vascular abnormalities (45).

MECHANICAL CIRCULATORY SUPPORT IN THE NEONATE

Although mechanical circulatory support has been used with success in adults with cardiopulmonary heart failure, the extension of these successes to the neonatal population has been limited. Two factors in particular make mechanical support challenging in this population: small patient size requires devices designed specifically for a pediatric population, and congenital cardiac disease with abnormal anatomy (e.g. concurrent biventricular failure with or without pulmonary valvular issues) complicates the application of mechanical support. However, in patients with cardiac or pulmonary dysfunction refractory to maximal medical therapy, mechanical circulatory support may be beneficial in certain circumstances (46):

- preoperative stabilization before operative repair
- postoperative support to allow for recovery of cardiac or pulmonary function, or both
- temporary support in patients not in need of cardiac repair whose cardiac or pulmonary function is expected to improve with time
- as a bridge to transplantation.

Two forms of mechanical circulatory support are currently available to neonates: ECMO and ventricular assist device (VAD). Similar to cardiopulmonary bypass in the operating room, essentially, ECMO consists of veno-arterial bypass with a membrane oxygenator (Figure 20-10). In neonatal patients with respiratory failure, many subgroups have survival with ECMO which exceeds 80% (47). Increasingly, ECMO has been used for postcardiotomy cardiopulmonary support in the pediatric cardiac surgical patient. However, in this application, survival in multicenter studies (of heterogenous patient populations and indications) is only 32 to 44%, although some institutions have reported survival exceeding 50% (46,48). Outcomes naturally vary depending upon the cardiac anatomy and the status of repair. Patients with biventricular physiology appear to have improved outcomes with ECMO when compared with those with single-ventricle physiology, and the management of aortopulmonary shunts (or patent ductus arterioses) during ECMO remains controversial (46).

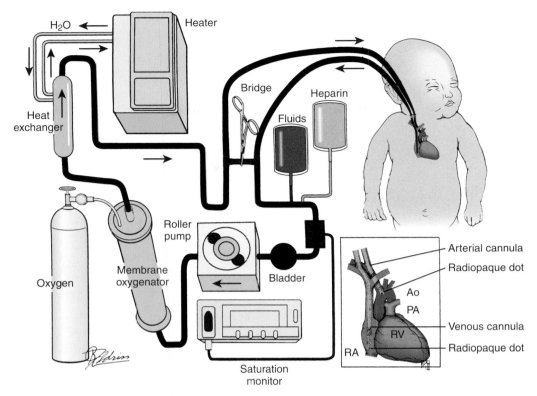

FIGURE 20–10 Extracorporeal membrane oxygenation (ECMO) uses veno-arterial bypass with a membrane oxygenator. This technique allows both hemodynamic and pulmonary support. ECMO systems generally consist of a silicone membrane oxygenator, a heat exchanger, a bladder, and a roller pump. Ao, aorta; PA, pulmonary artery; RA, right atrium; RV, right ventricle. *From Jacobs (46).*

Currently, few VAD options are available for neonates owing to their size constraints. Two devices have been used extensively in Europe for this indication, the MEDOS and Berlin Heart ventricular assist devices. The Berlin Heart (Berlin Heart AG) is a paracorporeal pulsatile, uni- or biventricular assist device that is available across several different sizes of pumps (Figure 20-11); for neonates, the 10 cc pumps are most often used. The pumps require inflow from the atrium (for right-sided assistance) or the ventricular apex (for left-sided support), as well as outflow (to either pulmonary artery, aorta, or both). Implantation requires cardiopulmonary bypass and often cardiac arrest. The cannulae for inflow and outflow exit the skin at the upper abdomen and are attached to two extracorporeal devices whose pumping mechanism is activated via pneumatic actuation from a separate console. The device requires systemic anticoagulation.

Until 2003, the Berlin Heart was largely unavailable in the USA, but more recently it has been allowed application under a compassionate use protocol with the Food and Drug Administration (FDA). Already, in 2005, nearly 28 devices have been implanted in the USA (personal communication). The time of device support is theoretically limitless; however, the ongoing risk of stroke or hemorrhage encourages weaning from device support (for reversible myocardial failure) or bridging to transplantation as soon as is physiologically possible. Several new devices are currently under development and investigation as part of an initiative by the National Heart, Lung and Blood Institute, with, it is hoped, clinical application by 2010.

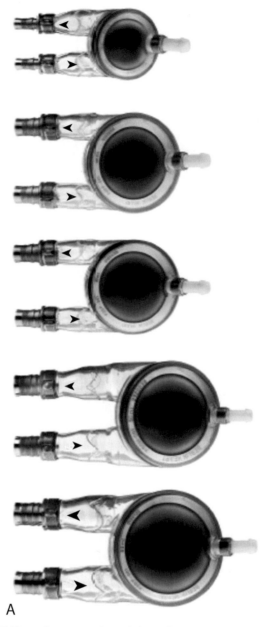

A

FIGURE 20–11 **(A)** The various pump sizes of the Berlin Heart EXCOR ventricular assist device. *Courtesy of the Berlin Heart AG.*

SUMMARY

The 50 years since the inception of intracardiac repair of congenital heart disease have resulted in remarkable changes in operative techniques and the perioperative management of these patients. Consequently, the preferred age at definitive repair has steadily decreased, resulting in a parallel decrease in the need for palliative procedures in the neonatal period. The coming years should yield further advances, particularly with regard to the use of mechanical circulatory support in neonates, refinements in surgical repair techniques for both short-term outcomes and long-term durability, as well as the development

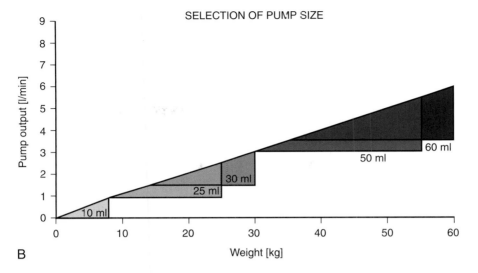

B

FIGURE 20-11 **(B)** Correlation between patient size and pump size, based on the cardiac output delivered by each pump. *Courtesy of Berlin Heart AG.*

of catheter-based solutions (isolated or in combination with open surgery) for early repair.

REFERENCES

1. Lewis FJ, Taufic M. Closure of atrial septal defects with the aid of hypothermia: experimental accomplishments and the report of one successful case. Surgery 1953;33:52–59.
2. Barrat-Boyes BG, Simpson M, Neutze JM. Intracardiac surgery in neonates and infants using deep hypothermia with surface cooling and limited cardiopulmonary bypass. Circulation 1971; 43:125–130.
3. Warden HE, Cohen M, Read RC, Lillehi CW. Controlled cross circulation for open intracardiac surgery: physiologic studies and results of creation and closure of ventricular septal defects. J Thorac Surg 1954;28:331–334; discussion 341–343.
4. Albus RA, Trusler GA, Izukawa T, Williams WG. Pulmonary artery banding. J Thorac Cardiovasc Surg 1984;88:645–653.
5. Backer CL, Mavroudis C. Palliative Operations. In Mavroudis D, Backer CL eds. Pediatric Cardiac Surgery, third edition. Philadelphia, PA Mosby 2003:160–170.
6. Blalock A, Taussig H. The surgical treatment of malformations of the heart in which there is pulmonary stenosis or pulmonary atresia. JAMA 1984;251:2123–2138.
7. Davis P, Turner-Gomes S, Cunningham K, Way C, Roberts R, Schmidt B. Precision and accuracy of clinical and radiological signs in premature infants at risk of patent ductus arteriosus. Arch Pediatr Adolesc Med 1995;149:1136–1141.
8. Gersony WM, Peckham GJ, Ellison RC, Miettinen OS, Nadas AS. Effects of indomethacin in premature infants with patent ductus arteriosus: results of a national collaborative study. J Pediatr 1983;102:895–906.
9. Hillman ND, Mavroudis C, Backer CL. Patent Ductus Arteriosus. In Mavroudis C, Backer CL eds. Pediatric Cardiac Surgery, third edition. Philadelphia, PA Mosby 2003:223–233.
10. Collett RW, Edwards JE. Persistent truncus arteriosus: a classification according to anatomic types. Surg Clin N Am 1949;29:1245–1270.
11. Chen JM, Glickstein JS, Davis RR, Mercando ML, Hellenbrand WE, Mosca RS, Quaegebeur JM. The effect of repair technique on postoperative right-sided obstruction in patients with truncus arteriosus. J Thorac Cardiovasc Surg 2005;129:559–568.
12. Mavroudis C, Backer CL. Truncus Arteriosus. In Mavroudis C, Backler CL, eds. Pediatric Cardiac Surgery, third edition. Philadelphia, PA: Mosby, 2003; 339–352.
13. Mitchell MB, Clarke DR. Isolated Right Ventricular Outflow Tract Obstruction. In Mavroudis C, Backler CL, eds. Pediatric Cardiac Surgery, third edition. Philadelphia, PA: Mosby, 2003; 361–382.
14. Hanley FL, Sade RM, Freedom RM, Blackstone EH, Kirklin JW. Outcomes in critically ill neonates with pulmonary stenosis and intact ventricular septum: a multiinstitutional study. Congenital Heart Surgeons Society. J Am Coll Cardiol 1993;22:183–192.
15. Castenada A, Jonas RA, Mayer JE Jr, Hanley FL. Pulmonary atresia with intact ventricular septum Cardiac Surgery of the Infant and Neonate. Philadelphia, PA WB Saunders 1994:235–247.

16. Lofland GK, McCrindle BW, Williams WG, Blackstone EH, Tchervenkov CI, Sittiwangkul R, Jonas RA. Critical aortic stenosis in the neonate: a multi-institutional study of management outcomes, and risk factors. Congenital Heart Surgeons Society. J Thorac Cardiovasc Surg 2001;121:10–27.

17. Tchervenkov CI, Chu VFm Shum-Tim D. Left Ventricular Outflow Tract Obstruction. In Mavroudis C, Backer CL, eds. Pediatric Cardiac Surgery, third edition. Philadelphia, PA: Mosby, 2003; 537–559.

18. Kohl T, Sharland G, Allan LD, et al. World experience of percutaneous ultrasound-guided balloon valvuloplasty in human fetuses with severe aortic value obstruction. Am J Cardiol 2000;85:1230–1233.

19. Ettedgui JA, Tallman-Eddy T, Neches WH, et al. Long-term results of survivors of surgical valvotomy for severe aortic stenosis in early infancy. J Thorac Cardiovasc Surg 1992; 104:1714–1720.

20. Justo RN, McCrindle BW, Benson LN, Williams WG, Freedom RM, Smallhorn JF. Aortic valve regurgitation after surgical versus percutaneous balloon valvotomy for congenital aortic valve stenosis. Am J Cardiol 1996;77:1332–1338.

21. Kouchoukos NT, Blackstone EH, Doty DB, Hanley FL, Karp RB. Cardiac Surgery, third edition. Philadelphia, PA Elsevier 2003.

22. Jonas RA, Quaegebeur JM, Kirklin JW, Blackstone EH, Daicoff G. Outcomes in patients with interrupted aortic arch and ventricular septal defect. A multiinstitutional study. Congenital Heart Surgeons Society. J Thorac Cardiovasc Surg 1994;107:1099–1109; discussion 1109–1113.

23. Sell JE, Jonas RA, Mayer JE, Blackstone EH, Kirklin JW, Castanada AR. The results of a surgical program for interrupted aortic arch. J Thorac Cardiovasc Surg 1988;96:864–877.

24. Serraf A, Lacour-Gayet F, Robotin M, Bruniaux J, Sousa-Uva M, Roussin R, Planche C. Repair of interrupted aortic arch: a ten-year experience. J Thorac Cardiovasc Surg 1996;112:1150–1160.

25. Jonas RA. Interrupted Aortic Arch. In Mavroudis C, Backler CL, eds. Pediatric Cardiac Surgery, third edition. Philadelphia, PA: Mosby, 2003; 273–282.

26. Checcia PA, Larsen R, Sehra R, Daher N, Gundry SR, Razzouk AJ, Bailey LL. Effect of a selection and postoperative care protocol on survival of infants with hypoplastic left heart syndrome. Ann Thorac Surg 2004;77:477–483; discussion 483.

27. Mahle WT, Spray TL, Wernovsky G, Gaynor JW, Clark BJ III. Survival after reconstructive surgery for hypoplastic left heart syndrome: a 15-year experience from a single institution. Circulation 2000;102:136–141.

28. Bando K, Turrentine MW, Sun K, et al. Surgical management of hypoplastic left heart syndrome. Ann Thorac Surg 1996;62:70–76.

29. Jenkins PC, Flanagan MF, Jenkins KJ, et al. Survival analysis and risk factors for mortality in transplantation and staged surgery for hypoplastic left heart syndrome. J Am Coll Cardiol 2000;36:1178–1185.

30. Griselli M, McGuirk SP, Stumper O, et al. Influence of surgical strategies on outcome after the Norwood procedure. J Thorac Cardiovasc Surg 2006;131:418–426.

31. Iannettoni MD, Bove EL, Mosca RS, et al. Improving results with first-stage palliation for hypoplastic left heart syndrome. J Thorac Cardiovasc Surg 1994;107:934–940.

32. Duncan BW, Rosenthal GL, Jones TK, Lupinetti FM. First-stage palliation of complex univentricular cardiac anomalies in older infants. Ann Thorac Surg 2001;72:2077–2080.

33. Andrews R, Tulloh R, Sharland G, et al. Outcome of staged reconstructive surgery for hypoplastic left heart syndrome following antenatal diagnosis. Arch Dis Child 2001;85:474–477.

34. Bartram U, Grunenfelder J, Van Praagh R. Causes of death after the modified Norwood procedure: a study of 122 postmortem cases. Ann Thorac Surg 1997;64:1795–1802.

35. Bove EL, Lloyd TR. Staged reconstruction for hypoplastic left heart syndrome. Contemporary results. Ann Surg 1996;224:387–394; discussion 394–395.

36. Forbess JM, Cook N, Roth SJ, Serraf A, Mayer JE Jr, Jonas RA. Ten-year institutional experience with palliative surgery for hypoplastic left heart syndrome. Risk factors related to stage I mortality. Circulation 1995;92:262–266.

37. Graziano JN, Heidelberger KP, Ensing GJ, Gomez CA, Ludomirsky A. The influence of a restrictive atrial septal defect on pulmonary vascular morphology in patients with hypoplastic left heart syndrome. Pediatr Cardiol 2002;23:146–151.

38. Jenkins PC, Flanagan MF, Sargent JD, et al. A comparison of treatment strategies for hypoplastic left heart syndrome using decision analysis. J Am Coll Cardiol 2001;38:1181–1187.

39. Chang RK, Chen AY, Klitzner TS. Clinical management of infants with hypoplastic left heart syndrome in the United States, 1988 – 1997. Pediatrics 2002;110:292–298.

40. Backer CL, Ilbawi MN, Ohtake S, et al. Transposition of the great arteries: a comparison of the results of the mustard procedure versus the arterial switch. Ann Thorac Surg 1989;48:10–14.

41. Laks H. The arterial switch procedure for the neonate: coming of age. Ann Thorac Surg 1989;48:3–4.

42. Kirklin JW, Blackstone EH, Tchervenkov CI, Castenada AR. Clinical outcomes after the arterial switch operation for transposition. Patient, support, procedure, and institutional risk factors. Congenital Heart Surgeons Society. Circulation 1992;86:1501–1515.

43. Yee ES, Turley K, Hsieh WR, Ebert PA. Infant total anomalous pulmonary venous connection: factors influencing timing of presentation and operative outcome. Circulation 1987;76:83–87.

44. Burroughts JT, Edwards JE. Total anomalous pulmonary venous connection. Am Heart J 1960;59:913–931.

45. Kirschbolm PM, Jaggers J, Ungerleider R. Total Anomalous Pulmonary Venous Connection. In Mavroudis C, Backler CL eds. Pediatric Cardiac Surgery, third edition. Philadelphia, PA Mosby 2003:612–624.

46. Jacobs JP. Pediatric Mechanical Circulatory Support. In Mavroudis C, Backler CL eds. Pediatric Cardiac Surgery, third edition. Philadelphia, PA Mosby 2003:778–792.

47. Ichiba S, Bartlett RH. Current status of extracorporeal membrane oxygentation for severe respiratory failure. Artif Organs 1996;20:120–123.

48. Walters HL III, Hakimi M, Rice MD, Lyons JM, Whittlesey GC, Klein MD. Pediatric cardiac surgical ECMO: multivariate analysis of risk factors for hospital death. Ann Thorac Surg 1954;60:329–336discussion 336–327.

49. Wright GE, Nowak CA, Goldberg CS, et al. Extended resection and end-to-end anastomosis for aortic coarctation in infants: Results of a tailored surgical approach. Am Thorac Surg 2005;80:1453–1459.

Chapter 21

MRI Evaluation of the Neonate with Congenital Heart Disease

Beth Feller Printz, MD, PhD

INTRODUCTION

Although transthoracic echocardiography is currently the standard first-line technique used for the diagnosis and evaluation of neonates with congenital heart disease, there are times when echocardiography cannot adequately delineate particular aspects of cardiac or vascular anatomy. Often this may be due to suboptimal acoustic windows or interference from adjacent air-filled structures. Diagnostic cardiac catheterization has traditionally been considered the second-line procedure of choice when echocardiography is insufficient in neonatal cardiac or vascular assessment. However, cardiac magnetic resonance imaging (MRI) has recently emerged as an important imaging modality with which to assess neonates and older children with congenital heart disease (1–6). MRI has three major advantages over catheterization: it is a non-invasive technique; there is no ionizing radiation exposure to which neonates are particularly susceptible; and there is no need for iodinated contrast agents (2). In particular, magnetic resonance angiography (MRA) using injection of gadolinium, a paramagnetic contrast medium that, in the short term, is safe to use in infants less than six months of age (7), can produce high-resolution angiographic imaging of systemic and pulmonary vasculature within a few minutes. Cardiac MRI with MRA has the additional advantage of producing three-dimensional (3-D) tomographic images of the heart, vascular structures, lungs, and bronchi.

Performance of cardiac MRI with MRA in neonates presents a series of technical and practical challenges to neonatologists and imaging physicians (pediatric cardiologists, radiologists, or both). Technically, cardiac MRI methods have been developed and optimized for patients who are relatively large, have good-sized vascular and cardiac structures, slow heart rates, and are able to hold their breath in order to decrease motion artifacts. A number of different MRI techniques are now standard for MRI assessment of older children and adults with congenital heart disease, such as the techniques used to quantify cardiac function and flow (3,6-8), but are currently not optimized for newborns owing to limitations in both spatial and temporal resolution. Fortunately, transthoracic echocardiography is usually sufficient to address these issues in neonates.

Imaging obtained by use of MRA with gadolinium injection is independent of heart rate and, with adequate motion suppression, can produce three-dimensional images of neonatal thoracic vasculature with millimeter resolution. Following injection into any peripheral vein, gadolinium rapidly circulates in the vascular structures and greatly enhances the image resolution of these structures. In less than one minute the entire 3-D thoracic vasculature may be assessed by MRA. The 3-D nature of the acquired data allows postprocessing to recreate images in any desired plane as well as the creation of 3-D surface-rendered models, which may be useful in the assessment of spatial relationships (9,10).

There are a number of practical issues that must be overcome when performing cardiac MRI or MRA in neonates. In order to optimize imaging of the neonate's very small thoracic vascular structures, motion artifact, including respiratory motion, must be kept to an absolute minimum. This is in contrast to MRI of the neonatal brain, where respiratory motion artifact does not typically impair image resolution. Some centers have found it adequate to perform cardiac MRI examinations in newborns and young children who are calm and free breathing (either merely sleeping after a feed or by use of moderate sedation) (11). However, most centers where neonatal cardiac MRI or MRA is routinely performed have found that a suspended-respiration technique produces the highest-quality images of their small vascular structures. Suspended respiration requires intubation for the cardiac MRI procedure, with the use of sedation and neuromuscular blockade. Periods of suspended respiration, from 10 sec to 60 sec, are used during scan acquisition, and have been shown to be well-tolerated, even in potentially unstable infants with complex heart disease (12). These neonates must therefore be ventilated and closely monitored using magnetic resonance-compatible cardiorespiratory devices whilst inside the bore of the magnet. All medication pumps, lines, and monitoring devices must be magnetic resonance-compatible, or connected via long extension tubing to pumps outside the MRI room itself. An appropriately sized MRI receiver coil is placed around the neonate, as well as blankets for thermoregulation and earplugs for sound suppression. For these reasons, patient preparation time often exceeds the time of the cardiac MRI or MRA scan itself. Recently, magnetic resonance-compatible incubators with integrated MRI receiver coils have been introduced in order to ameliorate some of the problems inherent in neonatal MRI, but these are not in widespread use (13).

Clinical indications for neonatal cardiac MRI and MRA are rapidly expanding, and may include delineation of pulmonary vascular anatomy, aortic arch and collateral vessel anatomy, assessment of abnormalities of systemic and pulmonary venous return, assessment of airway compression due to abnormal vascular structures, tumor classification, and assessment of cardiac fibrosis.

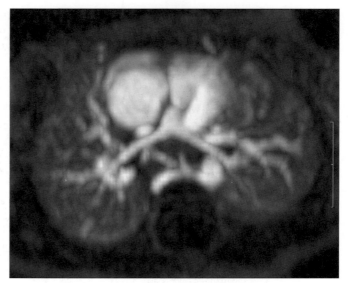

FIGURE 21–1 Newborn with tetralogy of Fallot and pulmonary atresia. Axial oblique submaximal intensity projection of three-dimensional (3-D) magnetic resonance angiography (MRA). Note the branch pulmonary arteries and visualization of aorta to pulmonary artery collateral vessels.

ASSESSMENT OF PULMONARY VASCULAR ANATOMY

Neonates with congenital heart disease commonly have abnormalities of the pulmonary arteries which may be difficult to evaluate adequately by transthoracic echocardiography. Cardiac MRI or MRA has been shown to identify accurately abnormalities of pulmonary vasculature when compared with invasive cardiac catheterization (14). For example, patients with tetralogy of Fallot may have isolated narrowing of a pulmonary artery or anomalous origin of the pulmonary artery from alternative structures (such as from the aorta or from collateral vessels which, in turn, originate from the aorta). Figure 21-1 illustrates an example of pulmonary artery visualization by use of MRA performed on a newborn with tetralogy of Fallot, pulmonary atresia, and multiple aorta to pulmonary artery collateral vessels.

Tetralogy of Fallot with absent pulmonary valve syndrome is a relatively rare condition in which the pulmonary arteries are often aneurysmally dilated and associated with neonatal bronchial compression; such infants are particularly well-suited for evaluation of both the airways and pulmonary vasculature by MRI (15,16). Cardiac MRI can also be useful in the postoperative assessment of neonates after palliative or definitive surgical repairs, such as after aorta-to-pulmonary artery shunt procedures.

ABNORMALITIES OF THE AORTIC ARCH

Many abnormalities of the aortic arch, such as critical coarctation of the aorta or aortic arch interruption, are diagnosed in the perinatal or neonatal period and may need intervention in the first few days of life. Transthoracic echocardiography may be adequate for diagnosis, but not uncommonly either the aortic arch itself, the branching pattern of the head vessels, or the anatomy of the ductus arteriosus may not be sufficiently well-visualized to enable surgical planning. MRI with MRA has been shown to be an excellent adjunct to echocardiography in assessment of aortic coarctation (17) and aortic arch interruption (18). Figure 21-2 demonstrates an example of reformatted MRA imaging in a newborn with long-segment hypoplasia of a left-sided aortic arch into which inserts a right-sided patent ductus arteriosus.

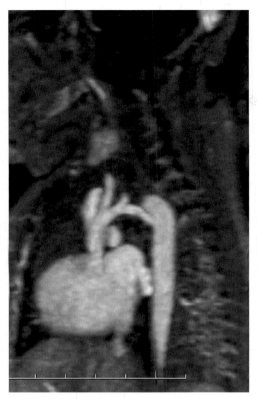

FIGURE 21–2 Reformatted image from three-dimensional (3-D) magnetic resonance angiography (MRA) of a newborn with a hypoplastic left-sided aortic arch and right-sided patent ductus arteriosus. This abnormality has produced a vascular ring (not shown in this image).

SYSTEMIC VENOUS ANOMALIES

Anomalies of the systemic veins may be associated with congenital heart disease, especially in association with heterotaxy syndrome. Abnormalities in systemic venous return may include interruption of the intrahepatic portion of the inferior vena cava, presence of bilateral superior vena cavae with or without the presence of a bridging vein and with normal drainage into the right atrium, bilateral superior vena cava with an unroofed coronary sinus and drainage of the left superior vena cava to the left atrium, right superior vena cava draining to the left atrium, and retro-aortic course of the innominate vein. Although many of these anomalies have no hemodynamic consequence, knowledge of systemic venous anatomy is essential to preoperative planning and during cannulation for cardiopulmonary bypass. Most of these anomalies can be detected accurately using echocardiography in the newborn period. However, in a small subset of patients, echocardiography may be inconclusive. Three-dimensional MRA provides excellent visualization of the entire systemic venous system with a single intravenous injection of gadolium (Figure 21-3) and is a useful noninvasive alternative to diagnostic cardiac catheterization (9).

PULMONARY VENOUS ANOMALIES

Anomalies of pulmonary veins may occur either in isolation or in association with other congenital heart defects. Partial (PAPVC) or total anomalous connection of the pulmonary veins (TAPVC) into a systemic vein is the most common pulmonary venous anomaly. Surgical treatment may be required in the newborn period for

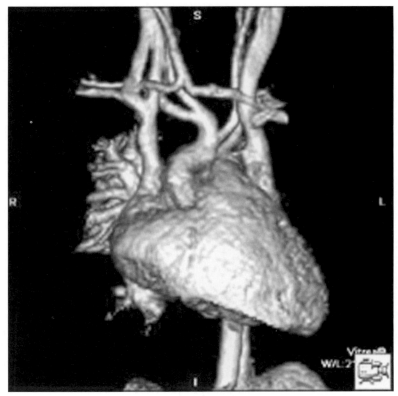

FIGURE 21–3 View from a surface-rendered three-dimensional (3-D) model of a 3-D magnetic resonance angiogram showing bilateral superior vena cavae with a small bridging vein.

TAPVC with obstruction or for milder forms with associated heart defects. The goals of preoperative evaluation are the accurate anatomic delineation of the anomalous pulmonary venous channel, along with its connections with the individual pulmonary veins and the presence of obstruction, if any. In most infants, this is accomplished by use of echocardiography. However, in infants with poor echocardiographic windows or with mixed type of anomalous pulmonary venous connection, echocardiographic evaluation may be insufficient for operative planning. Three-dimensional MRA is ideally suited for the evaluation of these anomalies since the entire systemic and pulmonary venous system is visualized with a single intravenous injection of contrast medium (Figure 21-4).

MRA is also useful in the evaluation of pulmonary venous stenosis or obstruction at the anastomotic site following surgical repair of TAPVC. In this setting, the location, severity, and length of the anatomic narrowing may be accurately defined. In addition, the identification of either dilatation or diffuse narrowing of the intrapulmonary pulmonary veins is useful in considering suitability for re-operation.

In infants with Scimitar syndrome, which is characterized by partial anomalous pulmonary venous return to the inferior vena cava with unilateral lung hypoplasia and systemic arterial supply to the hypoplastic lung (most commonly right-sided), 3-D MRA provides excellent visualization of the pulmonary venous anomaly (Figure 21-5) and the abnormal systemic arterial supply to the lung, in addition to providing an estimates of the degree of pulmonary hypoplasia (19).

HETEROTAXY SYNDROME

Many infants with complex congenital heart disease have abnormalities of visceral sidedness and arrangement that are grouped under the heterotaxy syndrome.

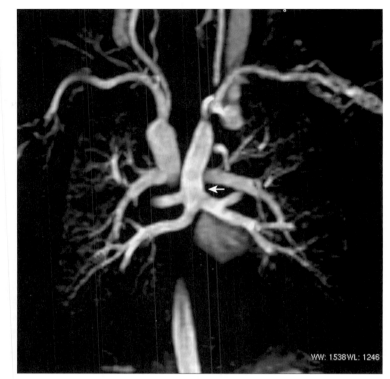

FIGURE 21–4 Coronal maximum intensity projection of a three-dimensional (3-D) magnetic resonance angiogram, demonstrating total anomalous pulmonary venous connection. All pulmonary veins join a confluence (arrow), which drains superiorly via a vertical channel into the left superior vena cava (not shown in image).

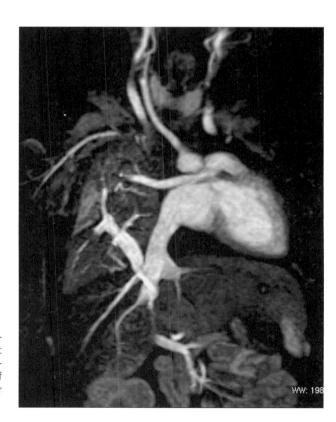

FIGURE 21–5 Coronal maximum intensity projection of a three-dimensional (3-D) magnetic resonance angiogram from an infant with scimitar syndrome showing anomalous connection of the right-sided pulmonary veins into the inferior vena cava.

In addition to assessment of abnormalities of the extracardiac thoracic vasculature, MRI can be useful in the assessment of abnormalities of the position and sidedness of the stomach, liver, spleen, intestines, and the mainstem bronchi (20).

ABNORMALITIES OF THE AIRWAY

Airway compression may be caused by abnormalities of the vasculature, such as vascular rings, left pulmonary artery sling, or compression by massively dilated pulmonary artery branches as in tetralogy of Fallot with absent pulmonary valve. MRI is especially well-suited to the evaluation of these abnormalities since it allows for evaluation of both the vascular abnormality and its effect on the airway (Figure 21-6 and Figure 21-7).

CARDIAC TUMORS

Tumors of the heart, although rare, may present in the newborn period. Although echocardiography may accurately identify the intracardiac extent of the tumor, the assessment of its extension into the mediastinum and relationship to other thoracic structures is often limited. MRI can be useful in evaluating the extent and spatial relationship of the tumor to surrounding structures. In addition, particular MRI imaging characteristics using T1- and T2-weighted sequences, first-pass perfusion, and delayed imaging following contrast injection can be used to predict the type of tumor (21) (Figure 21-8).

ASSESSMENT OF MYOCARDIAL VIABILITY AND PERFUSION

Imaging performed during first-pass of an intravenous contrast agent may be used to assess myocardial perfusion, while delayed imaging is useful in identifying myocardial fibrosis (22). Although there is limited application for these techniques

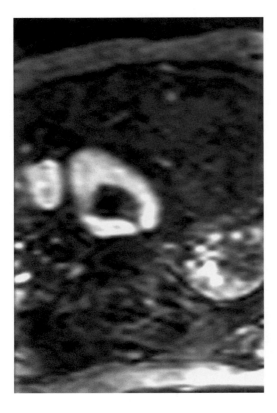

FIGURE 21–6 Axial maximum intensity projection of a three-dimensional (3-D) magnetic resonance angiogram from an infant with stridor, showing a double aortic arch with the two aortic arches encircling the trachea forming a vascular ring.

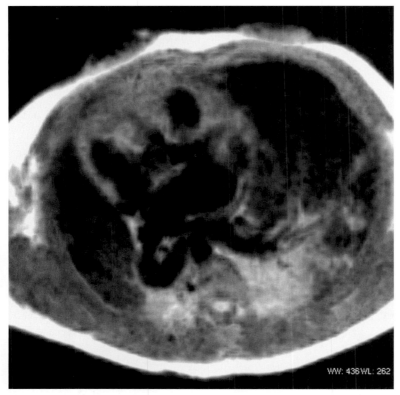

FIGURE 21–7 Axial black-blood image showing a left pulmonary artery sling. The left pulmonary artery arises from the right pulmonary artery and passes leftward posterior to the narrowed trachea. Also note dextrocardia due to associated scimitar syndrome.

in newborn infants, they can be useful in the assessment of tumors and in identifying endomyocardial fibrosis (Figure 21-9).

ASSESSMENT OF CARDIAC FUNCTION

MRI is the reference standard for the assessment of ventricular volume and systolic function in older children and adults. However, limited spatial and temporal resolution has precluded widespread use of this technique in newborn infants.

MEASUREMENT OF BLOOD FLOW

MRI phase velocity imaging can accurately measure blood flow in the cardiovascular system and may be used to measure accurately intracardiac shunt ratios (23), blood flow to each lung, and valve regurgitation. However, the small size of blood vessels limits the spatial resolution of this technique in newborn infants.

ACCURACY OF MRI EVALUATION OF CONGENITAL HEART DISEASE

The accuracy and utility of MRI evaluation of a wide spectrum of congenital heart disease in older children and adults has been demonstrated in several studies. Greil et al. (9) showed that gadolinum-enhanced 3-D MRA is capable of rapidly and accurately diagnosing a wide spectrum of pulmonary and systemic venous abnormalities. Compared with cardiac catheterization, 3-D MRA has also been shown to be

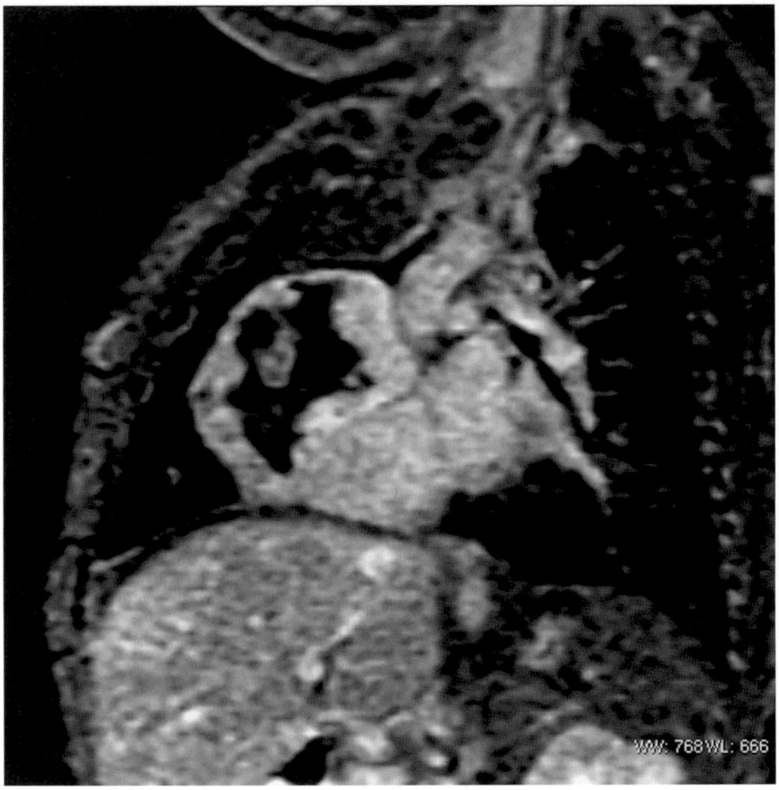

FIGURE 21–8 Oblique coronal maximum intensity projection of a three-dimensional (3-D) magnetic resonance angiogram from a newborn infant with a right atrial tumor. Avid contrast enhancement of the tumor wall is noted suggesting a vascular tumor with an avascular core. Histology showed a hemangioma.

an accurate technique for delineation of all sources of pulmonary blood supply in patients with complex pulmonary stenosis and atresia (14).

In infants, MRI has been shown to be an accurate and safe method to delineate the thoracic vasculature, evaluate possible airway compression, and characterize cardiac tumors (2). In young infants with Scimitar syndrome, we found that findings on MRA agreed with X-ray angiography, and that MRA image quality was excellent for the evaluation of the main and lobar pulmonary artery branches, lobar pulmonary veins, scimitar vein, and systemic–pulmonary collateral arteries (19). In another ongoing study at our institution, MRA performed on 28 consecutive young infants (median age six days) with complex congenital heart disease produced excellent-quality images in all infants when evaluated for visualization of the main and lobar pulmonary arteries, thoracic aorta, aorto–pulmonary collaterals, vena cavae, and visceral sidedness.

LIMITATIONS OF MRI IMAGING IN NEWBORNS

MRI imaging of small infants is inherently difficult related to limitations imposed by a low signal:noise ratio owing to small body size, rapid heart rate, and respiratory or motion artifacts. Most of these limitations can be overcome successfully with optimization of the acquisition parameters and with suspension of respirations during imaging (2). Whilst the visualization of extracardiac thoracic vessels is excellent, cine imaging of intracardiac structures is somewhat limited and may be better accomplished with echocardiography.

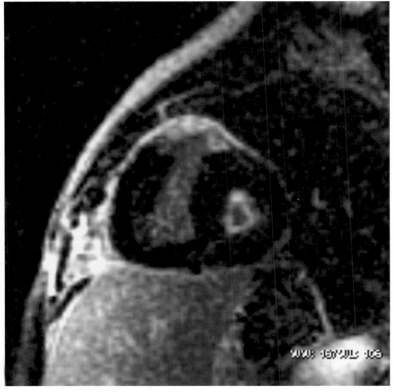

FIGURE 21–9 Delayed-enhancement image in the short-axis orientation from an infant with left ventricular hypoplasia showing delayed hyper-enhancement of the left ventricular endocardium suggesting endomyocardial fibroelastosis.

FUTURE DEVELOPMENTS

Several technical advances are likely in the near future. Improvements in pulse sequence and coil design with larger number of receiver channels are likely to allow faster imaging with improved signal:noise ratio, spatial, and temporal resolution. Improvements in MRI technology may allow scanning to be performed with free breathing and with minimal sedation (5). It may also be possible to perform interventional procedures under MRI guidance, thereby minimizing or even avoiding exposure to ionizing radiation (24).

REFERENCES

1. Chung T. Assessment of cardiovascular anatomy in patients with congenital heart disease by magnetic resonance imaging. Ped Cardiol 2000;21:18–26.
2. Tsai-Goodman B, Geva T, Odegard KC, Sena LM, Powell AJ. Clinical role, accuracy, and technical aspects of cardiovascular magnetic resonance imaging in infants. Am J Cardiol 2004;94:69–74.
3. Reddy GP, Higgins CB. Magnetic resonance imaging of congenital heart disease: evaluation of morphology and function. Seminars in Roentgenology 2003;38:342–351.
4. Razavi RS, Hill DL, Muthurangu V, et al. Three-dimensional magnetic resonance imaging of congenital cardiac anomalies. Cardiology in the Young 2003;13:461–465.
5. Sahn DJ, Vick GW III. Review of new techniques in echocardiography and magnetic resonance imaging as applied to patients with congenital heart disease. Heart 2001;86(Suppl. 2):II41–53.
6. Didier D, Ratib O, Beghetti M, Oberhaensli I, Friedli B. Morphologic and functional evaluation of congenital heart disease by magnetic resonance imaging. J Mag Res Imag 1999;10:639–655.
7. Marti-Bonmati L, Vega T, Benito C, et al. Safety and efficacy of Omniscan (gadodiamide injection) at 0.1 mmol/kg for MRI in infants younger than 6 months of age: phase III open multicenter study. Invest Radiol 2000;35:141–147.
8. Fogel MA. Assessment of cardiac function by magnetic resonance imaging. Pediatr Cardiol 2000;21:59–69.

9. Greil GF, Powell AJ, Gildein HP, Geva T. Gadolinium-enhanced three-dimensional magnetic resonance angiography of pulmonary and systemic venous anomalies. J Am Coll Cardiol 2002;39:335–341.

10. Sorensen TS, Pedersen EM, Hansen OK, Sorensen K. Visualization of morphological details in congenitally malformed hearts: virtual three-dimensional reconstruction from magnetic resonance imaging. Cardiology in the Young 2003;13:451–460.

11. Masui T, Katayama M, Kobauashi S, et al. Gadolium-enhanced MR angiography in the evaluation of congenital cardiovascular disease pre- and postoperative states in infants and children. J Mag Res Imag 2000;12:1034–1042.

12. Odegard KC, Dinardo JA, Tsai-Goodman B, Powell AJ, Geva T, Laussen PC. Anesthesia considerations for cardiac MRI in infants and small children. Ped Anesthes 2004;14:471–476.

13. Bluml S, Friedlich P, Erberich S, et al. MR imaging of newborns by using an MR-compatible incubator with integrated radiofrequency coils: initial experience. Radiology 2004;231:594–601.

14. Geva T, Greil GF, Marshall AC, Landzberg M, Powell AJ. Gadolinium-enhanced 3-dimensional magnetic resonance angiography of pulmonary blood supply in patients with complex pulmonary stenosis or atresia: comparison with x-ray angiography. Circulation 2002;106:473–478.

15. Frank H, Salzer U, Popow C, Stiglbauer R, Wolleneck G, Imhof H. Magnetic resonance imaging of absent pulmonary valve syndrome. Pediatr Cardiol 1996;17:35–39.

16. Taragin BH, Berdon WE, Printz BF. MRI in assessment of persistent bronchomalacia in absent pulmonary valve syndrome – with a review of the syndrome. Pediatr Radiol 2006;36:71–75.

17. Prince MR, Narasimham DL, Jacoby WT, et al. Three-dimensional gadolinium-enhanced MR angiography of the thoracic aorta. Am J Radiog 1996;166:1387–1397.

18. Roche KJ, Krinsky G, Lee VS, Rofsky N, Genieser NB. Interrupted aortic arch: diagnosis with gadolinium-enhanced 3D MRA. J Comp Ass Tomog 1999;23:197–202.

19. Khan MA, Torres AJ, Printz BF, Prakash A. Usefulness of magnetic resonance angiography for diagnosis of Scimitar syndrome in early infancy. Am J Cardiol 2005;96:1313–1316.

20. Geva T, Vick GW III, Wendt RE, Rokey R. Role of spin echo and cine magnetic resonance imaging in presurgical planning of heterotaxy syndrome. Comparison with echocardiography and catheterization. Circulation 1994;90:348–356.

21. Kiaffas MG, Powell AJ, Geva T. Magnetic resonance imaging evaluation of cardiac tumor characteristics in infants and children. Am J Cardiol 2002;89:1229–1233.

22. Prakash A, Powell AJ, Krishnamurthy R, Geva T. Magnetic resonance imaging evaluation of myocardial perfusion and viability in congenital and acquired pediatric heart disease. Am J Cardiol 2004;93:657–661.

23. Powell AJ, Tsai-Goodman B, Prakash A, Greil GF, Geva T. Comparison between phase-velocity cine magnetic resonance imaging and invasive oximetry for quantification of atrial shunts. Am J Cardiol 2003;91:1523–1525.

24. Razavi R, Hill DL, Keevil SF, et al. Cardiac catheterisation guided by MRI in children and adults with congenital heart disease. Lancet 2003;362:1877–1882.

Chapter 22

The Twin–Twin Transfusion Syndrome: Evolving Concepts

Jack Rychik, MD

Introduction

Characteristic Findings and Making the Diagnosis of Twin–Twin
Transfusion Syndrome

Mechanism and Pathophysiology of Twin–Twin Transfusion Syndrome

Spectrum of Cardiovascular Findings in Twin–Twin Transfusion Syndrome

Quantifying the Burden of Cardiovascular Impairment in TTTS

Strategies for the Treatment of Twin–Twin Transfusion Syndrome

Long-Term Issues and the Future

Acknowledgements

References

INTRODUCTION

Twin–twin transfusion syndrome (TTTS) is a disorder seen in 15% to 20% of monochorionic twin gestations (1,2). This disease process is increasingly recognized as the most important contributing factor to morbidity and mortality in twin gestations. If left untreated, its natural history results in death in at least one of the twins in 90% to 100% of cases. To date, our understanding of the pathophysiology of the disease is incomplete and the development of effective treatment strategies is still evolving. Recent data suggest that TTTS is primarily a circulatory derangement – a failure of partnership between the vascular systems of fetuses sharing the placenta. This failed circulatory arrangement results in consequences which set a course for cardiovascular decompensation that can be lethal if left unchecked and can have a significant long-term impact on cardiovascular health in survivors.

In this chapter, we will review our current understanding of TTTS, propose a score for characterizing the magnitude of cardiovascular perturbation seen in this disease, and discuss some of the questions that continue to challenge the investigators and clinical practitioners who deal with this intriguing condition.

CHARACTERISTIC FINDINGS AND MAKING THE DIAGNOSIS OF TWIN–TWIN TRANSFUSION SYNDROME

TTTS is suspected during pregnancy in the presence of monochorionic, diamniotic gestation in which there is a discrepant size between the fetuses of at least 10%, and in which there is oligohydramnios in the smaller and polyhydramnios in the larger fetus. Often the degree of oligohydramnios is so severe that the smaller twin appears to be "shrink-wrapped" in its own amniotic sac, with the amniotic membrane adhering tightly to it. With the larger twin exhibiting polyhydramnios, the smaller twin is pushed to a corner of the uterus, limiting its mobility – hence it is commonly referred to as a "stuck twin." Premature labor as a consequence of the polyhydramnios and maternal abdominal size is common. TTTS is to be distinguished from other causes of interfetal size discrepancy, such as intrauterine growth restriction, or the presence of congenital, genetic or chromosomal anomalies, or infection in the smaller twin.

The impact of TTTS on the outcome of affected twins can be quite considerable. The first historical report of TTTS dates from the seventeenth century, in which the twin sons of the mayor of Amsterdam, Jacob Dierkszon De Graeff were stillborn, one ruddy-colored and one very pale (3). The syndrome may result in the demise of the larger or smaller twin (4), serious neurological insult (5), and cardiovascular abnormalities (6–9). Death of one twin in a monochorionic system can subsequently lead to the rapid death of the partner twin. A mortal twin can act as a vascular low-resistance sink, which, through anastomotic intraplacental connections, leads to hypotension in the survivor. This "bleed" into the vascular system of the demised fetus can cause either death or neurological damage in the partner twin. In TTTS, the fetal neurological system can be seriously affected in a variety of ways, including the inherent primary disease process itself, the death of a co-twin resulting in hypotensive injury, or as a consequence of premature birth. Studies have demonstrated a high prevalence of morphological abnormalities when the brain is imaged, and an increased prevalence of neurocognitive impairment in survivors. Cardiovascular manifestations with the potential for long-term consequences are common in TTTS and will be discussed below.

In order to grade the severity of disease and to allow for rational analysis of treatment strategies and prognosis, Quintero and colleagues (10) developed a staging system for TTTS. The system is based upon a number of disease variables: presence of polyhydramnios (maximum vertical pocket >8 cm) in the larger twin and oligohydramnios (maximum vertical pocket of <2 cm) in the smaller twin; presence or absence of visualization of a bladder in the smaller twin; presence or absence of critically abnormal Doppler studies (defined as absent or reversed diastolic umbilical arterial flow, reverse flow in the ductus venosus, or umbilical venous pulsation); and presence or absence of hydrops. The staging system is listed in Table 22-1.

Although a number of criticisms of the system have been put forth, the Quintero score (10) has endured as a standard tool used in gauging the magnitude of disease present, and has been extensively applied in clinical trials of various treatment modalities. One limitation of the Quintero staging classification lies in its inability to discriminate between various degrees of cardiovascular derangement, with no consideration given to the absence, presence, or degree of recipient twin cardiomyopathy. This limitation led us to consider the development of a cardiovascular-based scoring system, which is discussed below.

Table 22–1 Quintero (10) Staging for Twin–Twin Transfusion Syndrome

Stage	Findings
I	Polyhydramnios or oligohydramnios sequence, but with visible bladder in smaller twin
II	Absent bladder in smaller twin
III	Abnormal Doppler studies
IV	Hydrops fetalis
V	Demise of one or both twins

MECHANISM AND PATHOPHYSIOLOGY OF TWIN–TWIN TRANSFUSION SYNDROME

The name "twin–twin transfusion syndrome" (TTTS) originates from the neonatal experience with this disease. Twins born with marked size discrepancy are often identified as presenting significant differences in hemoglobin, with the larger twin commonly manifesting polycythemia and the smaller twin anemia. This led to the belief that a simple *in utero* exchange of blood between the twins was the cause of this disorder. Current findings suggest that the pathophysiology is much more complex. Fetal blood sampling commonly demonstrates no significant difference in hemoglobin concentrations between twins with clinical manifestations of TTTS, hence a simple inter-twin blood "transfusion" is unlikely to be the sole cause.

The primary mechanism of TTTS is initiated by the presence of a placental vasculopathy. In monochorionic twins, placental vascular connections exist between the circulatory systems of each of the twins (Figure 22-1).

These connections consist of arterial-to-arterial (A–A) anastomoses, veno-venous (V–V) anastomoses, or arterial-to-venous (A–V) anastomoses (11). At both A–A and V–V anastomoses an even, bidirectional exchange of blood volume occurs between the circulations; however, the exchange at the A–V anastomoses are unidirectional, based on the pressure gradient. In the balanced state, the uneven exchange that occurs between A–V anastomoses is counterbalanced by equilibration at the A–A, and less often, V–V anastomoses. The foundations for TTTS are set when there is a paucity of adequate A–A connections to allow for inter-twin equilibration, hence A–V connections predominate resulting in a disequilibrium of placental flow from one fetus to the other (12). Hence, one twin becomes a "donor" while the other a "recipient" of transplacental blood flow. Consequently, the donor manifests hypovolemia and oliguria, resulting in oligohydramnios, while the recipient manifests hypervolemia and polyhydramnios. This is the triggering event for a complex cascade of physiological sequelae which follows.

Recent data looking at the renovascular systems of twin in TTTS has shed important light on this complex process (13). Immunohistochemistry studies have demonstrated the renin-angiotensin system to be upregulated in the donor twin; as the expected natural response to hypovolemia, this is not surprising. Angiotensin II released by the renin-angiotensin system in the donor increases vasoconstriction and water retention and thereby promotes maintenance of perfusion pressure. Partner recipient twins in the TTTS exhibit down-regulation of the

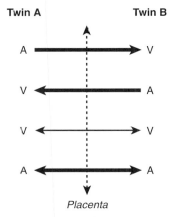

Placenta

FIGURE 22–1 Possible vascular connections between twins in a monochorionic system. Unidirectional flow occurs between A–V connections, with equilibration of flow occurring at V–V and A–A connections. The hatched line represents the vascular equator between the two fetal circulations. A, arterial; V, venous.

renin-angiotensin system, most likely as a consequence of the hypervolemia. However, serum levels of renin-angiotensin systems hormones, such as renin, are similar to that found in the donor. This suggests that the renin-angiotensin system hormones found in the recipient are not intrinsically produced, but, rather, are produced by the donor and delivered to the recipient through vascular connections. Hence, not only does the recipient receive an increase in volume, but also an increase in hormonal modulators that are typically released in response to low volume. These agents act as vasoconstrictors within the recipient, resulting in an increase in vascular resistance. In addition, other agents such as brain natriuretic peptide (14) and endothelin (15), hormonal modulators released in the presence of heart failure, are elevated in the amniotic fluid of recipient twins with hydrops. For the recipient twin partner a double insult takes place – an increase in *preload* and a paradoxical increase in *afterload*. This combination deleteriously affects the recipient cardiovascular system and is the cause of the cardiomyopathic changes seen in the recipient in TTTS.

SPECTRUM OF CARDIOVASCULAR FINDINGS IN TWIN–TWIN TRANSFUSION SYNDROME

Important changes take place in the cardiovascular system of fetuses in TTTS, with the potential for a wide spectrum of findings (6–9). The donor heart rarely manifests ostensible cardiac abnormalities on echocardiography, as the myocardium deals with a decrease in preload and an increase in afterload quite well. Systolic performance of the donor heart is preserved with no effect on valvular function. Ventricular cavity size and overall heart size is usually smaller than normal. Since the donor experiences an overall increase in systemic vascular resistance, analysis of placental vascular resistance by Doppler interrogation of the umbilical artery reveals an increase in the pulsatility index (a Doppler-derived measure of vascular resistance). This can be noted qualitatively by observing a low diastolic flow velocity or even absent or reversed flow at end-diastole in the spectral tracing of the umbilical artery (Figure 22-2). These findings suggest very high placental vascular resistance.

The recipient heart bears the brunt of the disease in TTTS. At first, and at an early stage, we may identify ventricular cavity dilation and mild ventricular hypertrophy. Mild atrioventricular valve regurgitation, probably as a consequence of cavity dilation, may be seen. Doppler flow patterns in the umbilical artery and vein are normal, and both systolic and diastolic ventricular performance is preserved. As the disease progresses ventricular wall thickening takes place, with a consequential negative effect on ventricular compliance and diastolic function. Of note, it has been observed that it is the right ventricle more than the left which typically manifests the majority of change in TTTS. As the ventricle hypertrophies, it becomes less compliant and Doppler parameters of ventricular filling begin to change. The normal twin peaks of inflow into the ventricle relating to passive filling (E wave) and active atrial filling (A wave) fuse into a single peak (Figure 22-3).

Ductus venosus flow during atrial contraction diminishes, often becoming absent or reversed in conditions of a very stiff, noncompliant right ventricle (Figure 22-4). Finally, further upstream the findings of pulsations in the umbilical vein may be seen, reflecting a severe degree of impediment to ventricular filling. As diastolic dysfunction progresses, ventricular systolic function is affected as well. Systolic ventricular dysfunction can be observed as a decrease in ventricular shortening fraction and a worsening of atrioventricular valve regurgitation, initially on the right and then progressing to the left side of the heart (Figure 22-5).

Ultimately, severe ventricular dysfunction and atrioventricular insufficiency lead to low cardiac output, development of hydrops, and fetal death. Barrea et al. (9) reviewed 28 twin pairs affected by TTTS and found cardiomegaly caused by right or

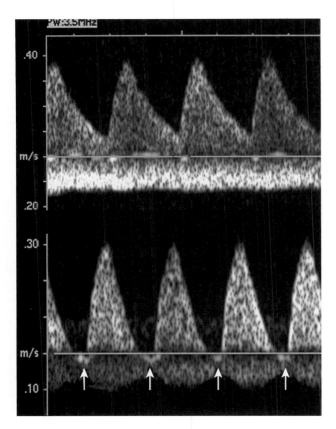

FIGURE 22–2 Doppler sampling in the umbilical cords of a donor twin (top panel) and a recipient twin (bottom panel). Umbilical arterial flow (pulsatile) is above the baseline, while umbilical venous flow is depicted below the baseline. Note the diminution in diastolic velocity in the donor umbilical artery flow as compared with the recipient. The arrows point out reversal of umbilical arterial flow in the donor twin (below the baseline) indicating that with systolic contraction and intended propulsion of blood forward into the placental circulation, there is a rebound wave of blood flow reversal during diastole. This strongly suggests a markedly elevated placental vascular resistance.

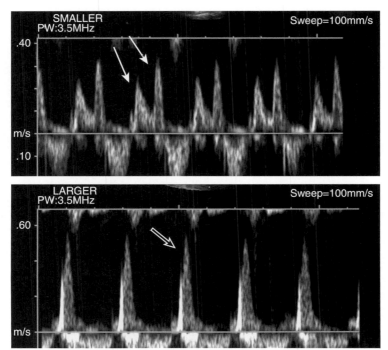

FIGURE 22–3 Doppler interrogation of flow across the tricuspid valve in a donor twin (top panel) and a recipient twin (bottom panel). The donor twin has a normal "double-peak" inflow pattern (solid arrows) representing flow during passive diastolic filling (first peak) and during atrial contraction (second peak). The recipient twin has a "single-peak" inflow pattern (open arrow) suggesting fusion of the diastolic phases into a single phase. This represents a poorly compliant and stiff ventricle. Note that often tachycardia may cause fusion of the double inflow peaks into a single peak; however, as may be seen in this case, the heart rate for the recipient is nearly identical to that of the donor twin, hence the appearance of a fusion wave suggests ventricular diastolic dysfunction and poor relaxation.

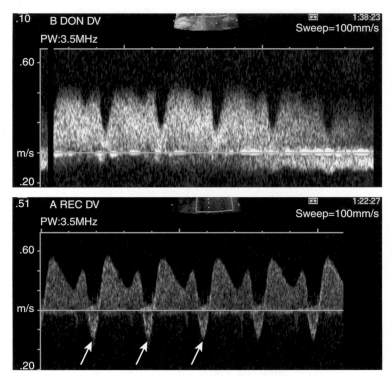

FIGURE 22–4 Doppler sampling in the ductus venosus of a donor twin (top panel) and recipient twin (bottom panel). The donor has a normal ductus venosus Doppler signal with continuous but phasic forward flow in the ductus venosus. The recipient ductus venosus Doppler signal displays reversal of flow with atrial contraction, suggesting a poorly compliant and stiff right ventricle (arrows in the bottom panel point to the reversal of flow with atrial contraction).

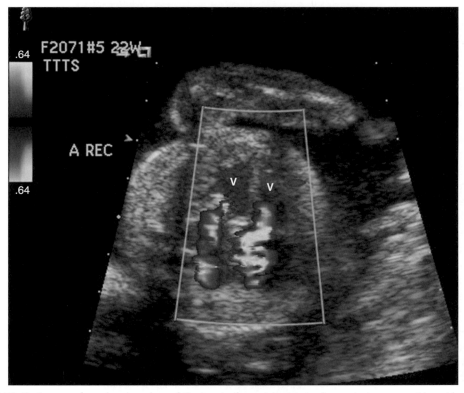

FIGURE 22–5 Apex up four-chamber view of the heart of a recipient twin demonstrates severe tricuspid and mitral regurgitation. V, ventricle.

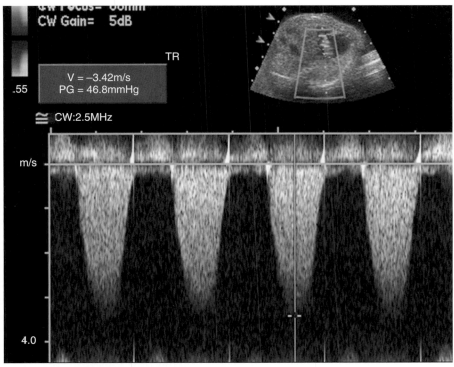

FIGURE 22–6 Spectral Doppler display of the tricuspid valve jet velocity of a fetus with recipient cardiomyopathy. The right ventricular pressure estimate from the peak velocity of the spectral Doppler display of tricuspid regurgitation is elevated at approximately 50 mmHg. PG, peak gradient; V, peak velocity.

left ventricular hypertrophy in 58% of recipient twins. Diastolic dysfunction of both right and left ventricles was present in two-thirds, and right ventricular systolic dysfunction with significant tricuspid regurgitation was seen in one-third, of the pairs. Progression of findings was associated with a higher perinatal mortality.

Right ventricular pressure estimates from the peak velocity of the tricuspid regurgitant jet in the recipient with TTTS will typically demonstrate very high intracavity pressures (Figure 22-6).

This finding further supports the notion that the recipient twin heart is stressed by the presence of increased vascular resistance and increased afterload as well as increased volume preload. The true blood pressure and ventricular cavity pressure in the human fetus is unknown. However, the typical peak systolic pressure for a newborn premature infant born at 24 weeks' gestation is known to be approximately 30–40 mmHg. The normal fetal heart in series with the low vascular resistance placenta should perhaps be less, but certainly no higher, than this blood pressure value noted in the premature infant. We have observed right ventricular pressures as high as 80–90 mmHg in the absence of any outflow tract obstruction, supporting the notion that an increase in vascular resistance is part of the pathophysiologic process resulting in the cardiomyopathy of TTTS seen in the recipient twin.

One intriguing phenomenon seen in TTTS is that of progressive development of right ventricular outflow tract obstruction in some recipient fetuses (8). This "acquired" right ventricular outflow tract obstruction is phenotypically identical to the congenital heart defect of pulmonary atresia or pulmonary stenosis with a hypoplastic, hypertrophied right ventricle. This phenomenon of development of selective right ventricle outflow tract obstruction in otherwise structurally normal hearts raises the question of whether a similar process leads to the development of some forms of congenital heart disease. It is enticing to speculate that perhaps a similar mechanism of hormonal conditions and altered load very early in gestation may be the cause of right-sided obstructive anomalies in the singleton fetus born with these forms of congenital heart disease (16). This speaks to the fundamental aspects of the mechanisms of formation of congenital heart disease. Alterations in blood flow and other extrinsic variables may potentially lead to the development of "acquired–congenital" heart disease at a period of time following completion of embryological formation of the human heart.

QUANTIFYING THE BURDEN OF CARDIOVASCULAR IMPAIRMENT IN TTTS

Gauging the magnitude of cardiovascular derangement in TTTS can be an important part of understanding the state of the disease that is present. A variety of noninvasive tools may be employed in evaluating the fetal cardiovascular system. One measure of the magnitude of ventricular dysfunction used in a variety of forms of congenital and acquired heart disease is the myocardial performance index (MPI) (17). The MPI is a ventricular geometry-independent measure of combined *systolic* and *diastolic* ventricular performance. By performing Doppler sampling of inflow and outflow across the ventricle, we can measure the time intervals relating to isovolumic contraction, isovolumic relaxation, and ventricular ejection (Figure 22-7).

The MPI is a measure of the ratio of combined isovolumic times to the ejection time. As global systolic and diastolic dysfunction worsens, MPI values increase progressively above normal. Raboisson and colleagues (18) used the MPI to assess ventricular performance status of recipient and donor twins with TTTS. Recipient twins exhibited higher MPI values relative to their donor partners. These authors also found that ventricular dysfunction in the recipient was so strongly characteristic of the TTTS that the MPI could reliably be used to distinguish between TTTS and other causes of twin size discrepancy, such as intrauterine growth restriction.

Our group has investigated the utility of various Doppler-derived measures of ventricular performance in order to help improve our understanding of the

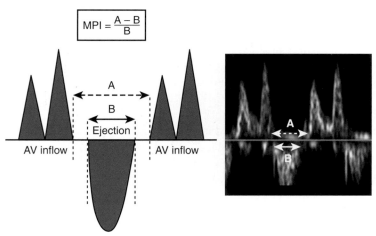

FIGURE 22–7 Pictorial display of calculation of the myocardial performance index. Time intervals are measured from cessation of atrioventricular valve flow to onset of atrioventricular valve flow (time A) and from onset of systolic semilunar valve flow to cessation of flow (ejection time, time B). Subtracting the time interval B from time interval A and indexing to time interval B provides for a measure of the ratio of combined isovolumic contraction and relaxation times to the ejection time. This ratio of isovolumic times to ejection reflects ventricular efficiency and performance. The lower the value the lower the isovolumic times needed for the ventricle to eject, which reflects an efficient and well-performing myocardium.

$$EF = (1.055 \times CSA \times VTIac) \times PSV/TTP$$

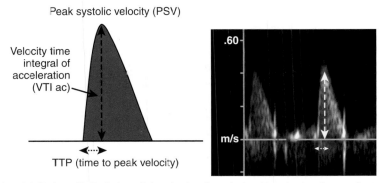

FIGURE 22–8 Pictorial display of calculation of the ejection force index. The ejection force reflects systolic ventricular performance and is derived from a formula which describes the mass of blood propelled forward during acceleration and is very preload-sensitive. A higher value corresponds to greater force exerted in ejecting the ventricular volume of blood during systole.

pathophysiology of TTTS as well as help stratify patients by severity of disease. Szwast et al. (19) applied the MPI and calculated ventricular ejection force and cardiac output in 22 twin pairs with TTTS. The ventricular ejection force describes the acceleration of blood across the pulmonic or aortic valve over a specific time interval, and is a reflection of systolic ventricular performance derived from Newton's laws (Figure 22-8). A higher value corresponds to a greater force exerted in ejecting the ventricular volume of blood during systole. The combined right and left ventricle cardiac output (CCO) is a measure of total blood flow through the fetal heart and is indexed to the estimated fetal weight in kilograms. The twin pairs were then compared to 36 age-matched singleton fetuses as normal control subjects. The findings are listed in Table 22-2.

Table 22–2   Summary of Results for the Twin-Donor versus Twin-Recipient versus Normal Control*

Variable	Twin-donor (*n* = 22)	Twin-recipient (*n* = 22)	Normal (*n* = 36)	P1, Twin-donor versus Twin recipient	P2, Twin-donor versus Normal control	P3, Twin-recipient versus Normal Contol
Gestational age (weeks)	22.3 ± 2.3	22.3 ± 2.3	22.9 ± 2.0	1	0.42	0.42
Fetal weight (kg)	0.42 ± 0.22	0.56 ± 0.21	0.64 ± 0.27	<0.001	<0.05	0.23
Right ventricular myocardial performance	0.38 ± 0.07	0.56 ± 0.09	0.24 ± 0.05	<0.001	<0.05	<0.001
Left ventricular myocardial performance	0.35 ± 0.07	0.54 ± 0.12	0.41 ± 0.05	<0.001	<0.05	<0.001
Right ventricular ejection force (mN)	2.5 ± 1.5	6.1 ± 4.0	5.4 ± 3.3	<0.001	<0.001	0.53
Left ventricular ejection force (mN)	2.0 ± 1.7	5.7 ± 3.2	4.6 ± 2.0	<0.001	<0.001	0.19
Combined cardiac output (cc/min·kg)	416 ± 74	568 ± 109	506 ± 86	<0.001	<0.001	<0.05

*The subgroup of the normal control population with a similar gestational age is used for statistical analysis. P values are sequentially recorded as: P1, Twin-donor versus Twin-recipient; P2, Twin-donor versus Normal Control; and P3, Twin-recipient versus Normal Control.
From Szwast A, Tian Z, McCann M, et al. Impact of altered loading conditions on verticular performance in fetuses with congenital cystic adenomatoid malformation and twin–twin transfusion syndrome. Ultrasound Obstet Gynecol 2007;30:40–46

In the donor twins, right ventricular and left ventricular MPI values were lower than the recipient twins, and lower still than normal control fetuses. Donor twins also had diminished right ventricular and left ventricular ejection forces compared with recipient twins, and diminished right ventricular and left ventricular ejection forces compared with normal control fetuses. Donor twins have lower CCO when compared with recipient twins and with normal control fetuses. These findings are consistent with the belief that donor twins are volume-depleted, but have preserved myocardial function. In contrast, the recipient twins had an abnormally elevated right ventricular and left ventricular MPI compared with normal fetuses, although there was no significant difference between left ventricular and right ventricular ejection forces in recipient twins compared with normal fetuses. Finally, recipient twins had elevated CCO compared with their donor counterparts and compared with normal controls. This suggests that in our group of recipient twins systolic function was still preserved as ejection forces were increased while diastolic dysfunction was present. Application of these Doppler-derived parameters will help to identify fetuses with diastolic dysfunction, before the onset of low cardiac output and hydrops, and may, therefore, be helpful in grading the magnitude of disease as the twin–twin transfusion process progresses.

An important goal is to provide a means for quantifying the cardiovascular burden present in TTTS. To that end we have identified and classified cardiovascular features to be considered (20). Table 22-3 lists these features and the values given to the various findings of the CHOP Cardiovascular Score for TTTS. The CHOP Cardiovascular Score is derived from echocardiographic data of a series of 150 twin pairs referred for TTTS and incorporates features describing ventricular dilation and hypertrophy, systolic function, valve regurgitation, and diastolic properties as described by Doppler indicators of ventricular compliance in the recipient twin, and umbilical arterial diastolic flow in the donor twin. Comparison of the CHOP Cardiovascular Score with the Quintero staging system demonstrates a significant degree of discrepancy between grades, which reflects the poor construction of the Quintero system to grade adequately subtle cardiovascular perturbations, which may be present in a progressive manner from the very outset of the disease (Figure 22-9).

Although right ventricular outflow tract obstruction is an end result in some cases of recipient cardiomyopathy in TTTS, we have observed situations in which there is reversed-size discrepancy between the pulmonary artery and the aorta. Whereas the pulmonary artery diameter is normally larger than the aorta by approximately 25%, some recipient fetuses exhibit an equal diameter between the pulmonary artery and aorta, or a pulmonary artery that is smaller than the aorta. We believe that this may reflect the spectrum of the disease, prior to the more severe finding of right ventricle outflow tract obstruction and pulmonary atresia. Altered compliance of the right ventricle can result in increased shunting from the right side across the foramen ovale to the left ventricle. In such a circumstance: with diminished flow on the right – but increased flow on the left – pulmonary artery growth is inhibited while aortic growth is enhanced. We have, therefore, included abnormal size discrepancy between the pulmonary artery and aorta in the CHOP Cardiovascular TTTS score.

The maximum score suggesting the most severe degree of cardiovascular impairment is 20/20. Currently, we apply this score in prospectively monitoring all fetuses with TTTS. In our original series, a wide spectrum of findings was present with ventricular dilation, dysfunction, hypertrophy, and abnormalities of diastolic filling properties seen most commonly (Figure 22-10).

In addition to the score, which is derived from qualitative parameters, we have been routinely measuring MPI values in the recipient and donor twins as a supplemental means of assessing myocardial function. Table 22-4 describes the

Table 22–3   CHOP Cardiovascular Score for Characterizing the Severity of Cardiovascular Perturbation in Twin–Twin Transfusion Syndrome

	Parameter	Finding	Numerical score
Donor	Umbilical artery	Normal	0
		Decreased diastolic flow	1
		Absent/reversed diastolic	2
Recipient	Ventricular hypertrophy	None	0
		Present	1
	Cardiac dilation	None	0
		Mild	1
		More than mild	2
	Ventricular dysfunction	None	0
		Mild	1
		More than mild	2
	Tricuspid valve regurgitation	None	0
		Mild	1
		More than mild	2
	Mitral valve regurgitation	None	0
		Mild	1
		More than mild	2
	Tricuspid valve inflow	Double-peak	0
		Single-peak	1
	Mitral valve inflow	Double-peak	0
		Single-peak	1
	Ductus venosus	All antegrade	0
		Absent diastolic flow	1
		Reverse diastolic flow	2
	Umbilical vein	No pulsations	0
		Pulsations	1
	Right-sided outflow tract	Pulmonary artery to aorta	0
		Pulmonary artery equals aorta	1
		Pulmonary artery more than aorta	2
		Right ventricular outflow obstruction	3
	Pulmonary regurgitation	None	0
		Present	1
Maximum total cardiovascular score			20 points

From Rychik J, Tian Z, Bebbington M, et al. The twin–twin transfusion syndrome: spectrum of cardiovascular abnormality and development of a cardiovascular score to assess severity of disease. Am J Obstet Gynecol 2007;197:392,e1–8.

findings of 150 twin pairs with TTTS with respect to the Doppler-derived measures of umbilical artery pulsatility index, middle cerebral artery index, ductus venosus flow, MPI for right and left ventricles as well as the parameters used to calculate the myocardial performance values. It is only through such a detailed and comprehensive characterization of the recipient and donor twins that we can appropriately gauge the effect of this disease, and the response of the cardiovascular system to various treatment strategies. Quantifying the degree of cardiovascular abnormality in the fetus with TTTS may also potentially be useful as a prognosticator of residual cardiovascular abnormalities after birth. These techniques will require further validation and analysis in a wide variety of cases. Early data suggests the score to be a valid method for assessing response to treatment, as score values decline after successful therapeutic intervention through laser photocoagulation (21).

STRATEGIES FOR THE TREATMENT OF TWIN–TWIN TRANSFUSION SYNDROME

A variety of treatment strategies have been proposed for TTTS. The serial removal of large volumes of amniotic fluid from the recipient (amnioreduction) has been

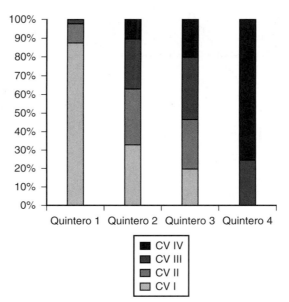

FIGURE 22–9 Bar graph demonstrating the relationship between the CHOP cardiovascular score and the Quintero staging system. Fetal twin pairs were graded for cardiovascular findings blinded to the Quintero designation, with score values broken down into quartiles (CV grade I, score 0–5; CV grade II, score 6–10; CV grade III, 11–15; CV grade IV, 16–20). Note the presence of severity discrepancy between the grading systems, as CV grades II or III are seen in at least 10% of Quintero Stage 1 patients, while a wide spectrum of CV grades is seen in the subsequent Quintero stages.

demonstrated to reduce morbidity and mortality (22). Initially employed as a means of creating comfort for the mother, it soon became apparent that serial amnioreduction exerts a positive effect on fetal outcome as well. This may be related to improved placental circulation after relief of placental vascular compression as well as prevention of preterm labor with the reduction in abdominal or uterine size. Creation of communication between the donor and recipient amniotic sacs has also been demonstrated to result in improved outcomes. Equilibration of amniotic volumes and pressure between the twins by creating a "micro-septostomy" may help; however, these communications commonly seal off, rendering this only a temporary intervention.

Ville and other workers (22–26) pioneered the concept of direct interruption of the initiating vascular anastomoses within the placental plate by percutaneous

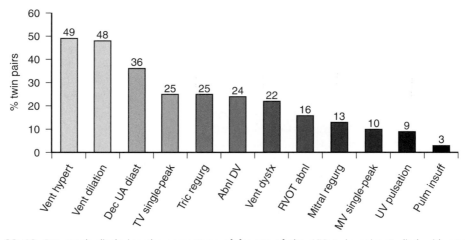

FIGURE 22–10 Bar graph displaying the percentage of fetuses of the 150 twin pairs studied with each of the cardiovascular parameters evaluated.

Table 22–4   Quantitative Parameters of Cardiovascular Function Evaluated in Both the Donor and Recipient Fetuses in 150 Twin Pairs with Twin–Twin Transfusion Syndrome

	Donor	Recipient	P value
Weight (gm)	399 (235)	527 (285)	<0.0001
Umbilical artery S wave peak velocity (cm/s)	29.2 (8.7)	41.7 (12.9)	<0.0001
Umbilical artery D wave peak velocity (cm/s)	4.7 (4.3)	9.78 (4.5)	<0.0001
Umbilical artery performance index	1.81 (0.8)	1.46 (0.4)	<0.0001
Middle cerebral artery S wave peak velocity (cm/s)	27.3 (8.1)	26.2 (8)	NS
Middle cerebral artery D wave peak velocity (cm/s)	5.1 (2.6)	5.1 (2.1)	NS
Middle cerebral artery performance index	1.79 (0.4)	1.70 (0.4)	NS
Ductus venosus A wave peak velocity (cm/s)	18.5 (6.8)	13.3 (16.7)	<0.01
Ductus venosus S wave peak velocity (cm/s)	51.1 (13)	53.3 (13.6)	NS
Ductus venosus A:S ratio	0.38 (0.12)	0.24 (0.31)	<0.001
Tricuspid valve closure-to-opening time (ms)	232 (18)	275 (32)	<0.0001
Pulmonary artery ejection time (ms)	169 (13)	169 (21)	NS
Right ventricle myocardial performance index	0.38 (0.11)	0.69 (0.47)	<0.0001
Mitral valve closure-to-opening time (ms)	222 (19)	263 (29)	<0.0001
Aorta ejection time (ms)	166 (15)	170 (17)	0.07
Left ventricle myocardial performance index	0.34 (0.12)	0.59 (0.28)	<0.0001

From Rychik J, Tian Z, Bebbington M, et al. The twin–twin transfusion syndrome: spectrum of cardiovascular abnormality and development of a cardiovascular score to assess severity of disease. Am J Obstet Gynecol 2007;197:392,e1–8.

laparoscopic laser techniques. Currently, this appears to be the most effective strategy for treating TTTS. In a large randomized trial of endoscopic laser photo-coagulation therapy versus serial amnioreduction (The Euro Foetus Consortium Trial (26)) laser therapy was identified as being superior as a first-line treatment at all stages of severity of the disease. As compared with the amnioreduction group, the laser group had a higher likelihood of survival of at least one twin (76% versus 56%) and a lower incidence of periventricular leukomalacia (6% versus 14%). Furthermore, surviving infants were more likely to be free of neurological complications at six months of age (52% versus 31%). Although laser therapy currently appears to be the more effective strategy, it is not a cure for the disease in all cases as significant morbidity and mortality affects large numbers of infants despite treatment. Further work is necessary to determine the appropriate candidates and the optimal timing for laser therapy.

LONG-TERM ISSUES AND THE FUTURE

There are a number of unanswered questions concerning TTTS and the associated cardiovascular changes which take place. Outcome studies looking at therapeutic effectiveness have focused on perinatal survival and neurologic outcome, with little focus on cardiovascular outcome. Which therapeutic interventions are most likely to result in cardiovascular improvement? Barrea and colleagues (9) demonstrated that, despite amnioreduction, cardiovascular changes may persist or even progress. The impact of laser therapy on cardiovascular changes and the ability to prevent progression of right ventricular outflow tract obstruction, cardiac failure, or hydrops has not yet been investigated. It is through the application of descriptive cardiovascular tools such as the CHOP Cardiovascular Score and other quantitative indices of function that we believe such questions may be addressed.

Many questions remain concerning the pathophysiology of TTTS. Why do some recipient twins severely affected manifest ventricular dysfunction and heart failure while others develop ventricular hypertrophy and right ventricular outflow tract obstruction? We speculate that it is not the severity of the disease alone that dictates this phenotype, but that inherent genetic factors play a role. It is well-recognized in the mature postnatal heart that the myocardial response to stressors is, to a degree, under genetic control (27). It is therefore reasonable to think that the fetal myocardial (host) response to a severe increase in preload (volume exchange) and afterload (hormonal modulators) may similarly be under genetic control. For some twin recipients the response to these stressors is cardiac hypertrophy, decompensation, and failure, while for others it is hypertrophy and development of right ventricular outflow tract obstruction. In fact, the latter may be a positive adaptive response, since few fetuses with right ventricle outflow tract obstruction experience fetal demise, unlike those who develop cardiac decompensation and hydrops. Variables such as the angiotensin converting enzyme (ACE) genotype or other myocardial genotypes may influence the phenotypic direction the recipient fetus will take. Angiotensin II can be a potent stimulant of myocardial hypertrophy in the mature heart; however, its direct myocardial affects are under complex genetic control (i.e. receptor type, density, and so on) (27–30). Might the phenotypic variability seen in the recipient twin in TTTS be a result of a genetically controlled inherent response to elevated levels of angiotensin II? The genetic determinants of myocardial hypertrophy in the fetus are currently unknown, but will likely explain this phenomenon.

The long term implications of cardiovascular disease in the fetus with TTTS are potentially significant. The "Barker hypothesis" proposes the concept of fetal origins of adult cardiovascular disease – "programming" of the heart and vascular system takes place during fetal life, setting the risk for the development of late diseases such as hypertension and atherosclerosis (31). Cheung and colleagues (32) demonstrated the impact of fetal TTTS on vascular dysfunction in infancy. TTTS donor twins at a mean of nine months of age exhibited diminished arterial distensibility as measured by abnormal pulse-wave velocity examination. Gardiner and colleagues (33) studied 27 twin pairs with TTTS after birth at a mean of 11 months of age and found that laser therapy altered, but did not abolish, these vascular abnormalities of arterial distensibility. Are the survivors of fetal TTTS at risk for significant cardiovascular difficulties as they grow into later childhood and into adults? What is the long-term cardiovascular burden of TTTS and to what degree do these patients carry added risk for cardiovascular disease as adults? These are intriguing questions, yet to be answered, and will undergo intense exploration in the coming years as more survivors of this disease grow into adulthood.

In summary, TTTS is a unique and complex disease process affecting monochorionic or diamniotic twins. The disease is primarily caused by a placental vasculopathy with resultant transfer of both volume as well as hormonal modulators through intraplacental vascular connections from donor to recipient twin. Morbidity and mortality remains high, but is improving substantially through the development of treatment strategies such as endoscopic laser photocoagulation. Complex changes take place within the cardiovascular system which contribute substantially to the outcome of this disease. Application of tools to better grade the degree of cardiovascular derangement will help in determining the efficacy of current treatment strategies. The long-term impact of TTTS on the postnatal and mature adult cardiovascular system is yet to be fully understood.

ACKNOWLEDGEMENTS

The author would like to acknowledge the work of Dr Zhiyun Tian for her contributions of thought as well as skillful imaging in the pursuit of improved understanding of the cardiovascular manifestations of twin–twin transfusion syndrome.

REFERENCES

1. Sebire NJ, Snijders RJ, Hughes K, Sepulveda W, Nicolaides KH. The hidden mortality of monochorionic twin pregnancies. Br J Obstet Gynaecol 1997;104:1203–1207.

2. Harkness UF, and Crombleholme TM. Twin-twin transfusion syndrome: where do we go from here? Semin Perinatol 2005;29:296–304.

3. Berger HM, de Waard F, Molenaar Y. A case of twin-to-twin transfusion in 1617. Lancet 2000;356:847–848.

4. Gonsoulin W, Moise KJ Jr, Kirshon B, Cotton DB, Wheeler JM, Carpenter RJ Jr. Outcome of twin–twin transfusion diagnosed before 28 weeks of gestation. Obstet Gynecol 1990;75:214–216.

5. Haverkamp F, Lex C, Hanisch C, Fahnenstich H, Zerres K. Neurodevelopmental risks in twin-to-twin transfusion syndrome: preliminary findings. Eur J Paediatr Neurol 2001;5:21–27.

6. Zosmer N, Bajoria R, Weiner E, Rigby M, Vaughan J, Fisk NM. Clinical and echographic features of in utero cardiac dysfunction in the recipient twin in twin–twin transfusion syndrome. Br Heart J 1994;72:74–79.

7. Simpson LL, Marx GR, Elkadry EA, D'Alton ME. Cardiac dysfunction in twin–twin transfusion syndrome: a prospective, longitudinal study. Obstet Gynecol 1998;92:557–562.

8. Lougheed J, Sinclair BG, Fung Kee Fung K, et al. Acquired right ventricular outflow tract obstruction in the recipient twin in twin-twin transfusion syndrome. J Am Coll Cardiol 2001;38:1533–1538.

9. Barrea C, Alkazaleh F, Ryan G, et al. Prenatal cardiovascular manifestations in the twin-to-twin transfusion syndrome recipients and the impact of therapeutic amnioreduction. Am J Obstet Gynecol 2005;192:892–902.

10. Quintero RA, Morales WJ, Allen MH, Bornick PW, Johnson PK, Kruger M. Staging of twin–twin transfusion syndrome. J Perinatol 1999;19:550–555.

11. Bajoria R, Wigglesworth J, Fisk NM. Angioarchitecture of monochorionic placentas in relation to the twin–twin transfusion syndrome. Am J Obstet Gynecol 1995;172:856–863.

12. Galea P, Jain V, Fisk NM. Insights into the pathophysiology of twin–twin transfusion syndrome. Prenat Diag 2005;25:777–785.

13. Mahieu-Caputo D, Meulemans A, Martinovic J, et al. Paradoxic activation of the renin-angiotensin system in twin–twin transfusion syndrome: an explanation for cardiovascular disturbances in the recipient. Pediatr Res 2005;58:685–688.

14. Bajoria R, Ward S, Chatterjee R. Natriuretic peptides in the pathogenesis of cardiac dysfunction in the recipient fetus of twin–twin transfusion syndrome. Am J Obstet Gynecol 2002;186:121–127.

15. Bajoria R, Sullivan M, Fisk NM. Endothelin concentrations in monochorionic twins with severe twin–twin transfusion syndrome. Hum Reprod 1999;14:1614–1618.

16. Clark EB, Hu N, Frommelt P, Vandekieft GK, Dummett JL, Tomanek RJ. Effect of increased pressure on growth in stage 21 chick embryos. Am J Physiol Heart Circ Physiol 19889;257:H55–H61.

17. Eicem BW, Edwards JM, Cetta F. Quantitative assessment of fetal ventricular function: establishing normal values of the myocardial performance index in the fetus. Echocardiography 2001;18:9–13.

18. Raboisson MJ, Fouron JC, Lamoureux J, et al. Early intertwin differences in myocardial performance during the twin-to-twin transfusion syndrome. Circulation 2004;110:3043–3048.

19. Szwast A, Tian Z, McCann M, et al. Impact of altered loading conditions on ventricular performance in fetuses with congenital cystic adenomatoid malformation and twin–twin transfusion syndrome. Ultrasound Obstet Gynecol 2007;30:40–46.

20. Rychik J, Tian Z, Bebbington M, et al. The twin–twin transfusion syndrome: spectrum of cardiovascular abnormality and development of a cardiovascular score to assess severity of disease. Am J Obstet Gynecol 2007;197:392, e1–e8.

21. Bebbington MW, Rychik J, Tian ZY, et al. The CHOP cardiovascular score for twin–twin transfusion the effect of treatment with selective laser ablation. Ultrasound Obstet Gynecol 2007;30(4):489 (abstract).

22. Mari G, Roberts A, Detti L, et al. Perinatal morbidity and mortality rates in severe twin–twin transfusion syndrome: results of the International Amnioreduction Registry. Am J Obstet Gynecol 2001;185:708–715.

23. Ville Y, Hyett J, Hecher K, Nicolaides K. Preliminary experience with endoscopic laser surgery for severe twin–twin transfusion syndrome. N Engl J Med 1995;332:224–227.

24. De Lia JE, Kuhlmann RS, Lopez KP. Treating previable twin–twin transfusion syndrome with fetoscopic laser surgery: outcomes following the learning curve. J Perinat Med 1999;27:61–67.

25. Hecher K, Diehl W, Zikulnig L, Vetter M, Hackeloer BJ. Endoscopic laser coagulation of placental anastomoses in 200 pregnancies with severe mid-trimester twin-to-twin transfusion syndrome. Eur J Obstet Gynecol Reprod Biol 2000;92:135–139.

26. Senat MV, Deprest J, Boulvain M, Paupe A, Winer N, Ville Y. Endoscopic laser surgery versus serial amnioreduction for severe twin-to-twin transfusion syndrome. N Engl J Med 2004;351:136–144.

27. Lips DJ, deWindt LJ, van Kraaij DJ, Doevendans PA. Molecular determinants of myocardial hypertrophy and failure: alternative pathways for beneficial and maladaptive hypertrophy. Eur Heart J 2003;24:883–896.

28. Yamazaki T, Komuro I, Yazaki Y. Role of the renin-angiotensin system in cardiac hypertrophy. Am J Cardiol 1999;83:53H–57H.

29. Sadoshima J, Izumo S. Molecular characterization of angiotensin II-induced hypertrophy of cardiac myocytes and hyperplasia of cardiac fibroblasts. Critical role of the AT1 receptor subtype. Circ Res 1993;73:413–423.

30. Sadoshima J, Xu Y, Slayter HS, et al. Autocrine release of angiotensin II mediates stretch-induced hypertrophy of cardiac myocytes in vitro. Cell 1993;75:977–984.

31. Barker DJ. Fetal origins of cardiovascular disease. Ann Med 1999;31(Suppl. 1):3–6.

32. Cheung YF, Taylor MJ, Fisk NM, Redington AN, Gardiner HM. Fetal origins of reduced arterial distensibility in the donor twin in twin–twin transfusion syndrome. Lancet 2000;355:1157–1158.

33. Gardiner HM, Taylor MJ, Karatza A, et al. Twin–twin transfusion syndrome: the influence of intrauterine laser photocoagulation on arterial distensibility in childhood. Circulation 2003;107:1906–1911.

Index

(Figure references in **bold**; table reference in *italics*)